Textbook of
Biomedical
Instrumentation

Textbook of Biomedical Instrumentation

K. N. SCOTT

A.K. MATHUR

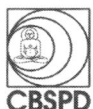

CBSPD

CBS Publishers & Distributors Pvt Ltd

New Delhi • Bengaluru • Chennai • Kochi • Kolkata • Lucknow • Mumbai
Hyderabad • Jharkhand • Nagpur • Patna • Pune • Uttarakhand

Textbook of
Biomedical
Instrumentation

ISBN: 978-81-239-1402-4 (PB)

ISBN: 978-81-239-1422-9 (HB)

First Edition: 2007
Reprint: 2007, 2013, 2019, 2023

Published by **Satish Kumar Jain** and produced by **Varun Jain** for

CBS Publishers & Distributors Pvt Ltd
4819/XI Prahlad Street, 24 Ansari Road, Daryaganj, New Delhi 110 002, India.
Ph: 011-23289259, 23266861
Website: www.cbspd.com
e-mail: delhi@cbspd.com

Corporate Office: 204 FIE, Industrial Area, Patparganj, Delhi 110 092
Ph: 011-4934 4934   Fax: 011-4934 4935
e-mail: publishing@cbspd.com; publicity@cbspd.com

Branches

- **Bengaluru:** Seema House 2975, 17th Cross, KR Road, Banasankari 2nd Stage, Bengaluru 560 070, Karnataka, India
  Ph: +91-80-26771678/79   Fax: +91-80-26771680   e-mail: bangalore@cbspd.com
- **Chennai:** 7, Subbaraya Street, Shenoy Nagar, Chennai 600 030, Tamil Nadu, India
  Ph: +91-44-26680620, 26681266   Fax: +91-44-42032115   e-mail: chennai@cbspd.com
- **Kochi:** 42/1325, 1326, Power House Road, Opp KSEB, Power House, Ernakulum Kochi 682 018, Kerala, India
  Ph: +91-484-4059061-65,67   Fax: +91-484-4059065   e-mail: kochi@cbspd.com
- **Kolkata:** 147, Hind Ceramics Compound, 1st Floor, Nilgunj Road, Belghoria, Kolkata-700056, West Bengal, India
  Ph: +033-25633055, 033-25633056   e-mail: kolkata@cbspd.com
- **Lucknow:** Basement, Khushnuma Complex, 7 Meerabai Marg (Behind Jawahar Bhawan),Lucknow-226001, UP, India
  Ph: +0522-4000032   e-mail: tiwari.lucknow@cbspd.com
- **Mumbai:** PWD Shed, Gala no 25/26, Ramchandra Bhatt Marg, Next to JJ Hospital Gate no. 2, Opp. Union Bank of India, Noorbaug, Mumbai-400009, Maharashtra, India
  Ph: 022-66661880/89   e-mail: mumbai@cbspd.com

Representatives

• Hyderabad	0-9885175004	• Jharkhand	0-9811541605	• Nagpur	0-9421945513
• Patna	0-9334159340	• Pune	0-9923910676	• Uttarakhand	0-9716462459

Printed at Sanjay Printer, Sahibabad, UP, India

Preface

During the last two decades, there has been a tremendous increase in the use of electronic equipment in the medical field for clinical and research purposes. In other words recent advances in medical field have been fuelled by instruments developed by the electronics and instrumentation engineers.

This textbook on BIOMEDICAL INSTRUMENTATION is essential reading for students, teachers, professionals, electronics and instrumentation engineers, researchers, involved with life sciences, microbiology, biotechnology, biochemical engineering and medical institutes and hospitals.

The textbook is divided into four sections. Section I deals with measuring, recording and monitoring instruments. Chapter 1 is devoted to fundamentals of medical instrumentation. A medical instrument performs a specific function in a biological system which may be the exact measurement of physiological parameters, such as, pressure, flow, voltage, current, pH, volume, weight, temperature and the rate of change of these parameters. Chapter 2 concentrates on bioelectric signals and electrodes. In order to measure and record potentials and hence current in the body, it is necessary to provide some interface between the body and the electronic measuring apparatus. The interface is carried out by biopotential electrodes. Chapter 3 deals with biomedical sensors which are used in clinical medicine and biological research for measuring a wide range of physiological variables. These are often called biomedical transducers and are the main building blocks of the diagnostic medical instrumentation found in physician's office, clinical laboratories and hospitals. Some biomedical sensors are also used in non-medical applications such as in environmental monitoring, bioprocessing and petrochemical industries. Amplifiers are an important part of modern instrumentation systems for measuring biopotential. Such measurements involve voltages that often are at the low levels, have high source impedance or both. These are also required to increase signal strength while maintaining high fidelity. Keeping this in mind, Chapter 4 focuses on biopotential amplifiers. Chapter 5 is devoted to biomedical recorders such as ECG and EEG (Electron encephalograph) and various others which are discussed in detail. Chapter 6 deal with the various types of patient monitors. These systems aid the nurses and medical persons to quickly gather information about the vital physiological parameters of the patient before, during and after operation and in the intensive care ward where patients condition is kept under constant surveillance. Chapter 7 deals with Biotelemetry. Telemetry systems are special cases of patient monitor system in which monitoring is done from remote location. This chapter explains the techniques and instrumentation for monitoring physiological data by telemetry in variety of situations and also includes transmission of biomedical signals over telephone lines, wireless for their study and analysis at a distant place.

Blood flow is one of the important physiological parameter and is also one of the difficult to measure. Cardiac out measurement details out the present state of art in this important area. Keeping this in mind Chapter 8 is devoted to cardiac output measurement. Chapter 9 concentrates on non-invasive optical monitoring. Non-invasive optical monitoring means the use of visible or near infrared light to directly assess the internal physiologic status of person without the need of extracting a blood of tissue sample or using a catheter.

Clinical laboratory is responsible for analysing patient specimens to provide information to aid in diagnosis of disease and to evaluate the effectiveness of therapy. The hospital department that performs these functions may also be called the department of clinical pathology or the department of laboratory medicine. Keeping this in view Chapter 10 deals with clinical laboratory instrumentation. Chapter 11 focuses on the hearing aids. The chapter presents hearing aid fundamentals, symptoms and causes of hearing disorders, design, systems and fitting procedures.

Section II is devoted to modern medical imaging systems. For many years, photographic film was the principal means for storing medical images. Computer's have provided a new means for storing, processing, transferring and displaying images. Chapter 12 deals with medical X-ray equipment. X-ray image is resolution limited by the dimension of the X-ray source and noise limited by the beam intensity. First use for computerised tomography, computer and digital image processing have engendered a revolution in the way medical images are produced and manipulated. Now it is possible to acquire data, perform mathematical operations to produce images, emphasise details or differences of images and store and retrieve images from remote sites all without film. Keeping this in mind Chapter 13 focuses on X-ray computed tomography. Chapter 14 concentrates on nuclear medical imaging systems. In contrast to X-ray, ultrasound and magnetic resonance, nuclear medicine imaging techniques do not produce an anatomical map of the body, but instead image the spatial distribution of radiopharmaceuticals introduced into the body. Chapter 15 explains magnetic resonance imaging which is a non-ionising technique with full three dimensional capabilities, excellent soft tissue contrast and high spatial resolution. Chapter 16 deals with ultrasound equipment. Ultrasonic equipment encompasses a large number of different instruments or devices that are diagnostic or therapeutic ultrasonic is also used for imaging internal organs non-invasively and use to apply massage and deep heat therapy to muscle tissue.

Section III focuses on therapeutic equipment. A wide variety of electric stimulators are used in patient care and research. They range from very low current, low duty cycle stimulators such as the cardiac pacemaker, to high current pulse stimulators, such as defibrillators. Chapter 17 concentrates on cardiac defibrillators. No medical device so clearly represents emergency and in some aspects, intensive care medicine as much as the defibrillator. These are electric shock devices that are used to correct fatal cardiac arrhythmias such as ventricular fibrillation and ventricular tachycardia. Chapter 18 is devoted to electrosurgical devices. These are electric devices to assist in surgical procedures by providing cutting and hemostasis (stop bleeding) are widely used in the operating room. Chapter 19 focuses on biomedical lasers. These are used for bloodless surgery and for coagulation of fine structures in the small and sensitive organs of the body. In other words these are used in control of bleeding through photocoagulation and heating. Chapter 20 deals with ventilators and humidifiers. Mechanical ventilators, which are often also called respirators, are used to artificially ventilate the lungs of the patients who are unable to naturally breathe from the atmosphere. Chapter 21 concentrates on implantable insulin delivery systems. Various drug delivery devices and new techniques of insulin administration are discussed in detail. Chapter 22 is devoted to essentials of anaesthesia delivery. The practice of anaesthesia includes more than just providing relief from pain. Chapter 23 concentrates on Lung, blood gas and dialysis machines.

Section IV focuses on special topics. Medical procedures usually expose the patient to more hazards than the typical home or work place, because in medical environments the skin and mucous membranes are frequently penetrated or altered and because there are many sources of potentially hazardous substances and energy forms that could injure either the patient or medical staff. These sources include fire, air, water, chemicals, drugs, microorganisms, noise, electricity, radiation from X-ray, ultrasound, microwaves and lasers, etc. Keeping this in mind, Chapter 24 deals with Hospital equipment safety, various safety measures adopted by patients, doctors and hospital staff are discussed in detail. Chapter 25 is devoted to computer application in biomedical instrumentation. The purpose of clinical laboratory is to analyse body fluids and tissues for specific substances of interest and to report the results in a form which is of value to clinicians in the diagnosis and treatment of disease. Keeping this in mind, Chapter 26 focuses on clinical laboratory: separation, spectral and nonspectral methods. A large tests have been developed to achieve this purpose.

Glossary and index have been provided at the end for quick reference. Diagrams, figures and tables supplement the text. All the topics have been covered in a coagent and lucid style to help the reader grasp the information quickly and easily.

K. N. Scott
A. K. Mathur

Contents

Section III
THERAPEUTIC EQUIPMENT

Section IV

SPECIAL TOPICS

SECTION I

Measuring, Recording and Monitoring Instruments

Chapter 1

Fundamentals of Medical Instrumentation

INTRODUCTION

The physical forms taken by most examples of medical devices, such as instruments, tools and machines, are illustrated by the block diagram in Fig. 1.1. Each switch position sets the instrument up in one of the physical forms as an instrument for measurement, for monitoring, for diagnosis of disease, for therapy of patients or for surgery. Most medical instruments fall into one of these categories.

A medical instrument performs a specific function on a biological system. The function may be the exact measurement of physiological parameters—pressure, flow, voltage, current, chemical pH, volume, weight, temperature—and rates of change of these parameters. In physiological systems, because the parameters often have small magnitudes or are otherwise difficult to process, a transducer (illustrated in Fig. 1.1) is necessary to transform the physiological signal into a form that can be read by the signal processor. The transducer may, for example, amplify voltages or pressures, select an appropriate parameter for measurement, provide a transitional medium or effect an impedance match of the biological system to the signal processor.

In physiological systems, measurable parameters cover a wide range. Voltages range from 1 microvolt (μV) to several millivolts (mV) and up to thousands of volts (V) of static charge. Frequencies range from DC to 20 kilohertz (kHz). The dynamic range of sound amplitudes is 100 decibels (dB) and above. Pressures range from 0.1 millimeter of mercury (mmHg) to approximately 1000 mmHg. Fluid flow rates rise to 25 litres per minute (litres/minute) and air flow up to 600 litres/minute. The need to maintain physiological stability and control feedback is illustrated by the relatively narrow temperature range in the human body, 90 to 104 degrees Fahrenheit (°F).

The output of a transducer should be a signal compatible with the signal processor illustrated in the Fig 1.1. This output may be a force or flow rate sufficient to move a gauge, a voltage of current that can deflect a meter needle, a sound capable of being amplified above ambient noise so it can be measured or an ionic concentration requiring further processing. For many signal processors (for example, those having digital components), the compatible signal is binary, typically either +5 or 0V. Only upon appropriately processed signals can the arithmetic and logical functions of microprocessors and digital circuits be performed.

The type of signal processing depends upon the function of the instrument—measurement, monitoring, diagnosis, therapy or surgery. The function is selected by a switch in the figure.

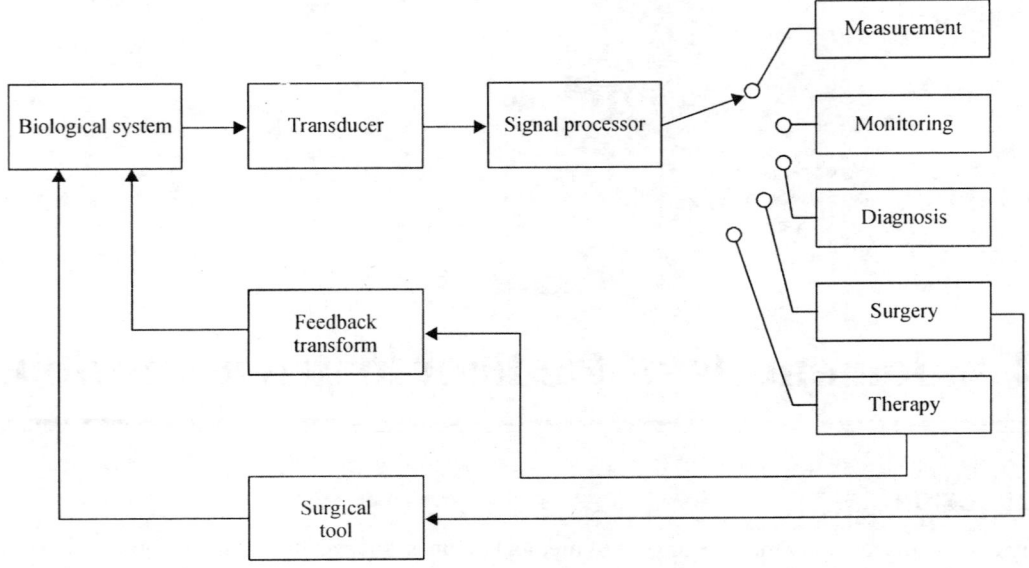

Fig. 1.1. A block diagram of a generalised medical instrument.

A common example of a measuring instrument is the thermometer. The transducer is the glass bulb and scale; the signal processor and monitor are the observer who records the measurement. Other examples of measuring devices are sphygmomanometers, electroencephalographs and electrocardiographs. A monitoring instrument represents a higher level of complexity in that it includes a memory, which can take the form of a paper strip recorder, a storage oscilloscope or a computer memory, which holds information for later use. An even higher level of sophistication is usually required for machine diagnosis. The diagnostic function may be performed by an instrument as simple as an alarm that warns of an excessive heart rate or as complex as a mainframe computer that processes symptoms and prescribes a health care programme.

In order for a medical instrument to be used in the performance of therapy, it must feedback a signal or force to the biological system, as indicated by the position of the feedback transform in Fig. 1.1. Therapy is applied by a crutch, for example, allowing a leg to heal while the patient remains ambulatory. More complex therapy may be applied by a biofeedback instrument such as a speech therapy device capable of deriving the information-bearing elements from speech and applying them to another sense such as sight or touch. Other therapeutic instrumentation may operate independently of physiological parameters in the system to which the therapy is applied. An example is an ultrasonic massager operated by a physical therapist. This is closely related to another category of instruments used in surgery and surgical procedures, namely invasive units, which penetrate the skin of the patient. These include electrosurgical knives, hypodermic needles and lasers.

The medical instruments illustrated in Fig. 1.1 are those that may be used in connection with the patient. Another category is assigned to laboratory instruments used to investigate and assess biological fluids and tissue. The measurement of pH is fundamental to the operation of many of these instruments, as are techniques for investigating particles in fluids.

MEDICAL INSTRUMENTS IMPORTANT CONSIDERATIONS

The fundamental purpose of tools is to enhance the capabilities of human beings by helping them to lift more weight, to move faster and more comfortably, to communicate over greater distances and to use the five senses more effectively.

Throughout history, as technology was developed, the number of human functions extended by the use of tools increased. Most recently, the introduction of computers has extended even our ability to think, particularly in calculating, analysing and storing large amounts of information.

Consider, for example, the sense of touch. The ancient Greeks used the technique of 'laying on of hands' to determine the size of organs, the nature of wounds and the extent of bodily growths; the technique is still used today. Modern instruments that extend the sense of touch include devices for massage, such as electrical current stimulators, automatic vibrators and ultrasonic therapy equipment. In the Tadoma method of speech therapy, the therapist places a hand on the speaker's face during speech training to feel where the sounds are placed. An electronic tactile vocoder can be used to extend the therapist's ability to locate these placements by amplifying these acoustic cues transferring them to other, more convenient cutaneous body sites.

One specific bit of information obtained by the sense of touch is a relative measure of body temperature. In this function, the thermometer extends the sense of touch, serving to quantify a measurement that has previously been only approximate.

Invention of the Thermometer

In 1603, the Italian scientist Galileo showed that a closed glass tube inserted in a container of water could be arranged so that the height of the water sucked into the tube by a partial vacuum varied with the temperature. In 1625, Santorio Santonio, a Slavic physician, constructed a similar device, which he used to measure the temperature in the human body. The problem with the instrument (Fig. 1.2a) was that the height of the water was also affected by the atmospheric pressure. This problem was solved a quarter of a century later when Ferdinand II, Grand Duke of Tuscany, sealed the water in a closed vessel to eliminate the effect of atmospheric pressure. The essentially modern thermometer shown in Fig. 1.2b was introduced by the Dutch instrument maker Gabriel D. Fahrenheit, who in the eighteenth century replaced the water with mercury and improved the instrument's accuracy. This thermometer is still widely used, although more recently liquid crystal thermometers have been adopted for special applications.

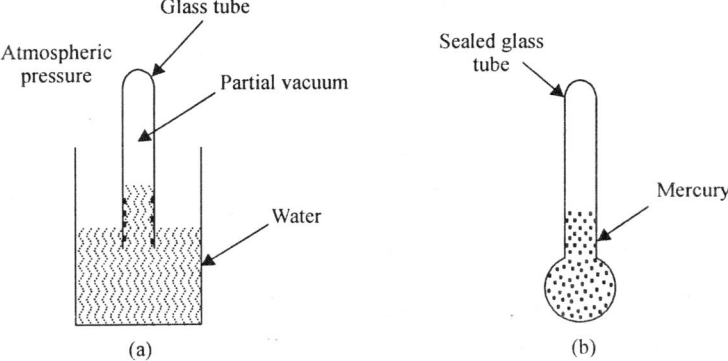

Fig. 1.2. Thermometer development.

Stethoscope and Hearing Enhancement

From the time of the ancient Greeks, physicians have used their hearing for diagnosis, such as in placing the ear against the chest or back to listen for the sounds of breathing and the heart. An early enhancement of this sense was achieved by the use of a 'hearing tube,' or stethoscope.

The stethoscope is a refinement of the hearing tube, attributed to Rene T. H. Laennec, a French physician who probably used it as much to avoid touching the bodies of his patients with his ear as to improve his ability to hear heart and breathing sounds. His device, a simple hollow tube, was designed to amplify sound, since it contained a taper (Fig. 1.3) that served to improve the coupling of chest to ear by the impedance matching principle.

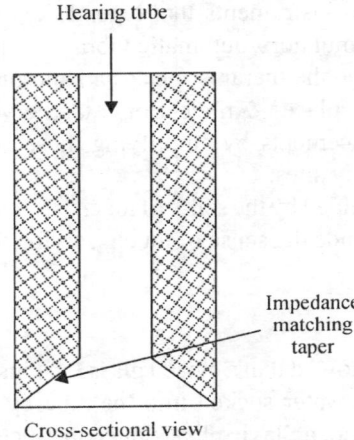

Hearing tube

Impedance matching taper

Cross-sectional view

Fig. 1.3. A stethoscope.

Measurand

The physical quantity, property or condition that the system measures is called the measurand. The accessibility of the measurand is important because it may be internal (blood pressure), it may be on the body surface (electrocardiogram potential), it may emanate from the body (infrared radiation) or it may be derived from a tissue sample (such as blood or a biopsy) that is removed from the body. Most medically important measurands can be grouped in the following categories: biopotential, pressure, flow, dimensions (imaging), displacement (velocity, acceleration and force), impedance, temperature and chemical concentrations. The measurand may be localised to a specific organ or anatomical structure.

Sensor

Generally, the term transducer is defined as a device that converts one form of energy to another. A sensor converts a physical measurand to an electric output. The sensor should respond only to the form of energy present in the measurand, to the exclusion of all others. The sensor should interface with the living system in a way that minimises the energy extracted, while being minimally invasive. Many sensors have a primary sensing element such as a diaphragm, which converts pressure to displacement. A variable-conversion element, such as a strain gauge, then converts displacement to an electric voltage. Sometimes the sensitivity of the sensor can be adjusted over a wide range by altering the primary sensing element. Many variable-conversion elements need external electric power to obtain a sensor output.

Signal Conditioning

Usually the sensor output cannot be directly coupled to the display device. Simple signal conditioners may only amplify and filter the signal or merely match the impedance of the sensor to the display. Often sensor outputs are converted to digital form and then processed by specialised digital circuits or a microcomputer. For example, signal filtering may reduce undesirable sensor signals. It may also average repetitive signals to reduce noise or it may convert information from the time domain to the frequency domain.

Output Display

The results of the measurement process must be displayed in a form that the human operator can perceive. The best form for the display may be numerical or graphical, discrete or continuous, permanent or temporary—depending on the particular measurand and how the operator will use the information.

Auxiliary Elements

A calibration signal with the properties of the measurand should be applied to the sensor input or as early in the signal-processing chain as possible. Many forms of control and feedback may be required to elicit the measurand, to adjust the sensor and signal conditioner and to direct the flow of output for display, storage or transmission. Control and feedback may be automatic or manual. Data may be stored briefly to meet the requirements of signal conditioning or to enable the operator to examine data that precede alarm conditions. Or data may be stored before signal conditioning, so that different processing schemes can be utilised. Conventional principles of communications can often be used to transmit data to remote displays at nurses' stations, medical center or medical data-processing facilities.

ALTERNATIVE OPERATIONAL MODES

Direct-Indirect Modes

Often the desired measurand can be interfaced directly to a sensor because the measurand is readily accessible or because acceptable invasive procedures are available. When the desired measurand is not accessible, we can use either another measurand that bears a known relation to the desired one or some form of energy or material that interacts with the desired measurand to generate a new measurand that is accessible. Examples include cardiac output (volume of blood pumped per minute by the heart), determined from measurements of respiration and blood gas concentration or from dye dilution; morphology of internal organs, determined from X-ray shadows and pulmonary volumes, determined from variations in thoracic impedance plethysmography.

Sampling and Continuous Modes

Some measurands—such as body temperature and ion concentrations—change so slowly that they may be sampled infrequently. Other quantities–such as the electrocardiogram and respiratory gas flow—may require continuous monitoring. The frequency content of the measurand, the objective of the measurement, the condition of the patient and the potential liability of the physician all influence how often medical data are acquired. Many data that are collected may go unused.

Generating and Modulating Sensors

Generating sensors produce their signal output from energy taken directly from the measurand, whereas modulating sensors use the measurand to alter the flow of energy from an external source in a way that affects the output of the sensor. For example, a photovoltaic cell is a generating sensor because it provides an output voltage related to its irradiation, without any additional external energy source. However, a photoconductive cell is a modulating sensor, to measure its change in resistance with irradiation, we must apply external energy to the sensor.

Analog and Digital Modes

Signals that carry measurement information are either analog, meaning continuous and able to take on any value within the dynamic range or digital, meaning discrete and able to take on only a finite number of different values. Most currently available sensors operate in the analog mode, although some inherently digital measuring devices have been developed. Increased use of digital signal processing has required concurrent use of analog-to-digital and digital-to-analog converters to interface computers with analog sensors and analog display devices. Also quasi-digital sensors, such as quartz-crystal thermometers, give outputs with variable frequency, pulse rate or pulse duration that are easily converted to digital signals.

The advantages of the digital mode of operation include greater accuracy, repeatability, reliability and immunity to noise. Furthermore, periodic calibration is usually not required. Digital numerical displays are replacing many analog meter movements because of their greater accuracy and readability. Many clinicians, however, prefer analog displays when they are determining whether a physiological variable is within certain limits and when they are looking at a parameter that can change quickly, such as beat-to-beat heart rate. In the latter case, digital displays often change numbers so quickly that they are very difficult and annoying to observe.

Real-Time and Delayed-Time Modes

Of course sensors must acquire signals in real time as the signals actually occur. The output of the measurement system may not display the result immediately, however, because some types of signal processing, such as averaging and transformations, need considerable input before any results can be produced. Often such short delays are acceptable unless urgent feedback and control tasks depend on the output. In the case of some measurements, such as cell cultures, several days may be required before an output is obtained.

MEDICAL MEASUREMENT CONSTRAINTS

The principal measurement and frequency ranges for each parameter are major factors that affect the design of all the instrument components shown in Fig. 1.1. To get a brief overview of typical medical parameter magnitude and frequency ranges, refer to Table 1.1. Shown here are approximate ranges that are intended to include normal and abnormal values. Most of the parameter measurement ranges are quite low compared with non-medical parameters. Note, for example, that most voltages are in the microvolt range and that pressures are low (about 100 mm Hg = 1.93 psi = 13.3 kPa). Also note that all the signals listed are in the audiofrequency range or below and that many signals contain DC and very low frequencies. These general properties of medical parameters limit the practical choices available to designers for all aspects of instrument design.

Many crucial variables in living systems are inaccessible because the proper measurand—sensor interface cannot be obtained without damaging the system. Unlike many complex physical systems, a biological system is of such a nature that it is not possible to turn it off and remove parts of it during the measurement procedure. Even if interference from other physiological systems can be avoided, the physical size of many sensors prohibits the formation of a proper interface. Either such inaccessible variables must be measured indirectly or corrections must be applied to data that are affected by the measurement process. The cardiac output is an important measurement that is obviously quite inaccessible.

Table 1.1. Medical and physiological parameters.

Parameter or measuring technique	Principal measurement, range of parameter	Signal frequency range, Hz	Standard sensor or method
Ballistocardiography (BCG)	0–7 mg	DC–40	Accelerometer, strain gauge
	0–100 μm	DC–40	Displacement (LVDT)
Bladder pressure	1–100 cm H_2O	DC–10	Strain-gauge manometer
Blood flow	1–300 ml/s	DC–20	Flowmeter (electromagnetic or ultrasonic)
Blood pressure, arterial			
Direct	10–400 mm Hg	DC–50	Strain-gauge manometer
Indirect	25–400 mm Hg	DC–60	Cuff, auscultation
Blood pressure, venous	0–50 mm Hg	DC–50	Strain gauge
Blood gases			
P_{O_2}	30–100 mm Hg	DC–2	Specific electrode, volumetric or manometric
P_{CO_2}	40–100 mm Hg	DC–2	Specific electrode, volumetric or manometric
P_{N_2}	1–3 mm Hg	DC–2	Specific electrode, volumetric or manometric
P_{CO}	0.1–0.4 mm Hg	DC–2	Specific electrode, volumetric or manometric
Blood pH	6.8–7.8 pH units	DC–2	Specific electrode
Cardiac output	4–25 litre/minute	DC–20	Dye dilution, Fick
Electrocardiography (ECG)	0.5–4 mV	0.01–250	Skin electrodes
Electroencephalography (EEG)	5–300 μV	DC–150	Scalp electrodes
(Electrocorticography and brain depth)	10–5000 μV	DC–150	Brain-surface or depth electrodes
Electrogastrography (EGG)	10–1000 μV	DC–1	Skin-surface electrodes
	0.5–80 mV	DC–1	Stomach-surface electrodes
Electromyography (EMG)	0.1–5 mV	DC–10000	Needle electrodes
Eye potentials			
EOG	50–3500 μV	DC–50	Contact electrodes
ERG	0–900 μV	DC–50	Contact electrodes
Galvanic skin response (GSR)	1–500 kΩ	0.01–1	Skin electrodes
Gastric pH	3–13 pH units	DC–1	pH electrode; antimony electrode
Gastrointestinal pressure	0–100 cm H_2O	DC–10	Strain-gauge manometer
Gastrointestinal forces	1–50 g	DC–1	Displacement system, LVDT
Nerve potentials	0.01–3 mV	DC–10000	Surface or needle electrodes

(Contd...)

Parameter or measuring technique	Principal measurement, range of parameter	Signal frequency range, Hz	Standard sensor or method
Phonocardiography (PCG)	Dynamic range 80 dB, threshold about 100 μPa	5–2000	Microphone
Plethysmography (volume change)	Varies with organ measured	DC–30	Displacement chamber or impedance change
Circulatory	0–30 ml	DC–30	Displacement chamber or impedance change
Respiratory functions			
Pneumotachography (flow rate)	0–600 litre/minute	DC–40	Pneumotachograph head and differential pressure
Respiratory rate	2–50 breaths/minute	0.1–10	Strain gage on chest, impedance, nasal thermistor
Tidal volume	50–1000 ml/breath	0.1–10	Above methods
Temperature of body	32–40°C 90–104°F	DC–0.1	Thermistor, thermocouple

Variables measured from the human body or from animals are seldom deterministic. Most measured quantities vary with time, even when all controllable factors are fixed. Many medical measurements vary widely among normal patients, even when conditions are similar. This inherent variability has been documented at the molecular and organ levels and even for the whole body. Many internal anatomical variations accompany the obvious external difference among patients. Large tolerances on physiological measurements are partly the result of interactions among many physiological systems. Many feedback loops exist among physiological systems and many of the interrelationships are poorly understood. It is seldom feasible to control or neutralise the effects of these other systems on the measured variable. The most common method of coping with this variability is to assume empirical statistical and probabilistic distribution functions. Single measurements are then compared with these norms.

Nearly all biomedical measurements depend either on some form of energy being applied to the living tissue or on some energy being applied as an incidental consequence of sensor operation. X-ray and ultrasonic imaging techniques and electromagnetic or Doppler ultrasonic blood flow-meters depend on externally applied energy interacting with living tissue. Safe levels of these various types of energy are difficult to establish, because many mechanisms of tissue damage are not well understood. A fetus is particularly vulnerable during the early stages of development. The heating of tissue is one effect that must be limited, because even reversible physiological changes can affect measurements. Damage to tissue at the molecular level has been demonstrated in some instances at surprisingly low energy levels.

Operation of instruments in the medical environment imposes important additional constraints. Equipment must be reliable, easy to operate and capable of withstanding physical abuse and exposure to corrosive chemicals. Electronic equipment must be designed to minimise electric-shock hazards. The safety of patients and medical personnel must be considered in all phases of the design and testing of instruments.

CLASSIFICATIONS OF BIOMEDICAL INSTRUMENTS

The study of biomedical instruments can be approached from at least four viewpoints. Techniques of biomedical measurement can be grouped according to the quantity that is sensed, such as pressure, flow or temperature. One advantage of this classification is that it makes different methods for measuring any quantity easy to compare.

A second classification scheme uses the principle of transduction, such as resistive, inductive, capacitive, ultrasonic or electrochemical. Different applications of each principle can be used to strengthen understanding of each concept; also, new applications may be readily apparent.

Measurement techniques can be studied separately for each organ system, such as the cardiovascular, pulmonary, nervous and endocrine systems. This approach isolates all important measurements for specialists who need to know only about a specific area, but it results in considerable overlap of quantities sensed and principles of transduction.

Finally, biomedical instruments can be classified according to the clinical medicine specialities, such as pediatrics, obstetrics, cardiology or radiology. This approach is valuable for medical personnel who are interested in specialised instruments. Of course, certain measurements—such as blood pressure—are important to many different medical specialities.

INTERFERING AND MODIFYING INPUTS

Desired inputs are the measurands that the instrument is designed to isolate. Interfering inputs are quantities that inadvertently affect the instrument as a consequence of the principles used to acquire and process the desired inputs. If spatial or temporal isolation of the measurand is incomplete, the interfering input can even be the same quantity as the desired input. Modifying inputs are undesired quantities that indirectly affect the output by altering the performance of the instrument itself. Modifying inputs can affect processing of either desired or interfering inputs. Some undesirable quantities can act as both a modifying input and an interfering input. An example of a modifying input is the orientation of the patient cables. If the plane of the cables is parallel to the AC magnetic filed, magnetically introduced interference is zero. If the plane of the cables is perpendicular to the AC magnetic field, magnetically introduced interference is maximal.

Compensation Techniques

The effects of most interfering and modifying inputs can be reduced or eliminated either by altering the design of essential instrument components or by adding new components designed to offset the undesired inputs. The former alternative is preferred when it is feasible, because the result is usually simpler. Unfortunately, designers of instruments can only rarely eliminate the actual source of the undesired inputs.

Inherent insensitivity

If all instrument components are inherently sensitive only to desired inputs, then interfering and modifying inputs obviously have no effect.

Negative feedback

When a modifying input cannot be avoided, then improved instrument performance requires a strategy that makes the output less dependent on the transfer function.

Usually the feedback device carries less power, so it is more accurate and linear. Less input-signal power is also needed for this feedback scheme, so less loading occurs. The major disadvantage of using this feedback principle is that dynamic instability leading to oscillations can occur.

Signal filtering

A filter separates signals according to their frequencies. Most filters accomplish this by attenuating the part of the signal that is in one or more frequency bands. A more general definition for a filter is 'a device or programme that separates data, signals or material in accordance with specified criteria'.

Filters may be inserted at the instrument input, at some point within the instrument or at the output of the instrument. In fact, the limitations of people's senses may be used to filter unwanted signal components coming from display devices. An example is the utilisation of flicker fusion for rapidly changing images from a real-time ultrasonic scanner.

Electronic filters are often incorporated at some intermediate stage within the instrument. To facilitate filtering based on differences in frequency, mixers and modulators are used to shift desired and/or undesired signals to another frequency range where filtering is more effective. Digital computers are used to filter signals on the basis of template-matching techniques and various time-domain signal properties. These filters may even have time or signal-dependent criteria for isolating the desired signal.

Output filtering is possible, though it is usually more difficult because desired and undesired output signals are superimposed. The selectivity needed may be easier to achieve with higher-level output signals.

Opposing inputs

When interfering and/or modifying inputs cannot be filtered, additional interfering inputs can be used to cancel undesired output components. These extra intentional inputs may be the same as those to be cancelled. In general, the unavoidable and the added opposing inputs can be quite different, as long as the two output components are equal so that cancellation results. The two outputs must cancel despite variations in all the unavoidable interfering inputs and variations in the desired inputs. The actual cancellation of undesired output components can be implemented either before or after the desired and undesired outputs are combined.

Biostatistics

The application of statistics to medical data is used to design experiments and clinical studies; to summarise, explore, analyse and present data; to draw inferences from data by estimation or hypothesis testing; to evaluate diagnostic procedures; and to assist clinical decision making.

Medical research studies can be observational studies, wherein characteristics of one or more groups of patients are observed and recorded or experimental intervention studies, wherein the effect of a medical procedure or treatment is investigated. The simplest observational studies are case-series studies that describe some characteristics of a group. These studies are without control subjects, in order only to identify questions for further research. Case-control observational studies use individuals selected because they have (or do not have) some outcome or disease and then look backward to find possible causes or risk factors. Cross-sectional observational studies analyse characteristics of patients at one particular time to determine the status of a disease or condition.

To enable purchasers to compare commercially available instruments and evaluate new instrument designs, quantitative criteria for the performance of instruments are needed. These criteria must clearly specify how well an instrument measures the desired input and how much the output depends on interfering and modifying inputs. Characteristics of instrument performance are usually sub-divided into two classes on the basis of the frequency of the input signals.

Accuracy

The accuracy of a single measured quantity is the difference between the true value and the measured value divided by the true value. This ratio is usually expressed as a per cent.

The accuracy usually varies over the normal range of the quantity measured, usually decreases as the full-scale value of the quantity decreases on a multirange instrument and also often varies with the frequency of desired, interfering and modifying inputs. Accuracy is a measure of the total error without regard to the type or source of the error. The possibility that the measurement is low and that it is high are assumed to be equal. The accuracy can be expressed as per cent of reading, per cent of full scale, ± number of digits for digital readouts or ±½ the smallest division on an analog scale. Often the accuracy is expressed as a sum of these.

Precision

The precision of a measurement expresses the number of distinguishable alternatives from which a given result is selected. For example, a meter that displays a reading of 2.434 V is more precise than one that displays a reading of 2.43 V. High-precision measurements do not imply high accuracy, however, because precision makes no comparison to the true value.

Resolution

The smallest incremental quantity that can be measured with certainty is the resolution. If the measured quantity starts from zero, the term threshold is synonymous with resolution. Resolution expresses the degree to which nearly equal values of a quantity can be discriminated.

Reproducibility

The ability of an instrument to give the same output for equal inputs applied over some period of time is called reproducibility or repeatability. Reproducibility does not imply accuracy. For example, a broken digital clock with an a.m. or p.m. indicator gives very reproducible values that are accurate only once a day.

Statistical control

The accuracy of an instrument is not meaningful unless all factors, such as the environment and the method of use, are considered. Statistical control ensures that random variations in measured quantities that result from all factors that influence the measurement process are tolerable. Any systematic errors or bias can be removed by calibration and correction factors, but random variations pose a more difficult problem. The measurand and/or the instrument may introduce statistical variations that make outputs unreproducible. If the cause of this variability cannot be eliminated, then statistical analysis must be used to determine the error variation. The estimate of the true value can be improved by making multiple measurements and averaging the results.

Static sensitivity

A static calibration is performed by holding all inputs (desired, interfering and modifying) constant except one. This one input is varied incrementally over the normal operating range, resulting in a range of incremental outputs. The static sensitivity of an instrument or system is the ratio of the incremental output quantity to the incremental input quantity.

Zero drift

Interfering and/or modifying inputs can affect the static calibration curve in several ways. Zero drift has occurred when all output values increase or decrease by the same absolute amount. The following factors can cause zero drift: manufacturing misalignment, variations in ambient temperature, hysteresis, vibration, shock and sensitivity to forces from undesired directions.

Sensitivity drift

When the slope of the calibration curve changes as a result of an interfering and/or modifying input, a drift in sensitivity results. Sensitivity drift causes error that is proportional to the magnitude of the input.

Input ranges

Several maximal ranges of allowed input quantities are applicable for various conditions. Minimal resolvable inputs impose a lower bound on the quantity to be measured. The normal linear operating range specifies the maximal or near-maximal inputs that give linear outputs.

The static linear range and the dynamic linear range may be different. The maximal operating range is the largest input that does not damage the instrument.

Input impedance

Because biomedical sensors and instruments usually convert non-electric quantities into voltage or current, we introduce a generalised concept of input impedance. This is necessary so that we can properly evaluate the degree to which instruments disturb the quantity being measured.

Generalised dynamic characteristics

Only a few medical measurements, such as body temperature, are constant or slowly varying quantities. Most medical instruments must process signals that are functions of time. It is this time-varying property of medical signals that requires us to consider dynamic instrument characteristics. Differential or integral equations are required to relate dynamic inputs to dynamic outputs for continuous systems.

Transfer functions

The transfer function for a linear instrument or system expresses the relationship between the input signal and the output signal mathematically.

ROLE OF ELECTRONIC CIRCUIT THEORY

To deal with instrumentation in detail, it is necessary to analyse it. The fundamental skill required by an engineer or service professional is the ability to analyse, to figure things out, to determine how a piece of equipment is supposed to work. This skill is essential both for engineering design and for troubleshooting of equipment. Probably the most comprehensive expression of the engineering analysis procedure is electronic circuit theory. This theory applies to electronic circuits, of course, but it also applies to fluid systems, pneumatic systems and mechanical machines, all of which are present in medical equipment. Strict analogies can be made to allow you to apply what you learn in circuit theory to those types of systems. To learn engineering analysis, it is helpful to study electrical circuits and electronics. Systems using these components are often the most complex and contain the largest number of components. If you become skilled in electrical and electronic circuit analysis, dealing with pneumatics, mechanics and fluids—of which many medical instruments are composed—will be much easier.

The variables in an electronic system are voltage and current. Physiological potentials arising from the heart, such as the electrocardiogram (ECG), are periodic and may be represented by sinusoidal. The general mathematical form of a voltage sinusoid is

$$v_1 = V_1 \cos(\omega t + \theta)$$

This voltage is defined by its frequency ω (in radians per second), its phase angle θ (in radians) and its peak magnitude V_1. In instrumentation such a signal is operated upon by elements such as resistors, R (in ohms, Ω), capacitors, C (in farads, F) and inductors, L (in henrys, H). Applications of these elements give rise to complicated current and voltage relations, some of which are described by differential equations that are usually unwieldy and difficult to solve. Fortunately, however, mathematical methods have been developed to transform differential equations into algebraic equations containing complex numbers. The process for solution of such equations is called AC circuit theory and it uses phasors.

Electrical circuits are structures composed of resistors, R, inductors, L and capacitors, C. The connections between these elements are called nodes. The voltage and current variables are created by ideal sources. An ideal voltage source, illustrated in Fig. 1.4, maintains the voltage, v_S, across the nodes, regardless of the current passing through it. In effect, it has an internal impedance of zero.

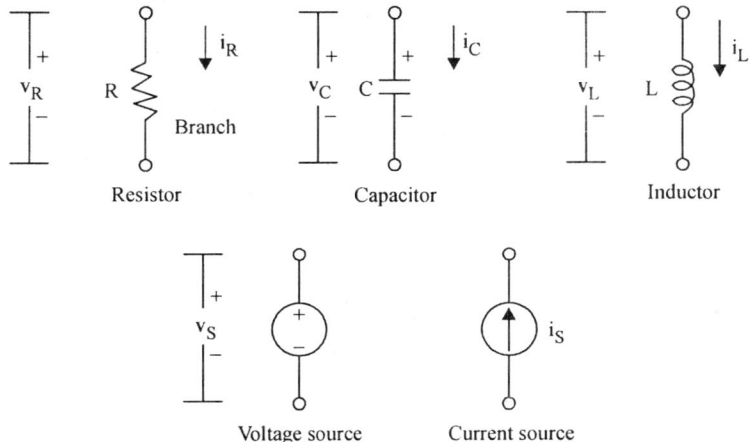

Fig. 1.4. The time domain representation of electrical circuit components.

The ideal current source maintains a current i_S regardless of the voltage across it. Its internal impedance approaches infinity.

AC Circuits

Alternating current circuit theory is based on the phasor expressions for sinusoidal steady state voltages and currents. A phasor is a complex-number representation of a circuit quantity, consisting of a real part, [Re] and an imaginary part, [Im]. Phasors are manipulated mathematically by complex-number algebra.

A set of phasor domain relationships that define R, L and C for sinusoidal steady state is as follows:

$$V_R = (R)I_R \qquad\qquad \text{... (1.1)}$$

$$V_L = (j\omega L)I_L \qquad\qquad \text{... (1.2)}$$

$$V_C = \left(\frac{1}{j\omega C}\right)I_C \qquad\qquad \text{... (1.3)}$$

where j is the imaginary number $\sqrt{-1}$ used in complex-number algebra and ω is the radian frequency. These relationships are basic to AC circuit theory. The quantities in parentheses are called resistance (R), inductive reactance ($j\omega L$) and capacitive reactance ($1/j\omega C$). Here the symbols R, L and C have the same meaning as previously indicated. Equations (1.1) through (1.3) are expressions of Ohm's law in the phasor domain.

Each of these equations has the following form, generally known as Ohm's law:

$$V = ZI \qquad \qquad \dots (1.4)$$

where V is the phasor voltage, I the phasor current and Z the impedance. These phasor quantities, V, I and Z are complex numbers containing real and imaginary parts. The impedance of a resistor in a series with a capacitor, for example, is given by

$$Z = R + \frac{1}{j\omega C}$$

expressed in rectangular form. The expression in polar form has the symbol

$$Z = |Z| \angle \theta$$

where $|Z|$ is the magnitude of the impedance and θ is the phase angle. Conversion between the rectangular form and the polar form is easily done with the aid of a hand-held scientific calculator. (It is assumed that most student have such calculators and will not have to do the conversion by hand).

The impedance of a resistor, a capacitor and an inductor connected in series is

$$Z = R + j\omega L + \frac{1}{j\omega C}$$

$$Z = R + j\left(\omega L - \frac{1}{\omega C} \right)$$

Since modern scientific programmable calculators accept and manipulate complex numbers directly, the effort required in calculations using impedance is minimal. The use of a calculator with these capabilities is strongly encouraged as an aid to performing calculations on medical instrument circuits. For example, plotting a complex impedance versus frequency is often practically impossible without a programmable calculator. One of the most widely used and most effective techniques for troubleshooting defective equipment involves voltage measurement at test points. Comparison of measured voltages with predicted voltages may reveal discrepancies that can be used as clues to locate defective parts or components.

Troubleshooting tip

Signal tracing may be done by measuring the voltage at a node and comparing it with the voltage calculated for it. Differences aid in locating troubles. To predict the voltage at one point in a circuit due to a known voltage elsewhere, it is often necessary to use circuit analysis. Circuit analysis in the phasor domain is the process by which one finds a circuit variable, such as listed in Table 1.2 in terms of the network component values or variables. In a fixed network, the variables R, L and C are often constant, while the radian frequency $\omega = 2\pi f$, where frequency, f, measured in Hertz, is variable. The current through a circuit branch or the voltage across the branch, is often computed as a function of frequency.

Table 1.2. Phasor domain components and variables.

Variables (units)	Components	Units
V (volts)	R, resistance	Ohms
I (amps)	$j\omega L$, inductive reactance	Vars
	$\dfrac{1}{j\omega C}$, capacitive reactance	Vars

In Fig. 1.5, each branch illustrates either a phasor source or impedance. Positive, conventional current travels in the direction of the current arrow and the positive voltage terminal is shown by the plus (+) sign. Capacitive reactance and inductive reactance are represented by imaginary numbers.

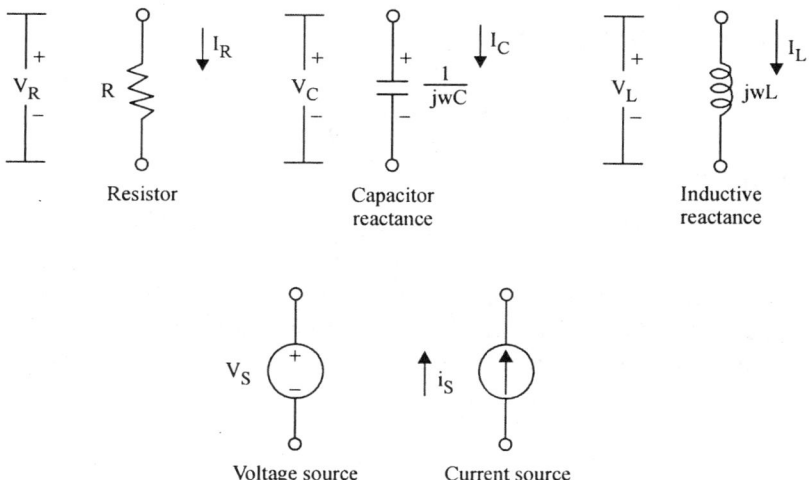

Fig. 1.5. Electrical circuit components in the phasor domain.

Phasor voltages across element branches and phasor currents entering (or leaving) the nodes are governed by Kirchhoff's laws.

Kirchhoff's current law (KCL): The complex-number sum of phasor currents entering a node equals zero. An equivalent statement of this law is: the complex number sum of phasor currents leaving a node equals zero. In Fig. 1.6a, each of the currents is defined as leaving the node. KCL then implies that

$$I_1 + I_2 + I_3 + I_4 + I_5 = 0$$

Kirchhoff's voltage law (KVL): The complex-number sum of phasor voltages drops or alternatively rises, around any closed loop of branches travelled in the same direction is zero. In Fig. 1.6b, applying KVL as current travels in the clockwise direction through the closed loop implies that

$$V_1 + V_2 + V_3 + V_4 + V_5 - V_S = 0$$

The plus (+) sign before V_1 through V_5 indicates that they are voltage drops. The minus (−) sign on V_S indicates that voltage rises occur as current travels through the branch going in the clockwise direction.

If V_{IN}, V_{OUT} and all of the circuit impedances are known quantities, the previous two equations can be solved simultaneously to find the node voltages V_1 and V_2. This would then be sufficient information to compute all branch currents by application of Ohm's law.

Voltage Division

Ohm's law and Kirchhoff's current and voltage laws are sufficient to enable one to compute the voltages and current in any R, L, C circuit. However, it is often convenient to use the voltage division principle as derived from Fig. 1.7. Applying KVL then gives.

$$V_{IN} = IZ_1 + IZ_2$$

Then, Ohm's law applied to Z_2 gives

$$I = \frac{V_{OUT}}{Z_2}$$

This current substituted into the first equation yields

$$V_{IN} = V_{OUT}\left(\frac{Z_1}{Z_2} + \frac{Z_2}{Z_2}\right)$$

Solving this for V_{OUT} gives

$$V_{OUT} = \frac{Z_2}{Z_1 + Z_2} V_{IN} \qquad\qquad \dots (1.6)$$

Equation (1.6) is an expression of the voltage division principle for impedances connected in series. An easy way to remember this widely used formula for voltage division is to think of the output voltage as being proportional to the load impedance over the sum of the impedances in series.

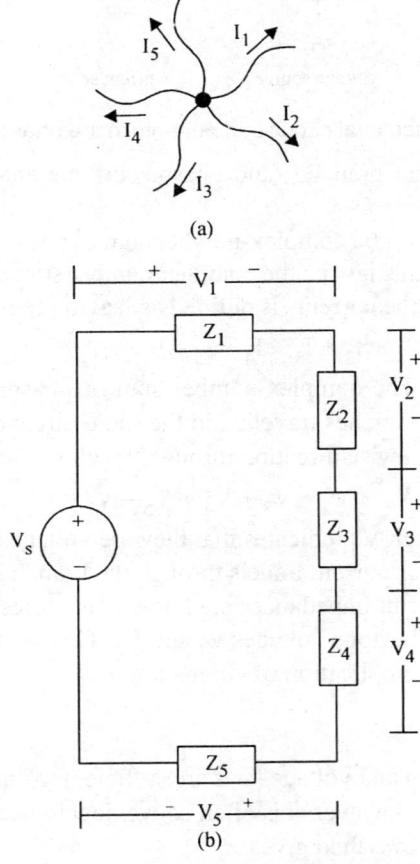

Fig. 1.6. (a) An illustration of KCL; and (b) an illustration of KVL.

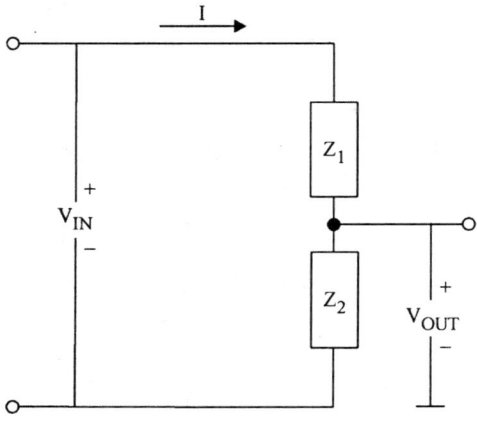

Fig. 1.7. A voltage divider.

Current Division

The current division principle is derived from Fig. 1.8. Here,

$$I_{IN} = \frac{V}{Z_2} + \frac{V}{Z_1}$$

and

$$V = I_{OUT}Z_1$$

Eliminating the voltage V between these two equations gives

$$I_{IN} = I_{OUT}\left(\frac{Z_1}{Z_2} + \frac{Z_1}{Z_1}\right)$$

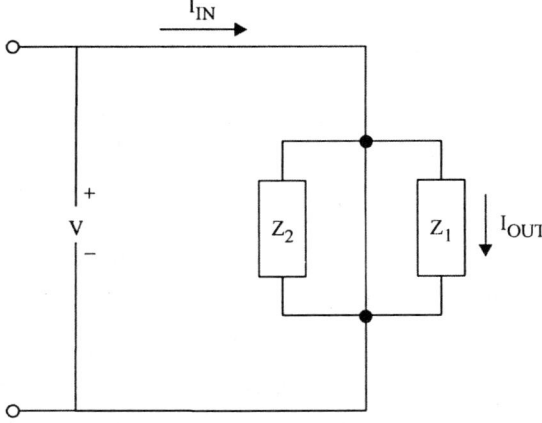

Fig. 1.8. A current divider.

Rearranging this gives the expression for the division of current between two impedance in parallel:

$$I_{OUT} = \frac{Z_2}{Z_1 + Z_2} I_{IN} \qquad \qquad ... (1.7)$$

An easy way to remember this widely used formula is to think of the current as being proportional to the opposite over the sum of the impedances in parallel.

Gain Function Analysis

The gain functions for voltage or current are defined from Fig. 1.9. The voltage gain A_V equals the ratio of output voltage V_{OUT} to input voltage V_{IN} computed as a function of R's, L's, C's and frequency f:

$$A_V = \frac{V_{OUT}}{V_{IN}}$$

Likewise, the current gain A_I is defined as the ratio of the output current to the input current or

$$A_I = \frac{I_{OUT}}{I_{IN}}$$

Calculation of either gain function, A_V or A_I, is accomplished by application of Kirchhoff's laws and Ohm's law to the circuit network.

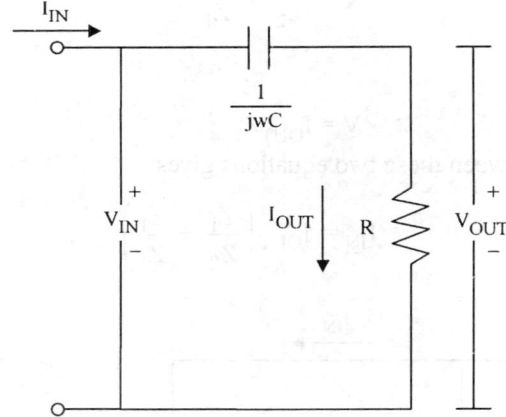

Fig. 1.9. Gain functions for voltage.

BJT Equivalent Circuit

In addition to R, L and C elements, electronic circuits contain various pn-junction semi-conductor devices, including semi-conductor diodes, bipolar junction transistors (BJTs) and integrated circuits. For use in electronic circuit analysis, the BJT can be represented as an equivalent circuit, consisting of R, L and C elements and an ideal current or voltage source. Bipolar junction transistors consist of three layers of semi-conductor material doped with impurities that make them either p-type or n-type. The circuit symbols for the BJT (Fig. 1.10) represent two types: the PNP and the NPN transistors. In Fig. 1.10a, I_B is the base current entering the base node B, I_C is the collector current entering the collector node C and I_E is the emitter current leaving the emitter node E of the NPN transistor.

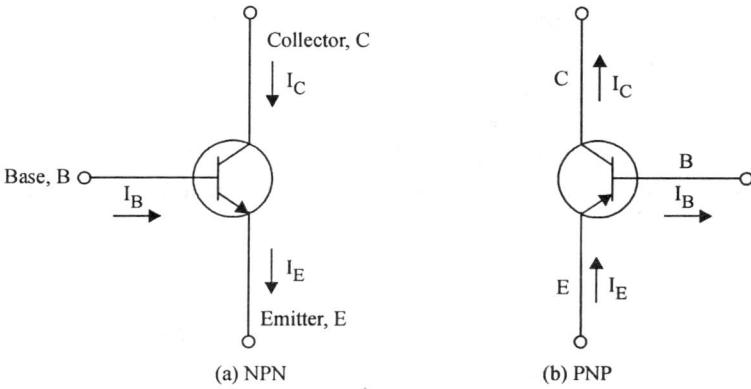

Fig. 1.10. (a) NPN; and (b) PNP transistor circuit symbols.

The characteristics of the transistor are described by the collector-to-emitter voltage, V_{CE} versus I_C. The curve plotting this voltage is shown in Fig. 1.11. Each of the family of curves is measured at a different value of base current: I_B, labeled I_{B0}, I_{B1}, I_{B2} and so on. In DC analysis of the transistor element, an important parameter usually specified by the manufacturer is the DC current gain, β_{DC}, defined as

$$\beta_{DC} = \frac{I_C}{I_B} \qquad \text{... (1.9)}$$

Applying Kirchhoff's current law to Fig. 1.10a yields

$$I_E = I_C + I_B$$

Combining these equations yields

$$I_E = (1 + \beta_{DC})I_B$$

Furthermore, when $\beta_{DC} \gg 1$, we have

$$I_E \approx \beta_{DC} I_B = I_C \qquad \text{... (1.10)}$$

Since the transistor is designed as a current gain device, the approximation $\beta_{DC} \gg 1$ often holds.

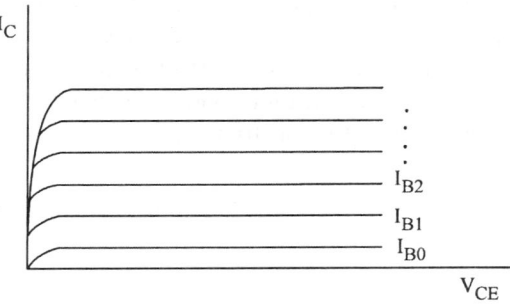

Fig. 1.11. The voltage-current characteristics of a BJT.

Because of the principle of superposition in electronic circuit theory, the analysis of the circuit due to the DC bias supply can be done separately from the analysis resulting from AC signal voltage. The AC analysis is performed using the small AC signal equivalent circuit given in Fig. 1.12.

In Fig. 1.12 the equivalent circuit parameters are defined as follows:

$\beta_{AC} = i_C/i_B$ is the AC current gain

r_e is the emitter resistance to AC currents

r_b is the base resistance to AC currents

r_c is the collector resistance to AC currents.

The lower case 'r' is used to indicate an AC equivalent circuit element. Capital 'R' designates the values of resistors in this text.

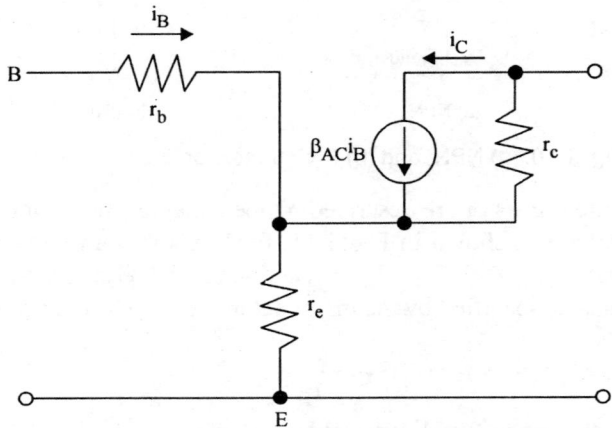

Fig. 1.12. A small signal AC equivalent circuit of a BJT.

DESIGN CRITERIA

Many factors affect the design of biomedical instruments. The factors that impose constraints on the design are of course different for each type of instrument. However, some of the general requirements can be categorised as signal, environmental, medical and economic factors.

Note that the type of sensor selected usually determines the signal-processing equipment needed, so an instrument specification includes more than just what type of sensor to use. To obtain a final design, some compromises in specifications are usually required. Actual tests on a prototype are always needed before final design decisions can be made. Changes in performance and interaction of the elements in a complex instrument often dictate design modifications. Good designs are frequently the result of many compromises throughout the development of the instrument.

Chapter 2

Bioelectric Signals and Electrodes

INTRODUCTION

A biopotential is an electrical voltage caused by a current flow of ions through biological tissue. The study of biopotentials is fundamental to the understanding of medical instrumentation. Several of the major types of equipment, including electrocardiographs and electroencephalographs, measure biopotentials from the surface of the body. Physicians use the data obtained from these instruments to assess the health of their patients. All professionals who work with medical instrumentation must understand the safety hazards associated with biopotentials. The primary hazard is electrical shock. Certain occurrences, called microshock, can cause a fatality at current levels as low as 20 microamps (μA). Corresponding dangerous voltages are on the order of millivolts (mV).

FUNDAMENTAL LAWS FOR CURRENT IN BIOLOGICAL TISSUE

The single cell is the unit from which living systems are built. Its complexity is illustrated by the fact that within its membrane hundreds of chemical reactions take place, many of which are not understood. You can observe a membrane potential, V_m, in living cells by inserting a microtip wire or conductor-filled glass electrode into a cell, as shown in Fig. 2.1. The value of V_m measured is usually about –90 mV.

The potential appearing across the cell membrane is the basis for the biopotentials measured on the body, including the electrocardiogram (ECG), electroencephalogram (EEG), electrooculogram, electro-retinogram and electromyogram (EMG). Notice here that the suffix 'gram', as in electrocardiogram, designates the potential itself, whereas the suffix 'graph', as in electrocardiograph, designates the instrument that measure or records the potential.

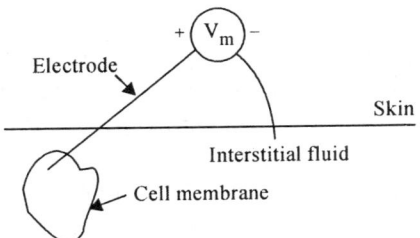

Fig. 2.1. A circuit for measuring cell membrane potential.

Whereas the particle producing electrical events in passive circuits is the free electron, the particle producing electrical events in biological tissue is the ion in an electrolyte solution. The rules governing these ionic events are (i) fick's law for diffusion; (ii) the drift equation; and (iii) the Einstein relation.

Fick's Law

Fick's law for diffusion states that if there is a high concentration [C] of particles in one region that are free to move, they will flow in a direction to equalise the concentration [C] throughout the region. Fick's law for diffusion holds for the diffusion of perfume molecules throughout a room, electrons in a doped semi-conductor or ions in an electrolyte. In one dimension, Fick's law is expressed as:

$$J = -D\frac{d[C]}{dx} \qquad \qquad ...(2.1)$$

for positive ions. The minus sign is dropped for negative ions. The current density, J, expressed in amperes per unit area, is caused by the concentration gradient. As illustrated in Fig. 2.2, [C] is the concentration of ions as a function of the distance, x, in units of moles per litre (mol/litre). (Recall that a mole is an amount of the substance in grams equal to the sum of the atomic weights of its constituent atoms). D is the diffusion constant, x is the position and [C] is a positive number.

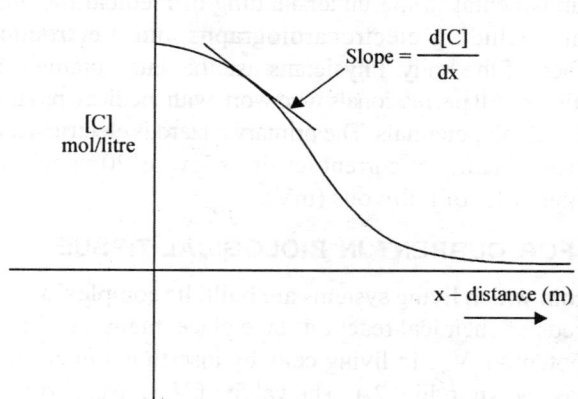

Fig. 2.2. An ionic concentration as a function of position.

In Fig. 2.2 the slope d[C] for x > 0 is negative; the ionic current flow is in the positive x direction, as indicated in Equation (2.1). A typical system of units is: [C] in moles per litre (mol/litre); x, meters (m); J, amperes per meter squared (A/m^2); and D, litre amperes per mole meter [(litre · A)/(mol · m)].

Particle Drift

In addition to the diffusion force acting on ions, there is a force due to electric fields acting as well. Charged particles such as ions in an electric field will move under the forces of electrical attraction and repulsion. The resulting ionic flow is called the drift current. Drift current is proportional to the voltage drop, V, the ion valence, Z and the concentration, [C]. Z is equal to the number of charges on the ion. The proportionality constant is called the mobility, μ. That is, the current density due to particle drift is given by:

$$J_{drift} = -\mu Z\frac{dV}{dx}[C] \qquad \qquad ...(2.2)$$

where μ is the mobility expressed in litre amperes per volt meter mole [(litre · A)/(V · m · mol)]; Z is valence; $E = -dv/dx$ is the electric field intensity in volts per meter (V/m); and [C] is the concentration of ions taken as a positive number in moles per litre (mol/litre). The two physical constants, mobility μ and the diffusion coefficient D, are related to each other by the Einstein relationship usually derived in the theory of solid-state pn-junction diodes. The Einstein relationship is:

$$\frac{D}{\mu} = \frac{kT}{q} \qquad \qquad \text{... (2.3)}$$

where k is Boltzmann's constant, q is the charge and T is the absolute temperature.

Equations (2.1) through (2.3) can be used to derive the membrane potential in biological cells. The following verbal description based on a physical interpretation of Fick's law, the drift equation and the Einstein relationship will help to explain how the biopotential arises and how it differs from other voltage-producing processes. It will also help to explain biopotential electrodes used in medical instrumentation.

Single-Cell Membrane Potential

The way in which the diffusion and drift processes give rise to a membrane potential is illustrated in Fig. 2.3. Here we see the hypothetical case of a 10 molar potassium chloride (KCl) solution outside a membrane and a 1 molar solution inside.

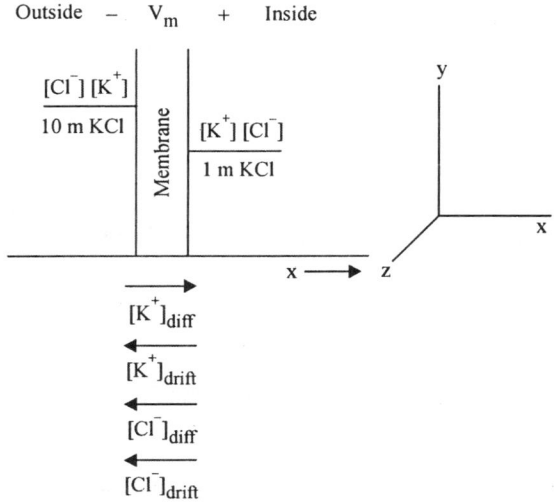

Fig. 2.3. Ionic currents due to drift and diffusion forces.

The x-y plane is shown. The y-z plane is perpendicular to the paper. The membrane separating the two KCl solutions is in the y-z plane. A high concentration of ions of $[K^+]$ and $[Cl^-]$ appears on the outside of the cell, while a low concentration appears on the inside. This means that the slope of the ionic concentrations is negative, since in both cases the concentration decreases as x increases. According to Fick's law, the negative chlorine ions $[Cl^-]$ flow from outside to inside, causing a diffusion current flowing to the left, as shown by the arrow in the Fig. 2.3; the arrow points in the direction of conventional positive-charge current flow. Likewise, the positive potassium ions $[K^+]$ diffuse from outside to inside, causing a conventional diffusion current flowing to the right, shown by the arrow pointing right in the figure. These positive ions collect on the inside of the membrane, thereby causing a voltage that is positive on the right and negative on the left. This voltage has a positive slope; it increases as x increases. In accordance with the drift equation, this voltage produces drift currents. The positive voltage repels the positive $[K^+]$ ions, causing a drift current indicated by the arrow pointing left, labelled $[K^+]_{drift}$. This voltage also attracts negative $[Cl^-]$ ions, moving them to the right across the membrane, producing a conventional current to the left, as indicated by the arrow pointing left, labelled $[Cl^-]_{drift}$. V_m, in this case, is assumed positive in the direction indicated in the Fig. 2.3. If V_m were predominantly determined by the negative ions in the electrolyte, it would be a negative number.

At equilibrium, which is the condition of a cell membrane at rest, the total current across the membrane must be zero. Otherwise the regions, no matter how large, would eventually fill, since ions are matter. Therefore, the total current is zero. That is,

$$J_{K\,(drift)} + J_{K\,(diff)} + J_{Cl\,(drift)} + J_{Cl\,(diff)} = 0$$

This condition leads to Goldman's equation, stated here as

$$V_m = -\frac{kT}{q} \ln\left(\frac{P_K[K^+]_i + P_{Cl}[Cl^-]_o}{P_K[K^+]_o + P_{Cl}[Cl^-]_i}\right)$$

where the subscript i indicates inside the cell, o designates outside and

k	=	Boltzmann's constant
T	=	absolute temperature (K)
q	=	the charge on a proton
P_K	=	the permeability of potassium
P_{Cl}	=	the permeability of chlorine
$[K^+]$	=	the concentration of potassium ions
$[Cl^-]$	=	the concentration of chlorine ions

Permeability is a measure of the ease with which ions pass through the cell membrane.

Resting Potential in a Cell

In a similar argument, we can extend the preceding equation for three ions as follows:

$$V_m = -\frac{kT}{q} \ln\left(\frac{P_K[K^+]_i + P_{Na}[Na^+]_i + P_{Cl}[Cl^-]_o}{P_K[K^+]_o + P_{Na}[Na^+]_o + P_{Cl}[Cl^-]_i}\right) \qquad \text{... (2.4)}$$

Goldman's equation specifies the cell membrane voltage for actual concentrations of potassium, chlorine and sodium. It shows that membrane potential depends strongly on temperature. Since the permeabilities of different cell types vary, the corresponding membrane potentials vary as well. This relationship is the basis for understanding many aspects of transducer behaviour, including surface electrodes. It also explains the behaviour of chemical electrodes used in clinical instrumentation.

In a living cell, when the approximations $P_{Na} \approx 0$ and $P_{Cl} \approx 0$ hold, Goldman's equation reduces to a simple form as

$$V_m = -\frac{kT}{q} \ln\left(\frac{[K^+]_i}{[K^+]_o}\right) \qquad \text{... (2.5)}$$

This is called the Nernst equation and it is often valid as an approximation to the Goldman equation.

Example 2.1. Suppose a frog skeletal muscle has the following ion concentrations and permeabilities of the membrane:

Ion	Inside (mmol/litre)	Outside (mmol/litre)	Permeability (cm/s)
Na^+	11	146	1.9×10^{-8}
K^+	150	4.35	2.1×10^{-6}
Cl^-	5	125	3.9×10^{-6}

Compute the membrane voltage from inside to outside the cell at 37°C (310 K).

Solution.

Boltzmann's constant k   = 1.38×10^{-23} J/K

An electronic charge q   = 1.602×10^{-19} C

The temperature T   =   310 K

Then

$$V_m = -0.0267 \ln \left(\frac{2.1(10^{-6})(150) + 3.9(10^{-6})(125) + 1.9(10^{-8})(11)}{2.1(10^{-6})(4.35) + 1.9(10^{-8})(146) + 3.9(10^{-6})(5)} \right)$$

$$= -86.5 \text{ mV}$$

Considering potassium, $[K^+]$ in this equation yields

$$V_m = -0.0267 \ln \left(\frac{[K^+]_i}{[K^+]_o} \right)$$

$$= -0.0267 \ln \left(\frac{150}{4.35} \right) = -94.5 \text{ mV}$$

These two results verify the idea that the resting potential in a cell is caused primarily by potassium flow. We see that if potassium is considered alone, the result is −94.5 mV, whereas if we also take into account Cl and Na, the result is −86.5 mV. The accuracy is improved by 9.2 per cent when all ions are accounted for. Under certain circumstances, the approximation given by the Nernst equation is better than this.

Action Potential and Muscle Contraction

Living cells are encased in a high-resistance membrane, which, at rest, has a potential caused by the flow of sodium and chlorine ions into the cell and potassium ions out of it. The resting potential, V_m, as computed by the Goldman (Eq. 2.4) normally has values between −50 mV and −100 mV. If the potential is raised across the membrane by about 20 per cent, then a stimulus threshold is exceeded and the cell membrane resistance changes, causing a change in the membrane potential. This new membrane potential, called the action potential, is shown in Fig. 2.4. As long as the action potential exists, the cell is said to be depolarised. In a tissue, the depolarisation disturbance of one cell is propagated to the next until the entire tissue depolarises. In muscle, where cells are situated in an orderly arrangement, the tissue contracts and becomes shorter in length after some delay following a depolarisation. A typical delay of 10 ms between the action potential depolarisation and the subsequent muscle twitch is indicated in the figure. A stimulus voltage generally does not affect a cell while it is changing its polarisation. The refractory period is the time duration of cell non-response to further stimuli. During the relative refractory period, a higher stimulus is required to re-initiate an action potential and the subsequent contraction of muscle.

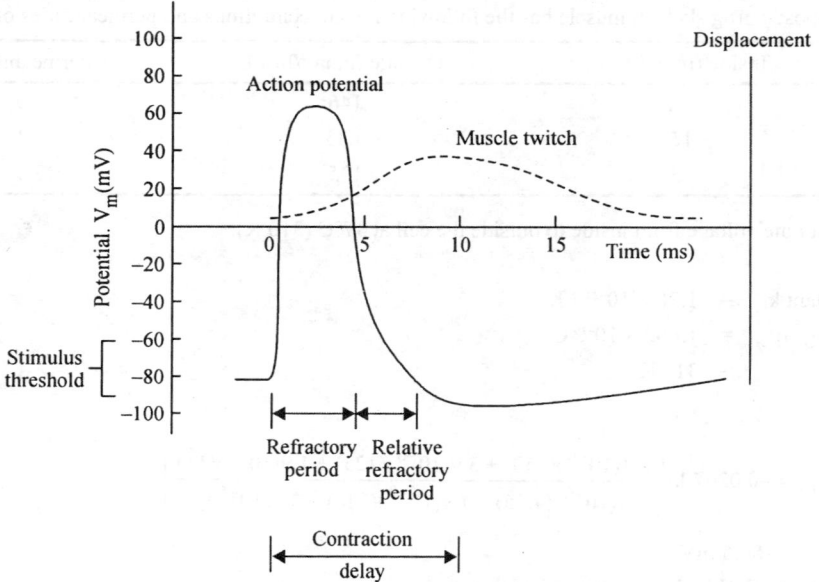

Fig. 2.4. The relationship between the action potential and muscle contraction.

BIOPOTENTIALS IN THE HEART

The electrical activity of the heart is integral to the operation of several types of medical instruments, including the electrocardiograph, the pacemaker and the defibrillator. Very small electrical disturbances can cause this vital organ to cease pumping blood necessary to sustain life.

The heart consists of two major smooth muscles, the atrium and the ventricle, which form a syncytium or fusion of cells, that conducts depolarisation from one cell to an adjacent cell. Because of ionic leakage in the smooth muscle membrane, the tissue of the heart depolarises spontaneously from its resting state and effectively oscillates or beats. The sinoatrial (SA) node beats at a rate of from 70 to 80 beats per minute (bpm) at rest; the atrioventricular (AV) node beats at 40 to 60 bpm and the bundle branch oscillates at 15 to 40 bpm.

The SA node normally determines the heart rate, since it beats at the fastest rate and cause stimulation of the other tissue before it reaches its self-pacing threshold. Thus, the SA node can be considered the heart's pacemaker. The path of the depolarisation of cells in a heart is illustrated in Fig. 2.5.

The depolarisation of the SA node spreads throughout the atrium and reaches the AV node in about 40 ms. Because of the low conduction velocity of the AV node tissue, it requires about 110 ms for the depolarisation to reach the bundle branches pointed out in the figure, called the Purkinje system. The ventricles then contract, the right ventricle forcing blood into the lungs, the left ventricle pushing blood into the aorta and subsequently through the circulation system. The contraction period of the heart is called systole.

The action potentials in the ventricle hold for 200 to 250 ms. This relatively long time allows the ventricular contraction to empty blood into the arteries. The heart then re-polarises during a rest period, called diastole. Then the cycle repeats.

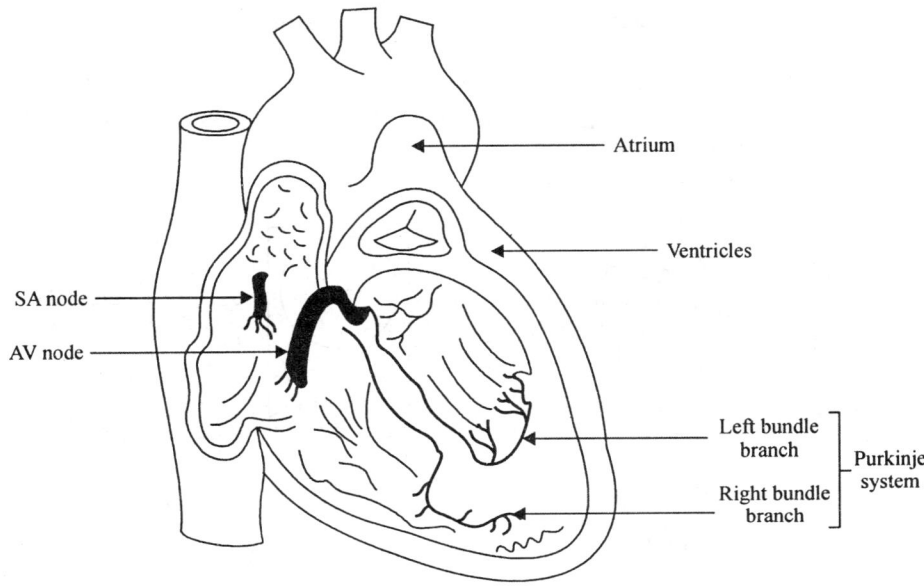

Fig. 2.5. The depolarisation path through the heart.

ELECTROCARDIOGRAM

During diastole, while the heart is at rest, all of the cells are polarised so that the potential inside each cell is negative with respect to the outside. Normally, depolarisation occurs first at the SA node, making the outside of the tissue negative with respect to the inside of the cells and also making it negative with respect to the tissue not yet depolarised. This imbalance results in an ionic current, I, causing the left arm (LA) to measure positive with respect to the right arm (RA), as illustrated in Fig. 2.6a. The resulting voltage is called the P-wave.

After about 90 ms, the atrium is completely depolarised and the ionic current measured by lead I reduces to zero. The depolarisation then passes through the atrioventricular node, causing a delay of about 110 ms. The depolarisation then passes into the right ventricular muscle, depolarising it and making it negative relative to the still-polarised left ventricular muscle, as illustrated in Fig. 2.6b. Again, the direction of I causes a plus-to-minus voltage from LA to RA called the R-wave.

The complete waveform in Fig 2.7 is called an electrocardiogram (ECG), with labels P, Q, R, S and T indicating its distinctive features. The P-wave arises from depolarisation of the atrium. The QRS complex arises from depolarisation of the ventricles. The magnitude of the R-wave within this complex is approximately 1 mV. The T-wave (Fig. 2.6c) arises from re-polarisation of the ventricle muscle. During the T-wave, partial re-polarisation of the cardiac muscle causes ionic currents and a corresponding ECG potential, as previously described for the R-wave. The U-wave that sometimes follows the T-wave is a second-order effect of uncertain origin and is of little diagnostic significance. The intervals, segments and complexes of the ECG are defined in Fig. 2.7. Typical durations are as follows:

Feature	Duration (ms)
QRS complex	70–110
R-R interval	600–1000

P-R interval	150 – 200
S-T interval	320

The QRS duration, P-R interval and S-T interval depend on the depolarisation rate of the heart and are relatively constant for an individual, regardless of his or her exercise level. The ranges above reflect individual differences in a normal population.

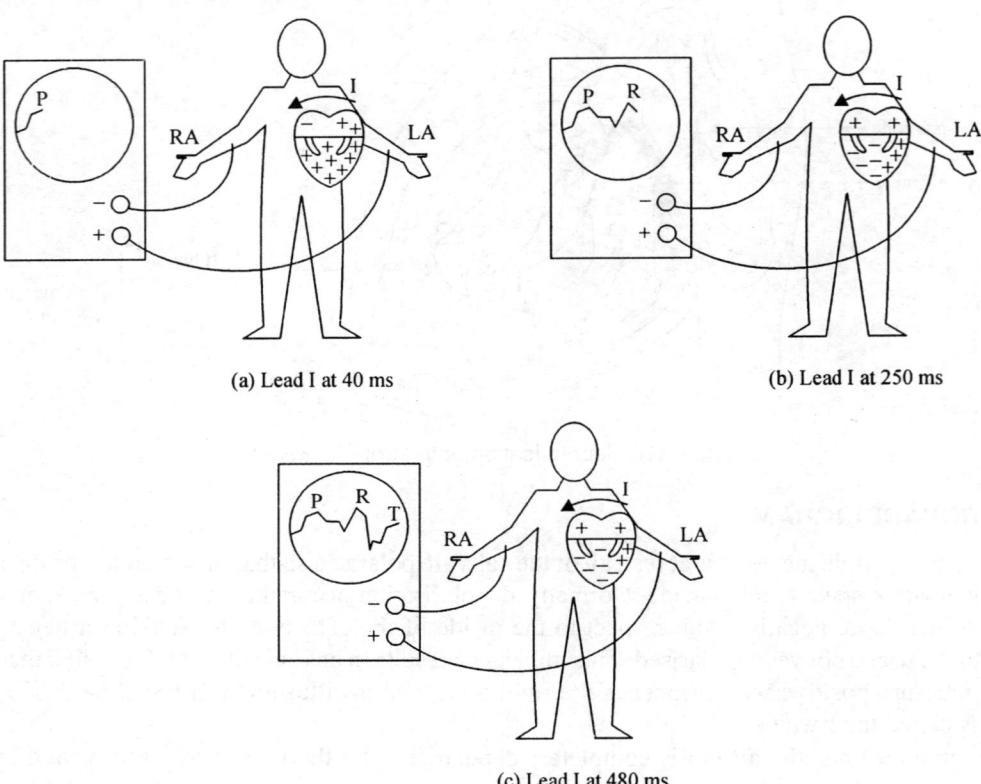

(a) Lead I at 40 ms (b) Lead I at 250 ms

(c) Lead I at 480 ms

Fig. 2.6. Ionic currents as the source of an electrocardiogram.

ELECTRICAL SHOCK

An understanding of electrical shock is important to everyone working with and around electrical equipment. Patients and hospital equipment users are especially susceptible to shock because they must make physical contact with the hardware.

The physiological effects of shock range from discomfort to injury to death, if the heart or respiratory system is affected. An electrical shock is an unwanted or unnecessary physiological response to current. Electrical shock may cause an unwanted cellular depolarisation and its associated muscular contraction or it may cause cell vapourisation and tissue injury. A cell is depolarised when the membrane potential is changed by approximately 20 per cent. The question is, how much current is required to create this threshold?

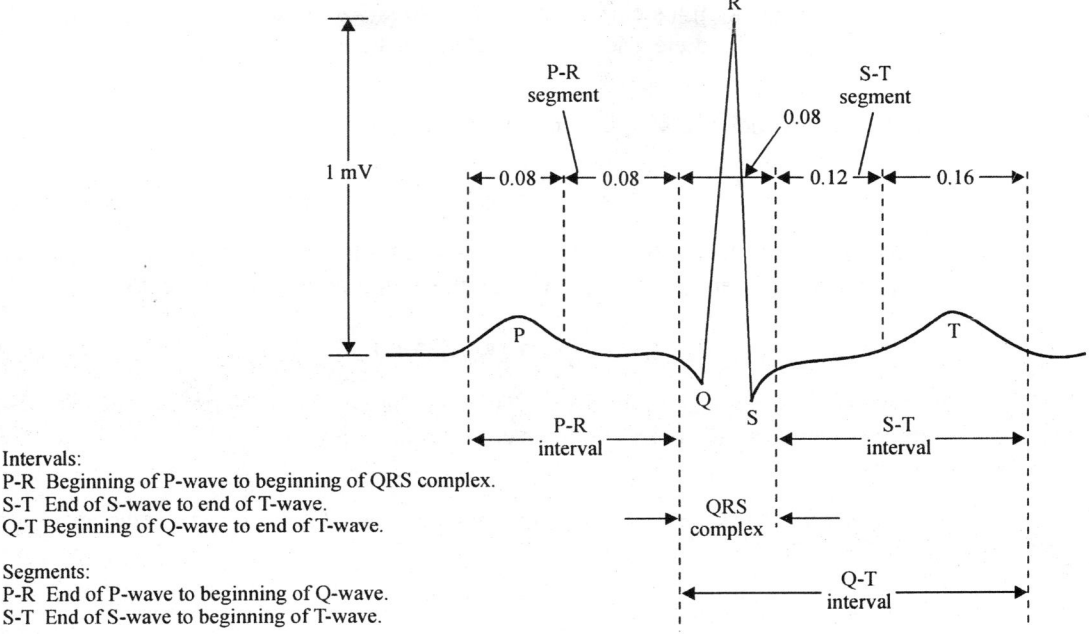

Intervals:
P-R Beginning of P-wave to beginning of QRS complex.
S-T End of S-wave to end of T-wave.
Q-T Beginning of Q-wave to end of T-wave.

Segments:
P-R End of P-wave to beginning of Q-wave.
S-T End of S-wave to beginning of T-wave.

Complex:
QRS Beginning of Q-wave to end of S-wave.

Durations:
Average durations shown on drawing, in seconds.

Fig. 2.7. ECG definitions.

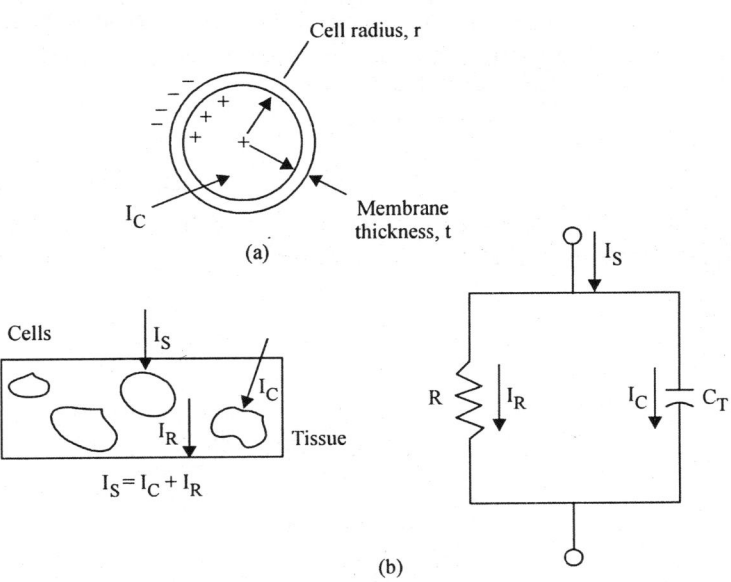

Fig. 2.8. A cell model illustrating high-frequency effects on cell membrane current.

To conveniently estimate the stimulus current in a cell, a spherical model (Fig. 2.8a) may be used. The cell membrane is modelled as a dielectric with dielectric constant ε,

$$\varepsilon = \varepsilon_0 \varepsilon_r$$

The capacitance of the sphere enclosed by the membrane is given by

$$C = \varepsilon \frac{Area}{t} = \varepsilon_0 \varepsilon_r \frac{4\pi r^2}{t} \qquad \ldots (2.7)$$

where $\varepsilon_0 = 8.85 \times 10^{-12}$ F/m, ε_r is the relative dielectric constant, t is the membrane thickness and r is the radius. The stimulus current I_C entering the cell to initiate the action potential is given by

$$I_C = \frac{V_{mt}}{Z} \approx V_{mt}(j2\pi fC) \qquad \ldots (2.8)$$

where V_{mt} is the threshold potential required to depolarise the cell. This approximation holds for frequencies, f, sufficiently high for the current I_s to be considered steady state and allows us to calculate the high-frequency effects.

Example 2.2. A cell membrane has a thickness t of 0.1 μm and a radius r of 10 μm. Assuming a relative dielectric constant ε_r of 2, compute the cell capacity C.

Solution.

$C = 2 (8.85 \times 10^{-12})4 (10 \times 10^{-6})^2\pi/(0.1 \times 10^{-6})$

$= 0.222$ pF

A model of tissue may be regarded as a set of cells in an interstitial fluid. The fluid is a conducting electrolyte, as shown in Fig. 2.8b, where I_S is the total stimulus current into the tissue, I_R is the component through the interstitial fluid and I_C is the sum of all currents entering the cells in the tissue.

Example 2.3. A tissue 1 cm² in area contains 450×10^6 cells with characteristics as described in Example 2.2. The conductance of the interstitial fluid is 1 siemens (mho) per square centimeter (Ω/cm²). Make an equivalent circuit for this tissue.

Solution. The total capacitance, C_T, is the sum of the capacitances of each cell from example 2.2. These capacitances are added because the reference is taken as the inside of the cell. Thus,

$$C_T = (450 \times 10^6) (0.22 \times 10^{-12})$$
$$= 100 \text{ μF/cm}^2$$

From this tissue model, we can also estimate the current levels necessary to produce an electrically induced muscle contraction. From Fig. 2.9, the stimulus threshold may be estimated at 20 mV. We can then use Equation (2.8) to estimate the stimulus current.

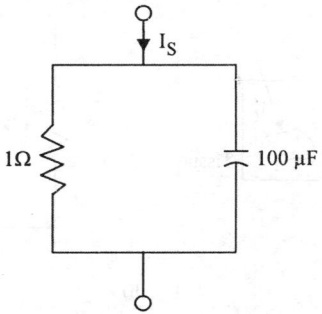

Fig. 2.9. An equivalent circuit of tissue passing high-frequency current.

Example 2.4. If the stimulus for an action potential in the individual cells of the tissue in Example 2.3 is 20 mV, compute the stimulus current necessary to depolarise all of the cells simultaneously at a frequency of 60 Hz. The syncytium of these cells may, for example, represent a muscle.

Solution.

$$I_s = (20/Z_T) \, (10^{-3})$$

and, from Fig. 2.9, the tissue impedance Z_T is

$$Z_T = 1/[1 + j2\pi \, (60) \, (10^{-4})]$$

Therefore,

$$|I_s| = |(20 \times 10^{-3}) \, [1 + j2\pi(60) \, (10^{-4})]| = 20 \text{ mA}$$

In this case a 20 mA current would cause an involuntary contraction of the muscle. This is consistent with let-go current given in the safety tips in Table 2.1 which lists the effects of arm-to-arm currents, applied as shown in Fig. 2.10. These are 60 Hz currents entering one hand and travelling through the vital organs of heart, respiration control center and brain. Similar effect would occur if the current passed from the right to left arm to a foot, from the hand to the head and from the head to a foot. In each case, currents could pass through the vital organs of respiration and the heart. Such currents, however, travelling from the bicep brachii to a hand or between two abdominal points, for example, would not cause the life-threatening effects of respiratory paralysis or heart failure, provided that the currents did not pass through these vital organs.

Table 2.1. Safety tips.

Electrical currents passing through surface electrodes from one arm to the other have serious physiological consequences. At 60 Hz, such currents above 5 mA are considered dangerous. Specific physiological effects are listed in the table.

Type of current	Current range (mA)	Physiological effect
Threshold	1–5	Tingling sensation
Pain	5–8	Intense or painful sensation
Let-go	8–20	Threshold of involuntary muscle contraction
Paralysis	>20	Respiratory paralysis and pain
Fibrillation	80–1000	Ventricular and heart fibrillation
Defibrillation	1000–10000	Sustained myocardial contraction and possible tissue burns

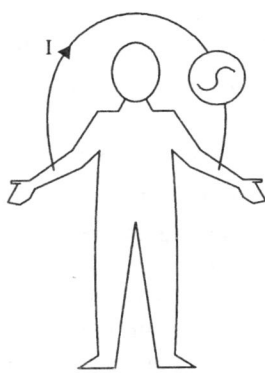

Fig. 2.10. Current passed from arm to arm, described in Table 2.1.

In general, the physiological effects of current on the body for several seconds range from a tingling sensation at 1 to 5 mA applied to the surface, to tissue injury due to burns when more than 1 A is applied. A surface current above 5 mA is considered dangerous because it may cause pain or injury (Table 2.1). Let-go current (8 to 20 mA) causes involuntary muscle contractions. It may, for example, prevent a person receiving such a current from releasing himself or herself from the source of shock. At 20 mA, widespread muscle contraction in the respiratory system and interference with respiratory control signals from the brain could prevent breathing and would lead to death if sustained. Above 80 mA, currents reach parts of the heart and cause ectopic beats to occur. If this happens at several sites on the heart simultaneously, the heart may begin to fibrillate. The SA node then loses control of the pacing so that the heart continues to flutter without pumping blood. The fluttering will continue until therapeutic action is taken to reverse it. One method of reversing it, called defibrillation, requires the application of a current exceeding 1 A across the thorax. This causes simultaneous contraction of all of the heart muscle. When the current is removed, the SA node is able to regain control and pace the heart normally.

In summary, it is clear that currents above 5 mA should be considered hazardous. Currents above 20 mA passing through a vital organ can be fatal. The electrical effects listed in Table 2.1 are called macroshocks because they are distributed over large areas. The thresholds listed are for current durations greater than 1 second. If the shock duration is reduced to 0.1 second, the fibrillation threshold increases ten times. This fact is used to design circuit interrupters to prevent injuries due to shock.

High-Frequency Effects

Although most electrical currents that might contact a patient are of low frequency (around 60 Hz), the effects of high frequencies cannot be ignored. Since electrosurgical scalpels operate at frequencies in the order of 500 kHz, the question arises as to whether a muscle contraction or heart fibrillation might be stimulated by a scalpel.

As frequency is increased in a conductor, the current tends to flow near the surface. This is called the skin effect. Compared with the effects of currents flowing within the human body, the skin effect does not seem important. On the other hand, the 500 kHz current generated by an electrosurgical unit (ESU) flows strongly in the core of the body.

We can look to the model of tissue in Fig. 2.8 for one of the more important reasons why currents cause less muscle contraction at ESU frequencies and so are less dangerous. The let-to current as a function of frequency is plotted in Fig. 2.11, indicating that it increases at high frequency. Example 2.5 interprets the data in Fig. 2.11 by showing that the current needed to create the threshold for the action potential on the cells increases according to the computed value in the figure.

Example 2.5. Extend the calculation in Example 2.4 and compute I_s as a function of frequency.

Solution.

$$I_s = 0.020 \,(1 + j2\pi f \times 10^{-4})$$
$$= 0.020 + j\, 1.26 \times 10^{-5}\, f$$

A calculation of I_s versus frequency is plotted as computed data in Fig. 2.11. For example, a frequency of 500 kHz produces $I_S = 6.3$ A. The conclusion from this calculation is that at 500 kHz it is necessary to drive 6.3 A into the tissue in order to reach the threshold for an action potential. Such high currents cause the cells to vapourise rather than depolarise. Therefore, the muscle would not contract at these current levels and electric shock manifested as muscle contractions or heart fibrillations would not occur. Thus, we would not expect an ESU to produce shock in patients from currents intended for surgical cutting.

Any shock hazard would come from stray currents at low frequency. ESUs are designed to eliminate such low-frequency currents.

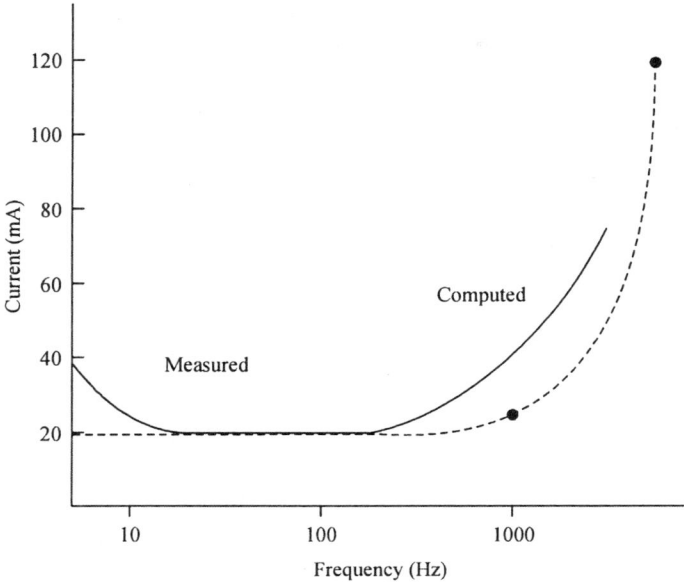

Fig. 2.11. An example let-go current measured from arm to arm as a function of frequency compared with Example 2.5 calculations.

Microshock and Macroshock

The electrical shock situations we have just described are called macroshock. A much subtler electrical shock situation (one that may sometimes be more dangerous because it is difficult to detect) is microshock. The two situations differ as indicated in the following definitions:

Macroshock: A physiological response to a current applied to the surface of the body that produces unwanted or unnecessary stimulation, muscle contractions or tissue injury.

Microshock: A physiological response to a current applied to the surface of the heart that results in unwanted stimulation, muscle contractions or tissue injury.

Microshock is most often caused when currents in excess of 10 µA flow through an insulated catheter to the heart, as illustrated in Fig. 2.12. The catheter may be an insulated, conductive-fluid–filled tube or a solid-wire pacemaker cable as illustrated in Fig. 2.12a. The microshock results because the current density at the heart can become high in the situation depicted there, in which the catheter is touching the heart. To produce macroshock, much larger current is required, because the current distributes itself throughout the body, as shown in Fig. 2.12b. Obviously, the current density at the heart is much lower in this case and more current is required to cause a shock. This accounts for the thousand-to-one ratio of macroshock current to microshock current levels.

RECORDING ELECTRODES

In order to be able to monitor the signals from intensive care patients reliably for extended periods, it is particularly important that detailed attention should have been given to both the type of electrode used and the site and nature of the attachment of the electrodes to the patient. The commonest electrical signal recorded is the electrocardiogram (ECG). Apart from visual inspection of the individual ECG complexes, use is often made of the ECG R-waves for triggering a heart rate meter. The R-R intervals and R-wave widths may also be used in conjunction with arrhythmia detection circuitry. Attention to the electrodes is important, since a badly attached electrode may give rise to intermittent bursts of AC mains frequency pick-up which can lead to erratic heart rate readings and possible false tachycardia alarms. An electrode which becomes detached from the patient will give rise to a large amount of mains pick-up (hum) which will obscure the cardioscope display of the ECG waveform and activate the tachycardia alarm. There is nothing like the frequent occurrence of false alarms for bringing a patient monitoring system into disrepute, hence the emphasis on electrodes.

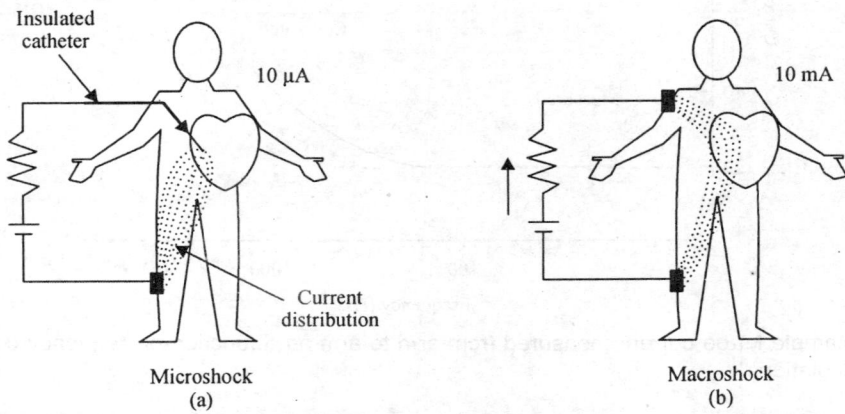

Fig. 2.12. The current density accompanying microshock versus that accompanying macroshock.

Requirements for Recording Electrodes

The electrodes normally used in patient monitoring are of the surface type and in various forms are used for the monitoring of the ECG, EEG and the impedance pneumogram. For the best quality recordings when the electrodes are placed on the skin it is necessary that the skin-electrode contact impedance should be stable and as low as possible. The contact impedances for individual electrodes should be as nearly equal as can be arranged. Any potential difference produced across the electrode–skin interface should also be as small as possible and should differ little from one electrode to another.

Recording electrodes are generally used in conjunction with a balanced amplifier having a differential input, i.e., two active input electrodes and an indifferent electrode (e.g., the Lead 1 ECG—right arm, left arm as the active electrodes and the right leg as the indifferent electrode). The amplifier will accept signals which are in anti-phase from the two active electrodes and will reject unwanted interference signals which are picked-up in-phase from the active electrodes.

The discrimination ratio DR between the wanted anti-phase bio-electric signals and the unwanted in-phase interference signals is given by DR = $(R_I/2)/(R_2 - R_1)$ where R_I is the total input impedance in ohms of the recording amplifier and R_1 and R_2 are the electrode–skin contact impedances of the two active recording electrodes. If R_I = 5 meg-ohms whilst R_1 = 6 k-ohms and R_2 = 4 k-ohms, then DR = 1250. DR is also known as the common mode rejection ratio (CMR).

The voltage picked-up from the recording electrodes consists of two main components. The first is the contact potential which is usually of the order of a fraction of a volt and normally is relatively constant. However, Flasterstein has reported that it is possible for corrosion effects occurring at electrodes to generate artefacts in an AC recording. Superimposed upon the standing contact potential is the bio-electrical signal. This can be up to 1000 times smaller in amplitude than the contact potential and will usually contain higher frequency components. In most applications, it is the higher frequencies which are of interest and hence an AC recording amplifier is used which will not pass the DC (or slowly varying) contact potential. In some cases the very low frequency content of the signal of interest makes it necessary to use a DC recording system. Examples of this occur with the bladder electromyogram which contains signal components down to 0.05 Hz and the DC electro-oculogram (EOG) where the signals arising from eye movements are approximately 200 micro-volts in amplitude. Noise and baseline shifts produced at the electrode–skin interface are generated because at the interface there is a transition from ionic current flow in the body tissues to an electronic flow in the connecting wire from the electrodes. To provide a stable baseline voltage, the electrode selected must have a stable and predictable potential with respect to the electrolyte with which it is in contact. In EEG and EOG recording where the signal amplitudes are small, it is usual to employ silver–silver chloride electrodes. These are reversible electrodes. Shackel attained mean DC drifts of less than 50 micro-volts per minute with suction cup silver–silver chloride electrodes.

Reversible Electrodes

The combination of a metal electrode and an electrolyte forms a half-cell which generates a DC potential whose magnitude depends on both the nature of the metal and the electrolyte. When the two recording electrodes are joined by a common electrolyte, they constitute two half-cells connected in series opposition. If the electrodes were identical, then the emf measured across the cell would be zero. However, when the electrodes are fabricated from different materials, a cell emf will exist since now each electrode will assume a different potential with respect to the electrolyte. The value of the cell emf will depend on the temperature, the ionic concentration in the electrolyte and the material of the electrodes.

In a reversible cell, changing the direction of the current flow through the cell will not affect the composition of the electrodes. A simple example consists of a pair of copper electrodes immersed in a copper sulphate solution. When current is not drawn from a reversible cell, the cell emf will be zero since each electrode will have acquired the same potential with respect to the electrolyte.

Silver–silver chloride electrodes

Tissue fluids contain a major proportion of sodium, potassium, chloride, bicarbonate and protein ions with chloride ions being the most widely distributed. Because they are reactive, sodium and potassium are unsuitable as electrode materials so that an insoluble chloride such as silver chloride is most suitable for choice as a stable electrode material. The approximation to reversibility is shown by the fact that potential differences of only fraction of a millivolt can exist between pairs of carefully prepared silver–silver chloride electrodes.

Silver–silver chloride electrodes are usually prepared by electrolysis. A pair of silver disks is suspended in a 5 per cent saline solution and the electrode to be chlorided is connected to the positive terminal of a 1.5 V battery, the other electrode being connected to the negative terminal. An electrode for EEG recording can be produced by passing current for about 30 seconds to form a layer of silver chloride upon the anode. Margerison recommended that re-chloriding should be performed when the current which flows between a pair of silver–silver chloride electrodes in saline exceeds one micro-ampere. Geddes and Baker recommend a maximum chloriding current density of 5 mA per cm^2 of electrode area and found that a chloride deposit of 100–500 mA per second per cm^2 of electrode area produced the lowest electrode–electrolyte impedance. Miller describes an electrolytic technique for the preparation of silver–silver chloride electrodermal electrodes and a suitable electrode paste.

Polarisation over-voltage

In a reversible cell, the electrodes do not change their composition when current flows through the cell in either direction. However, if this is not the case and the passage of current alters the electrode composition, a potential difference will build-up across the electrodes and alter the current. This effect is known as polarisation and the presence of the potential will aid current flow in one direction and reduce it in the other. The polarisation over voltage is the change in the open-circuit potential due to the current flow. It takes time to build-up and can cause distortions when recording pulses of the order of 2 mV in amplitude and 100 ms wide.

Electrodes for the Recording of the Electrocardiogram

Almost every patient monitoring system is concerned with the ECG and hence the choice of electrodes is a matter of general concern. The type of electrode utilised will depend very much on the circumstances. In screening clinics, the electrodes must be capable of being put on and taken off as quickly as possible and the person being examined is likely to be able to sit or lie still for the relatively short space of time required for the various ECG leads to be recorded. In this situation, conventional metal plate electrodes or multipoint electrodes are generally employed. Another example of where ECG electrodes need to be applied in a hurry consists of a portable monitor box carrying three electrodes which can be placed on the chest to pick-up the ECG if it is present and actuate the pointer of a meter.

In contrast, in an intensive care unit the patient will need to keep his ECG electrodes securely in place for at least 24 hours. He is likely to be restless and perspiring and the positioning of the electrodes on the chest must allow for the placement of DC defibrillator paddles in an emergency. Under these circumstances conventional limb electrodes are ruled out because, not only are their connection cables likely to get in the way, but excessive movement artefacts can occur with restless patients. Nearly all commercial patient monitoring systems currently employ light-weight stick-on disposable chest ECG electrodes.

Particularly in intensive care situations, it is necessary to ensure that a stable contact impedance can be maintained at the skin—electrode interface over a period of at least 24 hours. A loosely applied electrode can produce artefacts which will trigger heart rate alarms and cause endless inconvenience. It is also important to take precautions to minimise the chance of infection of irritation occurring beneath the electrodes as this will lead to the patient interferring with the electrode.

Electrode-skin contact impedance

The electrical impedance measured between any pair of sites in the body tissues lying beneath the skin is quite low, of the order of several tens of ohms. In comparison, the contact impedance between an electrode and the skin is relatively high and can be as much as tens of thousands of ohms. Grease at the skin surface plus the outer horny layer is responsible for the bulk of the contact impedance. In order to attain a contact impedance which is both stable and as small as possible, it is recommended that the skin at the electrode site should be first rubbed vigorously with an ether-meth mixture and a non-irritant conducting paste or jelly should be rubbed into the skin in order to produce a good physical contact with the electrode when it is held firmly in contact with the prepared site. Some degree of irritation nearly always occurs under an electrode and for this reason it is usually desirable to move the position of the electrode slightly at regular intervals of perhaps 24 hours. A simple method of obtaining the approximate value of the impedance lying between two recording electrodes is to first note the amplitude of the recorded signal, say an ECG, taken from across the electrodes in question. A decade resistance box is then placed across the electrodes and the box adjusted until the recorded signal amplitude has been halved. The resistance in the box is now equal to the impedance existing between the electrodes. This approach has been used to show that the impedance between the tips of a pair of fine wire EMG electrodes spaced 10 mm apart in the wall of the bladder was approximately 20000 ohms.

A more accurate technique is the arrangement shown in Fig. 2.13. It uses an alternating current to avoid changes in the contact impedance which could occur due to the direct current producing polarisation effects. The technique also allows the contact impedance to be measured at various frequencies. Since impedance measurements for stroke volume and tidal volume operate at radio frequencies, it is desirable to measure the electrode contact impedance at the signal frequency to be encountered in practice. The contact impedance can be simulated by an electrical network consisting of a parallel combination of resistors and capacitors and the impedance will fall with increasing frequency. For a normal ECG, the bulk of the signal energy will be concentrated below 30 Hz so that 10 Hz would be a convenient test frequency to use.

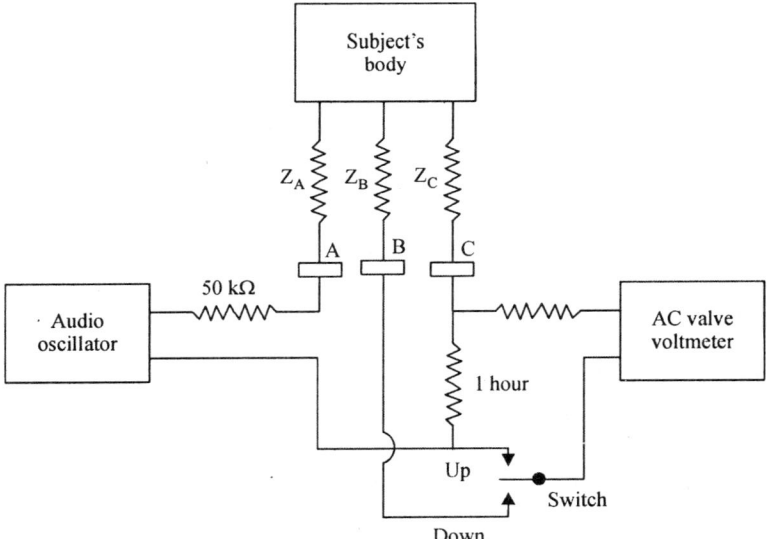

Fig. 2.13. Arrangement for measuring the skin-contact impedance of a recording electrode.

In Fig. 2.13, three electrodes are placed on the subject's skin, usually on the forearm. The test signal, from a sinewave oscillator, enters the subject at A and leaves at C returning to the oscillator via the 1000 ohm resistor. When the switch is up, a high resistance AC voltmeter reads the rms voltage developed across the 1000 ohm resistor. The oscillator output control is adjusted to produce a reading of 100 mV on the meter which is equivalent to a current of 0.1 mA. Once this has been set, the switch is placed in the down position and the meter reading noted. Assuming that the potential drop occurring across the tissue lying between A and C is negligible and that the meter draws a negligible input current, then for the current of 0.1 mA, each 1 mV corresponds to a 10 ohm contact impedance at electrode C. Figure 2.14 illustrates how the contact impedance varies with frequency for various types of ECG electrode.

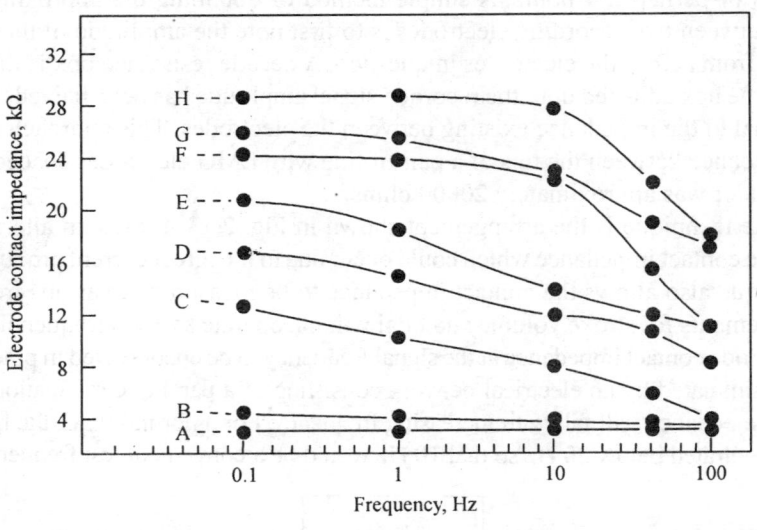

(A) Cup type electrode of Boter
(B) Sanborn plate electrode with redux paste.
(C) Newmark plate electrode over a conducting plastic sheet.
(D) Dry multi-point electrode.

(E) Dry multi-point suction electrode (chest).
(F) Self-adhesive multi-point chest electrode.
(G) Self-adhesive gauge electrode.
(H) Dry self-adhesive multi-point electrode.

Fig. 2.14. The variation of electrode-skin contact impedance with signal frequency.

The contact impedance of a standard limb electrode with jelly would be in the range 4000 to 6500 ohms whilst a dry multipoint electrode made from stainless steel nutmeg grater material would be about 9000 ohms and a disposable self-adhesive stainless steel gauge monitoring electrode with jelly would have a contact impedance of about 20000 ohms.

Electrodes for monitoring the ECG

Chest electrodes are nearly always employed for monitoring the ECG in intensive care situations and should be of a lightweight construction in order to minimise the problem of keeping them securely attached to the skin. Obviously, the cable attached to the electrode must be as light in weight as is feasible with the required degree of strength and the cable must be anchored to the patient's body so that it will not drag on the electrode.

ECG monitoring electrodes used with conventional apparatus are connected to the monitor by a wire for each electrode and are normally used with a conducting paste or jelly. Kahn and Boter showed that artefact signals can arise as a result of motion occurring at the interface between the metal electrode and the adjacent layer of jelly or paste. Both papers recommended the mounting of the electrode within a small, rigid, plastic cup which holds the jelly or paste. Because the electrode does not make a direct contact with the skin this is known as a floating electrode. The cup is provided with a flange so that it can be attached to the skin by the use of a double sided adhesive ring. A typical cup diameter would be 15 mm. In Boter electrode the side of the cup facing the patient is open, whereas in Kahn's (Beckman Instruments) the cup is closed except for some small holes on the skin side. This requires that the cup is filled with jelly through the holes by means of a syringe and needle. A period of about 30 minutes should be allowed for this type of electrode to attain a sufficiently low value of skin contact impedance. Before the elapse of this period significant amounts of hum may appear on the tracing. Thus when an ECG or other signal has to be recorded in a hurry this electrode should not be used. However, once it has settled in, the Kahn electrode gives excellent results with the minimum of motion artefacts. For example, it has been used to monitor the ECG's of swimmers.

It is attached to the skin by a double-sided adhesive paper ring and can be left in position for several days. Boter electrode is attached by means of a fabric ring and a special non-irritant glue. Rickles and Seal evaluated four long-term techniques for attaching transducers to the skin. Stomaseal was found to give the best results with a mean endurance time of 14.7 days on the male sternum.

A number of commercial patient monitoring systems employ plastic cup electrodes with a silver–silver chloride or silver disk inside the cup. For the best results, the grease on the skin should be removed with an ether-meth mixture or isopropyl alcohol and the outer horny layer of the skin abraded with pumice.

Another form of electrode commonly used in patient monitoring is disposable and consists of a piece of stainless steel gauge about 1 cm square placed at the center of a 4 cm × 4 cm piece of self-adhesive plaster. The skin site is first cleaned with an ether–meth mixture and vigorously rubbed. A small amount of electrode jelly is placed on the gauge and this is then pressed down firmly on to the skin.

Fluck and Burgess have described a disposable ECG electrode made from an ordinary press-stud which is mounted in a shallow plastic cup having a rim 35 mm in diameter. The electrode cable attaches to the press stud and the cup is filled with electrode jelly. 'Micropore' adhesive tape is used to hold the cup to the skin which has previously been shaved and cleaned with alcohol. Micropore plaster is recommended for holding down electrodes for extended periods as it is porous and allows perspiration to evaporate and hence reduced risk of inflammation. Russell and Thorne have discussed skin reaction occurring beneath plasters.

Albisser and others have produced an atraumatic electrode especially designed for cardiac monitoring with neonates. The disposable electrode consists of polythene band 102 mm long by 19 mm wide and 1 mm thick to which is cemented a folded paper electrode and the insulator of a lead wire assembly. One end of the band is provided with a pull-tab covering and adhesive upon which the band adheres during application in a bracelet fashion. A small quantity of saline or water is introduced under the plastic film to activate the electrode. The average interval for successive applications of saline was found in practice to be in excess of 10 hours.

Davis and Samuels designed a simple disposable salt-bridge oesophageal ECG electrode which could be constructed at the bedside. The unipolar electrode is made from a plastic nasogastric tube. It has proved to be particularly useful for picking-up P-waves.

Electrode jellies, creams and pastes

The earliest string galvanometer electrocardiographs employed low input impedance galvanometers and needed skin contact impedances of not more than a few thousand ohms. In order to meet this demand as reliably as possible, use was made of abrasive saline creams and jellies interposed between the skin and the electrodes. It is interesting to note that in a study on Frank vector ECG leads, Berson and Pipberger found that electrode skin contact impedances were extremely variable and unpredictable, ranging between 0 and 206 k-ohms at 10 Hz. In most instances, they decreased with the passage of time. Errors in Q, R, S and T-wave amplitudes measured using a digital computer occurred in 17 of the 24 patients as a result of skin-to-electrode contact impedances. As a result of these findings, Berson and Pipberger recommend that buffer amplifiers be employed in ECG recording whatever weighting networks are used between the electrodes and the recording device.

Because of the large variations in contact impedance which can occur with a range of patient's skins, the skin preparation had to be vigorous when earlier designs of low input impedance electrocardiographs were in use. Contact impedances of 3000 ohms or less can be obtained with the use of abrasive creams. Bell reported that the addition of crushed quartz to green soap reduced the contact impedance measured with soap alone beneath an electrode by a factor of three after rubbing.

With present-day ECG amplifiers having input impedances of more than two meg-ohms, satisfactory recordings can be made with electrode contact impedances in the range 10 to 20 k-ohms. Conventional stick-on electrodes are used in conjunction with a cream or jelly. When monitoring ECGs for periods of at least 24 hours, the choice of cream is important. It should be colourless and odourless. It must wet the surface of the body and should not contain soap. It must be of a bland nature and non-irritant. An average value for the specific resistance of electrode creams at 10 Hz is 100 ohm-cm.

Dry ECG electrodes

The multi-point electrode does not require any jelly and works well with conventional ECG recorders. Its points pierce the outer horny layer of the skin and within a few minutes a layer of perspiration has formed beneath the electrode and a contact impedance comparable with that found with plate electrodes and jelly occurs. The development of integrated circuit operational amplifiers has meant that a high input impedance voltage follower can actually be mounted on the rear side of an electrode to act as an input buffer amplifier. The electrodes are usually insulated and rely on a capacitive coupling to the patient's body. Hence, they do not require any conducting paste or jelly and they block any DC potential which may be present. The drying-out of the paste or jelly can be a problem with conventional electrodes when these are worn for extended periods. Richardson used aluminium oxide as the dielectric for their insulated electrodes, whilst Lagow chose tantalum oxide. David and Portnoy employed a dielectric of silver dioxide on a silicon substrate. A high input impedance pre-amplifier is required. David and Portnoy's amplifier had a 100 meg-ohm input impedance and an output impedance of approximately 5 ohms. A lower cut-off frequency of between 0.01 and 1 Hz is obtainable depending upon the nature of the material used for the dielectric and its thickness.

Placement of ECG monitoring electrodes

Three electrodes (two active and one indifferent) are normally placed on the chest for monitoring the ECG. When it is important to minimise motion artefacts from exercising or restless patients and a radio telemetry system is in use, two electrodes only may be used.

These are placed over the manubrium and the xiphisternum. Muscle activity is now reduced since the electrodes are located over bony structures. With this placement, Lewes and Hill obtained a clean ECG by radio telemetry from a subject running up and down a flight of 19 steps. The M–X lead is non-standard and is not recommended for diagnostic purposes.

Since the use of conventional limb electrodes is often unacceptable due to motion artefacts, Mason and Likar located electrode sites on the thorax which produced tracings similar to the conventional leads 1, 2 and 3. They placed two of their electrodes on the right and left chest below the clavicles with the third on the anterior axillary line halfway between the costal margin and the crest of the ileum.

For the ECG monitoring of post-cardiac surgery patients, a simulated lead 2 tracing can be obtained with the two active electrodes located at the top of the thorax close to each shoulder, the positive electrode being on the right and the indifferent electrode on a thigh. This arrangement leaves the surgical incision clear. Considerable attention has naturally been given to the placement of electrodes for the monitoring of the ECG in coronary care units. Here it is important to be able to recognise the presence of cardiac arrhythmias and to leave the area over the heart free for the possible application of DC defibrillator electrodes. Figure 2.15 shows the positions of electrodes designed to simulate lead 2. The negative electrode is placed at the second intercostal space to the right of the sternum, medial to the right pectoral muscle, the positive electrode is placed at the level of the lowest palpable rib on the left side, in the anterior axillary line; the indifferent (earth) electrode is placed at the second intercostal space to the left of the sternum, medial to the left pectoral muscle.

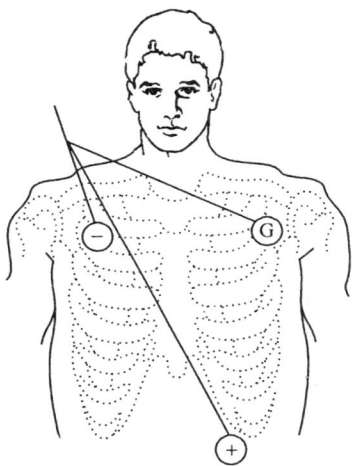

Fig. 2.15. Simulated Lead 2 placement of ECG monitoring electrodes.

In order to make the single lead monitoring for monitoring the ECG more useful, particularly for the identification of aberrant rhythms and blocks, Marriott and Fogg have designated three ECG leads, called by them MCL_1, M_3 and MCL_6, by placing the positive electrode as shown in Fig. 2.16. In each case the negative electrode is located at the outer fourth of the left clavicle and the indifferent (earth) electrode is located at the right shoulder. The praecordium is left clear for examination or for the application of defibrillator electrodes and the positioning of the electrodes also avoids hairy or mammary sites. The modified chest lead MCL_1 is obtained by placing the positive electrode at the usual V_1 site (fourth right interspace at the right sternal edge). Marriott and Fogg have found that the MCL_1 lead can be of value in distinguishing between the right or left ventricular origin of a premature beat and hence providing an early warning of the possible onset of ventricular fibrillation. In patients having pacing catheters in place, a shift in the pacing pattern from right ventricular to left ventricular could indicate an otherwise silent perforation of the right ventricular wall or septum by the catheter tip. Marriott and Fogg also advocate the MCL_1 lead for distinguishing between a right and left bundle branch block and for its value in anticipating a complete atrio-ventricular block. It has also been found useful in making the distinction between left ventricular ectopy and right bundle branch block in patients having a myocardial infarction. A minor disadvantage of the MCL_1 lead occurs in that both sinus and retrograde P-waves may be upright, biphasic or inverted. Thus P-wave polarity is of little diagnostic value with this lead. Re-location of the positive electrode to the left side of the abdomen given a modified lead 2 tracing in which retrograde

P-wave can be readily identified. Placement of the positive electrode at the usual V_6 position (MCL_6 lead) may prove helpful in distinguishing between left ventricular ectopy and right bundle branch block aberration.

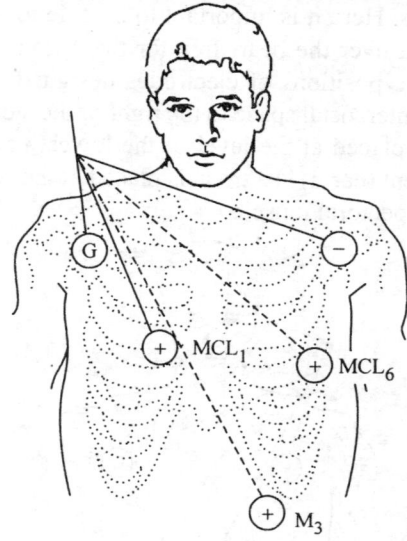

Fig. 2.16. Possible electrode placements for ECG arrhythmia monitoring.

Electrodes for Radio Frequency Impedance Measurements

With electrical impedance measurements for tidal and stroke volumes, it is essential to have a low, stable, electrode-skin contact impedance otherwise motion artefacts can obscure the wanted signal. In tidal volume measurement the thoracic impedance change per breath will be of the order of one fiftieth or less of the standing impedance across the chest and in stroke volume measurements it will be approximately one part in 250.

For tidal volume monitoring, Baker and Hill employed 10 mm diameter silver disk electrodes and conductive jelly, the electrodes being held in place by a rubber strap placed around the chest. Day and Lippit have described a long-term electrode system for both electrocardiograph and impedance pneumography. When the impedance system of Kubicek is used for the monitoring of stroke volume and limb blood flow changes, a most convenient form of electrode is a strip of aluminium approximately 6 mm wide mounted on a self-adhesive Mylar plastic strip. These electrodes are simple to apply in clinical intensive care situations and can be kept in place for more than 24 hours if required.

EEG Electrodes

In intensive care units dealing with patients having brain injuries it is common practice to monitor the electroencephalogram (EEG). The low amplitude (100 micro-volts or less) of the signal calls for low-noise, stable contact impedance electrodes. A frequently encountered type consists of a chlorided silver button about 10 mm in diameter and slightly domed. There is a hole in the center and a tag at one edge to which is attached a flexible connection wire. The electrode is stuck to a cleaned site on the scalp with collodion and electrode jelly is forced through the hole from a syringe by means of a blunt needle. The end of the needle is pressed lightly against the skin and rotated in order to penetrate the outer horny layer. The contact impedance between a pair of stick-on electrodes should not be in excess of

5000 ohms. Kahn's electrode is also suitable for EEG monitoring. The circuitry for recording the mean activity in certain EEG frequency bands has proved of value as a cerebral function monitor. In order to detect artefacts which can arise from loose electrodes, Prior continuously monitored the electrode contact impedance with a high frequency signal.

Placement of EEG monitoring electrodes

For the monitoring of cerebral function in cardiac surgery patients and in patients suffering from brain damage or a drug induced coma, Prior used a pair of silver–silver chloride electrodes attached with collodion to the parietal regions on both sides of the head after a preliminary separation of the hair and cleansing of the scalp. This site was chosen to reduce muscle and movement artefact and to minimise interference during nursing procedure. A third (earth) electrode is normally used.

For monitoring the EEG during routine surgery in order to study the action of anaesthetic and analgesic drugs, two temporal electrodes may be used with the indifferent electrode located on the left ear. This arrangement helps to avoid undue interference with patient's hair and enables the electrodes to be applied quickly in the anaesthetic room, but it may not be the most suitable for recording the alpha rhythm.

EMG Electrodes

In the case of patient monitoring during intensive care, it is unlikely that it will be necessary to record an EMG (electromyogram). However, in a number of situations, such as the investigation of bladder dysfunction, equipment which is used for patient monitoring may be utilised and EMG's recorded if the amplifiers are suitable and the display has a sufficient bandwidth. Lippold has described several types of surface electrode for picking-up the EMG activity from specific muscles. Lippold reported that the use of chlorided silver disks 2 to 10 mm in diameter held in place with sticking plaster was satisfactory. By covering the electrode with several layers of lint soaked in 10 per cent saline and placing a waterproof plaster on top, the electrode could be left in place for up to 12 hours without an appreciable change occurring in the skin contact impedance.

Fine insulated silver or copper wires can be inserted into specific sites such as the urethral or anal sphincters and the bladder and left in place for several hours in order to monitor the muscular activity. The wire (or a pair of wires) is fed down the lumen of a long needle and then bent back to give a small hook across the bevel. The tip of the wire is left bare. The needle is inserted into the muscle and gently withdrawn, leaving the tip of the wire in position. A light pull on the wire will bend the hook straight and cause the wire to be released at the termination of monitoring.

Foetal ECG Electrodes

A requirement exists in obstetrics for foetal scalp ECG electrodes. When labour is sufficiently far advanced that contact can be made directly with the foetal scalp, clip-on scalp electrodes can provide the best foetal ECG signal. Indirect abdominal surface ECG recordings from the mother are complicated by the presence of the material ECG and artefacts arising from uterine and bowel movements. The foetal scalp electrodes must be sterilisable and provide a firm contact with the minimum of trauma to the foetus. Hon and Klock describe suitable designs. Klock's electrode is gold plated and coated with silver–silver chloride and insulated with a polyamide material. It is claimed to have a good elasticity and pliability and to be suitable for multiple use.

Chapter 3

Biomedical Sensors

INTRODUCTION

Biomedical sensors are used in clinical medicine and biological research for measuring a wide range of physiological variables. They are often called biomedical transducers and are the main building blocks of diagnostic medical instrumentation found in physician's offices, clinical laboratories and hospitals. These sensors are routinely used *in vivo* to perform continuous invasive and noninvasive monitoring of critical physiological variables as well as *in vitro* to help clinicians in various diagnostic procedures. Some biomedical sensors are also used in nonmedical applications such as in environmental monitoring, agriculture, bioprocessing, food processing and the petrochemical and pharmacological industries.

Increasing pressures to lower health care costs, optimise efficiency and provide better care in less expensive settings without compromising patient care are shaping the future of clinical medicine. As part of this ongoing trend, clinical testing is rapidly being transformed by the introduction of new tests that will revolutionise the way physicians will diagnose and treat diseases in the future. Among these changes, patient self-testing and physician office screening are the two most rapidly expanding areas. This trend is driven by the desire of patients and physicians alike to have the ability to perform some types of instantaneous diagnosis and to move the testing apparatus from an outside central clinical laboratory closer to the point of care.

Biomedical sensors play an important role in a range of diagnostic medical applications. Depending on the specific needs, some sensors are used primarily in clinical laboratories to measure *in vitro* physiological quantities such as electrolytes, enzymes and other biochemical metabolites in blood. Other biomedical sensors for measuring pressure, flow and the concentrations of gases, such as oxygen and carbon dioxide, are used *in vivo* to follow continuously (monitor) the conditions of a patient. For real-time continuous *in vivo* sensing to be worthwhile, the target analytes must vary rapidly and most often unpredictably.

The need for accurate medical diagnostic procedures places stringent requirement on the design and use of biomedical sensors. Usually, the first step in developing a biomedical sensor is to assess *in vitro* the accuracy, precision, range, response time and drift of the sensor. Later, depending on the intended application, similar *in vivo* tests may be required to confirm the specifications of the device and to ensure that the measurement remains reliable and safe.

SENSOR CLASSIFICATIONS

Biomedical sensors are usually classified as physical, electrical or chemical depending on their specific applications. Biosensors, which can be considered a special sub-classification of biomedical sensors, refers to a group of sensors that have two distinct components: (i) a biological recognition element, such as a purified enzyme, antibody or receptor, which functions as a mediator and provides the selectivity that is needed to detect the analyte of interest; and (ii) supporting structure, which also acts as a transducer and is positioned in intimate contact with the biological component. The purpose of the transducer is to convert the biochemical reaction into a quantifiable measurement, typically in the form of an optical, electrical or physical signal.

Sensor Packaging

Packaging of certain biomedical sensors, primarily sensors for *in vivo* applications, is an important consideration during the design, fabrication and use of the device. The sensor must be safe and remain functionally reliable. In the development of implantable biosensors, an additional key issue is the long operational lifetime and biocompatibility of the sensor. Whenever a sensor comes into contact with body fluids, the host itself may affect the function of the sensor or the sensor may affect the site in which it is implanted. For example, protein absorption and cellular deposits can alter the permeability of the sensor packaging that is designed to both protect the sensor and allow free chemical diffusion of certain analytes between the body fluids and the biosensor. Improper packaging of implantable biomedical sensors could lead to drift and a gradual loss of sensor sensitivity over time. Furthermore, inflammation of tissue, infection or clotting in a vascular site may produce harmful adverse effects. Hence, the materials used in the construction of the sensor's outer body must be nonthrombogenic and nontoxic since they play a critical role in determining the overall performance and longevity of an implantable sensor. One convenient strategy is to utilise various polymeric covering materials and barrier layers to minimise leaching of potentially toxic sensor components into the body. It is also important to keep in mind that once the sensor is manufactured, common sterilisation practices by stream, ethylene oxide, or gamma radiation must not alter the chemical diffusion properties of the sensor packaging material.

This chapter will examine the operating principles of different types of biomedical sensors including examples of invasive and noninvasive sensors for measuring biopotentials and other physical and biochemical variables encountered in different clinical and research applications.

BIOPOTENTIAL MEASUREMENTS

Biopotential measurements are made using different kinds of specialised electrodes. The function of these electrodes is to couple the ionic potentials generated inside the body to an electronic instrument. Biopotential electrodes are generally classified either as noninvasive (skin surface) or invasive (e.g., microelectrodes or wire electrodes).

Electrolyte/Metal Electrode Interface

When a metal is placed in an electrolyte (i.e., an ionisable) solution, a charge distribution is created next to the metal/electrolyte interface as illustrated in Fig. 3.1. This localised charge distribution causes an electric potential called a half-cell potential, to be developed across the interface between the metal and the electrolyte solution. The half-cell potentials of several important metals are listed in Table 3.1. Note that the hydrogen electrode is considered to be the standard electrode against which the half-cell potentials of other metal electrodes are measured.

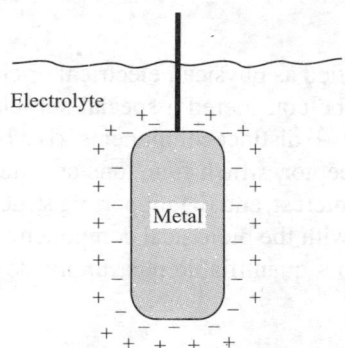

Fig. 3.1. Distribution of charges at a metal/electrolyte interface.

Table 3.1. Half-cell potentials.

Primary metal and chemical reaction			Half-cell potential
Al	→	$Al^{3+} + 3e^-$	−1.706
Cr	→	$Cr^{3+} + 3e^-$	−0.744
Cd	→	$Cd^{2+} + 2e^-$	−0.401
Zn	→	$Zn^{2+} + 2e^-$	−0.763
Fe	→	$Fe^{2+} + 2e^-$	−0.409
Ni	→	$Ni^{2+} + 2e^-$	−0.230
Pb	→	$Pb^{2+} + 2e^-$	−0.126
H_2	→	$2H^+ + 2e^-$	−0.000 (Standard by definition)
Ag	→	$Ag^+ + e^-$	0.799
Au	→	$Au^{3+} + 3e^-$	1.420
Cu	→	$Cu^{2+} + 2e^-$	0.340
$Ag + Cl^-$	→	$AgCl + 2e^-$	0.223

Example 1.1. Silver and aluminium electrodes are placed in an electrolyte solution. Calculate the current that will flow through the electrodes if the equivalent resistance of the solution is equal to 2 kΩ.

Solution:

$$0.799 - (-1.706) = 2.505 \text{ V}$$
$$2.505 \text{ V}/2 \text{ k}\Omega = 1.252 \text{ mA}$$

ECG Electrodes

Examples of several types of noninvasive biopotential electrodes used primarily for ECG recording are shown in Fig. 3.2.

Rigid metal plate electrodes, which are usually made from an alloy of zinc, nickel and copper, are usually used for short-term recording of biopotentials from the skin. These electrodes are attached to the skin either by an elastic strap (Fig. 3.2a) or a double-sided peel-off adhesive tape. A thin layer of electrolyte gel must be applied between the metal and the skin in order to establish good electrical contact with the skin during the recording of electrical potential from the body. The main ingredients of these electrolytes are water and additional ionic salts, such as sodium chloride and potassium chloride.

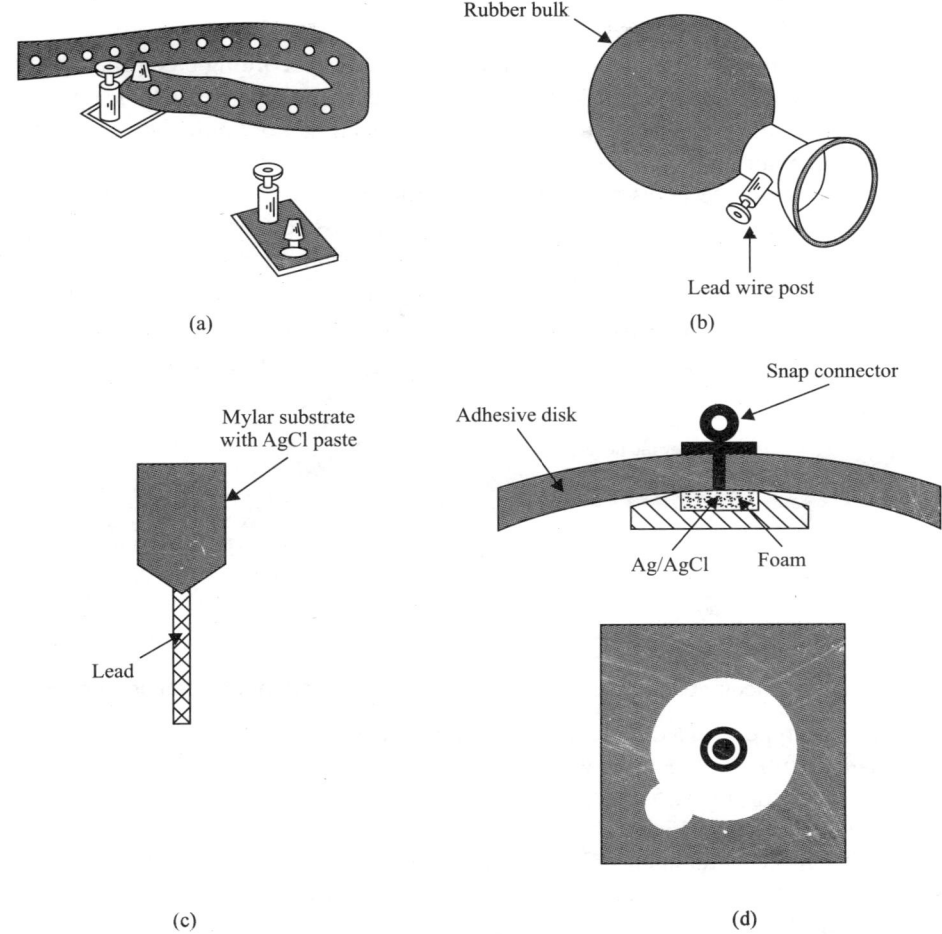

Fig. 3.2. Biopotential skin surface ECG electrodes: (a) Rigid metal plate electrode and attachment strap; (b) suction-type metal electrode; (c) flexible Mylar electrode; and (d) disposable snap-type Ag/AgCl electrode.

Suction electrodes (Fig. 3.2b) are very convenient as ECG chest leads since they can be easily moved from one location to another. These electrodes are attached to the skin by using a rubber suction bulb to create a vacuum inside the hollow metallic cup. A third type of biopotential sensor is a flexible electrode made of certain types of polymers or elastomers that are made electrically conductive by the addition of a fine carbon or metal powder. These electrodes are available with prepared AgCl gel for quick and easy application to the skin (Fig. 3.2c). The fourth and most common type of biopotential electrode is the 'floating' silver/silver chloride electrode (Ag/AgCl) which is formed by electrochemically depositing a very thin layer of silver chloride onto a silver electrode (Fig. 3.2d). These electrodes are recessed and imbedded in foam that has been soaked with an electrolyte paste and provides good electrical contact with the skin. The electrolyte saturated foam is also known to reduce motion artifacts which could be produced, for example, during stress testing when the layer of the skin moves relative to the surface of the Ag/AgCl electrode. This motion artifact could cause large interference in the recorded biopotential and in extreme cases, could severely degrade the measurement.

Electromyographic Electrodes

A number of different types of biopotential electrodes are used in recording electromyographic (EMG) signals from different muscles in the body. The shape and size of the recorded EMG signals depends on the electrical property of these electrodes and the recording location. For noninvasive recordings, proper skin preparation, which normally involves cleansing the skin with alcohol, or the application of a small amount of an electrolyte paste helps to minimise the impedance of the skin-electrode interface and improve the quality of the recorded signal considerably. The most common electrodes used for surface EMG recording and nerve conduction studies are circular discs, about 1 cm in diameter, that are made of silver or platinum. For direct recording of electrical signals from nerves and muscle fibres, a variety of percutaneous needle electrodes are available as illustrated in Fig. 3.3.

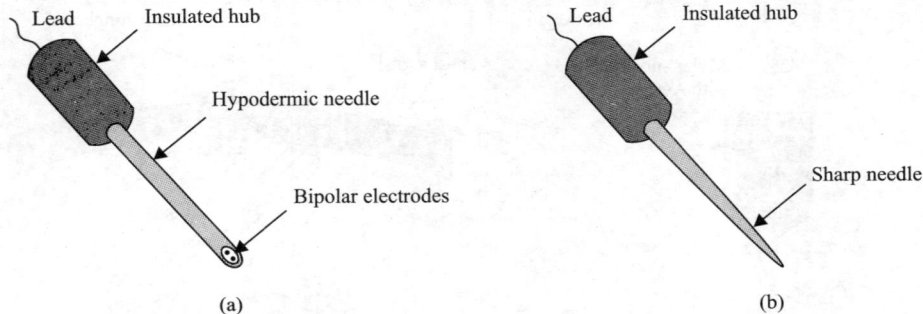

Fig. 3.3. Intramascular biopotential electrodes; (a) bipolar; and (b) unipolar configuration.

The most common type of needle electrode is the concentric bipolar electrode shown in Fig. 3.3a. This electrode is made from thin metallic wires encased inside a larger canula or hypodermic needle. The two wires serve as the recording and reference electrodes. Another types of percutaneous EMG electrode is the unipolar needle electrode (Fig. 3.3b). This electrode is made of a thin wire that is mostly insulated by a thin layer of Teflon except for about 0.3 mm near the distal tip. Unlike a bipolar electrode, this electrode requires a second unipolar reference electrode to close the electrical circuit. The second recording electrode is normally placed either adjacent to the recording electrode or attached to the surface of the skin.

Electroencephalographic Electrodes

The most commonly used electrodes for recording signals from the brain [electroencephalograms (EEG)] are cup electrodes and subdermal electrodes. Cup electrodes are made of platinum or tin approximately 5–10 mm in diameter. These cups are filled with a conducting electrolyte gel and are attached to the scalp with an adhesive tape. Subdermal EEG electrodes are basically fine platinum or stainless-steel needle electrodes, about 10 mm long by 0.5 mm wide, which are inserted under the skin to provide a better electrical contact.

Microelectrodes

A microelectrode is a biopotential electrode with an ultra-fine tapered tip that can be inserted into individual biological cells. These electrodes serve an important role in recording action potentials from single cells and are commonly used in neuro-physiological studies. The tip of these electrodes must be small with respect to the dimensions of the biological cell to avoid cell damage and at the same time sufficiently strong to penetrate the cell wall. Figure 3.4 illustrates the construction of three typical types of microelectrodes; glass micropipettes, metal microelectrodes and solid-state microprobes.

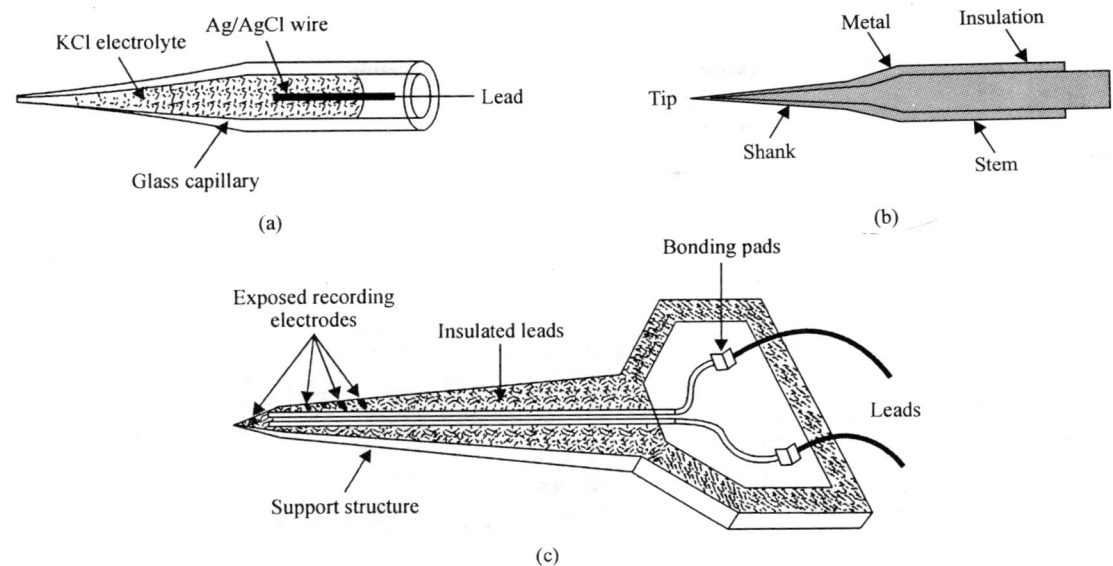

Fig. 3.4. Biopotential microelectrodes; (a) capillary glass micro-electrode; (b) insulated metal microelectrode; and (c) solid-state multisite recording microelectrode.

In Fig. 3.4a, a hollow glass capillary tube, typically 1 mm in diameter, a heated and softened in the middle inside a small furnace and then quickly pulled apart from both ends. This process creates two similar microeletrodes with an open tip that has a diameter in the order of 0.1–10 μm. The larger end of the glass tube (the stem) is then filled with a 3 M KCl electrolyte solution. A small piece of Ag/AgCl wire is inserted through the stem to provide an electrical contact with the electrolyte solution. When the tip of the microelectrode is inserted into an electrolyte solution, such as the intracellular cytoplasm of a biological cell, ionic current can flow through the fluid junction at the tip of the microelectrode. This establishes a closed electrical circuit between the Ag/AgCl wire inside the microelectrode and the biological cell.

A different kind of microelectrode made from a small-diameter strong metal wire (e.g., tungsten or stainless steel) is illustrated in Fig. 3.4b. The tip of this microelectrode is usually sharpened to a diameter of a few micrometers by an electrochemical etching process. The wire is then insulated up to its tip.

Solid-state microfabrication techniques commonly used in the production of integrated circuits can be used to produce microprobes for multichannel recordings of biopotentials or for electrical stimulation of neurons in the brain or spinal cord. An example of such a microsensor is shown in Fig. 3.4c. This probe consists of a precisely micromachined silicon substrate with four exposed recording sites. One of the major advantages of this fabrication techniques is the ability to mass produce very small and highly sophisticated microsensors with highly reproducible electrical and physical properties.

PHYSICAL MEASUREMENTS

Displacement Transducers

Inductive displacement transducers are based on the inductance L of a coil given by:

$$L = n^2 G \mu \qquad \qquad ...(3.1)$$

where G is a geometric form constant, n is the number of coil turns and μ is the permeability of the magnetically susceptible medium inside the coil. These types of transducers measure displacement by changing either the self-inductance of a single coil or the mutual inductance coupling between two or more stationary coils, typically by the displacement of a ferrite or iron core in the bore of the coil assembly. A widely used inductive displacement transducer is the linear variable differential transformer (LVDT) illustrated in Fig. 3.5.

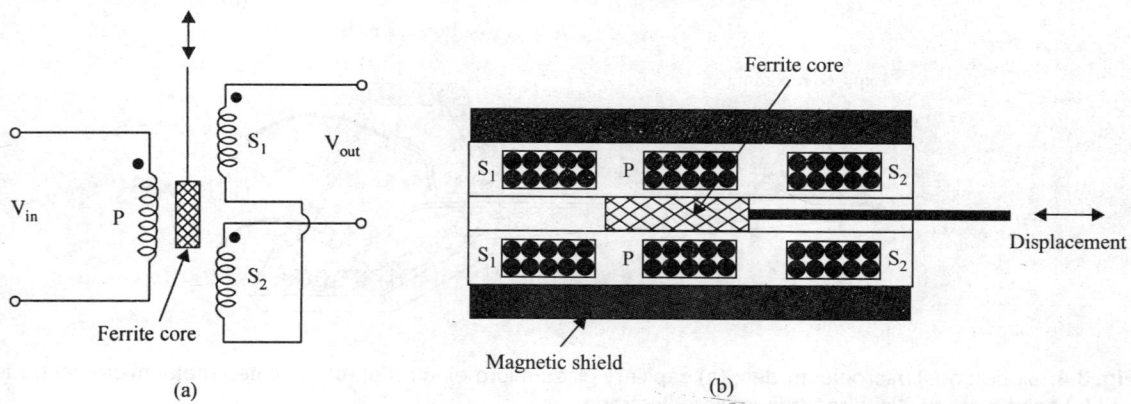

(a)   (b)

Fig. 3.5. LVDT transducer; (a) electric diagram; and (b) cross-section.

This device is essentially a three-coil mutual inductance transducer that is composed of a primary coil details; (P) and two secondary coils (S_1 and S_2) connected in series but in opposite polarity in order to achieve a wider linear output range. The mutual inductance coupled between the coils is changed by the motion of a high-permeability slug. The primary coil is usually excited by passing an AC current. When the slug is centered symmetrically with respect to the two secondary coils, the primary coil induces an alternating magnetic field on the secondary coils. This produces equal voltages (but of opposite polarities) across the two secondary coils. Therefore, the positive voltage excursions from one secondary coil will cancel out the negative voltage excursions from the other secondary coil, resulting in a zero net output voltage. When the core moves toward one coil, the voltage induced in that coil is increased in proportion to the displacement of the core while the voltage induced in the other coil is decreased proportionally, leading to a typical voltage-displacement diagram as illustrated in Fig. 3.6.

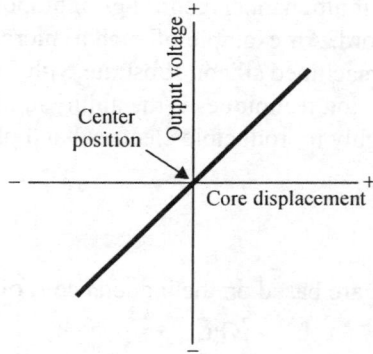

Fig. 3.6. Output voltage versus core displacement of a typical LVDT transducer.

Since the voltages induced in the two secondary coils are out of phase, special phase-sensitive electronic circuits must be used to detect both the position and the direction of the core's displacement. Blood flow through an exposed vessel can be measured by means of an electromagnetic flow transducer. It is used extensively in research studies to measure blood flow in major blood vessels near the heart, including the aorta at the point where it exits from the heart.

Consider a blood vessel of diameter l filled with blood flowing with a uniform velocity u. If the blood vessel is placed in a uniform magnetic field $\vec{B}$ that is perpendicular to the direction of blood flow, the negatively charged anion and positively charged cation particles in the blood will experience a force $\vec{F}$, which is normal to both the magnetic field and blood flow directions and is given by

$$\vec{F} = q\,(\vec{u} \times \vec{B}) \qquad \text{... (3.2)}$$

where, q is the elementary charge (1.6×10^{-19} C). As a result, these charged particles will be deflected in opposite directions and will move along the diameter of the blood vessels according to the direction of the force vector $\vec{F}$. This movement will produce an opposing force $\vec{F}_0$ that is equal to

$$\vec{F}_0 = q\,\vec{E} = q\left(\frac{V}{l}\right) \qquad \text{... (3.3)}$$

where, $\vec{E}$ is the net electrical field produced by the displacement of the charged particles and V is the potential produced across the blood vessel. At equilibrium, these two forces will be equal. Therefore, the potential difference, V, is given by

$$V = Blu \qquad \text{... (3.4)}$$

and is proportional to the velocity of blood through the vessel.

Example 3.2. Calculate the voltage in a magnetic flow probe if the probe is applied across a blood vessel with a diameter of 0.5 cm and the flow rate of blood is 5 cm/s. Assume that the magnitude of the magnetic fluid is 1.5×10^{-5} tesla (T).

Solution:

From Eq. (3.4),

$$V = Blu = (1.5 \times 10^{-5}\ \text{T})\ (0.5\ \text{cm})\ (5\ \text{cm/s}) = 37.5\ \mu V$$

Practically, this device consists of a clip-on probe that fits snugly around the blood vessel as illustrated in Fig. 3.7. The probe contains electrical coils to produce an electromagnetic field transverse to the direction of blood flow.

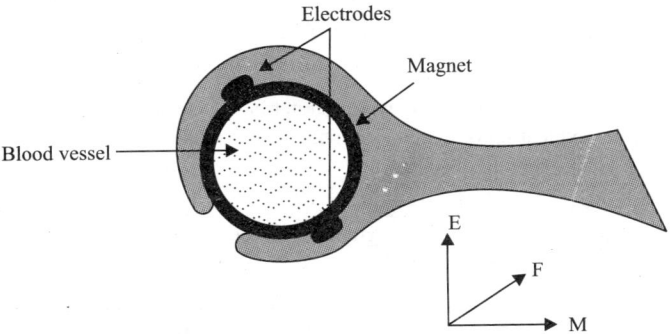

Fig. 3.7. Electromagnetic blood-flow probe.

The coil is usually excited by an AC current. A pair of very small biopotential electrodes are attached to the housing and rest against the wall of the blood vessel to pick up the induced potential. The flow-induced voltage is an AC voltage at the same frequency as the excitation voltage. Using an AC method instead of DC excitation helps to remove any offset potential error due to the contact between the vessel wall and the biopotential electrodes.

A potentiometer is a resistive-type transducer that converts either linear or angular displacement into an output voltage by moving a sliding contact along the surface of a resistive element. Figure 3.8 illustrates linear and angular-type potentiometric transducers. A voltage, V_i is applied across the resistor R. The output voltage, V_0 between the sliding contact and one terminal of the resistor is linearly proportional to the displacement. Typically, a constant current source is passed through the variable resistor and the small change in output voltage is measured by a sensitive voltmeter using Ohm's law (i.e., $I = V/R$).

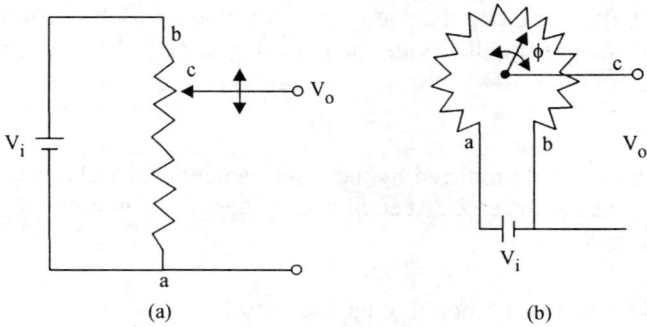

(a)   (b)

Fig. 3.8. Linear translational (a) an angular; (b) displacement transducers.

In certain clinical situations, it is desirable to measure changes in the peripheral volume of a leg when the venous outflow of blood from the leg is temporarily occluded by a blood pressure cuff. This volume-measuring method is called plethysmography and can indicate the presence of venous clots in the legs. The measurement can be performed by wrapping an elastic resistive transducer around the leg and measuring the rate of change in resistance of the transducer as a function of time. This change corresponds to relative changes in the blood volume of the leg. If a clot is present, it will take more time for the blood stored in the leg to flow out through the veins after the temporary occlusion is removed. A similar transducer can be used to follow a patient's breathing patterns by wrapping the elastic band around the chest.

An elastic resistive transducer consists of a thin elastic tube filled with an electrically conductive material as illustrated in Fig. 3.9.

Example 3.3. A 10-cm long elastic resistive transducer with a stretching resistance of 0.5 kΩ is wrapped around the chest. Assume the chest diameter during exhalation is 33 cm. Calculate the resistance of the transducer after it has been applied to the chest.

Solution:

After the transducer is stretched around the chest, its length will increase from 10 to 103.7 cm. Assuming that the cross-sectional area of the transducer remains unchanged after it is stretched, the resistance will increase to

$$R_{stretched} = 0.5 \times \left(\frac{103.7}{10}\right) = 5.18 \text{ k}\Omega$$

Strain gauges are displacement-type transducers that measure change in the length of an object as a result of an applied force.

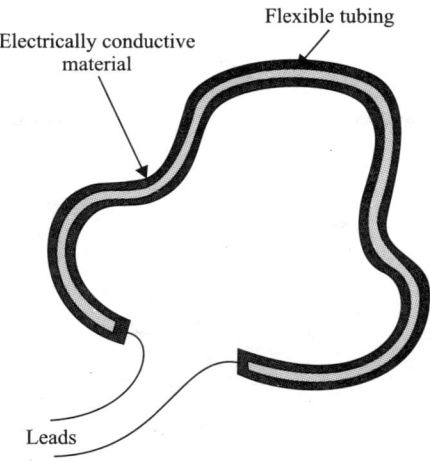

Electrically conductive
material

Flexible tubing

Leads

Fig. 3.9. Elastic resistive transducer.

These transducers produce a resistance change that is proportional to the fractional change in the length of the object, also called strain, S, which is defined as

$$S = \frac{\Delta l}{l} \qquad \qquad ... (3.5)$$

where Δl is the fractional change in length and l is the initial length of the object. Examples include resistive wire elements and certain semiconductor materials.

Example 3.4. Calculate the strain in a metal wire gauge for a fractional change in resistance of 10 per cent.

Solution:

Combine Eq. 3.5 and 3.11 to obtain

$$\frac{\Delta R}{R} = \frac{2\Delta l}{l} = 2S$$

$$\frac{0.1}{2R} = S$$

$$\frac{0.05}{R} = S$$

Strain gauges typically are classified into two categories, bonded or unbonded. A bonded strain gauge has a folded thin wire cemented to a semiflexible backing material, as illustrated in Fig. 3.10.

An unbonded strain gauge consists of multiple resistive wires (typically four) stretched between fixed and movable rigid frames. In this configuration, when a deforming force is applied to the structure, two of the wires are stretched and the other two are shortened proportionally. This configuration is used in blood pressure transducers and is illustrated in Fig. 3.11. In this arrangement, a diaphragm is coupled directly by an armature to a movable frame that is inside the transducer.

Blood in a peripheral vessel is coupled through a thin fluid-filled (saline) catheter to a disposable dome that is sealed by the flexible diaphragm. Changes in blood pressure during the pumping action of the heart apply a force on the diaphragm that causes the movable frame to move from its resting position. This movement causes the strain gauge wires to stretch or compress and results in a cyclical change in resistance that is proportional to the pulsatile blood pressure measured by the transducer.

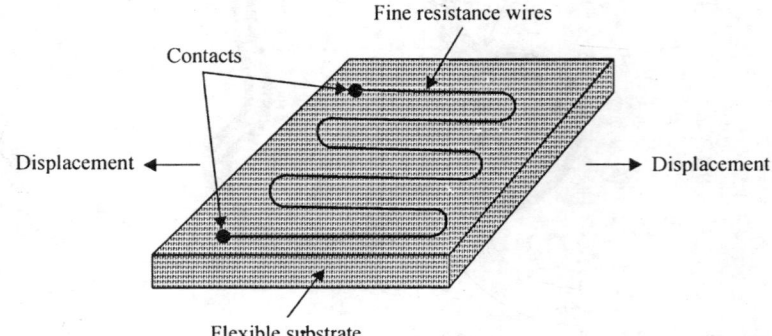

Fig. 3.10. Bonded-type strain gauge transducer.

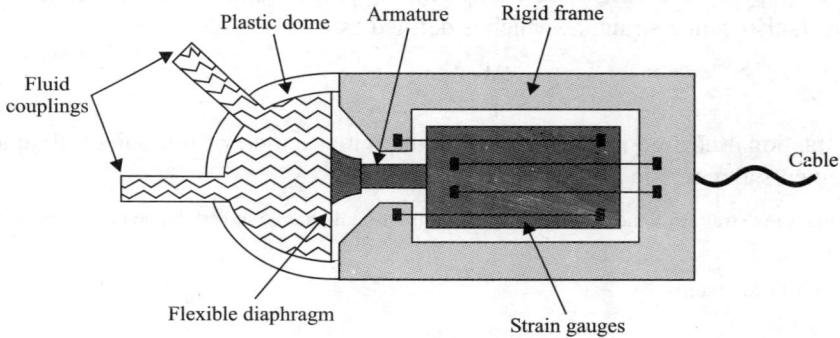

Fig. 3.11. Resistive strain gauge (unbonded type) blood pressure transducer.

In general, the change in resistance of a strain gauge is typically quite small. In addition, changes in temperature can also cause thermal expansion of the wire and subsequently lead to large changes in the resistance of a strain gauge. Therefore, very sensitive electronic amplifiers with special temperature compensation circuits are used in most applications.

The capacitance C between two equal-size parallel plates of cross-sectional area A separated by a distance d is given by:

$$C = \varepsilon_0 \varepsilon_r \left(\frac{A}{d} \right) \qquad \qquad ... (3.6)$$

where ε_0 is the dielectric constant of free space (8.85×10^{-14} F/cm) and ε_r is the relative dielectric constant of the insulating material placed between the two plates. The method that is most commonly used to measure displacement in capacitance transducers involves changing the separation distance d between a fixed and a movable plate as illustrated in Fig. 3.12.

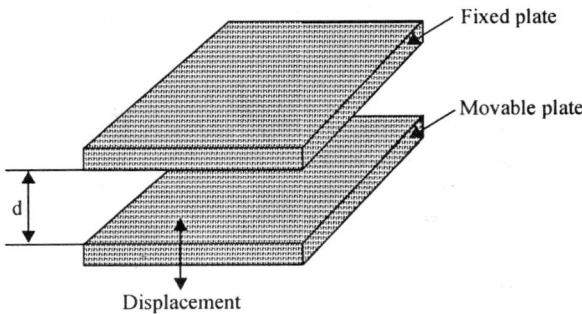

Fig. 3.12. Capacitive displacement transducer.

Example 3.5. Two metal plates with an area of 3 cm² and separation distance of 0.1 mm are used to form a capacitance transducer. If the material between the two plates has a dielectric constant of 2×10^{-2}, calculate the capacitance of the transducer.

Solution:

$$C = \varepsilon_0 \varepsilon_r \frac{A}{d} = (8.85 \times 10^{-14} \text{ F/cm} \times 2 \times 10^{-2} \times 3 \text{ cm}^2)/0.01 \text{ cm} = 0.53 \text{ pF}$$

Capacitive displacement transducers can be used to measure respiration of movement of a patient by attaching multiple transducers to a mat that is placed on a bed. A capacitive displacement transducer can also be used as a pressure transducer by attaching the movable plate to a thin diaphragm that is in contact with a fluid or air. By applying a voltage across the capacitor and amplifying the small AC signal generated by the vibrations of the diaphragm, it is possible to obtain a signal that is proportional to the applied external pressure source.

Piezoelectric transducers are used extensively in cardiology to listen to heart sounds (phonocardiography), in automated blood pressure measurement and for measurement of physiological forces and accelerations. They are also commonly employed in generating ultrasonic waves (high-frequency sound waves typically above 20 kHz) which are used for measuring blood flow or imaging internal soft structures in the body.

A piezoelectric transducer consists of a small crystal (usually quartz) that contracts if an electric field (usually in the form of a short voltage impulse) is applied across its plates as illustrated in Fig. 3.13. Conversely, if the crystal is mechanically strained, it will generate a small electric potential. Besides quartz several other ceramic materials, such as barium titanate and lead zirconate titanate, are also known to produce a piezoelectric effect.

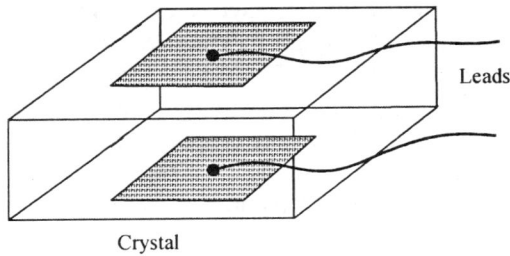

Fig. 3.13. Ultrasonic transducer.

The piezoelectric principle is based on the phenomenon that when an asymmetrical crystal lattice is distorted by an applied force F, the internal negative and positive charges are reoriented. This causes an induced surface charge Q on the opposite sides of the crystal. This charge is directly proportional to the applied force and is given by:

$$Q = kF \qquad \text{... (3.7)}$$

where, k is a proportionality constant for the specific piezoelectric material. By assuming that the piezoelectric crystal acts like a parallel plate capacitor, the voltage across the crystal, V, is given by

$$V = \frac{Q}{C} \qquad \text{... (3.8)}$$

where, C is the equivalent capacitance of the crystal.

Example 3.6. Derive a relationship for calculating the output voltage across a piezoelectric transducer that has a thickness, d and an area A, in terms of an applied force, F.

Solution: The capacitance of a piezoelectric transducer can be approximated by Eq. (3.6). Equation (3.8) is combined with the relationships given by Eq. (3.7) and (3.8) to give

$$V = \frac{Q}{C} = \frac{kF}{C} = \frac{kFd}{\varepsilon_0 \varepsilon_r A}$$

Since the crystal has an internal leakage resistance, any steady charge produced across its surface will eventually be dissipated. Consequently, these piezoelectric transducers are not suitable for measuring a steady or low-frequency DC force. Instead, they are used either as variable force transducers or as mechanically resonating devices to generate high frequencies (typically from 1 to 10 MHz) either in crystal-controlled oscillators or as ultrasonic pulse transducers.

Piezoelectric transducers are commonly used in biomedical applications to measure the thickness of an object or in noninvasive blood pressure monitors. For instance, if two similar crystals are placed across an object (e.g., a blood vessel), one crystal can be excited to produce a short burst of ultrasound. The time it takes for this sound to reach the other transducer can be measured. Assuming that the velocity of sound propagation in soft tissue, c_t, is known (typically 1540 m/s), the time, t, it takes the ultrasonic pulse to propagate across the object can be measured and used to calculate the separation distance, d, of the two transducers from the following relationship

$$d = c_t \, t \qquad \text{... (3.9)}$$

Airflow Transducers

One of the most common airflow transducer is the Fleish pneumotachometer illustrated in Fig. 3.14. The device consists of a straight short tube section with a fixed screen obstruction in the middle that produces a slight pressure drop as the air is passed through it. The pressure drop created across the screen is measured by a differential pressure transducer. The signal produced by the pressure transducer is proportional to the velocity of the air. The tube is normally cone shaped to generate a laminar flow pattern. A small heater heats the screen so that water vapour does not condense on it over time and produce an artificially high pressure drop. Fleish pneumotachometers are used to monitor volume, flow and breathing rates of patients on mechanical ventilators.

Temperature Measurement

Body temperature is one of the most tightly controlled physiological variables and one of the four basic vital signs used in the daily assessment of patients. The interior (core) temperature in the body is remarkably constant, about 37°C for a healthy person and is normally maintained within ±0.5°C. Therefore, elevated body temperature is a sign of disease or infection, whereas a significant drop in skin temperature may be a good clinical indication of shock.

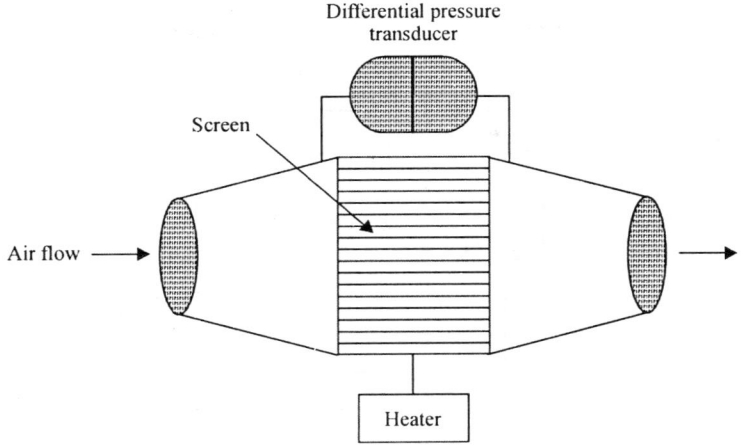

Fig. 3.14. Fleish airflow transducer.

There are two distinct areas in the body where temperature is measured routinely—the surface of the skin under the armpit and inside a body cavity such as the mouth or the rectum. The two most commonly used devices to measure body temperature are thermistors, which require direct contact with the skin or mucosal tissues and noncontact thermometers, which measure body core temperature inside the auditory canal. Thermistors are temperature-sensitive transducers made of compressed sintered metal oxide (such as nickel, manganese or cobalt) that change their resistance with temperature. Commercially available thermistors range in shape from small beads to large disks as illustrated in Fig. 3.15.

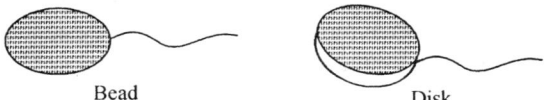

Bead   Disk

Fig. 3.15. Common forms of thermistors.

Mathematically, the resistance-temperature characteristic of a thermistor can be approximated by

$$R_T = R_0 \ \exp\left[\beta\left(\frac{1}{T} - \frac{1}{T_0}\right)\right]$$ ... (3.10)

where, R_0 is the resistance at a reference temperature T_0, (in degree K), R_T is the resistance at temperature T (in degrees K) and β is a material constant, typically between 2500 and 5500 k. A typical resistance-temperature characteristics of a thermistor is shown in Fig. 3.16. Note that unlike metals and conventional resistors which have a positive temperature coefficient (as the temperature increases, the resistance increases), thermistors have a nonlinear relationship between temperature and resistance and a negative temperature coefficient. Increasing the temperature decreases the resistance of the thermistor.

Examples 3.7. A thermistor with a material constant β of 4500 K is used as a thermometer. Calculate the resistance of this thermistor at 25°C. Assume that the resistance of this thermistor at body temperature (37°C) is equal to 85 Ω.

Solution: Using the resistance-temperature characteristics of a thermistor (Eq. 3.10) gives

$$R_T = 85 \exp\left[4500\left(\frac{1}{298} - \frac{1}{310}\right)\right] = 152.5 \ \Omega$$

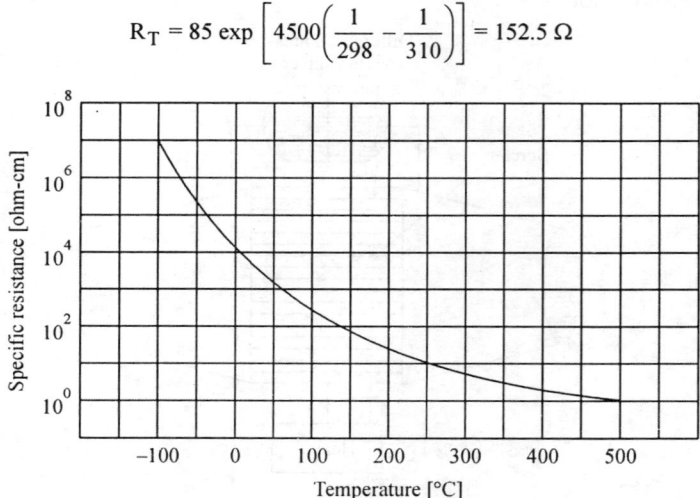

Fig. 3.16. Resistivity versus temperature characteristics of a typical thermistor.

The size and mass of a thermistor probe in a medical thermometer must be small in order to give a rapid response time to temperature variations. The probe is normally covered with very thin sterile plastic that is also disposable to prevent cross-contamination between patients.

A thermistor sensor is utilised in a thermodilution technique for measuring cardiac output (the volume of blood ejected by the heart each minute) as illustrated in Fig. 3.17. The technique involves the bolus injection of a cold indicator solution, usually a saline solution kept at 0–5°C, via a pulmonary artery catheter. The catheter is inserted into either the femoral or jugular veins. The tip of the flexible catheter is passed through the right side of the heart into the pulmonary artery with the aid of a small inflatable balloon. The cold liquid mixes with the venous blood in the right atrium of heart and causes the blood to cool slightly. The cooled blood is ejected by the right ventricle into the pulmonary artery, where it contacts a thermistor located in the wall near the tip of a Swan-Ganz catheter. The thermistor measures the change in blood temperature as the blood passes on to the lungs. An instrument measures the extent of blood cooling which is inversely proportional to cardiac output.

Noncontact thermometer measures the temperature of the ear canal wall near the tympanic membrane, which is known to track the core temperature by about 0.5–1.0°C. Basically, as illustrated in Fig. 3.18, infrared radiation from the tympanic membrane is channelled to a heat-sensitive detector through a metal waveguide that has a gold-plated inner surface for better reflectivity. The detector, which is either a thermopile or a pyroelectric sensor that converts heat flow into an electric current, is normally maintained in a constant temperature environment to minimise inaccuracies due to fluctuation in ambient temperature. A disposable speculum is used on the probe to protect patients from cross-contamination.

BLOOD GASES AND PH SENSORS

Measurements of arterial blood gases (pO_2 and pCO_2) and pH are frequently performed on critically ill patients in both the operating room and the intensive care unit and are used by physicians to determine the need for adjusting mechanical ventilation or administering pharmacological agents.

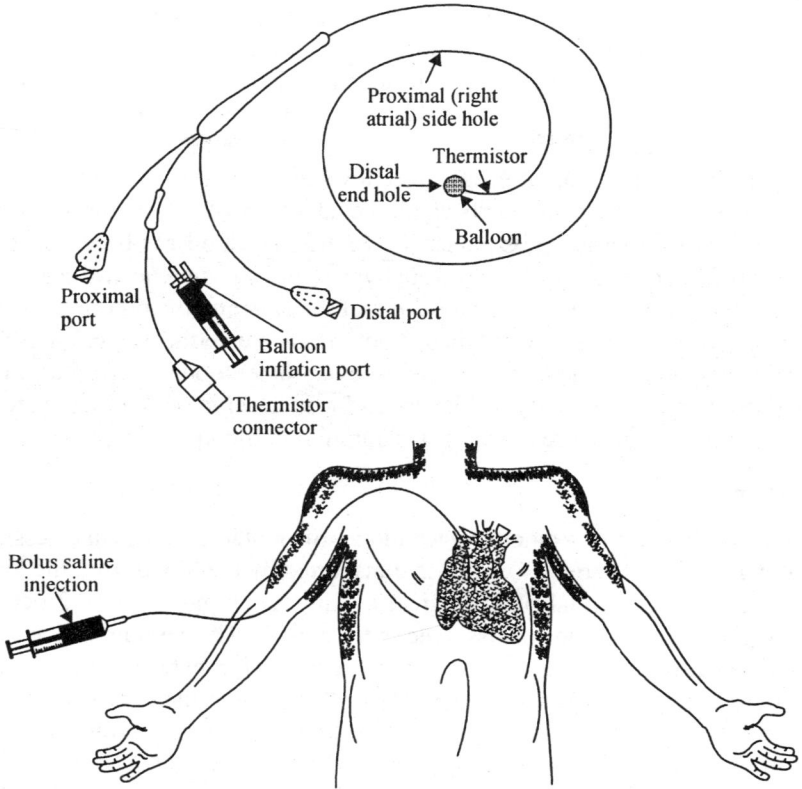

Fig. 3.17. A Swan-Ganz thermodilution catheter.

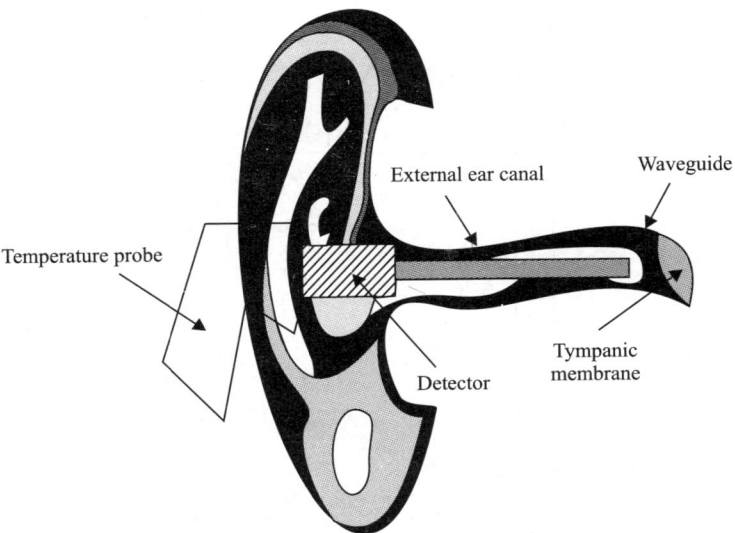

Fig. 3.18. Non-contact-type infrared ear thermometer.

These measurements provide information about the respiratory and metabolic imbalances in the body and reflect the adequacy of blood oxygenation and CO_2 elimination.

Traditionally, blood gas analysis has been performed by withdrawing blood from a peripheral artery. The blood sample is then transported to a clinical laboratory for analysis. The need for rapid test results in the management of unstable, critically ill patients has led to the development of newer methods for continuous noninvasive blood gas monitoring. This allows the physician to follow trends in the patient's condition as well as receive immediate feedback on the adequacy of certain therapeutic interventions.

Noninvasive sensors for measuring O_2 and CO_2 in arterial blood are based on the discovery that gases, such as O_2 and CO_2, can easily diffuse through the skin. Diffusion occurs due to a partial pressure difference between the blood in the superficial layers of the skin and the outermost surface of the skin. This concept has been used to develop two types of noninvasive electrochemical sensors for monitoring pO_2 and pCO_2 transcutaneously. Furthermore, the discovery that blood changes its colour depending on the amount of oxygen chemically bound to the haemoglobin in the erythrocytes has led to the development of several optical methods to measure the oxygen saturation in blood.

Oxygen Measurement

A quantitative method for measuring blood oxygenation is of great importance in assessing the circulatory and respiratory conditions of a patient. Oxygen is transported by the blood from the lungs to the tissues in two distinct states. Under normal physiological conditions, approximately 2 per cent of the total amount of oxygen carried by the blood is dissolved in the plasma. This amount is linearly proportional to the blood pO_2. The remaining 98 per cent is carried inside the erythrocytes in a loose reversible chemical combination with haemoglobin (Hb) as oxyhemoglobin (HbO_2). Thus, there are two options for measuring blood oxygenation—either using a pO_2 sensor or measuring oxygen saturation (the relative amount of HbO_2 in the blood) by means of an oximeter. A polarographic pO_2 sensor, also widely known as a Clark electrode, is used to measure the partial pressure of O_2 gas in a sample of air or blood. The measurement is based on the principle of polarography as illustrated in Fig. 3.19.

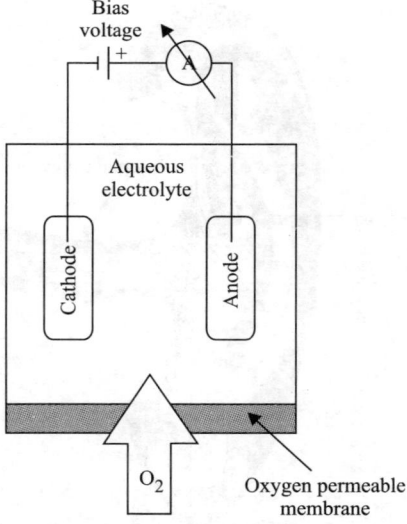

Fig. 3.19. Principle of a polarographic Clark-type pO_2 sensor.

The electrode utilises the ability of O_2 molecules to react chemically with H_2O in the presence of electrons to produce hydroxyl (OH^-) ions. This electrochemical reaction, called an oxidation/reduction or redox reaction, requires an externally applied constant polarising (bias) voltage source of about 0.6 V.

Oxygen is reduced (consumed) at the surface of a noble metal (e.g., platinum or gold) cathode (the electrode connected to the negative side of the voltage source) according to the following chemical reaction:

$$O_2 + 2H_2O + 4e^- \leftrightarrow 4OH^-$$

In this reduction reaction, an O_2 molecule takes four electrons and reacts with two water molecules, generating four hydroxyl ions. The resulting OH^- ions migrate and react with a reference Ag/AgCl anode (the electrode connected to the positive side of the voltage source), causing a two-step oxidation reaction to occur as follows:

$$Ag \leftrightarrow Ag^+ + e^-$$
$$Ag^+ + Cl^- \leftrightarrow AgCl_{\downarrow}$$

In this oxidation reaction, silver from the electrode is first oxidised to silver ions and electrons are liberated to the anode. These silver ions are immediately combined with chloride ions to form silver chloride that precipitates on the surface of the anode. The current flowing between the anode and the cathode in the external circuit produced by this reaction is directly (i.e., linearly) proportional to the number of O_2 molecules constantly reduced at the surface of the cathode. The electrodes in the polarographic cells are immersed in an electrolyte solution of potassium chloride and surrounded by an O_2-permeable Teflon or polypropylene membrane that permits gases to diffuse slowly into the electrode. Thus, by measuring the change in current between the cathode and the anode, the amount of oxygen that is dissolved in the solution can be determined.

With a rather minor change in the configuration of a polarographic pO_2 sensor, it is also possible to measure the pO_2 transcutaneously. Figure 3.20 illustrates a cross section of a Clark-type transcutaneous pO_2 sensor. This sensor is essentially a standard polarographic pO_2 electrode that is attached to the surface of the skin by double-sided adhesive tape.

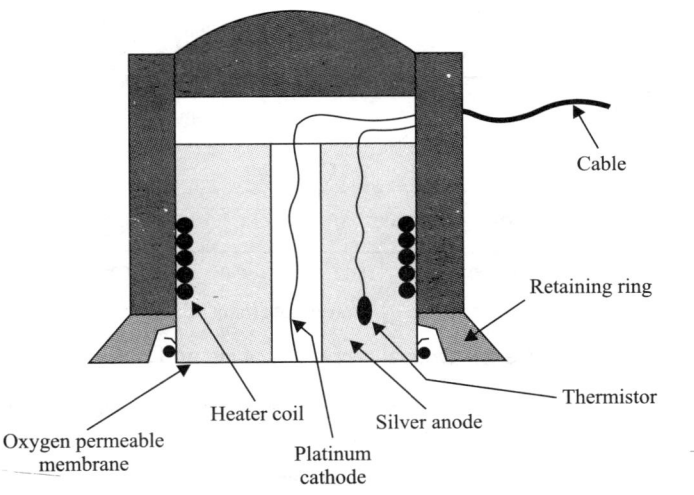

Fig. 3.20. Transcutaneous pO_2 sensor.

It measures the partial pressure of oxygen that diffuses from the blood through the skin into the Clark electrode similar to the way it measures the pO_2 in a sample of blood. However, since the diffusion of O_2 through the skin is normally very low, a miniature heating coil is incorporated into the housing of the electrode to cause gentle vasodilatation (increased local blood flow) of the capillaries in the skin. By raising the local skin temperature to about 43°C, the pO_2 measured by the transcutaneous sensor approximates that of the underlying arterial blood. This electrode has been used extensively in monitoring newborn babies in the intensive care unit. However, as the skin becomes thicker and matures in adult patients, the gas diffusion properties of the skin change significantly and cause large errors and inconsistent readings. Various methods for measuring the oxygen saturation, SO_2 (the relative amount of oxygen carried by the haemoglobin in the erythrocytes), of blood *in vitro* or *in vivo* in arterial blood (S_aO_2) or mixed venous blood (S_vO_2), have been developed. These methods, referred to as oximetry, are based on the light absorption properties of blood and in particular, the relative concentration of Hb and HbO_2 since the characteristic colour of deoxygenated blood is blue, whereas fully oxygenated blood has a distinct bright red colour.

The measurement is performed at two specific wavelengths; a red wavelength, λ_1, where there is a large difference in light absorbance between Hb and HbO_2 (e.g., approximately 660 nm) and a second wavelength, λ_2, in the near-infrared region of the spectrum, typically chosen between 805 and 960 nm. The second wavelength can be either isobestic (a region of the spectrum around 805 nm where the absorbance of light is independent of blood oxygenation) or around 940–960 nm, where the absorbance of Hb is slightly smaller than that of HbO_2. Figure 3.21 shows the optical absorption spectra of blood in the visible and near-infrared region.

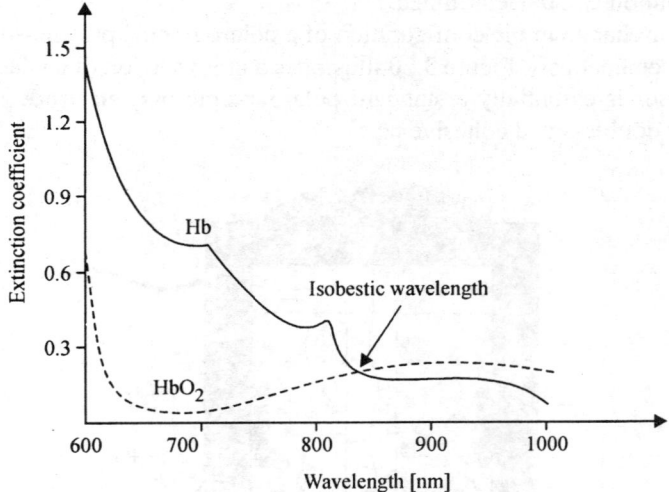

Fig. 3.21. Optical properties of Hb and HbO_2.

The measurement is based on Beer–Lamber's law that relates the transmitted light power, P_t to the incident light power, P_0, according to the following relationship:

$$P_t = P_0 \times 10^{-abc} \qquad \qquad \dots (3.11)$$

where a is a wavelength-dependent constant called the extinction coefficient (or molar absorptivity) of the sample, b is the light path length through the sample and c is the concentration of the sample.

Assuming for simplicity that (i) $\lambda_1 = 660$ nm and $\lambda_2 = 805$ nm (i.e., isobestic); (ii) the hemolysed blood sample (blood in which the erythrocytes have been ruptured, i.e., the haemoglobin has been released and uniformly mixed with the plasma) consists of a two-component mixture of Hb and HbO_2; and (iii) the total light absorbance by the mixture of these two components is additive, a simple mathematical relationship can be derived for computing the oxygen saturation of blood:

$$SO_2 = A - B\left[\frac{OD(\lambda_1)}{OD(\lambda_2)}\right] \qquad \ldots (3.12)$$

where A and B are two coefficients that are functions of the specific absorptivity of Hb and HbO_2, OD is defined as the optical density, i.e., $\log_{10}(1/T)$ (where T is the light transmission given by P_t/P_0) and SO_2 is defined as $C_{HBO_2}/(C_{HB} + C_{HBO_2})$.

The measurement of SO_2 in blood can be performed either *in vitro* or *in vivo*. *In vitro* measurement using a bench-top oximeter requires a sample of hemolysed blood, usually drawn from a peripheral artery. The sample is then injected into an optimcal cuvette (a parallel-wall glass container) which holds the sample while it is being illuminated sequentially by light from an intense white source after proper wavelength selection using narrow-band optical filters.

SO_2 can also be measured *in vivo* using a pulse oximeter. Noninvasive optical sensors for measuring S_aO_2 by a pulse oximeter consists of a pair of small and inexpensive light emitting diodes (LEDs)—typically a red LED around 660 nm and an infrared LED around 960 nm—and a single, highly sensitive silicon photodetector. These components are mounted inside a reusable spring-loaded clip or a disposable adhesive wrap. The sensor is usually attached either to the fingertip or earlobe such that the tissue is sandwiched between the light source and the photodetector. Electronic circuits inside the pulse oximeter generate signals to turn on the two LEDs in a sequential manner and synchronously measure the photodetector output when the corresponding LEDs are activated. Pulse oximetry relies on the detection of the photoplethysmographic signal, as illustrated in Fig. 3.22. This signal is caused by changes in arterial blood volume associated with periodic contractions of the heart during systole.

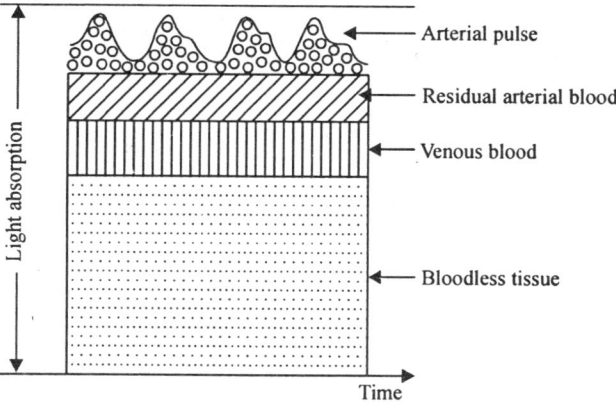

Fig. 3.22. Time dependence of light absorption by a peripheral vascular tissue bed illustrating the effect of arterial pulsation.

The magnitude of this signal depends on the amount of blood ejected from the heart into the peripheral vascular bed with each cardiac cycle, the optical absorption of the blood, skin and tissue and the wavelength used to illuminate the blood. S_aO_2 is derived by analysing the magnitude of the red and infrared photo-plethysmograms measured by the photodetector. Electronic circuits separate the photopletysmogram into its pulsatile (AC) and nonpulsatile (DC) signal components. An algorithm inside the pulse oximeter performs a mathematical normalisation by which the AC signal at each wavelength is divided by the corresponding DC component that results mainly from the light absorbed by the bloodless tissue, residual arterial blood when the heart is in diastole, venous blood and skin pigmentation. Since it is assumed that the AC portion in the photoplethysmogram results only from the arterial blood component, this scaling process provides a normalised red/infrared ratio, R, which is highly dependent on the colour of the arterial blood (i.e., S_aO_2) but is largely independent of the volume of arterial blood entering the tissue during systole, skin pigmentation, skin thickness and vascular structure. Hence, the instrument does not need to be recalibrated for measurements on different patients. The mathematical relationship between S_aO_2 and R is programmed by the manufacturer into the pulse oximeter.

pH Electrodes

pH describes the balance between acid and base in a solution. Acidic solutions have an excess of hydrogen ions (H^+), whereas basic solutions have an excess of hydroxyl ions (OH^-). In a dilute solution, the product of these ion concentrations is a constant (1.0×10^{-14}). Therefore, the concentration of either ion can be used to express the acidity or alkalinity of a solution. All neutral solutions have a pH of 7.0.

The measurement of blood pH is fundamental to many diagnostic procedures. In normal blood, pH is maintained under tight control and is typically approximately 7.40 (slightly basic). By measuring the pH of the blood, it is possible to determine whether the lungs are removing sufficient CO_2 gas from the body or how well the kidneys regulate the acid-base balance.

A pH electrode essentially consists of two separate electrodes: a reference electrode and an active (indicator) electrode as illustrated in Fig. 3.23. The two electrodes are typically made of an Ag/AgCl wire dipped in a KCl solution and encased in a glass container. A salt bridge, which is essentially a glass tube containing an electrolyte enclosed in a membrane that is permeable to all ions, maintains the potential of the reference electrode at a constant value regardless of the solution under test. Unlike the reference electrode, the active electrode is sealed with hydrogen-impermeable glass except at the tip. The reference electrode may also be combined with the indicator electrode in single glass housing.

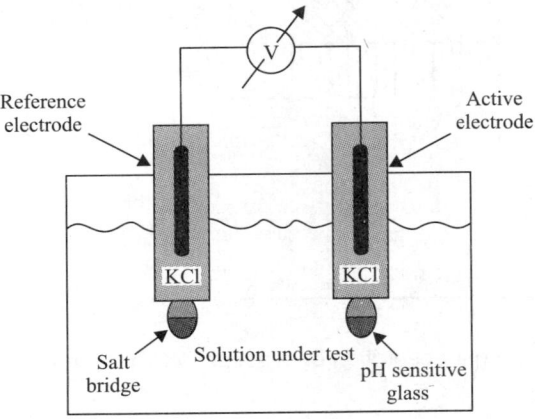

Fig. 3.23. Principle of pH electrode.

The boundary separating two solutions has a potential proportional to the hydrogen ion concentration of one solution and at a constant temperature of 25°C, is given by:

$$V = -59 \text{ mV} \times \log_{10} [H^+] + C \qquad \text{... (3.13)}$$

where, C is a constant. Since pH is defined as

$$pH = -\log_{10} [H^+] \qquad \text{... (3.14)}$$

the potential of the active pH electrode V is proportional to the pH of the solution under test and is equal to

$$V = 59 \times pH + C \qquad \text{... (3.15)}$$

The value of C is usually compensated for electronically when the pH electrode is calibrated by placing the electrode inside buffer solutions with known pH values.

Carbon Dioxide Sensors

Electrodes for measurement of partial pressure of CO_2 in blood or other liquids are based on measuring the pH as illustrated in Fig. 3.24. The measurement is based on the observation that, when CO_2 is dissolved in water, it forms a weakly dissociated carbonic acid (H_2CO_3) that subsequently forms free hydrogen and bicarbonate ions according to the following chemical reaction:

$$CO_2 + H_2O \leftrightarrow H_2CO_3 \leftrightarrow H^+ + HCO_3^-$$

As a result of this chemical reaction, the pH of the solution is changed. This change generates a potential between the glass pH and a reference (e.g., Ag/AgCl) electrode that is proportional to the negative logarithm of the pCO_2.

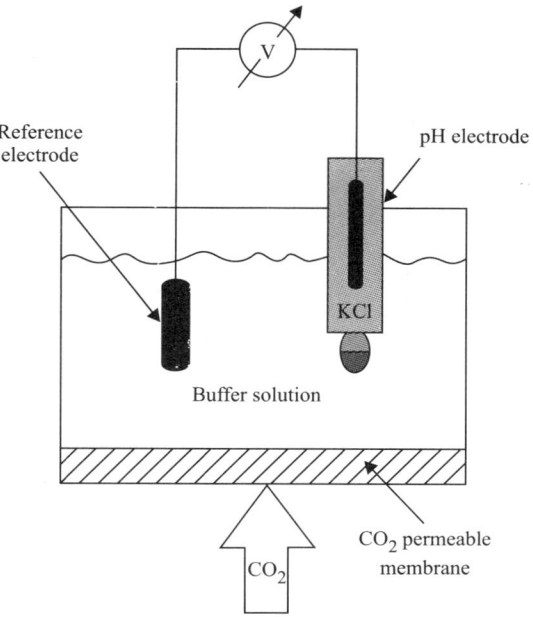

Fig. 3.24. Principle of a pCO_2 electrode.

BIOANALYTICAL SENSORS

The number of analytes that can be measured with electrochemical sensors can be increased significantly by adding biologically specific mediators (reagents that either undergo reactions or act as catalysts) to the semipermeable membrane structure. Several biosensors that have been constructed and used mainly for research applications have different enzymes and micro-organisms as the primary sensing elements. Although these biosensors have been used successfully *in vitro* to demonstrate unique medical and industrial applications, further technical improvements are necessary to make these sensors robust and reliable enough to fulfill the demanding requirements of routine analytical and clinical applications. Examples of some interesting sensor designs are given in the following sections.

Enzyme-Based Biosensors

Enzymes constitute a group of more than 2000 proteins having so-called biocatalytic properties. These properties give the enzymes their unique and powerful ability to accelerate chemical reactions inside biological cells. Most enzymes react only with specific substrates even though they may be contained in a complicated mixture with other substances. It is important to keep in mind, however, that soluble enzymes are very sensitive to both temperature and pH variations and they can be inactivated by many chemical inhibitors. For practical biosensor applications, these enzymes are normally immobilised by insolubilising the free enzymes via entrapment into an inert and stable matrix such as starch gel, silicon rubber or polyacrylamide. This process is important to ensure that the enzyme retains its catalytic properties and can be reusable.

The action of specific enzymes can be utilised to construct a range of different biosensors. A typical example of an enzyme-base sensor is a glucose sensor that uses the enzyme glucose oxidase. An immobilised enzyme which acts as a catalyst, such as glucose oxidase (g.o.), is commonly used to detect glucose by measuring electrochemically either the amount of hydrogen peroxide (H_2O_2) or gluconic acid produced or the amount of oxygen consumed according to the following reaction:

$$\text{Glucose} + O_2 \xleftrightarrow{\text{g.o.}} \text{gluconic acid} + H_2O_2$$

Biocatalytic enzyme-based sensors generally consist of an electrochemical gas-sensitive transducer or an ion-selective electrode with an enzyme immobilised in or on a membrane that serves as the biological mediator. The analyte diffuses from the bulk sample solution into the biocatalytic layer where an enzymatic reaction takes place. The electroactive production that is formed (or consumed) is usually detected by an ion-selective electrode. A membrane separates the basic sensor from the enzymes if a gas is consumed (such as O_2) or is produced (such as CO_2 or NH_3). Although the concentration of the bulk substrate drops continuously, the rate of consumption is usually negligible. The decrease is detected only when the test volume is very small or when the area of the enzyme membrane is large enough. Thus, this electrochemical analysis is nondestructive and the sample can be reused. Measurements are usually performed at a constant pH and temperature either in a stirred medium solutions or in a flowthrough solution.

Microbial Biosensors

A number of microbial sensors have been developed mainly for on-line control of biochemical processes in various environmental, agricultural, food and pharmaceutical applications. Microbial biosensors typically involve the assimilation of organic compounds by the micro-organisms, followed by a change in respiration activity (metabolism), or the production of specific electrochemical active metabolites, such as H_2, CO_2 or NH_3 that are secreted by the micro-organism.

A microbial biosensor is composed of immobilised micro-organisms that serve as specific recognition elements and an electrochemical or optical sensing device that is used to convert the biochemical signal into an electronic signal that can be processed. The operation of a microbial biosensor is a five-step process; (i) the substrate is transported to the surface of the sensor; (ii) the substrate diffuses through the membrane to the immobilised micro-organism; (iii) a reaction occurs at the immobilised organism; (iv) the products formed in the reaction are transported through the membrane to the surface of the detector; and (v) the products are measured by the detector.

Examples of microbial biosensors include ammonia (NH_3) and nitrogen dioxide (NO_2) sensors that utilise nitrifying bacteria as the biological sensing component. Ammonia biosensors are based on nitrifying bacteria, such as *Nitrosomonas* sp., that use ammonia as a source of energy and oxidise ammonia as follows:

$$NH_3 + 1.5O_2 \xrightarrow[\textit{Nitrosomonas sp.}]{} NO_2 + H_2O + H^+$$

The oxidation process proceeds at a high rate and the amount of oxygen consumed by the immobilised bacteria can be measured directly by a polarographic oxygen electrode placed behind the bacteria.

Nitric oxide (NO) and NO_2 are the two principal pollution gases of nitrogen in the atmosphere. The principle of a NO_2 biosensor is shown in Fig. 3.25. When a sample of NO_2 gas diffuses through the gas-permeable membrane, it is oxidised by the *Nitrobacter* sp. bacteria as follows:

$$2NO_2 + O_2 \xrightarrow[\textit{Nitrosomonas sp.}]{} 2NO_3$$

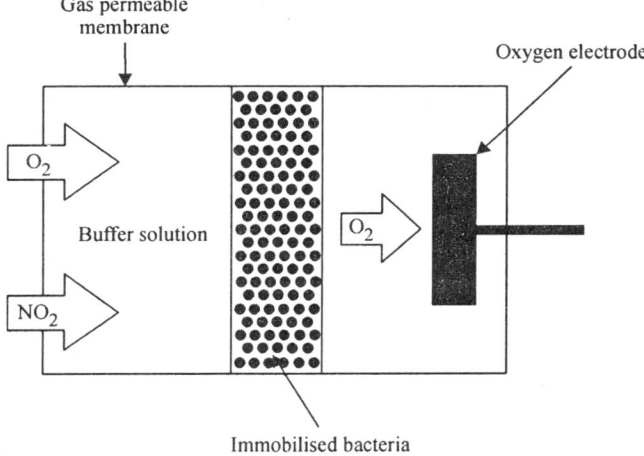

Fig. 3.25. Principle of a NO_2 microbial-type biosensor.

Similar to an ammonia biosensor, the consumption of O_2 around the membrane is determined by an electrochemical oxygen electrode.

The use of microbial cells in electrochemical sensors offers several advantages over enzyme-based electrodes, the principal one being the increased electrode lifetime of several weeks. On the other hand, microbial sensors may be less favourable compared with enzymes electrodes with respect to specificity and response time.

OPTICAL BIOSENSORS

Optical Fibres

Optical fibres are used to transmit light from one location to another. They are made from two concentric and transparent glass or plastic materials as illustrated in Fig. 3.26. One is known as the core and the second layer, which serves as a coating material, is called the cladding.

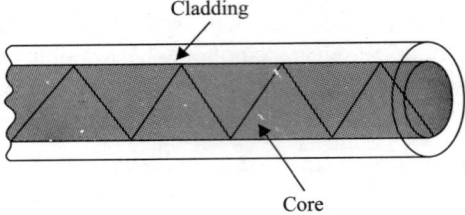

Fig. 3.26. Principle of optical fibres.

The core and cladding of an optical fibre have a different index of refraction, n. The index of refraction is a number that expresses the ratio of the light velocity in free space to its velocity in a specific material. For instance, the refractive index for air is equal to 1.0, whereas the refractive index for water is equal to 1.33. Assuming that the refractive index of the core material is n_1 and the refractive index of the cladding is n_2 ($n_1 > n_2$), Snell's law gives

$$n_1 \sin\phi_1 = n_2 \sin\phi_2 \qquad \text{... (3.16)}$$

where ϕ is the angle of incidence as illustrated in Fig. 3.27.

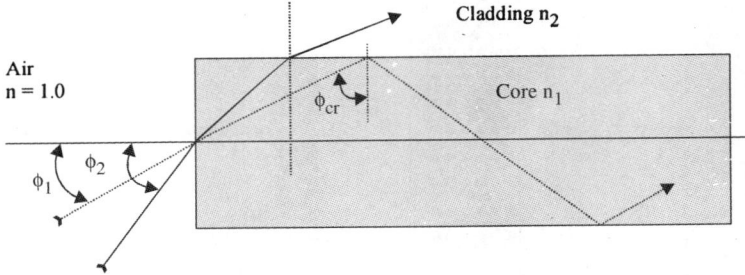

Fig. 3.27. Optical fibre illustrating the incident and refracted light rays. The solid line shows the light ray escaping from the core into the cladding. The dashed line shows the ray undergoing total internal reflection inside the core.

Accordingly, any light passing from a lower refractive index to a higher refractive index is bent toward the line that is perpendicular to the interface of the two materials. For small incident angles, ϕ_1, the light ray enters the fibre core and bends inwards at the first core/cladding interface. For larger incident angles, ϕ_2, the ray exceed a minimum angle required to bend it back into the core when it reaches the corecladding boundary. Consequently, the light escapes into the cladding. By setting $\sin\phi_2 = 1.0$, the critical angle, ϕ_{cr}, is given by

$$\sin \phi_{cr} = \frac{n_2}{n_1} \qquad \text{... (3.17)}$$

Any light rays that enter the optical fibre with incidence angle greater than ϕ_{cr} are internally reflected inside the core of the fibre by the surrounding cladding. Conversely, any entering light rays with incidence angles smaller than ϕ_{cr} escape through the cladding and are therefore not transmitted by the core.

Example 3.8. Assume that a beam of light passes from a layer of glass with a refractive index of $n_1 = 1.47$ into a second layer of glass with a refractive index of $n_2 = 1.44$. Using Snell's law, calculate the critical angle for the boundary between these two glass layers.

Solution.

$$\phi_{cr} = \arcsin\left(\frac{n_2}{n_1}\right) = \arcsin\ (0.9796)$$

$$\phi_{cr} = 78.4°$$

Therefore, light that strikes the boundary between these two glasses at an angle greater than 78.4° will be reflected back into the first layer.

Sensing Mechanisms

Optical fibres can be used to develop a whole range of sensors for biomedical applications. These sensors are small, flexible and free from electrical interference. They can produce an instantaneous response to microenvironment that surround their surface.

Commercial fibre optic sensors for blood gas monitoring became available during the past decade. While many different approaches have been taken, they all have some features in common as illustrated in Fig. 3.28. First, all sensors are interfaced with an optical module. The module supplies the excitation light, which may be from a monochromatic source such as diode laser or from a broadband source (e.g., quartz-halogen) that is filtered to provide a narrow bandwidth of excitation. Typically, two wavelengths of light are used: One wavelength is sensitive to changes in the species to be measured, whereas the other wavelength is unaffected by changes in the analyte concentration. This wavelength serves as a reference and is used to compensate for fluctuations in source output and detector stability. The light output from the optic module is coupled into a fibre optical cable through appropriate lenses and an optical connector.

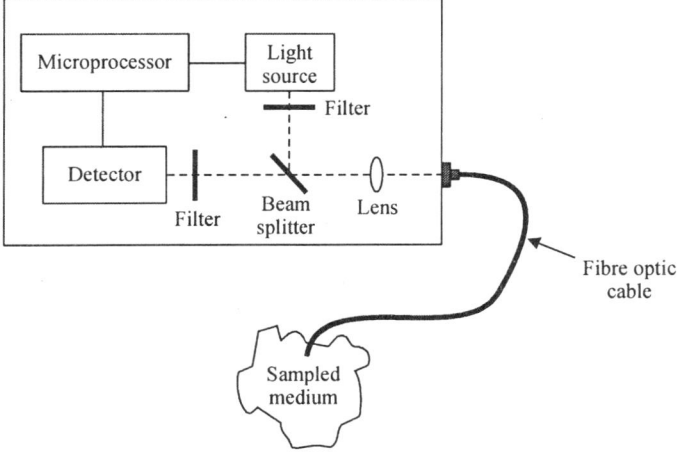

Fig. 3.28. General principle of a fibre optic-based sensor.

Several sensing mechanisms can be utilised to construct optical fibre sensor. In fluorescence-based sensors, the incident light excites fluorescence emission, which changes in intensity as a function of the concentration of the analyte to be measured. The emitted light travels back down the fibre to the monitor where the light intensity is measured by a photodetector. In other types of fibre optic sensors, the light-absorbing properties of the sensor chemistry change as a function of analyte chemistry. In the absorption-based design, a reflective surface near the tip or some scattering material within the sensing chemistry itself is usually used to return the light back through the same optical fibre.

Indicator-Mediated Fibre Optic Sensors

Since only limited number of biochemical substances have an intrinsic optical absorption or fluorescence property that can be measured directly with sufficient selectivity by standard spectroscopic methods, indicator-mediated sensors have been developed to use specific reagents that are immobilised either on the surface or near the tip of an optical fibre. In these sensors, light travels from a light source to the end of the optical fibre where it interacts with a specific chemical or biological recognition element. These transducers may include indicators and ion-binding compounds (ionophores) as wells as a wide variety of selective polymeric materials. After the light interacts with the biological sample, it returns through either the same optical fibre (in a single-fibre configuration) or a separate optical fibre (in a dual-fibre configuration) to a detector, which correlates the degree of a light attenuation with the concentration of the analyte.

Typical indicator-mediated sensor configurations are shown schematically in Fig. 3.29. The transducing element is a thin layer of chemical material that is placed near the sensor tip and is separated from the blood medium by a selective membrane. The chemical-sensing material transforms the incident light into a return light signal with a magnitude that is proportional to the concentration of the species to be measured. The stability of the sensor is determined by the stability of the photosensitive material that is used and also by how effective the sensing material is protected from leaching out of the probe. In Fig. 3.29a the indicator is immobilised directly on a membrane positioned at the end of the fibre. An indicator in the form of a powder can also be physically retained in position at the end of the fibre by a special permeable membrane as illustrated in Fig. 3.29b or a hollow capillary tube as illustrated in Fig. 3.29c

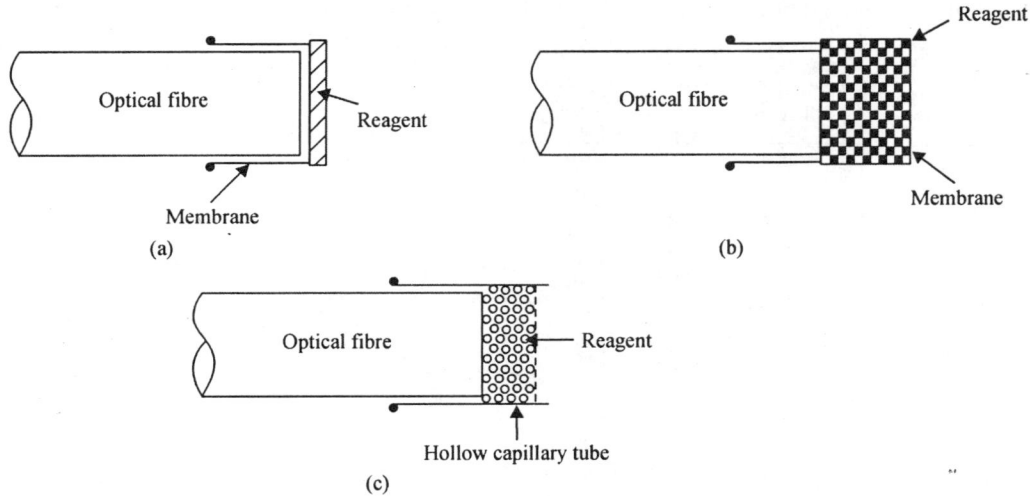

Fig. 3.29. Different indicator-mediated fibre optic sensor configurations.

Optical fibres have been used to construct immunoassay biosensors. The principle for this relies on the propagation of light along the optical fibre. When light travels along the fibre, it is not just confined to the core region. A small fraction (referred to as an evanescent wave) penetrates a characteristic distance (typically on the order of the one wavelength or less) beyond the core boundary into the surrounding cladding. The evanescent wave is attenuated exponentially, typically following Beer–Lamber's law. This concept has been exploited to construct several biosensors in which a portion of the cladding near the distal tip of an optical fibre has been removed and replaced by an optically absorbing compounds. The light, which propagates inside the optical fibre core, undergoes several multiple internal reflections along the sides of the unclad portion of the fibre tip. Usually, an optically reflecting material is coated on the distal tip of the fibre to divert the beam back through the same fibre where it is detected by a sensitive photodetector. In some designs, a stable fluorophore can be used instead of an absorbing material. The excitation light, which is typically generated either by a stable laser source or by a combination of a broadband light source and a narrow-width optical filter, is absorbed by the fluorophore and emits a detectable fluorescent light at a slightly higher wavelength than the excitation light. This concept provides improved sensitivity because narrow-width optical filters can be used to separate the incident light from the fluorescent light components that reach the photodetector.

Evanescent-type biosensors can be used in immunological diagnostics to detect antibodyantigen binding. Figure 3.30 shows a conceptual diagram of an immunoassay biosensor.

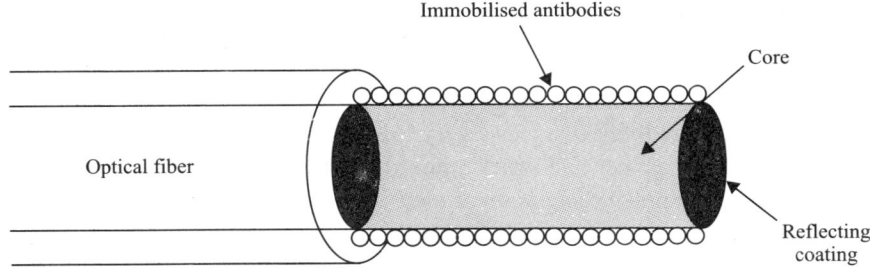

Fig. 3.30. Principle of a fibre optic immunoassay biosensor.

The immobilised antibody on the surface of the unclad portion of the fibre captures the antigen from the sample solution, which is normally introduced into a small flowthrough chamber where the fibre tip is located. The sample solution is then removed and labelled antibody is added into the flow chamber. A fluorescent signal is excited and measured when the labelled antibody binds to the antigen that is already immobilised by the antibody.

Chapter 4

Biopotential Amplifiers

INTRODUCTION

Biopotential amplifiers are a crucial component in many medical and biological measurements and largely determine the quality and information content of the measured signals. The extremely wide range of necessary specifications with regard to bandwidth, sensitivity, dynamic range, gain, common mode rejection ratio (CMRR) and patient safety leaves only little room for the application of general purpose biopotential amplifiers and mostly requires the use of special purpose amplifiers.

Biosignals are recorded as potentials, voltages and electrical field strengths generated by nerves and muscles. The measurements involve voltages at very low levels, typically ranging between 1 μV and 100 mV, with high source impedances and superimposed high level interference signals and noise. The signals need to be amplified to make them compatible with devices such as displays, recorders or A/D converters for computerised equipment. Amplifiers adequate to measure these signals have to satisfy very specific requirements. They have to provide amplification selective to the physiological signal, reject superimposed noise and interference signals and guarantee protection from damages through voltage and current surges for both patient and electronic equipment. Amplifiers featuring these specifications are known as biopotential amplifiers. Basic requirements and features, as well as some specialised systems are discussed below.

BASIC AMPLIFIER REQUIREMENTS

The basic requirements that a biopotential amplifier has to satisfy are:
1. The physiological process to be monitored should not be influenced in any way by the amplifier.
2. The measured signal should not be distorted.
3. The amplifier should provide the best possible separation of signal interferences.
4. The amplifier has to offer protection of the patient from any hazard of electrical shock.
5. The amplifier itself has to be protected against damages that might result from high input voltages as they occur during the application of defibrillators or electrosurgical instrumentation.

A typical configuration for the measurement of biopotentials is shown in Fig. 4.1. Three electrodes, two of them picking up the biological signal and the third providing the reference potential, connect the subject to the amplifier. The input signal to the amplifier consists of five components: (i) the desired biopotential; (ii) undesired biopotentials; (iii) a power line interference signal of 60 Hz (50 Hz in some

74

countries) and its harmonics; (iv) interference signals generated by the tissue/electrode interface; and (v) noise.

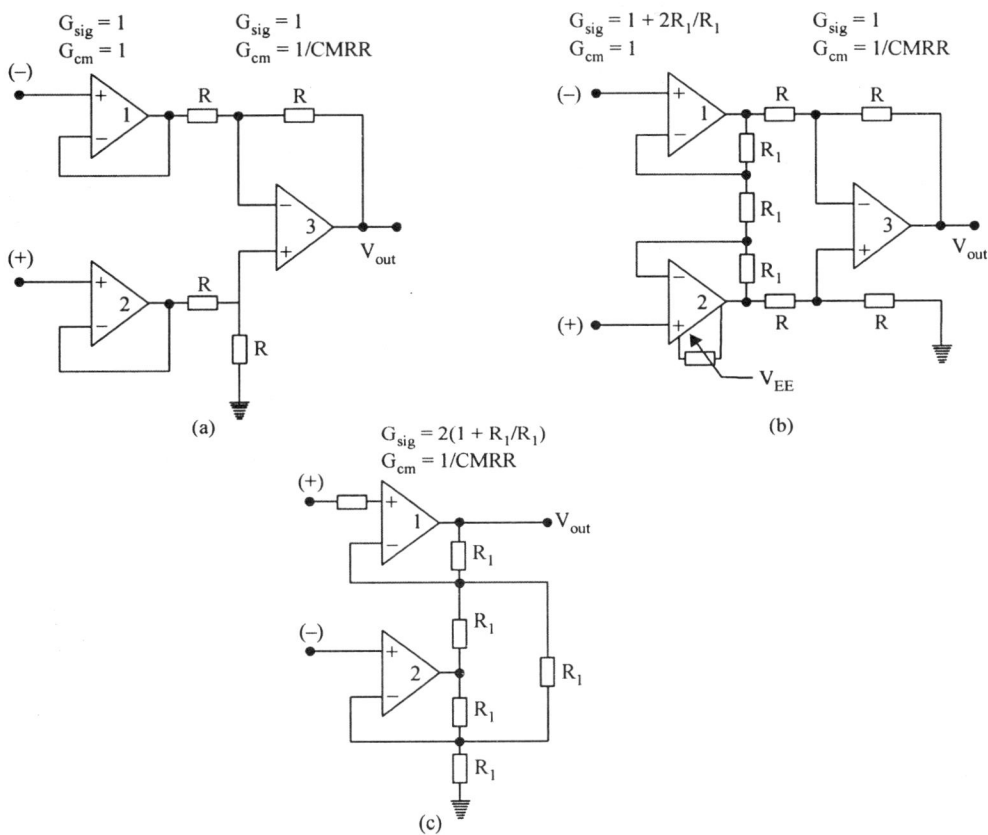

(a)

(b)

(c)

Fig. 4.1. Typical configuration for the measurement of biopotentials. The biological signal V_{biol} appears between the two measuring electrodes at the right and left arm of the patient and is fed to the inverting and the non-inverting inputs of the differential amplifier. The right leg electrode provides the reference potential for the amplifier with a common mode voltage V_c as indicated.

Proper design of the amplifier provides rejection of a large portion of the signal interferences. The main task of the differential amplifier as shown in Fig. 4.1 is to reject the line frequency interference that is electrostatically or magnetically coupled into the subject. The desired biopotential appears as a voltage between the two input terminals of the differential amplifier and is referred to as the differential signal. The line frequency interference signal shows only very small differences in amplitude and phase between the two measuring electrodes, causing approximately the same potential at both inputs and thus appears only between the inputs and ground and is called the common mode signal. Strong rejection of the common mode signal is one of the most important characteristics of a good biopotential amplifier.

The common mode rejection ratio (CMRR) of an amplifier is defined as the ratio of the differential mode gain over the common mode gain. As seen in Fig. 4.1, the rejection of the common mode signal in a biopotential amplifier is both a function of the amplifier CMRR and the source impedances Z_1 and Z_2. For the ideal biopotential amplifier with $Z_1 = Z_2$ and infinite CMRR of the differential amplifier, the output voltage is the pure biological signal amplified by G_D, the differential mode gain: $V_{out} = G_D \cdot V_{biol}$. With finite CMRR, the common mode signal is not completely rejected, adding the interference term $G_D \cdot V_c/$CMRR to the output signal. Even in the case of an ideal differential amplifier with infinite CMRR, the common mode signal will not completely disappear unless the source impedances are equal. The common mode signal V_c causes currents to flow through Z_1 and Z_2. The related voltage drops show a difference if the source impedances are unequal, thus generating a differential signal at the amplifier input which, of course, is not rejected by the differential amplifier. With amplifier gain G_D and input impedance Z_{in}, the output voltage of the amplifier is:

$$V_{out} = G_D V_{biol} + \frac{G_D V_c}{CMRR} + G_D V_c \left(1 - \frac{Z_{in}}{Z_{in} + Z_1 - Z_2}\right) \quad \dots (4.1)$$

The output of a real biopotential amplifier will always consists of the desired output component due to a differential biosignal, an undesired component due to incomplete rejection of common mode interference signals as a function of CMRR and an undesired component due to source impedance unbalance allowing a small proportion of a common mode signal to appear as a differential signal to the amplifier. Since source impedance unbalances of 5000 to 10000 Ω, mainly caused by electrodes, are not uncommon and sufficient rejection of line frequency interferences requires a minimum CMRR of 100 dB, the input impedance of the amplifier should be at least 10^9 Ω at 60 Hz to prevent source impedance unbalances from deteriorating the overall CMRR of the amplifier. State-of-the-art biopotential amplifiers provide a CMRR of 120 to 140 dB.

In order to provide optimum signal quality and adequate voltage level for further signal processing, the amplifier has to provide a gain of 100 to 50,000 and needs to maintain the best possible signal-to-noise ratio. The presence of high level interference signals not only deteriorates the quality of the physiological signals, but also restricts the design of the biopotential amplifier. Electrode half-cell potentials, for example, limit the gain factor of the first amplifier stage since their amplitude can be several orders of magnitude larger than the amplitude of the physiological signal. To prevent the amplifier from going into saturation, this component has to be eliminated before the required gain can be provided for the physiological signal. A typical design of the various stages of a biopotential amplifier is shown in Fig. 4.2. The electrodes which provide the transition between the ionic flow of currents in biological tissue and the electronic flow of current in the amplifier, represent a complex electrochemical system. The electrodes determine to a large extent the composition of the measured signal. The pre-amplifier represents the most critical part of the amplifier itself since it sets the stage for the quality of the biosignal. With proper design, the pre-amplifier can eliminate or at least minimise, most of the signals interfering with the measurement of biopotentials.

In addition to electrode potentials and electromagnetic interferences, noise—generated by the amplifier and the connection between biological source and amplifier—has to be taken into account when designing the preamplifier. The total source resistance R_s, including the resistance of the biological source and all transition resistances between signal source and amplifier input, causes thermal voltage noise with a root mean square (rms) value of:

$$E_{rms} = \sqrt{4kTR_sB} \text{ (volt)} \quad \dots (4.2)$$

where,

k = Boltzmann constant
T = absolute temperature

R_s = resistance in Ω
B = bandwidth in Hz

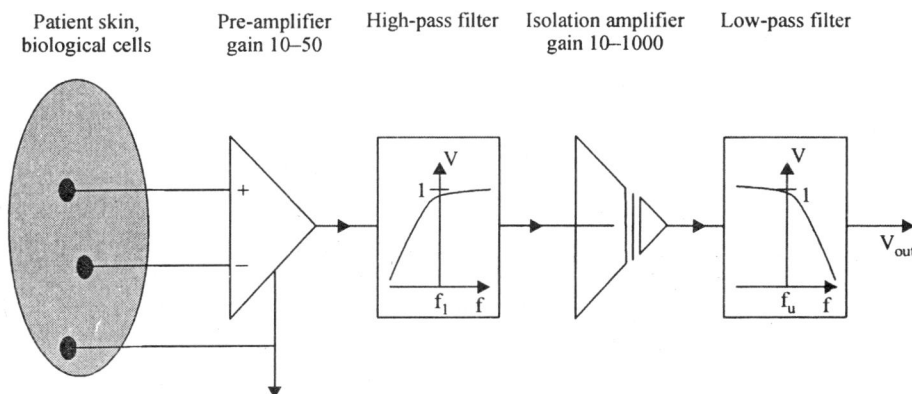

Fig. 4.2. Schematic design of the main stages of a biopotential amplifier. Three electrodes connect the patient to a pre-amplifier stage. After removing DC and low-frequency interferences, the signal is connected to an output low-pass filter through an isolation stage which provides electrical safety to the patient, prevents ground loops and reduces the influence of interference signals.

Additionally, there is the inherent amplifier noise. It consists of two frequency-dependent components, the internal voltage noise source e_n and the voltage drop across the source resistance R_s caused by an internal current noise generator i_n. The total input noise for the amplifier with a bandwidth of $B = f_2 - f_1$ is calculated as the sum of its three independent components:

$$E_{rms}^2 = \int_{f_1}^{f_2} e_n^2 df + R_s^2 \int_{f_1}^{f_2} i_n^2 df + 4kTR_sB \qquad \text{... (4.3)}$$

High signal-to-noise ratios thus require the use of very low noise amplifiers and the limitation of bandwidth. Current technology offers differential amplifiers with voltage noise of less than $10\ nV/\sqrt{Hz}$ and current noise less than $1\ pA/\sqrt{Hz}$. Both parameters are frequency dependent and decrease approximately with the square root of frequency. The exact relationship depends on the technology of the amplifier input stage. Field effect transistor (FET) pre-amplifiers exhibit about five times the voltage noise density compared to bipolar transistors but a current noise density that is about 100 times smaller.

The purpose of the high-pass and low-pass filters in Fig. 4.2 is to eliminate interference signals like electrode half-cell potential and pre-amplifier offset potentials and to reduce the noise amplitude by the limitation of the amplifier bandwidth. Since the biosignal should not be distorted or attenuated, higher order sharp-cutting linear phase filters have to be used. Active Bessel filters are preferred filter types due to their smooth transfer function. Separation of biosignal and interference is in most cases incomplete due to the overlap of their spectra.

The isolation stage serves the galvanic decoupling of the patient from the measuring equipment and provides safety from electrical hazards. This stage also prevents galvanic currents from deteriorating the signal-to-noise ratio especially by preventing ground loops. Various principles can be used to realise the isolation stage. Analog isolation amplifiers use either transformer, optical or capacitive couplers to transmit the signal through the isolation barrier. Digital isolation amplifiers use a voltage/frequency converter to digitise the signal before it is transmitted easily by optical or inductive couplers to the output frequency/voltage converter. The most important characteristics of an isolation amplifier are low leakage current, isolation impedance, isolation voltage (or mode) rejection (IMR) and maximum safe isolation.

Interferences

The most critical point in the measurement of biopotential is the contact between electrodes and biological tissue. Both the electrode offset potential and the electrode/tissue impedance are subject to changes due to relative movements of electrode and tissue. Thus, two interference signals are generated as motion artifacts: the changes of the electrode potential and motion-induced changes of the voltage drop caused by the input current of the pre-amplifier. These motion artifacts can be minimised by providing high input impedances for the pre-amplifier, usage of non-polarised electrodes with low half-cell potentials such as Ag/AgCl electrodes and by reducing the source impedance by use of electrode gel. Motion artifacts, interferences from external electromagnetic fields and noise can also be generated in the wires connecting electrodes and amplifier. Reduction of these interferences is achieved by using twisted pair cables, shielded wires and input guarding.

Recording of biopotentials is often done in an environment that is equipped with many electrical systems which produce strong electrical and magnetic fields. In addition to 60 Hz power line frequency and some strong harmonics, high frequency electromagnetic fields are encountered. At power line frequency, the electric and magnetic components of the interfering fields can be considered separately. Electrical fields are caused by all conductors that are connected to power, even with no flow of current. A current is capacitively coupled into the body where it flows to the ground electrode. If an isolation amplifier is used without patient ground, the current is capacitively coupled to ground. In this case, the body potential floats with a voltage of up to 100 V towards ground. Minimising interferences requires increasing the distance between power lines and the body, use of isolation amplifiers, separate grounding of the body at a location as far away from the measuring electrodes as possible and use of shielded electrode cables.

The magnetic field components produce eddy currents in the body. The amplifier, the electrode cable and the body form an induction loop that is subject to the generation of an interference signal. Minimising this interference signal requires increasing the distance between the interference source and patient, twisting the connecting cables, shielding of the magnetic fields and re-locating the patient to a place and orientation that offers minimum interference signals. In many cases, an additional narrow band-rejection filter (notch filter) is implemented as an additional stage in the biopotential amplifier to provide sufficient suppression of line frequency interferences.

In order to achieve optimum signal quality, the biopotential amplifier has to be adapted to the specific application. Based on the signal parameters, both appropriate bandwidth and gain factor are chosen. Fig. 4.3 shows an overview of the most commonly measured biopotentials and specifies the normal ranges for amplitude and bandwidth.

A final requirement for biopotential amplifiers is the need for calibration. Since the amplitude of the biopotential often has to be determined very accurately, there must be provisions to easily determine the gain or the amplitude range referenced to the input of the amplifier.

For this purpose, the gain of the amplifier must be well calibrated. In order to prevent difficulties with calibrations, some amplifiers that need to have adjustable gain use a number of fixed gain settings rather than providing a continuous gain control. Some amplifiers have a standard signal source of known amplitude built in that can be momentarily connected to the input by the push of a button to check the calibration at the output of the biopotential amplifier.

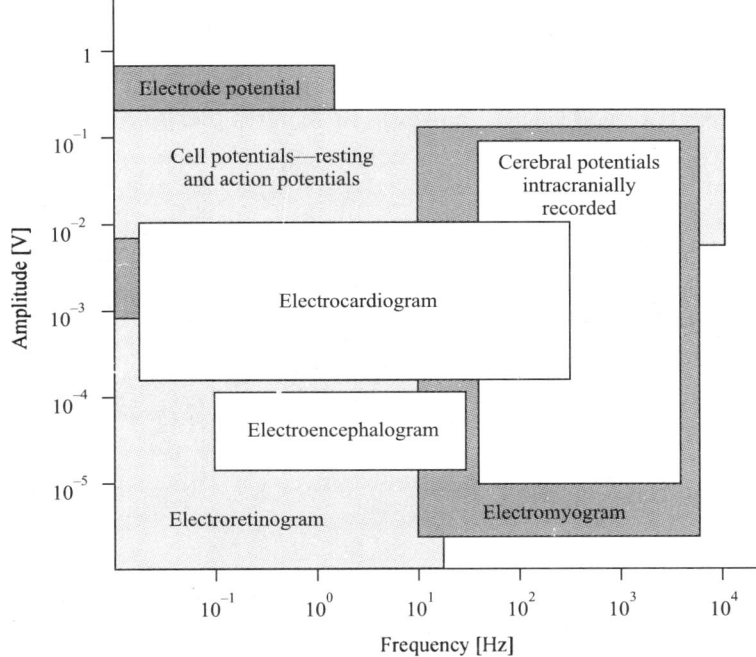

Fig. 4.3. Amplitudes and spectral ranges of some important biosignals. The various biopotentials completely cover the area from 10^{-6} V to almost 1 V and from DC to 10 kHz.

SPECIAL CIRCUITS

Instrumentation Amplifier

An important stage of all biopotential amplifiers is the input pre-amplifier which substantially contributes to the overall quality of the system. The main tasks of the pre-amplifier are to sense the voltage between two measuring electrodes while rejecting the common mode signal and minimising the effect of electrode polarisation overpotentials. Crucial to the performance of the pre-amplifier is the input impedance which should be as high as possible. Such as differential amplifier cannot be realised using a standard single operational amplifier (op-amp) design since this does not provide the necessary high input impedance. The general solution to the problem involves voltage followers, or non-inverting amplifiers, to attain high input impedances. A possible realisation is shown in Fig. 4.4a. The main disadvantage of this circuit is that it requires high CMRR both in the followers and in the final op-amp. With the input buffers working at unity gain, all the common-mode rejection must be accomplished in the output amplifier, requiring very precise resistor matching. The circuit in Fig. 4.4b eliminates this disadvantage. It represents the standard instrumentation amplifier configuration. The two input op-amps provide high differential gain and unity common-mode gain without the requirement of close resistor matching. The differential output from the first stage represents a signal with substantial relative reduction of the common-mode signal and is used to drive a standard differential amplifier which further reduces the common-mode signal. CMRR of the output op-amp as well as resistor matching in its circuit are less critical than in the follower type instrumentation amplifier. Offset trimming for the whole circuit can be done at one of the input op-amps. Complete instrumentation amplifier integrated circuits based on this standard instrumentation amplifier configuration are available from several manufacturers. All components except R_1, which determines the gain of the amplifier and the potentiometer for offset trimming are contained on the integrated circuit chip. Figure 4.4c shows another configuration that offers high input impedance with only two op-amps. For good CMRR, however, its requires precise resistor matching.

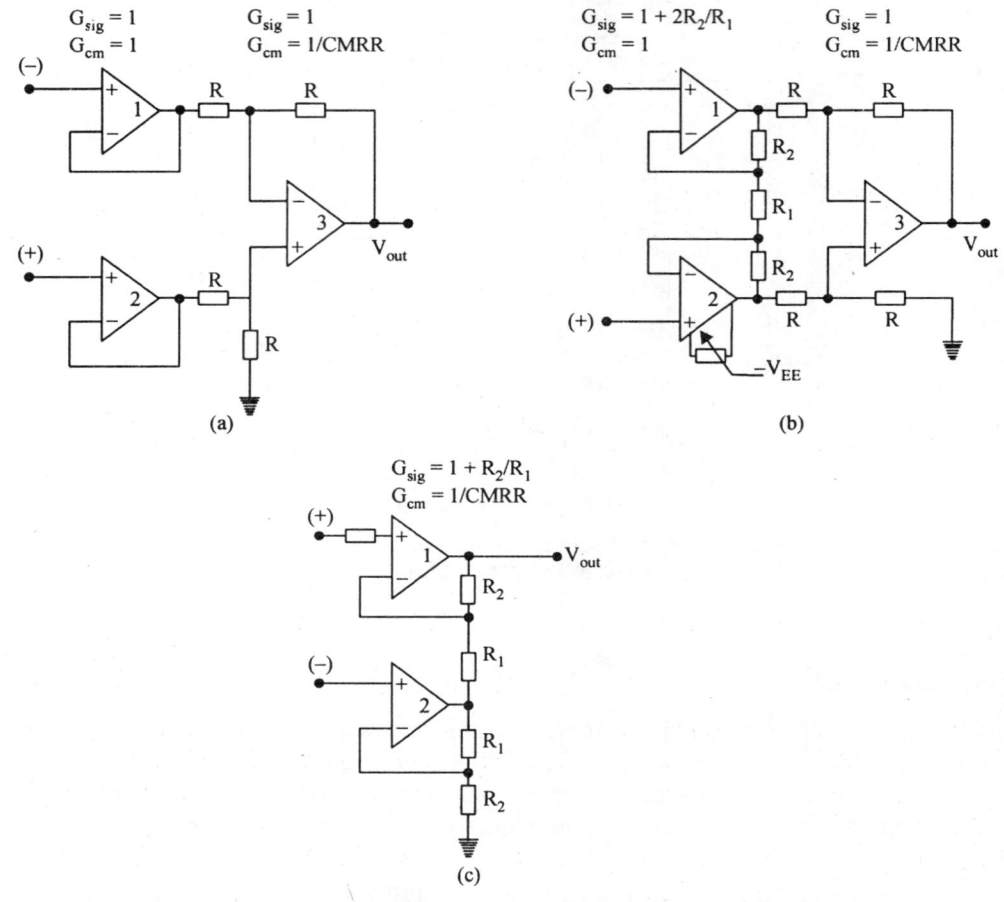

Fig. 4.4. Circuit drawings for three different realisations of instrumentation amplifiers for biomedical applications. (a) voltage follower input stage; (b) improved, amplifying input stage; and (c) and 2-op-amp version.

In applications where DC and very low frequency biopotentials are not to be measured, it would be desirable to block those signal components at the pre-amplifier inputs by simply adding a capacitor working as a passive high-pass filter. This would eliminate the electrode offset potentials and permit a higher gain factor for the pre-amplifier and thus a higher CMRR. A capacitor between electrodes and amplifier input would, however, result in charging effects from the input bias current. Due to the difficulty of precisely matching capacitors for the two input leads, they would also contribute to an increased source impedance unbalance and thus reduce CMRR. Avoiding the problem of charging effects by adding a resistor between the pre-amplifier inputs and ground as shown in Fig. 4.5a also results in a decrease of CMRR due to the diminished and mismatched input impedance. A 1 per cent mismatch for two 1 MΩ resistors can already create a –60 dB loss in CMRR. The loss in CMRR is much greater if the capacitors are mismatched, which cannot be prevented in real systems. Nevertheless, such realisations are used where the specific situation allows. In some applications, a further reduction of the amplifier to a two-electrode amplifier configuration would be convenient, even at the expense of some loss in the CMRR. Figure 4.6 shows a pre-amplifier design working with two electrodes and providing AC coupling as proposed by Pallas-Areny.

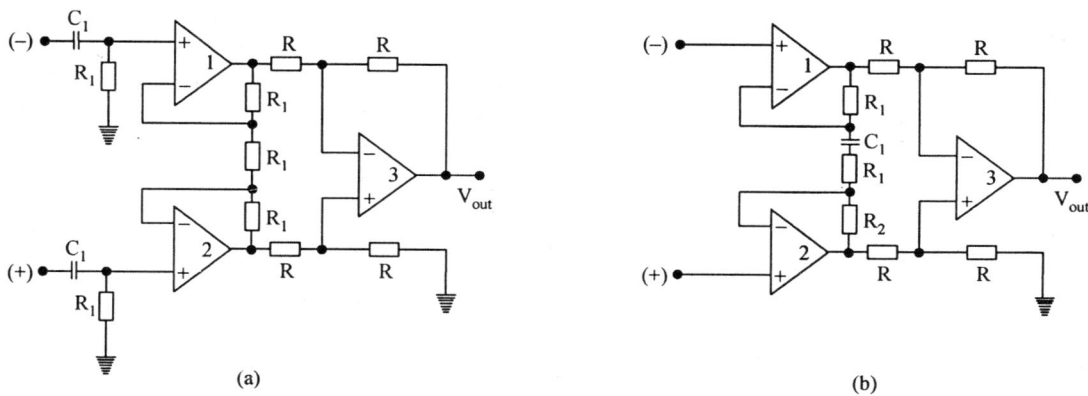

(a)   (b)

Fig. 4.5. AC coupled instrumentation amplifier designs. (a) The classical design using an RC high-pass filter at the inputs; (b) and a high CMRR 'quasi-high-pass' amplifier as proposed by Lu.

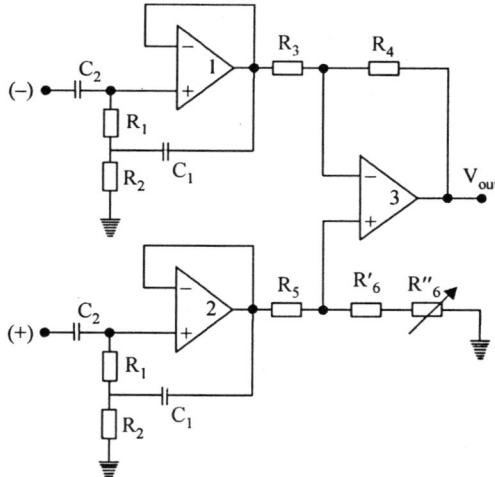

Fig. 4.6. Composite instrumentation amplifier based on an AC-coupled first stage. The second stage is based on a one op-amp differential amplifier which can be replaced by an instrumentation amplifier.

A third alternative of eliminating DC and low frequencies in the first amplifier stage is a directly coupled quasi-high-pass amplifier design, which maintains the high CMRR of DC coupled high input impedance instrumentation amplifiers. In this design, the gain determining resistor R_1 (Fig. 4.5a) is replaced by a first order high-pass filter consisting of R_1 and a series capacitor C_f. The signal gain of the amplifier is

$$G = 1 + \frac{2R_2}{R_1 + \dfrac{1}{j\omega C}} \qquad \dots (4.4)$$

Thus, DC gain is 1, while the high frequency gain remains at $G = 1 + 2R_2/R_1$. A realisation using an off-the-shelf instrumentation amplifier (Burr-Brown INA 118) operates at low power (0.35 mA) with low offset voltage (11 μV typical) and low input bias current (1 nA typical) and offers a high CMRR of 118 dB at a gain of $G = 50$. The very high input impedance (10 GΩ) of the instrumentation amplifier renders it insensitive to fluctuations of the electrode impedance. Therefore, it is suitable for bioelectric measurements using pasteless electrodes applied to unprepared, i.e., high impedance skin.

The pre-amplifier, often implemented as a separate device which is placed close to the electrodes or even directly attached to the electrodes, also acts as an impedance converter which allows the transmission of even weak signals to the remote monitoring unit. Due to the low output impedance of the pre-amplifier, the input impedance of the following amplifier stage can be low and still the influence of interference signals coupled into the transmission lines is reduced.

Isolation Amplifier and Patient Safety

Isolation amplifiers can be used to break ground loops, eliminate source ground connections and provide isolation protection to patient and electronic equipment. In a biopotential amplifier, the main purpose of the isolation amplifier is the protection of the patient by eliminating the hazard of electric shock resulting from the interaction among patient, amplifier and other electric devices in the patients's environment specifically defibrillators and electrosurgical equipment. It also adds to the prevention of line frequency interferences.

Isolation amplifies are realised in three different technologies: transformer isolation, capacitor isolation and opto-isolation. An isolation barrier provides a complete galvanic separation of the input side, i.e., patient and pre-amplifier, from all equipment on the output side. Ideally, there will be no flow of electric current across the barrier. The isolation-mode voltage is the voltage which appears across the isolation barrier, i.e., between the input common and the output common (Fig. 4.7). The amplifier has to with stand the largest expected isolation voltages without damage. Two isolation voltages are specified for commercial isolation amplifier: (i) the continuous rating; and (ii) the test voltage.

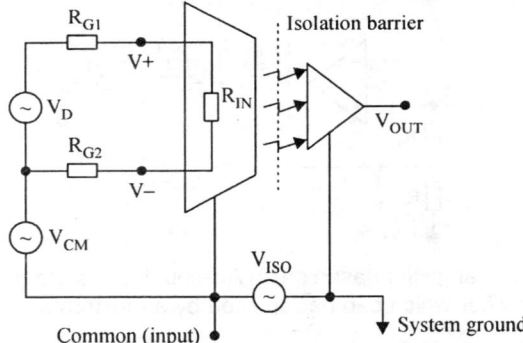

Fig. 4.7. Equivalent circuit of an isolation amplifier. The differential amplifier on the left transmits the signal through the isolation barrier by a transformer, capacitor or an opto-coupler.

To eliminate the need for longtime testing, the device is tested at about two times the rated continuous voltage. Thus, for a continuous rating of 2000 V, the device has to be tested at 4000 to 5000 V for a reasonable period of time. Since there is always some leakage across the isolation barrier, the isolation mode rejection ratio (IMRR) is not infinite. For a circuit as show in Fig. 4.7, the output voltage is:

$$V_{out} = \frac{G}{R_{G1} + R_{G2} + R_{IN}} \left[V_D + \frac{V_{CM}}{CMRR} \right] + \frac{V_{ISO}}{IMRR} \qquad \text{... (4.5)}$$

where, G is the amplifier gain, V_D, V_{CM} and V_{ISO} are differential, common-mode and isolation voltages, respectively and CMRR is the common mode rejection ratio for the amplifier.

Typical values of IMRR for a gain of 10 are 140 dB at DC and 120 dB at 60 Hz with a source unbalance of 5000 Ω. The isolation impedance is approximately 1.8 pF $\parallel$ 10^{12} Ω.

Transformer coupled isolation amplifiers perform on the basis of inductive transmission of a carrier signal that is amplitude modulated by the biosignal. A synchronous demodulator on the output port reconstructs the signal before it is fed through a Bessel response low-pass filter to an output buffer. A power transformer, generally driven by a 400 to 900 kHz square wave, supplies isolated power to the amplifier.

Optically coupled isolation amplifiers can principally be realised using only a singal LED and photodiode combination. While useful for a wide range of digital applications, this design has fundamental limitations as to its linearity and stability as a function of time and temperature. A matched photodiode design, as used in the Burr-Brown 3650/3652 isolation amplifier, overcomes these difficulties. Operation of the amplifier requires an isolated power supply to drive the input stages. Transformer coupled low leakage current isolated DC/DC converters are commonly used for this purposes. In some particular applications, especially in cases where the signal is transmitted over a longer distance by fibre optics, e.g., ECG amplifiers used for gated magnetic resonance imaging, batteries are used to power the amplifier. Fibre optic coupling in isolation amplifiers is another option that offers the advantage of higher flexibility in the placement of parts on the amplifier board.

Biopotential amplifiers have to provide sufficient protection from electrical shock to both user and patient. Electrical-safety codes and standards specify the minimum safety requirements for the equipment, especially the maximum leakage currents for chassis and patient leads and the power distribution system.

Special attention to patient safety is required in situations where biopotential amplifiers are connected to personal computers which are more and more often used to process and store physiological signals and data. Due to the design of the power supplies used in standard PCs permitting high leakage currents— an inadequate situation for a medical environment—there is a potential risk involved even when the patient is isolated from the PC through an isolation amplifier stage or optical signal transmission from the amplifier to the computer. This holds especially in those cases where, due to the proximity of the PC to the patient, an operator might touch patient and computer at the same time or the patient might touch the computer. It is required that a special power supply with sufficient limitation of leakage currents is used in the computer or that an additional, medical grade isolation transformer is used to provide the necessary isolation between power outlet and PC.

Surge Protection

The isolation amplifiers described in the preceding paragraph are primarily used for the protection of the patient from electric shock. Voltage surges between electrodes as they occur during the application of a defibrillator or electrosurgical instrumentation also present a risk to the biopotential amplifier. Biopotential amplifiers should be protected against serious damage to the electronic circuits. This is also part of the patient safety since defective input stage could otherwise apply dangerous current levels to the patient. To achieve this protection, voltage limiting devices are connected between each measuring electrode and electric ground. Ideally, these devices do not represent a shunt impedance and thus do not lower the input impedance of the pre-amplifier as long as the input voltage remains in a range considered safe for the equipment. They appear as an open circuit. As soon as the voltage drop across the device reaches a critical value V_b, the impedance of the device changes sharply and current passes through it to such an extent that the voltage cannot exceed V_b due to the voltage drop across the series resistor R as indicated in Fig. 4.8.

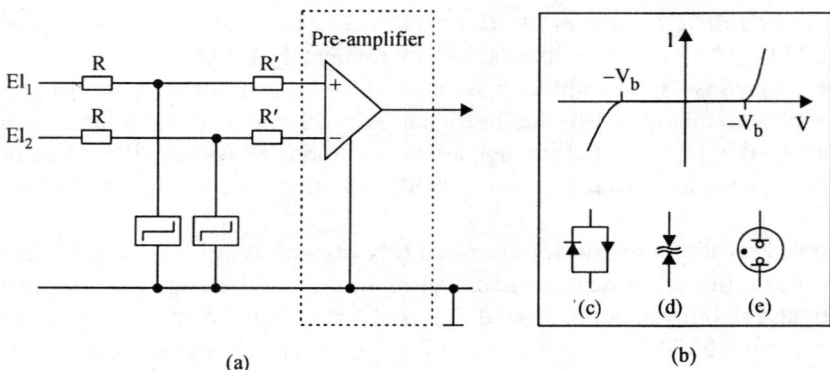

(a) (b)

Fig. 4.8. Protection of the amplifier input against high-voltage transients. The connection diagram for voltage-limiting elements is shown in panel (a) with two optional resistors R' at the input. A typical current-voltage characteristic is shown in panel; (b) voltage-limiting elements shown are the anti-parallel connection of diodes; (c) anti-parallel connection of Zener diodes; (d) and gas-discharge tubes (e).

Devices used for amplifier protection are diodes, Zener diodes and gas-discharge tubes. Parallel silicon diodes limit the voltage to approximately 600 mV. The transition from non-conducting to conducting state is not very sharp and signal distortion begins at about 300 mV which can be within the range of input voltages depending on the electrodes used. The breakdown voltage can be increased by connecting several diodes in series. Higher breakdown voltages are achieved by Zener diodes connected back to back. One of the diodes will be biased in the forward direction and the other in the reverse direction. The breakdown voltage in the forward direction is approximately 600 mV, but the breakdown voltage in the reverse direction is higher, generally in the range of 3 to 20 V, with a sharper voltage-current characteristic than the diode circuit.

A preferred voltage-limiting device for biopotential amplifiers is the gas-discharge tube. Due to its extremely high impedance in the non-conducting state, this device appears as an open circuit until it reaches its breakdown voltage. At the breakdown voltage which is in the range of 50 to 90 V, the tube switches to the conducting state and maintains a voltage that is usually several volts less than the breakdown voltage. Though the voltage maintained by the gas-discharge tube is still too high for some amplifiers, it is low enough to allow the input current to be easily limited to a safe value by simple circuit elements such as resistors like the resistors R' indicated in Fig. 4.8a. Preferred gas discharge tubes for biomedical applications are miniature neon lamps which are very inexpensive and have a symmetric characteristic.

Input Guarding

The common mode input impedance and thus the CMRR of an amplifier can be greatly increased by guarding the input circuit. The common mode signal can be obtained by two averaging resistors connected between the outputs of the two input op-amps of an instrumentation amplifier as shown in Fig. 4.9. The buffered common-mode signal at the output of op-amp 4 can be used as guard voltage to reduce the effects of cable capacitance and leakage.

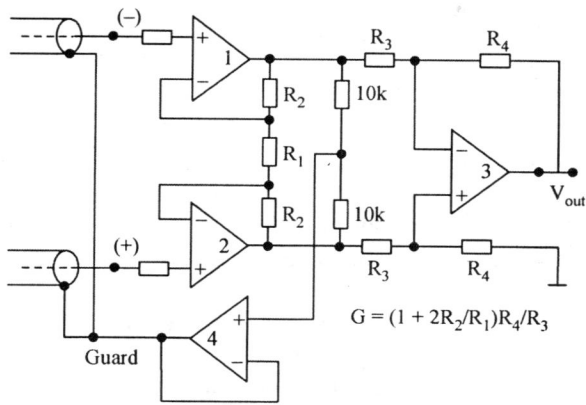

$$G = (1 + 2R_2/R_1)R_4/R_3$$

Fig. 4.9. Instrumentation amplifier providing input guarding.

In many modern biopotential amplifiers, the reference electrode is not grounded. Instead, it is connected to the output of an amplifier for the common mode voltage, op-amp 3 in Fig. 4.10, which works as an inverting amplifier. The inverted common mode voltage is fed back to the reference electrode. This negative feedback reduces the common-mode voltage to a low value. Electrocardiographs based on this principle are called driven-right-leg systems replacing the right leg ground electrode of ordinary electrocardiographs by an actively driven electrode.

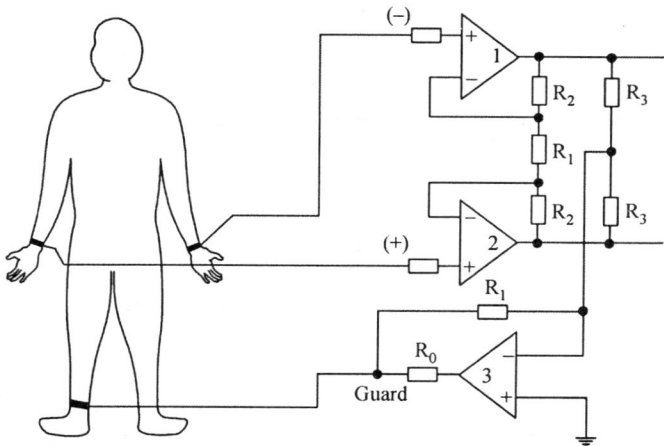

Fig. 4.10. Driven-right-leg circuit reducing common-mode interference.

Dynamic Range and Recovery

With an increase of either the common mode or differential input voltage there will be a point where the amplifier will overload and the output voltage will no longer be representative for the input voltage. Similarly, with a decrease of the input voltage, there will be a point where the noise components of the output voltage cover the output signal to a degree that a measurement of the desired biopotential is no longer possible. The dynamic range of the amplifier, i.e., the range between the smallest and largest possible input signal to be measured, has to cover the whole amplitude range of the physiological signal of interest. The required dynamic range of biopotential amplifiers can be quite large. In an application like fetal monitoring for example, two signals are recorded simultaneously from the electrodes which are quite different in their amplitudes: the fetal and the maternal ECG. While the maternal ECG shows an amplitude of up to 10 mV, the fetal ECG often does not reach more than 1 μV. Assuming that the fetal ECG is separated from the composite signal and fed to an analog/digital converter for digital signal processing with a resolution of 10 bit (signed integer), the smallest voltage to be safely measured with the biopotential amplifier is 1/512 μV or about 2 nV vs. 10 mV for the largest signal or even up to 300 mV in the presence of an electrode offset potential. This translates to a dynamic range of 134 dB for the signals alone and 164 dB if the electrode potential is included in the consideration. Though most applications are less demanding, even such extreme requirements can be realised through careful design of the biopotential amplifier and the use of adequate components. The penalty for using less expensive amplifiers with diminished performance would be a potentially severe loss of information.

Transients appearing at the input of the biopotential amplifier, like voltage peaks from a cardiac pacemaker or a defibrillator, can drive the amplifier into saturation. An important characteristic for the amplifier is the time it takes to recover from such overloads. The recovery time depends on the characteristics of the transient, like amplitude and duration, the specific design of the amplifier, like bandwidth and the components used. Typical biopotential amplifiers may take several seconds to recover from severe overload. The recovery time can be reduced by disconnecting the amplifier inputs at the discovery of a transient using an electronic switch.

Passive Isolation Amplifiers

Increasingly, biopotentials have to be measured within implanted devices and need to be transmitted to an external monitor or controller. Such applications include cardiac pacemakers transmitting the intracardiac ECG and functional electrical stimulation where, e.g., action potentials measured at one eyelid serve to stimulate the other lid to restore the physiological function of a damaged lid at least to some degree. In these applications, the power consumption of the implanted biopotential amplifier limits the life-span of the implanted device. The usual solution to this problem is an inductive transmission of power into the implanted device that serves to recharge an implanted battery. In applications where the size of the implant is of concern, it is desirable to eliminate the need for the battery and the related circuitry by using a quasi passive biopotential amplifier, i.e., an amplifier that does not need a power supply.

The function of passive telemetric amplifiers for biopotentials is based on the ability of the biological source to drive a low power device such as a FET and the sensing of the biopotentials through inductive or acoustic coupling of the implanted and external devices. In an inductive system, a FET serves as a load to an implanted secondary LC-circuit which is stimulated inductively by an extracorporal oscillator (Fig. 4.11). Depending on the special realisation of the system, the biopotential is available in the external circuit from either an amplitude or frequency-modulated carrier-signal. The input impedance of the inductive transmitter as a function of the secondary load impedance Z_2 is given by:

$$Z_1 = j\omega L_1 + \frac{(\omega M)^2}{Z_2 + j\omega L_2} \qquad \qquad ...\ (4.6)$$

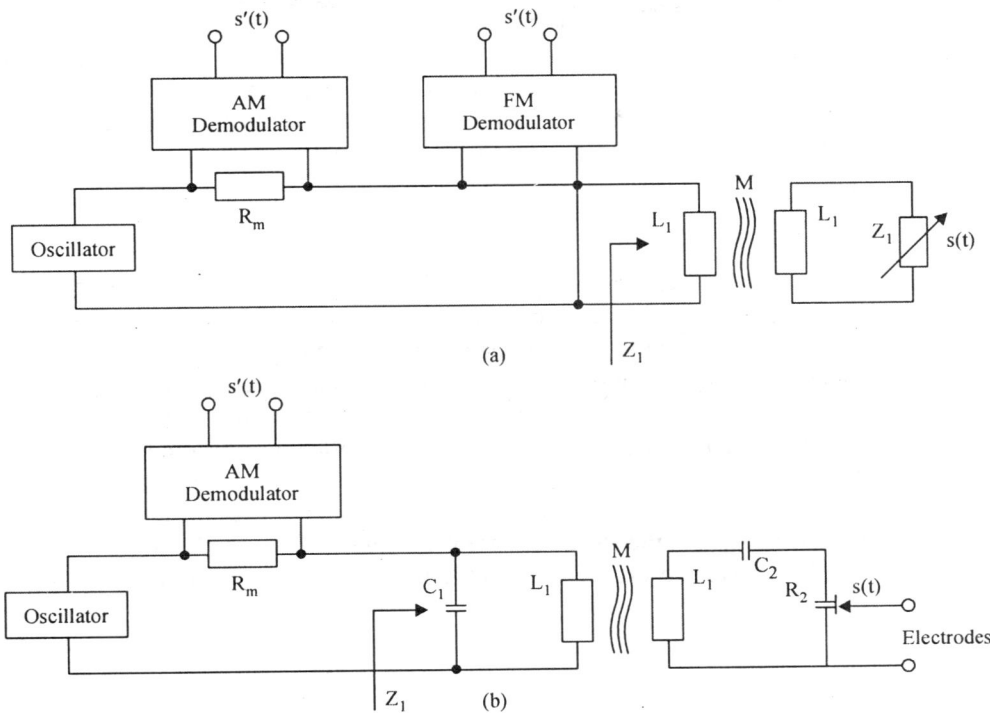

Fig. 4.11. The passive isolation amplifier can be operated without the need for an isolated power supply. The biological source provides the power to modulate the load impedance of an inductive transformer. As an easy realisation shown in panel (b), a FET can be directly connected to two electrodes. The source-drain resistance changes as a linear function of the biopotential which is then reflected by the input impedance of the transformer.

In an amplitude-modulate system, the resistive part of the input-impedance Z_1 must change as a linear function of the biopotential. The signal is obtained as the envelope of the carrier signal, measured across a resistor R_m. A frequency-modulated system is realised when the frequency of the signal generator is determined at least in part by the impedance Z_1 of the inductive transmitter. In both cases, the signal-dependent changes of the secondary impedance Z_2 can be achieved by a junction-FET. Using the field effect transistor as a variable load resistance changing its resistance in proportion to the source-gate voltage which is determined by the electrodes of this two-electrode amplifier, the power supplied by the biological source is sufficient to drive the amplifier. The input impedance can be in the range of 10^{10} Ω.

Optimal transmission characteristics are achieved with AM systems. Different combinations of external and implanted resonance circuits are possible to realise in an AM system, but primary parallel with secondary serial resonance yields the best characteristics. In this case, the input impedance is given by:

$$Z_1 = \frac{1}{j\omega C_1} + \left(\frac{L_1}{M}\right)^2 . R_2 \qquad \dots (4.7)$$

The transmission factor $(L_1/M)^2$ is optimal since the secondary inductivity, i.e., the implanted inductivity, can be small, only the external inductivity determines the transmission factor and the mutual inductivity should be small, a fact that favours the loose coupling that is inherent to two coils separated by skin and tissue. There are, of course, limits to M which cannot be seen from Equation (4.7). In a similar fashion, two piezoelectric crystals can be employed to provide the coupling between input and output.

This 2-lead isolation amplifier design is not limited to telemetric applications. It can also be used in all other applications where its main advantage lies in its simplicity and the resulting substantial cost savings as compared to other isolation amplifiers which require additional amplifier stages and an additional isolated power supply.

Digital Electronics

The ever increasing density of integrated digital circuits together with their extremely low power consumption permits digitising and pre-processing of signals already on the isolated patient-side of the amplifiers, thus improving signal quality and eliminating the problems normally related to the isolation barrier, especially those concerning isolation voltage interferences and long-term stability of the isolation amplifiers. Digital signal transmission to a remote monitoring unit, a computer system or computer network can be achieved without any risk of picking up transmission line interferences, especially when implemented with fibreoptical cables.

Digital techniques also offer an easy means of controlling the front-end of the amplifier. Gain factors can be easily adapted and changes of the electrode potential resulting from electrode polarisation or from interferences which might drive the differential amplifier into saturation can easily be detected and compensated.

Chapter 5

Biomedical Recorders

INTRODUCTION

The electrocardiograph is a widely used medical instrument that measures biopotential differences arising from electrical activity of the heart muscle. It usually uses surface electrodes and it requires high-input-impedance differential amplifiers and compensation for common-mode voltage inputs. The electrocardiograph is designated with the initials ECG, as is the electrocardiogram, a record of the data. In terms of the electrical signal, the ECG has a magnitude of about 1 mV at the electrode surface. In terms of signal processing, the significant features of the ECG data are the feature durations, polarities and magnitudes. The basic ECG machine picks up minute voltage on the surface of patient's skin that are generated by the heart. The function of ECG machine is to draw the waveform of that amplitude versum time function on a strip of special graph paper.

The weak bioelectric potential picked up and displayed by the ECG machine are generated by the cells of the heart. These cells, as well as many other types of cells in the body, can be viewed as a form of miniature biological 'battery'. Under normal circumstances, both sodium (Na) and potassium (K) are found on each side of the cell wall or membrane. In Fig. 5.1 only one element is shown on each side because the normal relative concentrations of the two are so radically different. In-side the cell, for example, the fluid has a concentration of potassium that is approximately 30 times that of sodium. On the outside, on the other hand, the concentration of sodium is approximately 10 times that of potassium. These concentration gradients produce an electrical potential difference across the cell wall of about −90 millivolts (mV), with the inside being the negative reference point.

When the heart cells is stimulated, the nature of its membrane wall changes so that it becomes more permeable to sodium ions. This allows sodium ions to rush into the cell in an attempt to neutralise the imbalance in concentrations. The voltage drop across the cell wall during this period (Fig. 5.2) switches rapidly from −90 mV to +20 mV. At this point the cell is said to be depolarised. The characteristics of the cell wall then change back to the pre-stimulus condition. During this period, called the re-polarisation period, the membrane potential gradient drops back to its −90 = mV resting level. Once the cell is triggered by a stimulus, it will go through this cycle completely and cannot be re-triggered until after it is re-polarised. The cells of the heart generate an electrical current from the cell depolarisations as it beats. The vector sum of these currents can be picked up as voltage drops across various points on the surface of the skin (Fig. 5.3).

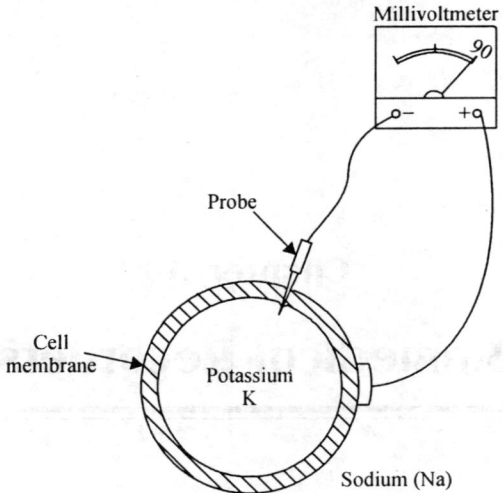

Fig. 5.1. One element shown on each side.

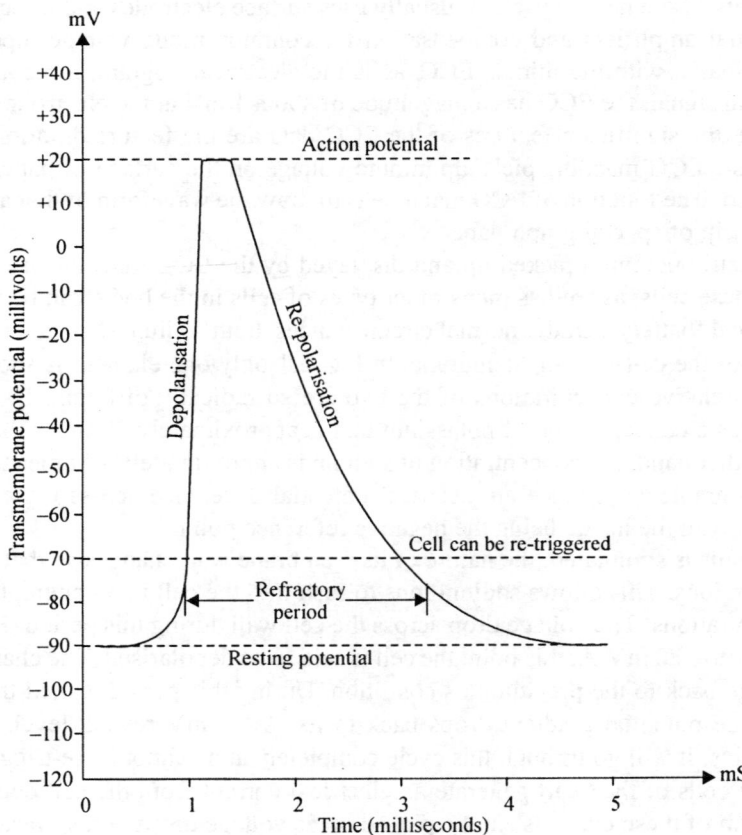

Fig. 5.2. Voltage drop across the cell wall.

Different views of the heart's electrical activity result in different waveforms and these are obtained from different points on the patient's body. Each of these views is called a 'lead' in ECG terminology. The reason why so many different views of the heart's electrical activity are desired by medical staff is that it helps them diagnose disease conditions more accurately. A multiplicity of views assists them in localising and analysing the areas that are diseased.

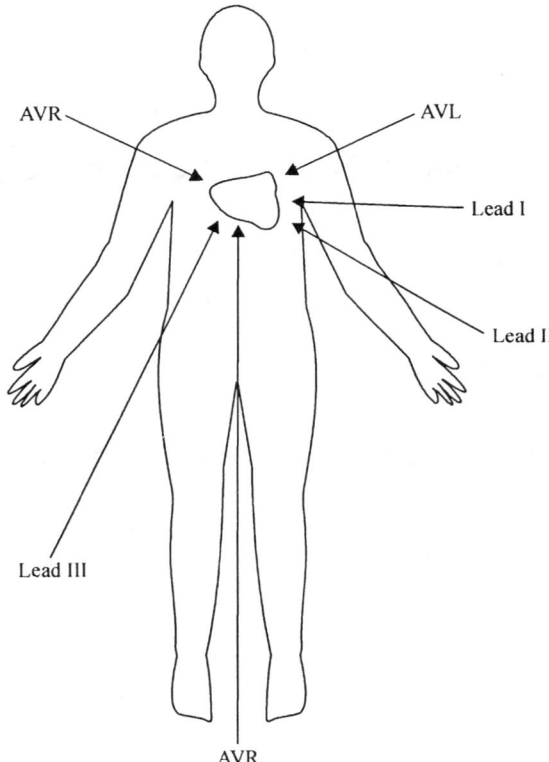

Fig. 5.3. Vector sum of currents and voltage drop across various points.

Figure 5.4 shows the major features of one of the classic ECG waveforms, called 'lead I' in medical terminology. Here we see the major amplitude features of the waveform and the standardised alphabetical letters normally used to identify these features.

The first feature, on the leaf, is called the P-wave and it corresponds to the pumping of the atria. Following the P-wave is a sharp spike corresponding to the beating of the ventricles (i.e., the 'power stroke' of the heart) and this is called the QRS complex. The QRS complex generally has the highest amplitude (on the order of 1 mV) of all features in the lead I display. Its major property, however, is the fast rise and fall times and rapid slope reversal. This, incidentally, indicates a high-frequency content of the waveform compared with its fundamental frequency in the 1 Hz region. The normally accepted frequency spectrum of the ECG waveform is 0.05 to 100 Hz (which is also the frequency response required of instruments that reproduce the waveform). The relative waveform amplitudes compared with a 1 mV calibration pulse are shown in Fig. 5.5.

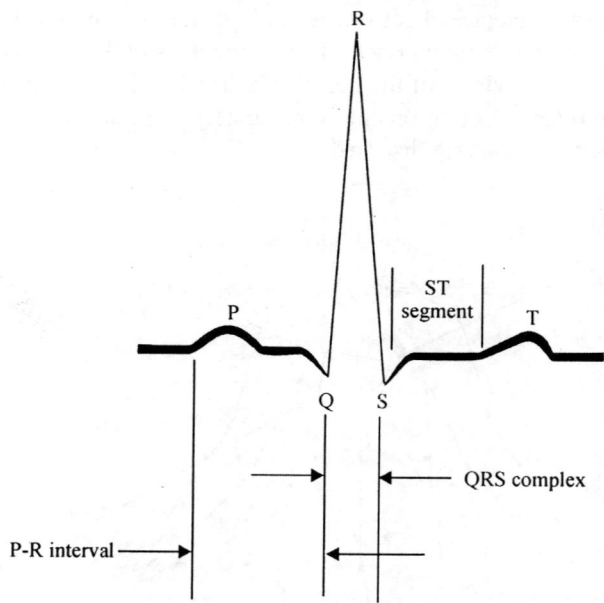

Fig. 5.4. Major features of classic ECG waves.

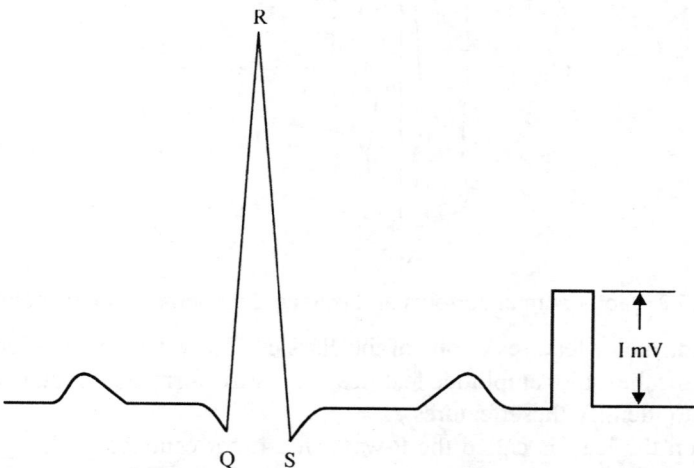

Fig. 5.5. Relative waveform amplitudes compared with a 1 mV calibration pulse.

The basic waveform acquisition system from a typical ECG machine is shown in Fig. 5.6. Wires from a patient cable are connected through a lead selector siwtch to the inputs of a differential amplifier. This amplifier usually has a push-pull output that is then used to drive a permanent magnet moving coil (PMMC) galvanometer pen assembly. The pen draws the vertical component of the waveform on a special graph paper that is passed under the pen tip at a fixed rate (in most cases 25 mm/sec). Figures 5.7, 5.8 and 5.9 shows the common ECG leads. In all cases, the common or reference ground point is the patient's right leg.

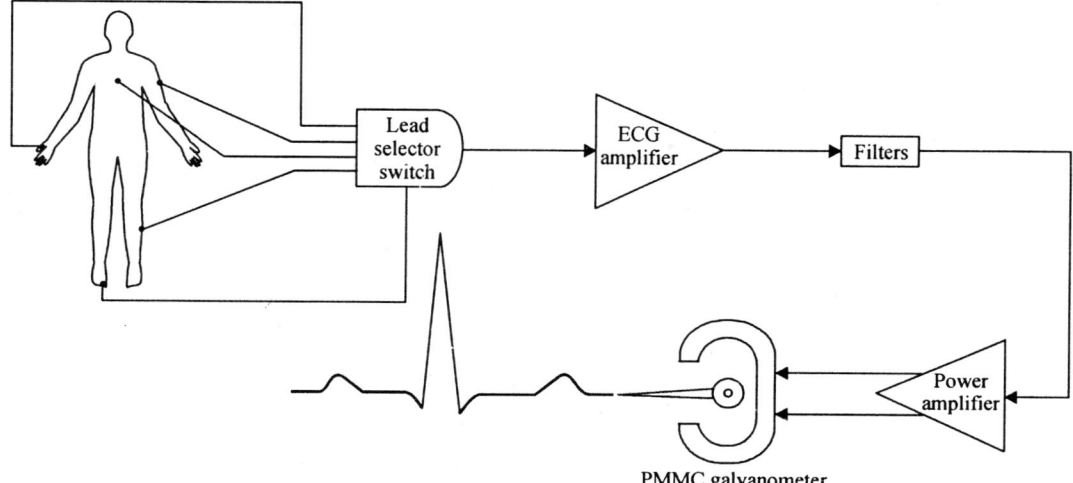

Fig. 5.6. Basic waveform acquisition system from ECG machine.

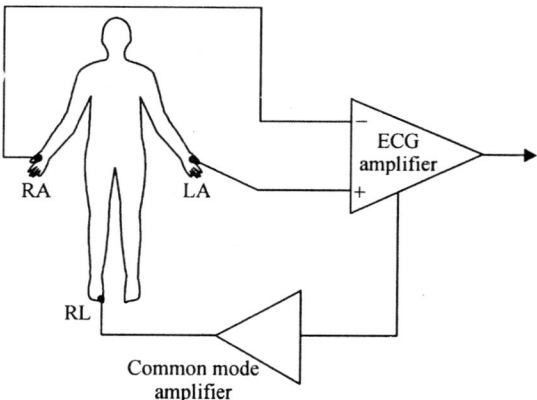

Fig. 5.7. Common ECG lead I.

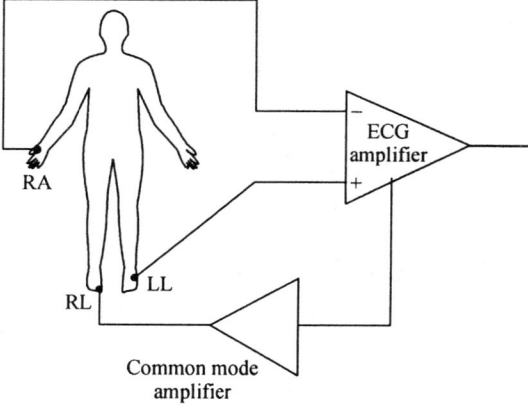

Fig. 5.8. Common ECG lead II.

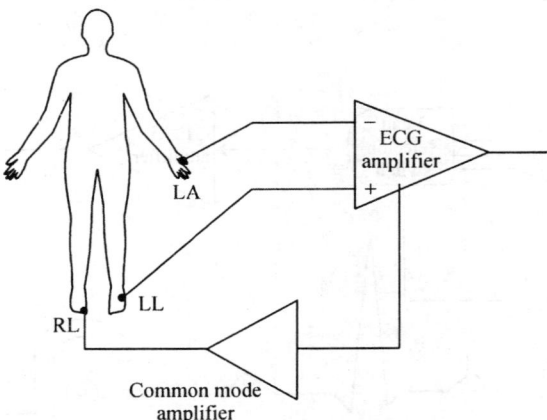

Fig. 5.9. Common ECG lead III.

The three simplest leads are the bipolar limb lead, designated I, II and III. These are known collectively as the Einthoven triangle leads because of the triangle formed by the right arm, left arm and left leg (against a right leg reference).

Three more leads are called either the augmented or unipolar limb leads, which are designated by the letters AVR, AVL and AVF. These leads are created by summing currents from two of the limbs in a resistor network and measuring them relative to the third limb electrode.

The last set of common standard leads are the V leads (V1 through V6). These leads are taken by summing currents from all three limbs in a resistor network and then measuring them against signals picked up from one of six standard positions on the patient's chest.

Each wire on an ECG patient cable is colour coded so that it won't be connected to the wrong place. This colour code is

      RA—white
      LA—black
      RL—green
      LL—red
      Chest—brown

ECG MACHINE OPERATION

Figure 5.10 is a simplified drawing of a typical ECG machine drive mechanism. Such devices are actually part of a larger family of instruments known collectively as strip-chart recorders. The most common single-channel, one-trace paper used in ECG recording is 50 mm wide and is divided into 1 mm and 5-mm squares to form a kind of graph paper. The paper is usually stored in a special compartment is either roll or Z-fold form. Three different mechanisms are used in normal clinical ECG machines. The three forms are thermal writer, ink pen writer ('ink slingers') and dot matrix writer.

In repairing ECG machines you will note that few drive motors ever go bad. However, there are a large number of idler rollers and a large (but somewhat smaller) number of drive rollers found bad in these machines. Rollers in machines located in high-use areas can be expected to wear out in a predictable period of time. The usual symptoms are a drive roller that seems to turn normally yet the paper moves either not at all or only haltingly.

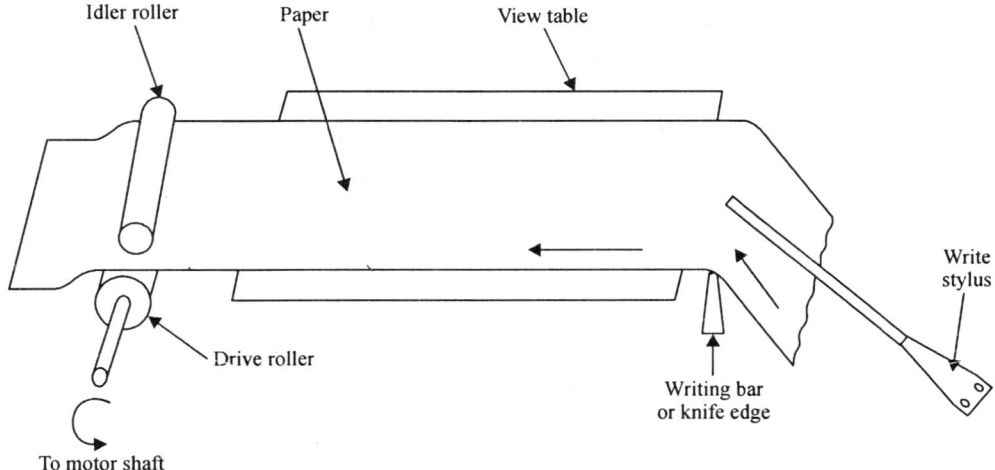

Fig. 5.10. Simplified diagram of a typical ECG machine driven mechanism.

Another common problem area is the write stylus. There are actually two types encountered in older ECG machines: ink and thermal. The dot matrix type is found on some modern machines. It is the thermal, by far, which is most frequently seen in ECG machines. Both, however, are subject to a variety of assorted faults. You can expect pens to clog with dried ink (especially if not used for several days) and thermal types to burn out. Both types of stylus are very delicate and will easily bend if allowed to slam against the high or low-end mechanical stops or travel limits. This may occur if too high an amplitude signal is applied to the input, which is often the result of pulling the cable electrodes off the patients before turning the machine off or to an inactive condition. Expect to replace a lot of styluses.

Still another mechanical defect is poor paper tension. Normal functioning ECG machines will produce a nice clean trace. When paper tension across the knife edge is reduced, either by a machine mechanical defect or improper paper loading by the operator, the paper strip chart will be allowed to skew under the tip of the stylus and a smeared trace is produced. In fact, it is the drag of the pen on the paper surface that tends to aggravate the skewing effect. Although the fault may be either mechanical or human failure, it is very common for the nurse, doctor or monitoring technician using the machine to complain of a worn-out or bad stylus. For the sake of doing a good job, the new technician should examine each machine before automatically replacing the stylus.

Interfering voltages applied to the input of the ECG machine may tend to obscure the real waveform and render it unreadable. Anomalies on the tracing that represent either machine errors or voltages present but not generated by the patient's heart are called artifacts. Most of the time, artifacts can be easily diagnosed and corrected by the operator. In some cases, however, artifacts will be referred to an electronics person for correction. You will, therefore, see both machine defects and user errors causing various artifacts. Thus, learn to recognise and correct some of the more common ECG artifacts.

The ECG is designed to measure and to record electrocardiograms, such as those illustrated in Fig. 5.11 for the surface potential measured between two arms of a patient. The distinctive features, labelled P, Q, R, S and T, vary considerably among subjects. Average amplitudes at the electrodes are given in Table 5.1 for these distinctive features at standard body site connections of the ECG. The ECG amplitude depends on the electrode connection sites and on the size and physical condition of the patient.

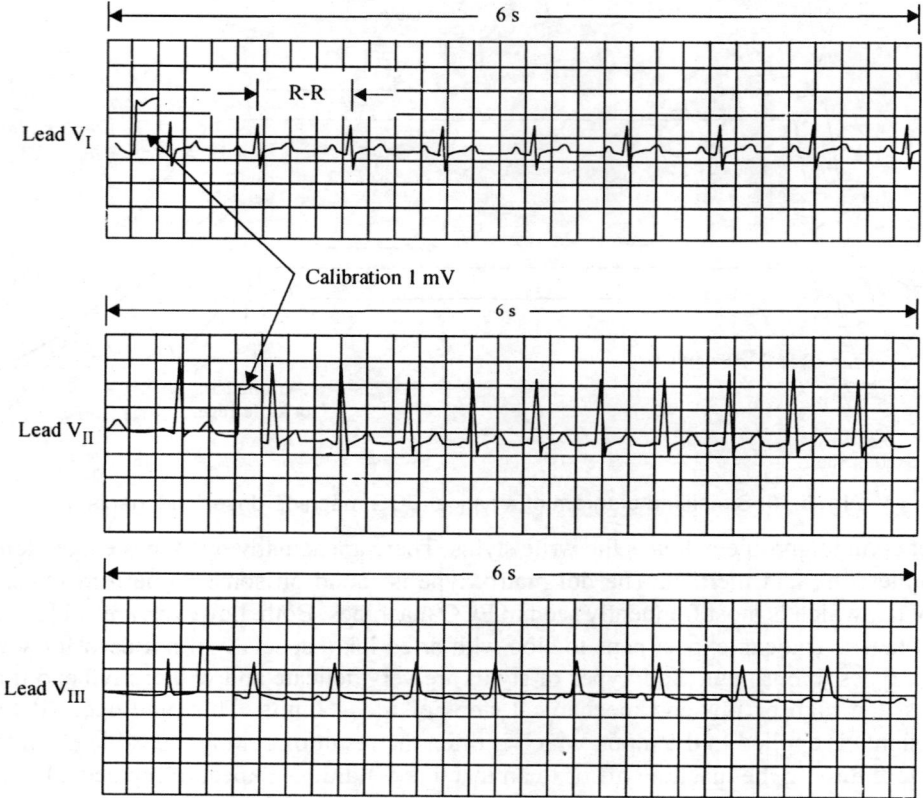

Fig. 5.11. A normal ECG for the standard lead connections V$_I$, V$_{II}$ and V$_{III}$.

Table 5.1. Amplitudes of ECG waves for standard lead connections.

Wave	*Lead voltage magnitudes [nominal (range)]*		
	V$_I$ (mV)	*V$_{II}$ (mV)*	*V$_{III}$ (mV)*
P	0.07 (0.01 to 0.12)	0.01 (0 to 0.19)	0.04 (0.0 to 0.13)
Q	0.03 (0 to 0.16)	0.03 (0 to 0.18)	0.04 (0 to 0.28)
R	0.53 (0.07 to 1.13)	0.71 (0.18 to 1.68)	0.38 (0.03 to 1.31)
S	0.10 (0 to 0.36)	0.12 (0 to 0.49)	0.12 (0 to 0.55)
T	0.22 (0.06 to 0.42)	0.26 (0.06 to 0.55)	0.05 (0.0 to 0.3)

Important clinical variables from ECG waveforms include the magnitude and polarity of these features, as well as their relative time duration. Variations from these norms may indicate illness. For example, an extended P-R interval indicates prolonged conduction time of the atrioventricular (AV) node and may be diagnosed as an AV block. A widening of the QRS complex may be due to a bundle block, which may result from improper conduction in the nerve fibre. An elevated S-T may indicate that a myocardial infarction has occurred and a negative-polarity T-wave may be due to coronary insufficiency. Other distinctive features of the ECG important in disease diagnosis are QRS voltage amplitude; polarity, the time duration; the R-R interval, which is the reciprocal of the pulse rate and T-wave amplitude.

The pulse rate BPM is usually expressed in beats per minute (bpm), given by

$$BPM = \frac{60}{R-R} \quad (bpm) \qquad \ldots (5.1)$$

where R-R is the period of the ECG in seconds. Normal heart rate is between 60 and 100 bpm at rest. An excessive rate is called tachycardia and a rate below normal is called bradycardia. Abnormal waveforms indicative of these conditions appear in Fig. 5.12. Heart fibrillation can be detected by observation of the ECG. Ventricular fibrillation, a critical and potentially fatal condition, is indicated by loss of the QRS complex. The missing QRS means that the ventricle is not contracting and blood circulation is severely impaired. The ECG waveform of the fibrillating heart is illustrated in the figure as well. The waveform has distinctive high frequency components that are used in automatic machine diagnosis of this condition. Atrial fibrillation, which is less serious, is indicated by a loss of the P-wave on the ECG. In this case and in the case of atrial flutter, the QRS is still present and blood circulation is maintained.

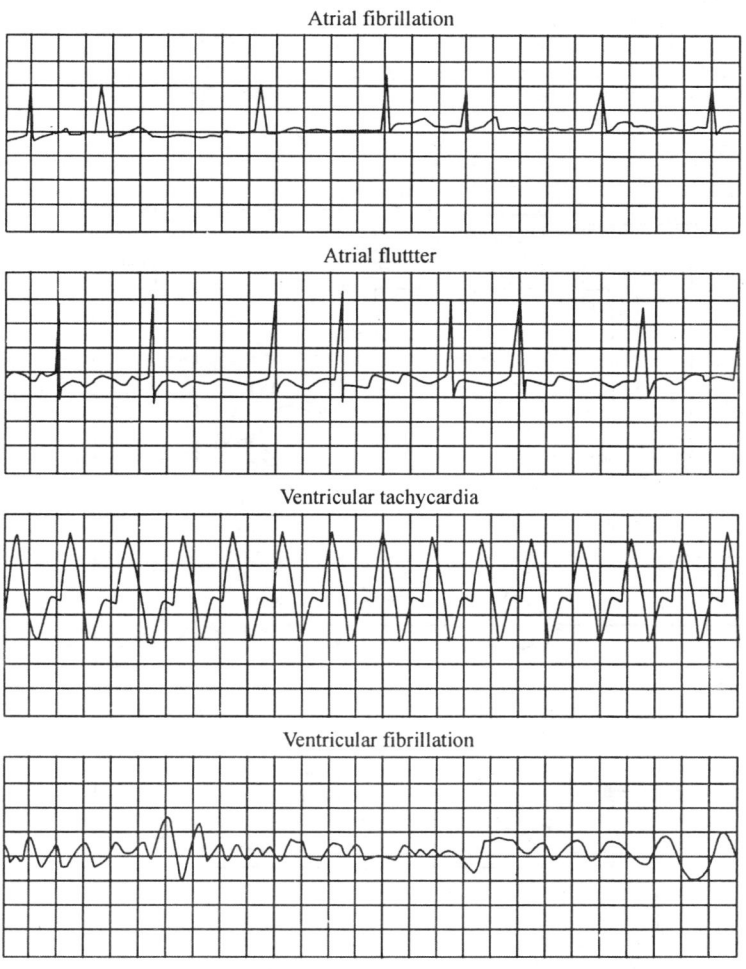

Fig. 5.12. Abnormal cardiograms.

Ectopic beats originate from a place other than the sinoatrial (SA) node. An ectopic beat in the ventricle causes an extra R-wave, indicative of a premature ventricular contraction (PVC). PVCs are easier to detect than ecotopic beats originating in the atrium, which are called premature atrial contractions (PACs). PVCs may be detected by monitoring the R-R interval of an ECG waveform.

ECG BLOCK DIAGRAM

An ECG device, as illustrated in Fig. 5.13, amplifies an ECG signal and displays it on an output unit. Representative specifications on the unit are as follows:

Input impedance	5 MΩ
Frequency response	± 0.5 dB (0.14 Hz to 25 Hz)
	3 dB (to 100 Hz)

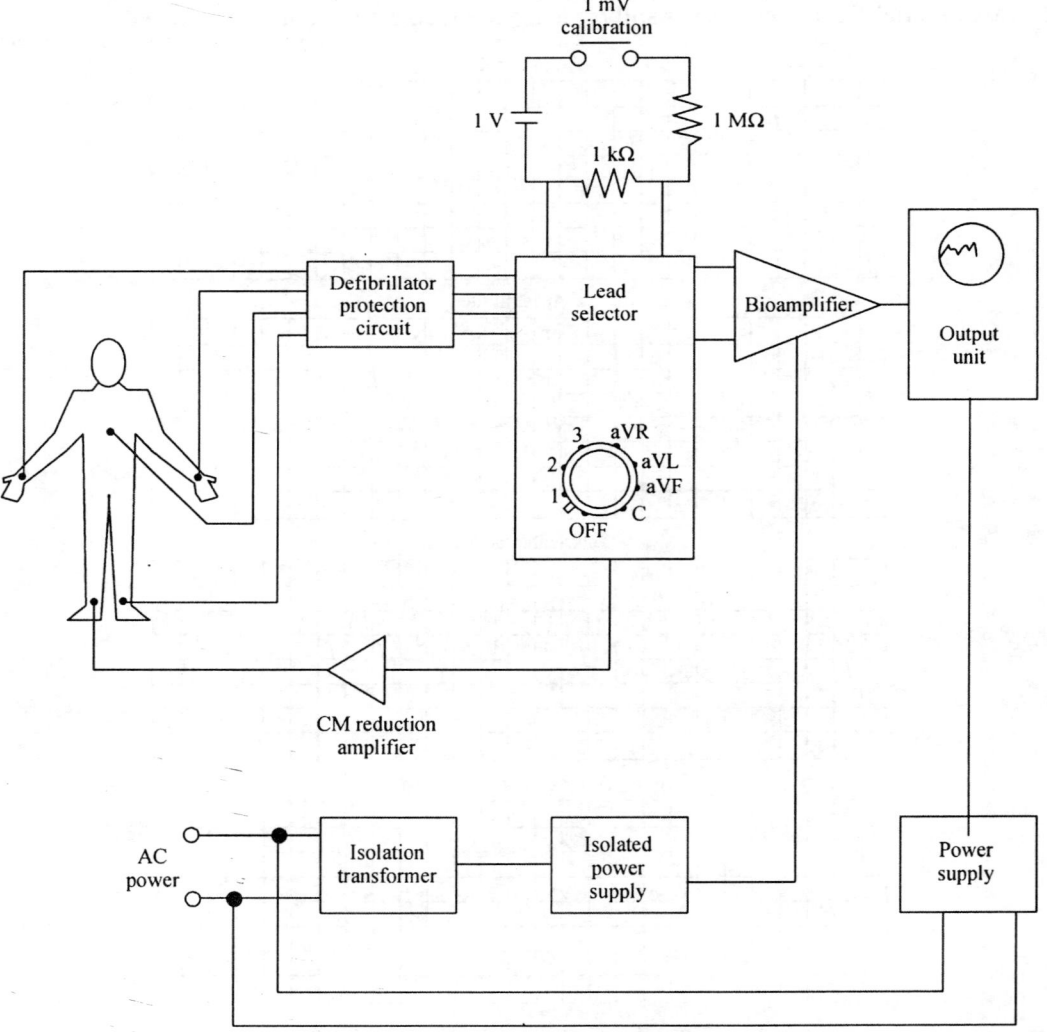

Fig. 5.13. A simplified block diagram of an ECG.

The ECG device processes the biopotential signal into a form suitable for the output unit. Often the data is presented graphically as in Fig. 5.12, on a strip chart recorder:

Normal rate   25 mm/s

High rate   100 mm/s

In its path through the instrument, the biopotential from the surface electrodes passes through a defibrillator protection circuit. One configuration of this circuit consists of neon gas tubes that fire when a pulse from a defibrillator is present. The defibrillator pulse may exceed 1000 V, which has the capability of destroying the bioamplifier. Various combinations of the ECG leads can be selected for configurations. A 1 mV calibration pulse is used to calibrate the bioamplifier by enabling the technician to observe the output and adjust the scale so that a known deflection corresponds to a 1 mV input signal. This calibration switch also provides a handy troubleshooting aid. If it works properly, it is clear that the electronics beyond it to the output is working and that a failure, if present, has occurred before it is in the signal path. Troubleshooting tips for this section of the equipment is shown in Table 5.2.

Table 5.2. Sources of interference in an ECG trace.

Possible artifacts	Check the following:
Base line with no wave form	Trace switch ON and gain control set high enough? Re-adjust as required. Select appropriate lead.
	Lead wires and patient cable fully inserted into proper receptacle?
	Cable or lead wires damaged? (Check with a lead continuity tester.)
Base line wander	Patient moving excessively? Secure lead wires and cable to patient.
	Caused by patient's respiration? Reposition electrodes.
	Electrodes dry? Re-prep skin and apply fresh moist electrodes.
	Static build-up around patient? Check with engineering.
AC noise	Gain set too high? Re-adjust as required.
	Unit in diagnostic mode? Select monitoring mode.
	Electrodes dry? Re-prep skin and apply fresh moist electrodes.
	Patient cable entwined with cables of other electrical devices? Separate patient cable from all other cables.
Intermittent signal	Connections not tight and properly secured (electrode to lead, lead to cable, cable to monitor)? Ensure proper connection.
	Electrodes dry? Re-prep skin and apply fresh moist electrodes.
	Cable or lead wires damaged? Check with continuity tester.
	Low battery in telemetry transmitter? Replace with fresh battery.
Low amplitude ECG signal	Gain set too low? Re-adjust as required.
	Skin properly prepared? Abrade skin.
	Is it the patient's normal complex? Check with 12 lead electrocardiogram.

Since the patient leads of an ECG are connected through relatively low impedance electrodes and are positioned on the skin across the heart, it is necessary to avoid the macroshock resulting from currents exceeding 10 mA. If the patient is wearing an external pacemaker or the patient's heart is catheterised, a microshock hazard exists and patient-level currents must be maintained below 10 μA. This is done by providing bias power to the amplifier through an isolation transformer, which drives an isolated power supply, as shown in Fig. 5.13. Because the electronic power requirements are low, a rechargeable battery may also be used. The output unit, consisting of a paper chart recorder or a cathode-ray-tube screen, requires high power and often requires an electronic power supply. This power supply does not require the same degree of isolation as the bioamplifier because it normally does not contact the patient. Detailed circuitry that may be used in these blocks is described in subsequent sections.

A variation on the ECG instrumentation illustrated in Fig. 5.14 uses a differential amplifier to measure the ECG of a fetus. The lead on the mother's chest referenced in a Wilson connection measures her ECG, called M. The mother's ECG will be stronger and at a lower rate than the ECG of the fetus. An electrode on the abdomen will measure both M and the fetus ECG, called F.

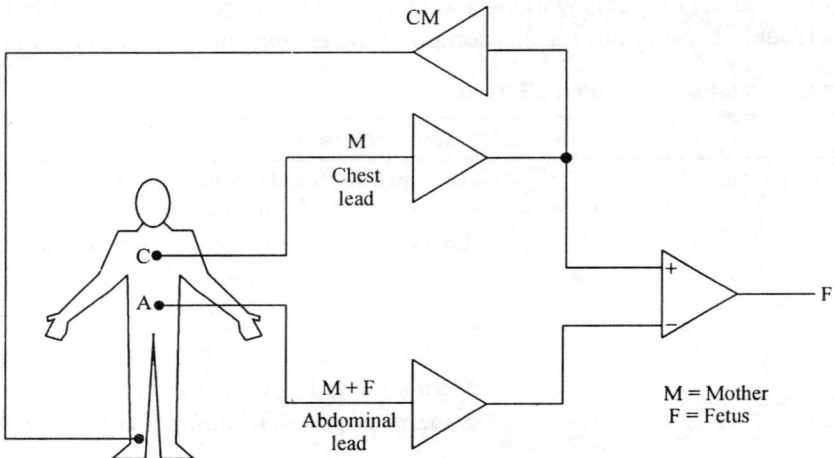

Fig. 5.14. A block diagram of a fetal ECG.

The differential amplifier then takes the difference (M + F) – M = F. Its output thus measures the ECG of the fetus, because the mother's ECG M, is subtracted away.

Certain abnormalities of the heart, such as PVCs, may occur only when the body is under a physical stress such as exercise, which makes demands for higher cardiac output. To simulate these conditions in the clinical environment and to obtain a record for diagnosis, stress testing ECG instrumentation is used. The patient walks on a treadmill at a controlled rate and vital parameters, including the ECG blood pressure and heart rate, are monitored and recorded. Signal processing in the instrumentation should be designed to eliminate or compensate for, artifacts due to skeletal muscle contraction and electrode motion.

It is important to be aware of PVCs or other abnormal episodes in ill patients. To detect these, the ECG leads are attached permanently so that the patient can carry on normal activities. In the 1940s Norman Holter introduced the idea of recording the ECG on a tape recorder at slow speed and playing it back at high speed, so that 24 hours of ECG could be viewed in as little as 12 minutes by a trained observer. These devices are called Holter monitors. However, because use of the tape recorder is time-consuming and there are mechanical difficulties associated with it, hand-held computers have been developed that store only the critical episodes for review at a later time. These devices are small enough to be worn conveniently by the ambulatory patient. They contain a solid-state memory that receives data all day. The data may then be reviewed by the physician at a convenient time.

ECG hard-copy display devices often use a thermal stylus that leaves a trace on heat-sensitive paper. Modern units use dot-matrix displays. A temporary record for real-time viewing, using a liquid-crystal display surface, is convenient for battery-operated devices. The display has low power drain, so the batteries last a long time.

ECG LEAD CONNECTIONS

The electrocardiogram (ECG) voltages measured from the four human limbs, in either a standard connection, an augmented lead connection or a Wilson lead connection, among others.

The standard biopotential polarities in Fig. 5.15 show voltage V_I, the voltage drop from the left arm (LA) to the right arm (RA); V_{II}, the drop from the left leg (LL) to the right arm (RA) and lead voltage V_{III}, the drop from the left leg to the left arm. Kirchhoff's voltage law (KVL) applied to the figure yields

$$V_I = V_{II} - V_{III} \qquad\qquad ... (5.2)$$

Historically, the closed path RA to LA to LL and back to RA has been called the Einthoven triangle. It should be noted that the values in Table 5.1 are not consistent with Equation (5.2) because they are averages taken over a group of subjects. Equation (5.2) applies to the ECG waveforms taken at one time on one individual.

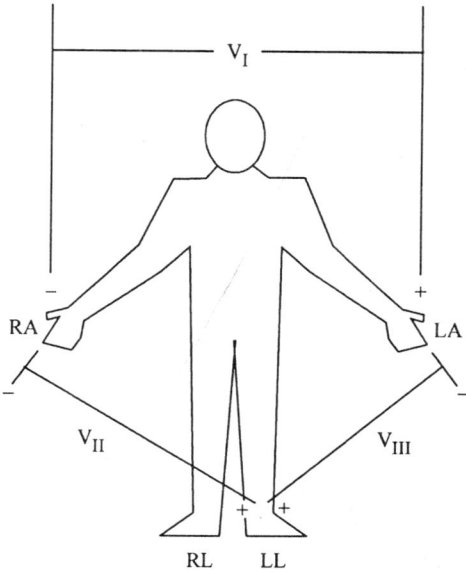

Fig. 5.15. Standard ECG lead connections.

Example voltages as measured by the connection at leads I, V_I and the lead II connection, V_{II}, are shown in Fig. 5.16.

Example 5.1 From the ECG lead I and lead II traces in Fig. 5.16, compute the following:

    1. The P-R interval.

    2. The QRS complex duration.

    3. The heart rate.

    4. The lead III, V_{III}, voltage as a function of time.

Solution: The P-R time = 0.16 second; the QRS duration = 90 ms; the heart rate = 60 bpm. To compute V_{III} note that $V_{III} = V_{II} - V_I$ in Fig. 5.15; V_{III} is plotted in Fig. 5.16.

The ECG potentials are measured with colour-coded leads according to the convention:

White – right arm
Black – left arm
Green – right leg
Red – left leg
Brown – chest

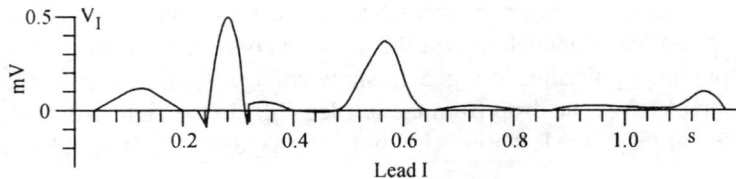

Lead I

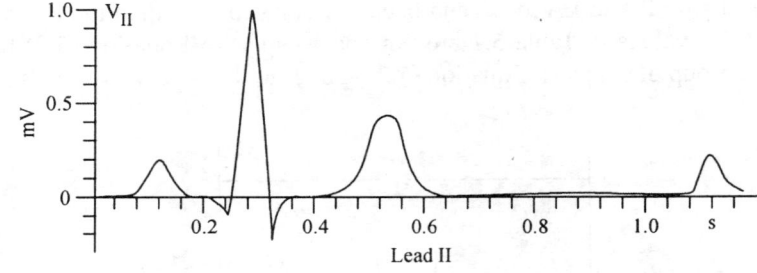

Lead II

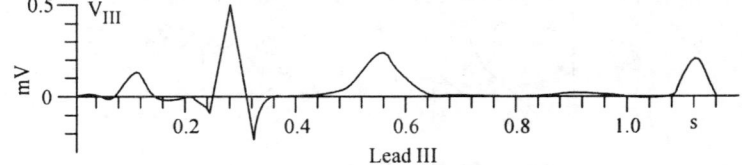

Lead III

Fig. 5.16. ECG lead voltage V_{III} is computed from V_I and V_{II}.

The standard voltage V_I is measured by connecting the left arm to the positive, non-inverting terminal and the right arm to the negative, inverting terminal of the differential amplifier. The common-mode, CM, voltage compensation is connected to the right leg as shown in Fig. 5.17a. Similarly, the lead connections for the standard voltage V_{II} and V_{III} are given in parts (b) and (c) of the figure.

Augmented ECG Lead Connections

For certain lead connections, a small increase in the ECG voltage can be realised by use of augmented lead connections, called augmented voltage right arm (aVR), augmented voltage left arm (aVL) and augmented voltage foot (aVF), illustrated in Fig. 5.18. All resistors have the same value R, which is made small compared to the input resistance of the measurement amplifier. In order to calculate the augmented voltages from standard lead voltages, the following relations are obtained from Fig. 5.18 by application of KVL:

$$aVR = -V_I - \frac{V_{III}}{2}$$

... (5.3)

$$aVL = -V_I - \frac{V_{II}}{2} \qquad \ldots (5.4)$$

$$aVF = -V_{II} - \frac{V_I}{2} \qquad \ldots (5.5)$$

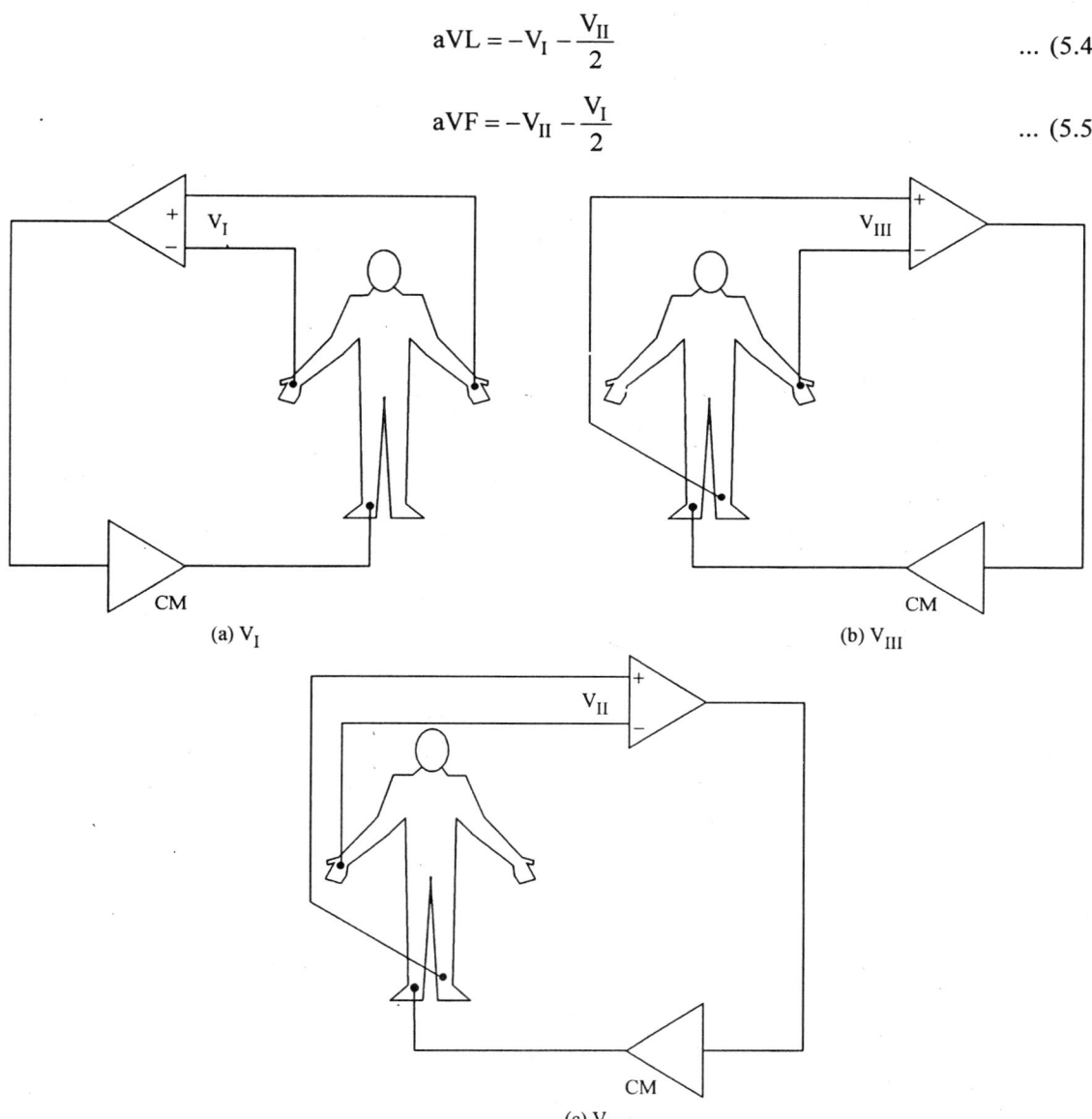

Fig. 5.17. The standard ECG connections to the bioamplifier and common-mode reduction amplifier.

Chest Lead Connection

To make chest lead ECG measurements, the chest lead, C, is applied to the non-inverting terminal of the differential amplifier, as shown in Fig. 5.19. The reference is taken from the node of a wye connection of resistors, called the Wilson central terminal. The end-nodes of the Wilson connection are made to the right arm, left arm and left leg, respectively.

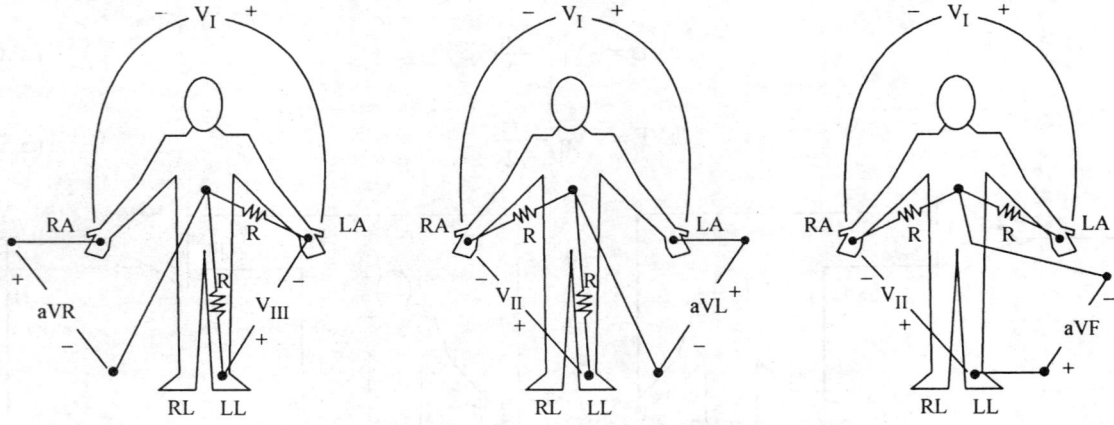

Fig. 5.18. Augmented lead connections for an ECG.

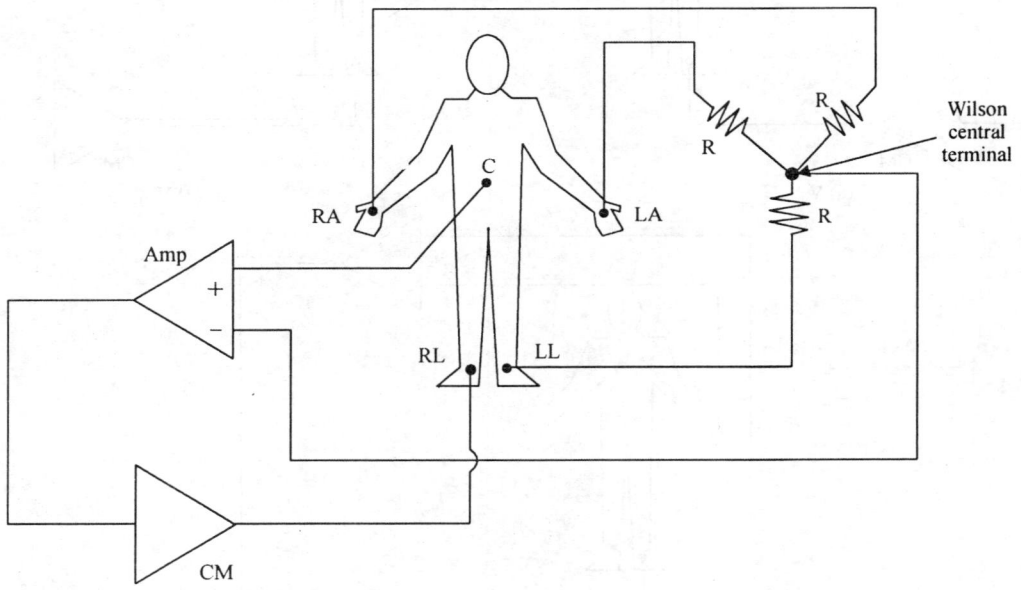

Fig. 5.19. Chest lead connections to an ECG.

The shape of the ECG from the chest lead depends strongly on the anatomical position. Six chest voltages are measured as the voltage drops from the chest lead to the Wilson central terminal. The chest lead positions, shown in Fig. 5.20 for these voltages, are:

V_1 – Fourth intercostal space, on the right sternal margin.
V_2 – Fourth intercostal space, on the left sternal margin.
V_3 – Midway between V_2 and V_4.
V_4 – Fifth intercostal space on the mid-clavicular line.
V_5 – Same level as V_4, on the anterior axillary line.
V_6 – Same level as V_4, on the mid-axillary line.

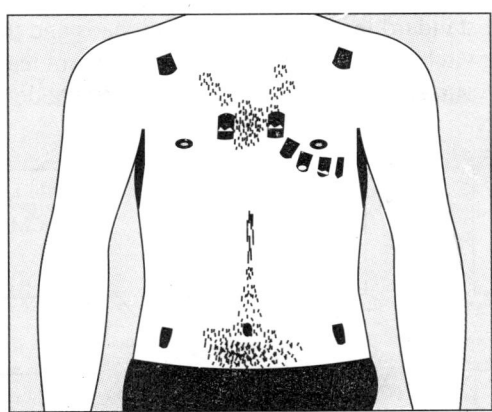

Fig. 5.20. Chest lead electrode positions V_1 through V_6. The limb connections are made through the four corners of the torso.

Example ECG wave shapes taken from these positions are shown in Fig. 5.21. The R-wave is strongly negative in V_1 and V_2 positions, because the chest lead straddles the right and left sides of the heart there. V_6 is similar to the standard V_I lead, because it is close to the left arm used in the V_I measurement. The strong dependency of the chest voltages on position makes it possible to identify the regions of the heart that may be abnormal by observing the chest lead ECG. If, for example, leads V_1 and V_2 were to read normal while the others were abnormal, this would be evidence that the injured region is near the left side of the heart.

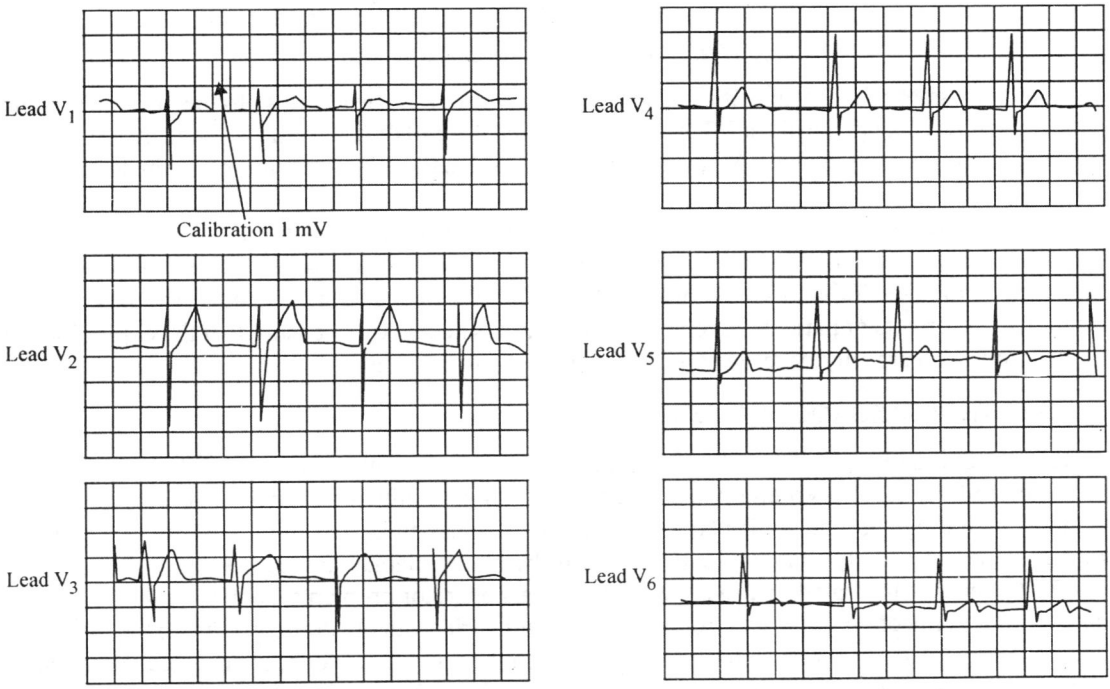

Fig. 5.21. Dependency of the chest lead ECG waveforms upon position.

In order to select among the standard leads, the augmented leads and the chest leads, the front panel of an ECG has a lead selector switch. This switch connects the patient leads to either the non-inverting amplifier terminal (+), the inverting terminal (–) or the common-mode reduction circuit connection (CM), as indicated in Fig. 5.22.

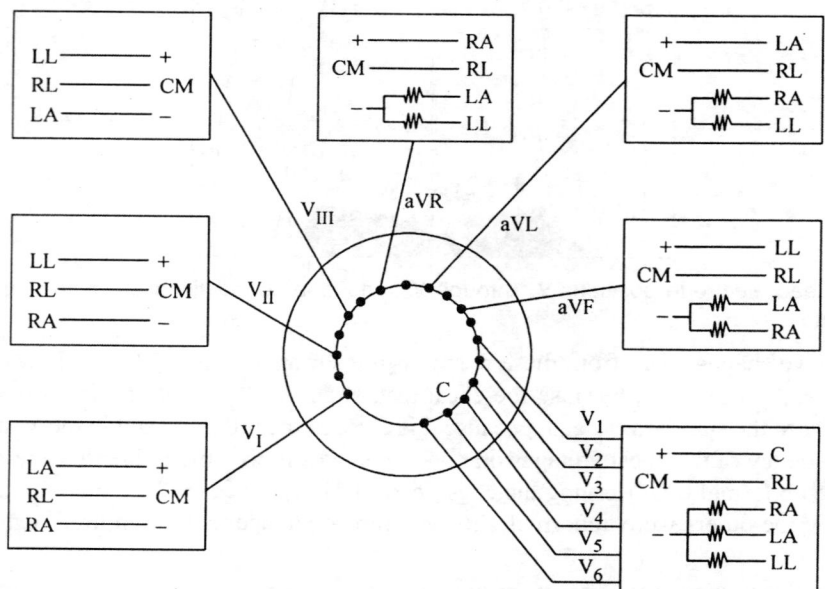

Fig. 5.22. A lead selector switch schematic.

In order to diagnose the P-wave, it is an advantage to position the leads close to the atrium. This may be achieved with an oesophageal lead. This lead is attached to a pill that is swallowed and then positioned in the oesophagus next to the heart. X-ray may be used to aid in the exact positioning of the lead near the heart.

As already discussed, proper attachment of electrodes to the patient is crucial to accurate ECG waveforms. User errors or ECG operator errors are often traced to inadequate electrode gel application or poor connection (see Table 5.2.). Adhesive, pre-gelled electrodes tend to standardise the collection and minimise the effects of patient movement. However, it is necessary to ensure that the expiration date of the electrodes is carefully observed, since the gel tends to dry out.

UNIT-LEVEL TROUBLESHOOTING: ECGs

Troubleshooting of an ECG is done at the unit level. It is assumed that from a system-level perspective, all other possibilities have been eliminated and it has been determined that there is a fault in the ECG instrument, including the patient leads and electrodes. Unless there is obvious physical damage or overheating, the most likely source of symptoms will be on the display device.

The ECG trace, as indicated in Table 5.2, often reveals operator problems, such as maladjustment of the gain or poor connection of the electrodes to the patient. Dried-out electrode gel due to the use of out-of-date pre-gelled electrodes or due to their being left on the patient too long, is an especially common problem. Visual inspection is usually sufficient to find this problem. Frayed or broken wires can be traced with an ohmmeter. A blank ECG trace can be caused by a blown fuse or an inoperative power supply. Suggested steps to take to remedy ECG trace artifacts are given in Table 5.2.

Proper placement of leads is especially important in ECGs such as the fetal monitor, the Holter monitor and the stress tester. In the case of the fetal monitor, the site of the abdominal lead depends upon the position of the fetus. Both the Holter and stress-testing monitors have leads attached to ambulatory patients and are thus subject to more movement, gel depletion and abuse than usual.

After lead problem and operator errors have been eliminated as a source of trouble, circuit-board-level troubleshooting should be pursued with the aid of a block diagram, such as in Fig. 5.13. The block diagram for a specific piece of equipment is available in the maintenance manual provided by the manufacturer. Referring to the figure, you would move logically from the input to the output, in a signal tracing procedure. To check the defibrillator protection circuit, you might interview the operator to determine if a defibrillator has recently been used. This problem would probably be specific to the channels being used and could be further isolated with the lead selector switch shown in the figure. For example, if the defibrillator protection lead opens in the RA lead, the lead selector switch on positions 1 and 2 would yield a faulty trace. However, switch position 3 should be normal. This is verified by referring to Fig. 5.15 and noting that the RA lead is not used when V_{III} is measured.

A failure in the CM reduction amplifier in the block diagram would increase the 60-~ hum on every channel of the ECG. Such a symptom could imply that the bioamplifier had a failure or became unbalanced and needed calibration. If 60-~ hum appears on only one channel, it is probable that the corresponding lead has lost its shielding or is improperly placed on the patient.

A distinction between a fault in the isolated power supply in the block diagram and a fault in the non-isolated power supply can be found by observing the output unit. If, for example, an output trace exists but there is no ECG signal, the isolated section of the power supply could be at fault.

Circuit-Board Swapping

After an instrument problem has been isolated by relating symptoms to the block diagram, the problem can be fixed by replacing the board containing the block. Circuit-board swapping should never be done blindly, however or without careful investigation, as it is possible to damage an expensive circuit board in the process. For example, if the problem in the ECG is an overvoltage in the power supply that blows out components on the circuit board, then installing a new board could obviously damage it. To avoid, this, check power supply voltages before considering circuit-board swapping.

Careful circuit-board swapping can be cost effective because it reduces equipment downtime. Furthermore, the old board can be easily shipped to the manufacturer, who can more economically trace the component problem and repair the board.

ELECTROENCEPHALOGRAPH

The electroencephalograph (EEG) is designed to measure the electrical activity of the brain, commonly called brain waves, by means of electrodes attached to the skull of a patient. The brain waves are the summation of neural depolarisations in the brain due to stimuli from the five senses as well as from the thought processes. On the surface of the brain, these voltages are on the order of 10 mV; but typical EEG electrodes measure the electrical activity propagated through skull bone and attenuated to levels from 1 to 100 μV, primarily in the frequency range from 0.5 to 3000 Hz. These potentials vary as a function of position over the surface of the skull, making it necessary for the EEG operator to select sets of electrodes grouped around the frontal, parietal, temporal or occipital lobes of the brain.

Electroencephalograph (EEG) Electrodes

In electroencephalography, electrodes are placed in standard positions on the skull in an arrangement along a line drawn on the skull from the root of the nose, the nasion, to the inion ossification or bump on the occipital lobe. The first mark is placed 10 per cent of the distance along this line and others are arranged at 20 per cent intervals, hence the name 10–20 system. A similar line is placed from one auricular (or ear) crease to the other. A third line goes around the circumference of the skull. A representative electrode arrangement placed at intersections of these lines is illustrated in Fig. 5.23, where the first letter of the electrode designation F stands for frontal lobe, C for central sulcus, P for parietal lobe and O for occipital lobe on the skull. P_g is the nasopharyngeal point and A is on the ear lobe.

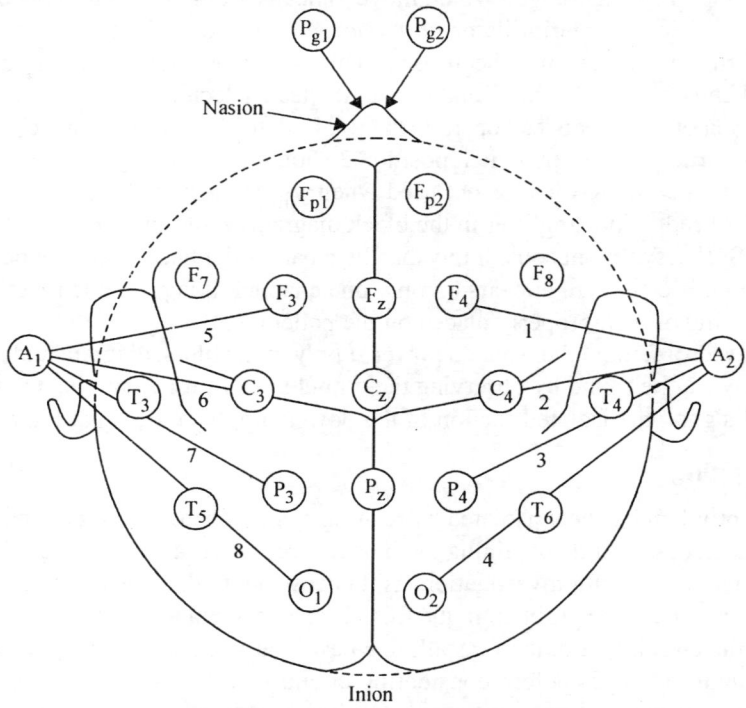

Fig. 5.23. EEG electrode positions on the scalp.

Electrode problems arise because of hair, which tends to increase the contact resistance. Surface electrodes may be made of silver, silver oxide disks from 1 to 3 mm in diameter. A conductive paste is used to lower the electrode resistance below 10 kΩ and to compensate for hair interference. The electrode may be covered with gauge and held with an adhesive such as collodion cement. To lower its resistance further, the skin may be abraded, but this introduces discomfort. Another method for reducing the electrode resistance employs a needle called a sphenoidal electrode, which breaks the skin and carries with it the danger of infection. The reference electrode may be attached to regions of negligible brain wave activity such as the ear lobe or inserted into the nostrils. The nostril or nasopharyngeal, electrode has a silver ball tip to reduce the contact resistance. If the skull is open during surgery, an electrocorticographic electrode, consisting of a cotton wick soaked in saline solution, may be placed on the brain to monitor electrical activity. Several different types of EEG electrodes are illustrated in Fig. 5.24.

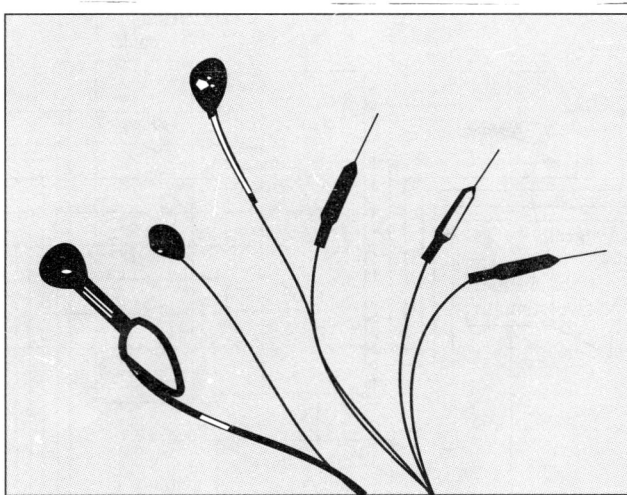

Fig. 5.24. Example of ECG electrodes showing needle, surface and ear-clip electrodes.

An EEG Block Diagram

The signal path through the EEG is perhaps best understood by Fig. 5.25. The cable from the electrodes to the eight-channel selector has 21 leads and is vulnerable to breaks in the leads or shielding. It is also affected by 60-~ interference. The electrodes are attached to the EEG in groups of eight, called a montage of electrodes. A representative montage is already illustrated in Fig. 5.23. In that case, the right-brain electrodes are referenced to the right ear, which serves as a reference point and the left-brain electrodes are referenced to the left ear. The brain wave activity in the ear lobe is very small and it serves as an adequate reference point for EEG studies. It is often more comfortable for the patient to have the electrode attached to the ear rather than to the nostril.

Voltage measurements may also be taken between adjacent electrodes; this is called the bipolar connection. Or the measurements may be taken from one of the electrodes to a common point developed by a resistor circuit; this is called a Wilson network or a unipolar connection and is illustrated in Fig. 5.26. In that case, each electrode is measured with respect to the same voltage. The voltage value at the reference usually cannot be computed because of insufficient data, but it is enough to know that each electrode is measured with respect to the same voltage.

The 60-~ interference is reduced by employing differential amplifiers with more than an 80 dB common-mode rejection ratio (CMRR), as already discussed by use of 60-~ notch filters. The notch filter can introduce phase distortion and reduce the gain, but its effect is minimised by the fact that the most important EEG signals have frequencies below 30 Hz. For very precise or experimental measurements, it is sometimes best to place the EEG in a room covered by a ferrous metal screen, which will shield it from 60-~ radiation as well as any other frequency.

Because of the high internal impedance of the brain wave source, the input impedance of the differential amplifiers should exceed 10 MΩ to prevent loss of signal amplitude. The gain needs to be around 10^6 to produce voltages near 1 V, which are required to drive the display recorder or imaging scope.

According to Fig. 5.25, the voltage output from the differential amplifiers may either be applied directly to the eight-channel display through the filter bank or it may be stored as data on a tape recorder or in a computer memory for further processing.

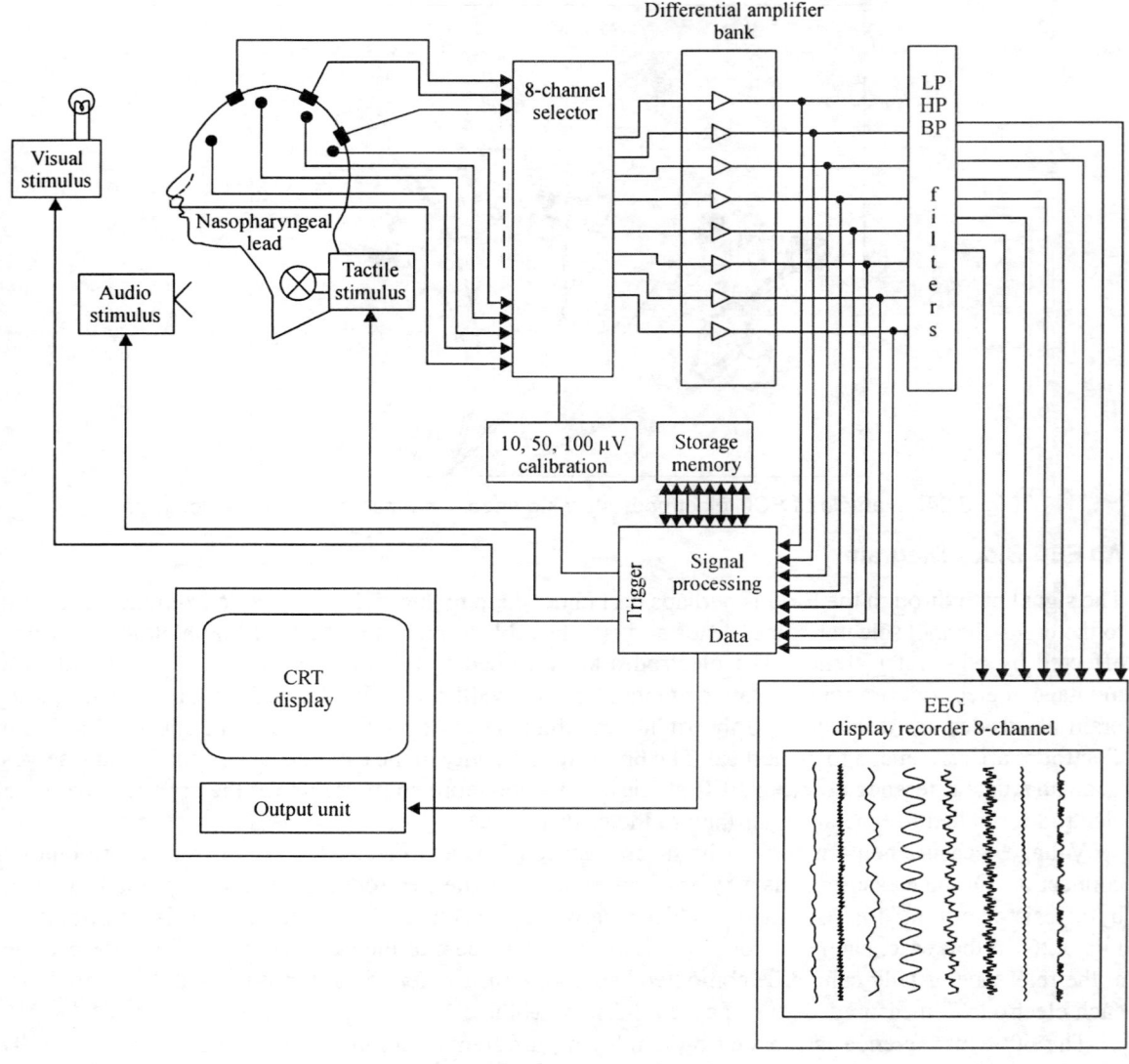

Fig. 5.25. An EEG block diagram.

The filter bank may contain high-pass, low-pass or band-pass filters and it enables the operator to select upper and lower frequency cut-offs. The appropriate filters are chosen in order to select frequency components of the brain wave significant in diagnosis of disease. The clinically significant bands are given approximately as follows:

delta:	below 4 Hz
theta:	4 to 8 Hz
alpha:	8 to 13 Hz
beta:	above 13 Hz

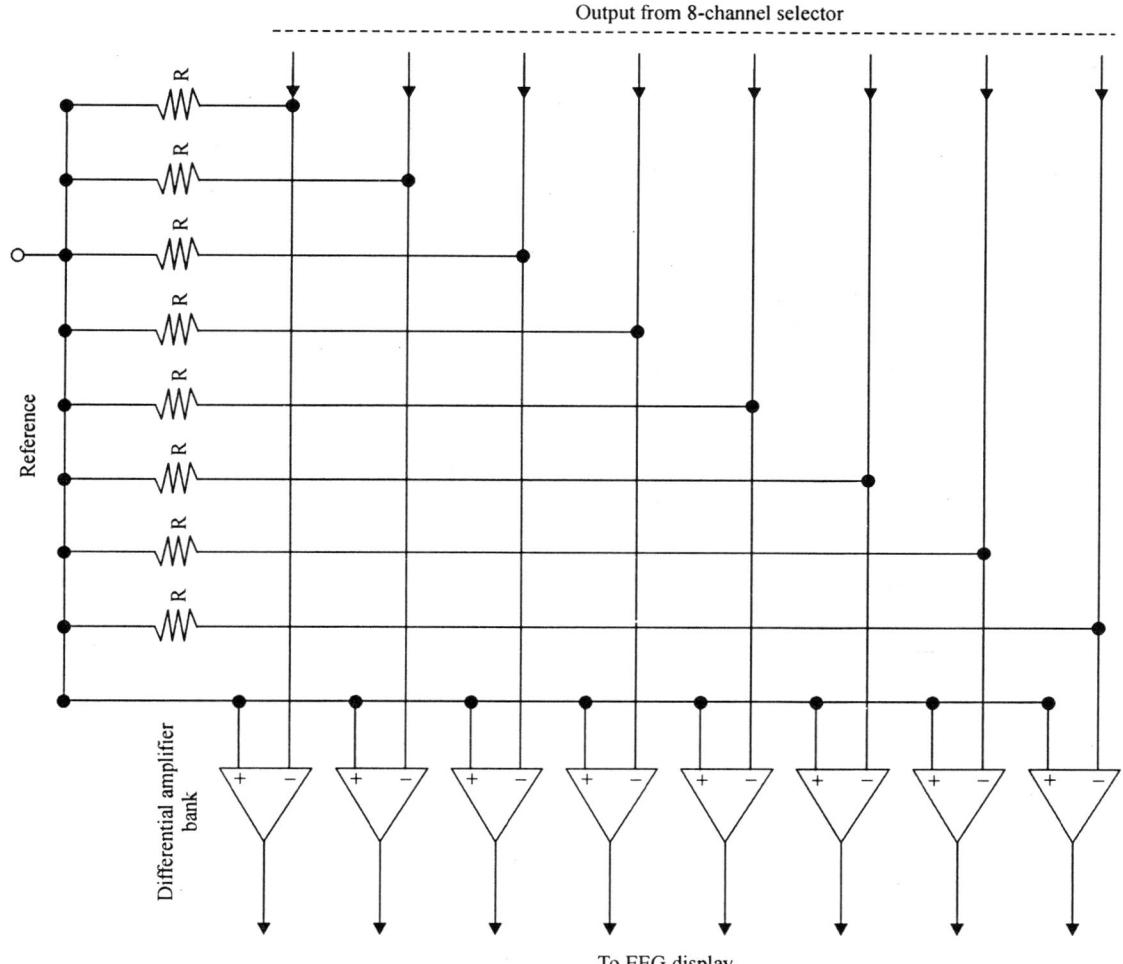

Fig. 5.26. A Wilson network.

Electroencephalograms

The brain waves of normal individuals range from low-frequency, nearly periodic waves with a large delta component in deep sleep, to high-frequency, non-coherent beta waves measured on the frontal lobe channels during vigorous mental activity, as illustrated in Fig. 5.27. A relaxed state is characterised by alpha waves from the occipital lobe channels. A visually evoked response is easily measured by opening and closing the eyes, as indicated in Fig. 5.27. This figure illustrates the fact that brain waves in normal individuals vary significantly with electrode position and with mental state.

Abnormal brain waves may indicate either a pathological state in the patient or the presence of some artifact introduced by the instrument. Such artifacts may be due to improper use of the instrument, especially at the electrode interface or they may be due to instrumentation problems. Some examples are given in Table 5.3.

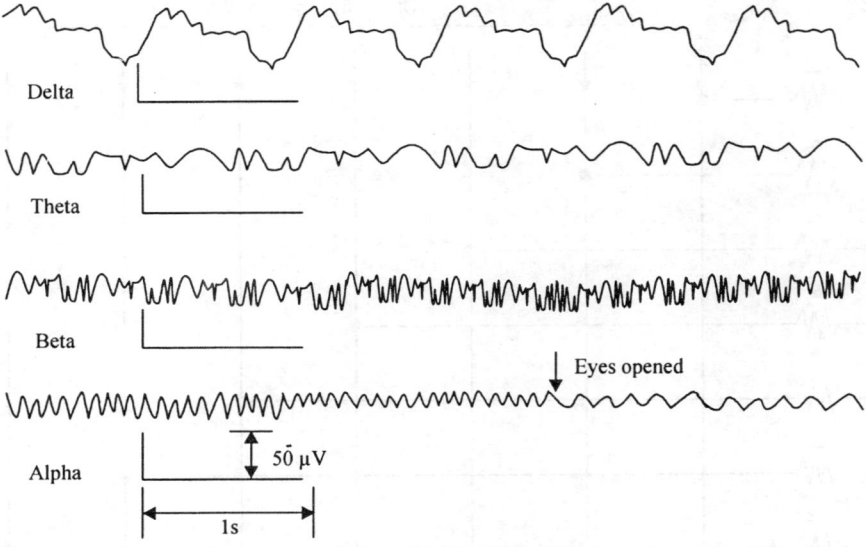

Fig. 5.27. Example EEG waves. The vertical scale is 50 µV and the horizontal scale is 1 s. The alpha wave is taken with eyes closed then opened where indicated by the arrow.

Table 5.3. Troubleshooting tips for EEGs.

Abnormalities in the EEG waveform may be due to artifacts categorised as follows:

Artifacts due to electrode problems may result from

Improper positioning

Poor contact

Poor electrode in the cap holding them

Dried-out gel

Oozing of tissue fluids in needle electrodes

Frayed connections

Sweating

Artifacts due to physiological interference may result from

The heart ECG

Tongue and facial movement

Eye movement

Skeletal muscle movement

High scalp impedance

Breathing

Artifacts due to electrical interference (EI) may result from:

60-~ common-mode interference

Radio frequency interference due to use of an electrical surgical unit

Defibrillation

Presence of pacemakers and neural stimulators

EEGs in Diagnosis

The purpose of the EEG is to help physicians diagnose disease. The pathological states or diseases most commonly diagnosed using the EEG are brain death, brain tumours, epilepsy, multiple sclerosis and sleep disorders. The advent of modern life-sustaining equipment, such as respirators and the need for donor organs for transplant operations have changed the legal definition of death. The sustained absence of EEG signals is a clinical measure of brain death and can be used in deciding whether to transplant a heart, liver or lung or whether to shut down life-sustaining equipment such as kidney dialyser, ventilator or an artificial heart pump.

The EEG is widely used in diagnosing both generalised epilepsy and partial epilepsy. One form of generalised epilepsy is characterised by grand mal seizures, in which large electrical discharges are produced from the entire brain that last from a few seconds to several minutes. It may also be accompanied by skeletal muscle twitches and jerks. Evidence of 'grand mal' seizures usually appears on all channels of the EEG. A less severe form of generalised epilepsy (but still 'generalised' in that it affects the entire brain) is characterised by petit mal seizures, during which strong delta waves are produced for 1 to 20 seconds. Partial epilepsy affects only part of the brain and therefore is visible on fewer channels of the EEG.

It is important that patients with epilepsy have a warning that a seizure is about to occur, so that they can take medication and avoid injury or other inconveniences. Warnings of a seizure occur as vigorous electrical activity in particular foci in the brain, which would be recorded on the appropriate channel of an EEG. If the foci are in the temporal lobe, the patient would hear a sound; if in the occipital lobe, the patient would see flashes and if in the motor area, the patient may experience muscle jerks. These are sensory warnings of an event that could develop into a grand mal seizure resulting in an extended stupor.

Transient signals due to epilepsy that do not result in physical seizures are important in diagnosis and treatment of the disease. To find such transients is tedious if not nearly impossible for a clinical technician unaided by instrumentation. One method of surveying large amounts of EEG data is to record it on magnetic tape at a low speed and play it back rapidly, at perhaps 60 times the original speed.

The availability of inexpensive minicomputers makes it feasible to search for particular patterns in the EEG, such as high-intensity bursts and store them in memory for later review by a physician diagnosing their meaning (Fig. 5.25). Such techniques make ambulatory monitoring of epilepsy patients a technical possibility. Without computer storage and signal processing capability, the amount of data produced would overwhelm a human observer.

The effect of either visual, audio or tactile stimuli upon the electroencephalogram of a patient is of clinical value in the diagnosis of disease.

Filters

There are many types of medical instruments in which it is necessary to select the frequency components of the input signal. For example, in the electroencephalograph, various brain states, such as the alert state, the sleep state and the deep sleep state, produce distinctive frequency bands. In the EEG, theta waves in the frequency band 4 to 8 Hz indicate sleep, while beta waves in the frequency band 13 to 22 Hz indicate a high state of alertness. Filters may be used to direct these frequency bands to different channels to facilitate signal processing and disease diagnosis. In this case, filtering is essential to the diagnostic function of the instrument. In almost all monitoring, filtering is useful in reducing noise and often in reducing the effects of 60-~ interference. In general, filters are used for either frequency selection or frequency rejection. An ideal filter is one that passes the desired signal without either amplitude or phase distortion and completely rejects any unwanted or unnecessary signals.

Classification of filters

Filters may be classified as either low-pass, high-pass, band-pass or band-reject, as illustrated in Fig. 5.28 in diagrams called Bode plots. Each filter has one or more cut-off frequencies, f_C and a pass-band gain, often given in decibels (dB) as a function of frequency. The attenuation outside the pass-band as a function of frequency is called the filter roll-off and is often linear as a function of the logarithm of frequency (log f).

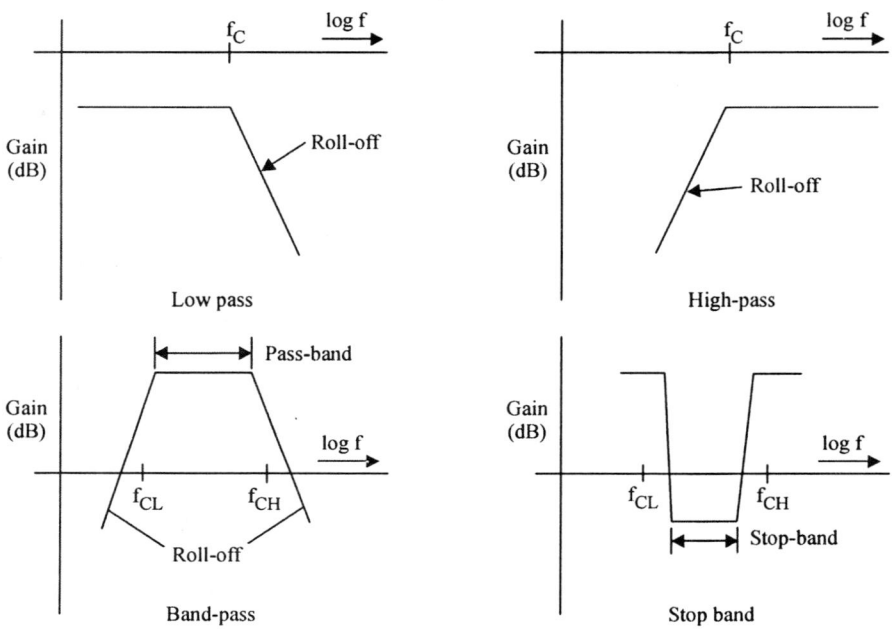

Fig. 5.28. Filter Bode plots for low-pass, high-pass, band-pass and stop-band filters.

The figures of merit in filters are primarily measures of filter gain and frequency characteristics. The terms that specify these figures of merit are defined as follows:

Filter gain

The filter gain, A_V, is the ratio of the output voltage of the filter to the input voltage. The gain is often expressed in decibels and is calculated from the formula $A_{dB} = 20 \log A_V$.

High-frequency cut-off

The high-frequency cut-off, f_{CH}, is usually taken as higher frequency above which the gain remains 3 dB below the filter pass-band given.

Low-frequency cut-off

The low-frequency cut-off, f_{CL}, is the lower frequency below which the gain remains more than 3 dB below the filter pass-band gain.

Filter bandwidth

The filter bandwidth, BW, is the difference between the low and high filter cut-off frequencies as calculated by the formula:

$$BW = f_{CH} - f_{CL} \qquad \qquad ...(5.6)$$

Band-pass filter resonant frequency

This resonant frequency, f_R, is the frequency midway between f_{CH} and f_{CL} on a logarithmic scale, given by the formula

$$\log f_R = (\log f_{CH} + \log f_{CL})/2$$
$$= \tfrac{1}{2} \log f_{CH} \, f_{CL}$$

Therefore, the resonant frequency is defined by the formula

$$f_R = \sqrt{f_{CH} \, f_{CL}} \qquad \qquad ...(5.7)$$

Band-pass filter quality

The filter with the highest quality, Q, is the one that gives the purest tone at the output. A mathematical definition consistent with this is given by the formula

$$Q = \frac{f_R}{BW} \qquad \qquad ...(5.8)$$

since this indicates that the narrower the band of the filter, the higher the Q.

Bode asymptote

A Bode asymptote is a straight line drawn on a semi-log plot of the filter gain A_{dB} versus the logarithm of the frequency. The line begins at a point defined by the filter pass-band gain and the cut-off frequency, either f_{CH} or f_{CL}. The line is then drawn to the asymptote of the high-frequency or low-frequency gain values, A_{dB}, for the low-pass case.

Filter roll-off

The slope of the Bode asymptote on a semi-log scale is called the filter roll-off and is measured in decibels per octave (dB/octave). A frequency an octave above another is double that frequency. The units decibels per decade (dB/decade), where a decade frequency is ten times the initial frequency, are also often used to describe the roll-off.

Filter order

The order N of the filter determines the slope of the filter roll-off. Ideally, the filter orders correspond to the formula

$$Roll\text{-}off = 6 \text{ N dB/octave}$$

which is equivalent to 20 N dB/decade. This formula generates a table of values as follows:

Filter order	Roll-off (dB/octave)
1	6
2	12
3	18
4	24

Chapter 6

Patient Monitoring Systems

INTRODUCTION

Patient monitoring systems consist of sensors for signal acquisition, a means for processing the information collected, computation capabilities and outputs consisting of alarms, video displays and hard copy for record-keeping. Such systems are in hospital locations that are involved with the critically ill: coronary care units, operating rooms, operating room recovery areas, critical care areas and the emergency room. This chapter describes the essentials of patient monitoring systems and their functions.

The first patient monitoring system consisted of physicians and nurses moving from patient to patient. Information was collected by stethoscope, mercury thermometer, pulse-rate measurements by clock, visual observations of the patient and asking a lot of questions. The processing of the data was based upon experience and association. The output usually consisted of instructions written on a sheet of paper. As medical knowledge increased, is patient monitoring system became inadequate because the rate of processing information had to increase.

Critically ill people must have their cardiac function assessed in as detailed a manner as possible. Respiratory status needs to be known as thoroughly as possible. Warnings need to be provided for impending congestive heart failure. Processing of large amounts of data must be accomplished in real time to provide alarms and meaningful information. The following knowledge, at least, is needed.

1. Electrocardiograph waveform and heart rate.
2. Blood pressure waveform with systolic, diastolic and mean pressures.
3. Respiratory waveform and rate.
4. Pulmonary and systemic pressures.
5. Cardiac output.
6. Temperature.
7. Blood gases, partial pressures of oxygen and carbon dioxide.
8. Rates of change of certain parameters.
9. Trend information.
10. Arrhythmia events for some heart patients.

Many pieces of information may be required from a critically ill patient. Eight such patients, not an uncommon situation, provide a flood of information that must be processed immediately to provide useful information and generate appropriate alarms. The data needed to properly manage these patients require that immediate information be rendered to the medical staff. The classical methods and instruments have given way to sophisticated sensors, microprocessor-based instrumentation and data-based management and computer systems. When these new tools are integrated in an installation, they establish a modern patient monitoring system.

MODERN SYSTEM

This device situated at the bedside of the individual patients collects ECG signal. Waveforms were displayed on a simple oscilloscope. Meters displayed average values and alarms were provided when the average value became too high or too low. Information could also be sent to a central station. Thus it was not necessary for nurses to continually be near the patient's bedside. In some cases it became possible for fewer nurses to manage a given number of patients. In many cases, though, the nursing staff did not decrease in size but was able to better manage and care for the critically ill.

Increasing medical knowledge has created additional demands on patient monitoring systems. Signals must be processed so that computations can be made. For some patients, it is necessary to detect heart arrhythmias. More sophistication was needed in the collection and processing of the ECG waveform to differentiate between pace pulses (from implanted pacemakers) and the underlying ECG information. Computational capabilities are needed for determining cardiac output and providing certain blood gas information. These are but a few examples of the current needs to process information. The human observer lacks the capacity to collect and evaluate copious amounts of information in a given time span. New patient monitoring systems require high-speed signal processing and computational capabilities as well as high-quality video displays and hard-copy outputs with annotations suitable for use by the medical staff.

One version of a modern patient monitoring system has each bedside unit connected to a central controller. Radiating from this central controller are branches to each of the bedside instruments. The controller grants permission for a bedside to 'talk' at a fixed time. The bedside then sends its data to the controller and the controller re-transmits the data to one or more other bedside units and the central station. A nurse at a given patient's bedside can call up information from any other patient and a nurse at the central station can monitor all information from all patients. This 'star' topology places each instrument on a separate branch, allowing the controller to isolate a single point failure by logically amputating a malfunctioning branch. The remainder of the network is unaffected. A controller failure does not impair individual bedside monitors. Bedside equipment, as well as central station equipment, can be connected and disconnected while this network is running, with no concern for transient disruption.

ARRHYTHMIA MONITORING SYSTEM

Conventional monitoring systems require continual user vigilance to detect certain cardiac arrhythmias that are usually of the transient nature but, at the same time, can present significant information with respect to the patient's heart condition. One alternative is to post human monitors in front of the display that presents the ECG waveforms and ask them to note each abnormal event. The task is tedious and due to human limitations, presents the possibility of overlooking important events. The computerised arrhythmia monitoring system is able continuously to review the ECG waveform of several patients simultaneously. Its algorithm recognises and identifies, to some level of accuracy, individual arrhythmias. The events can be plotted against time. Logs can show the frequency of occurrence of given events. Such systems may have waveform retrieval capability and printout of stored information.

The systems function by means of instructions stored in memory. These instructions, known as algorithms, divide that task into detection, classification and alarm. Some algorithms extract features in a manner roughly similar to the mental processes of a human observer; others use a template to match or cross-correlate data with waveforms considered to be normal. Deviations from this normal waveform are analysed; classification follows and alarms are provided for various arrhythmia events, based upon seriousness and frequency of occurrence.

Detection and classification are difficult tasks, especially so since attempts are being made to duplicate the complex pattern recognition system involved in the human brain. Arrhythmia systems are not perfect and the designer's task is to find a practical way to make the false-positive and false-negative rates approach zero. A compromise involves having as low false-positive rate as feasible without generating so many false-positive alarms that the user finds the system too difficult to use. On the other hand, the task is also to drive the false-negative rate to zero. Approaching zero errors require large amounts of memory, long processing times and algorithms not yet perfected. Users of these systems are aware that they are not ideal; but even with this lack of perfection, these systems have proven to be quite helpful in that they do pick up more arrhythmias than does continuous monitoring by human observers.

SAFETY

For the critically ill patient there is much concern about the small amounts of energy at power-line frequencies that may enter the heart and possibly cause ventricular fibrillation. Some hearts react unfavourably to currents in the range of 20 μA rms and lower (at power-line frequencies), whereas other patients are not susceptible even to milliampere currents that directly enter the heart.

The heart is one of the most sensitive organ to electric current. Since it depends for its function on periodic, highly organised muscle contractions controlled by internally generated electrical stimuli, small periodic currents through the heart can derange the organised patterns. If the current is of sufficient strength through a given area of the heart, some of the muscle cells are captured by the unwanted stimuli and act out of the sequence that would normally cause an effective heart contraction. If a group of cells becomes disorganised, the effect propagates to neighbouring cells that also become disorganised. This chain reaction can, in a relatively short time, result in most of the heart cells assuming a random, chaotic activity instead of the synchronised action necessary for useful pumping of the blood. This random activity referred to as ventricular fibrillation, defeats the heart's ability to pump blood and is fatal unless corrected within a few minutes.

MEASUREMENT OF CARDIAC OUTPUT AND STROKE VOLUME

A knowledge of the cardiac output is important in seriously ill patients, for example those in haemorrhagic shock or those who have suffered a cardiac arrest and been re-suscitated. The circumstances of an intensive care unit demand that cardiac output can be measured as quickly and conveniently as possible and several determinations may be required for a particular patient. Since it requires a knowledge of the patient's oxygen consumption and the difference between the oxygen contents of his arterial and mixed venous blood, it is not feasible to employ the well-known Fick method. The most accurate alternative methods are the indicator dilution methods using indocyanine green dye or cool saline, but those require access to arterial blood. For this reason, the radionuclide method is often used, plus the fact that an analysis of the right and left heart components of the isotope dilution curve can lead to information concerning the central blood volume and transit times. For the routine monitoring of patients, an urgent need exists for techniques capable of following stroke volume changes on a beat-by-beat basis by non-invasive means. Possible techniques are the pressure pulse contour method, the ultrasonic Doppler shift technique and the electrical impedance method.

Principles of the Indicator Dilution Method

A small amount of an indicator substance in solution, such as a dye or cool saline, is injected into a large vein or preferably into the right side of the heart itself. The indicator is passed rapidly through the right heart, the pulmonary circulation and the left heart and then into the systemic circulation. By this time it is assumed to be perfectly mixed with the blood. The appearance of the bolus of indicator is usually detected in a peripheral artery by means of the suitable detection system. The electrical output from the detector is taken to a chart recorder and produces a dilution curve as shown in Fig. 6.1. The indicator is injected as bolus and the appearance time of several seconds elapses before the signal from the detector commences to increase to a maximum and then diminishes. The appearance time corresponds with that required for the fastest particles of indicator to travel to the detector via the shortest route. In the case when the indicator is a dye, before the detector signal has time to return to its baseline value, a fraction of the injectate will have passed through some of the peripheral vessels and returned a second time through the heart. Because of this the dilution curve describes a second (recirculation) peak. The presence of this peak complicates the calculation of the cardiac output. It occurs with dye or radioactive indicators, but not with cool saline which has attained blood temperature by the time it has passed through the heart a second time. From a knowledge of the amount of indicator injected and the area under the dilution curve without recirculation, it is possible to calculate the cardiac output. The calculation will be illustrated for the dye, radio nuclide and cool saline methods. The measurement of the area under the dilution curve can be time-consuming (10 to 15 minutes) if performed manually from the chart recording. This is too long for routine work in intensive care situations and has resulted in the use of algorithms and calculators for this application.

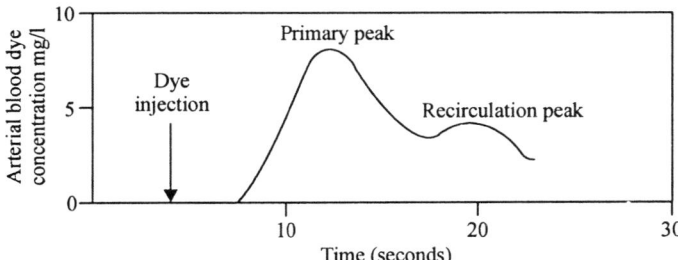

Fig. 6.1. A dye dilution curve.

Assuming that the indicator is injected in the form of a bolus, that the cardiac output is constant and that perfect mixing of the indicator with blood occurs, then it can be shown that the concentration of the indicator in the blood leaving the heart falls off with time in a simple exponential fashion. The fact that the downslope of the dilution curve is a simple exponential shape under normal conditions makes it easy to allow for the effects of recirculation where this occurs. In essence the approach relies on being able to distinguish sufficient of the exponential downslope in order to be able to predict the time course of the downslope during the presence of recirculation. However, in patients with low cardiac outputs which give rise to flattened dilution curves or in patients having a marked degree of valvular incompetence in which the recirculation peak occurs early, there may be insufficient exponential downslope available. As a result, approximate methods of calculating the area under the curve may have to be used which only require a knowledge of the area under the initial portion of the curve from the appearance to the peak concentration.

Dye dilution method

The dye usually employed is indocyanine green and it has the advantage that it absorbs light in the 800 nm region of the spectrum which is an isobestic point, i.e., where both oxygenated and reduced haemoglobin exhibit the same value of optical absorption. As a result, it is not necessary to have the patient breathe oxygen during the recording of the dilution curve as was necessary with some of the blue dyes previously used for cardiac output determination. Indocyanine green dye is cleared rapidly from the circulation so that repeated cardiac output determinations are possible, only approximately 3 per cent of the dose remaining in the circulation 20 minutes after the injection.

A suitable two-wavelength densitometer for measuring the dye concentration in blood is that of Sutterer and Wood. The optical arrangement of the densitometer is shown in Fig. 6.2 and the spectral response of its two photocells is given in Fig. 6.3. The 800 nm isobestic point is already used for measuring the dye concentration which means it cannot be employed for the monitoring of non-specific blood optical density changes such as flow velocity changes in the cuvette. Hence Sutterer and Wood used a dichroic mirror to reflect light in the region of 800 nm to one photocell whilst simultaneously transmitting light of shorter and longer wavelengths to a second photocell. As the transmission by blood of wavelengths shorter and longer than 800 nm is influenced in opposite directions by changes in the blood oxygen saturation, it is possible by a suitable choice of the optical filters and the spectral response of the compensating photocell to make the response of the photocell to these wavelengths cancel. Hence the response of the second photocell is unaffected by oxygen saturation changes and it can be used to compensate for non-specific effects. Light from the filament lamp is passed through the cuvette L and is then split by the dichroic mirror and falls on the compensating (C) and dye detection (IR) photocells. Each photocell is located behind an optical filter.

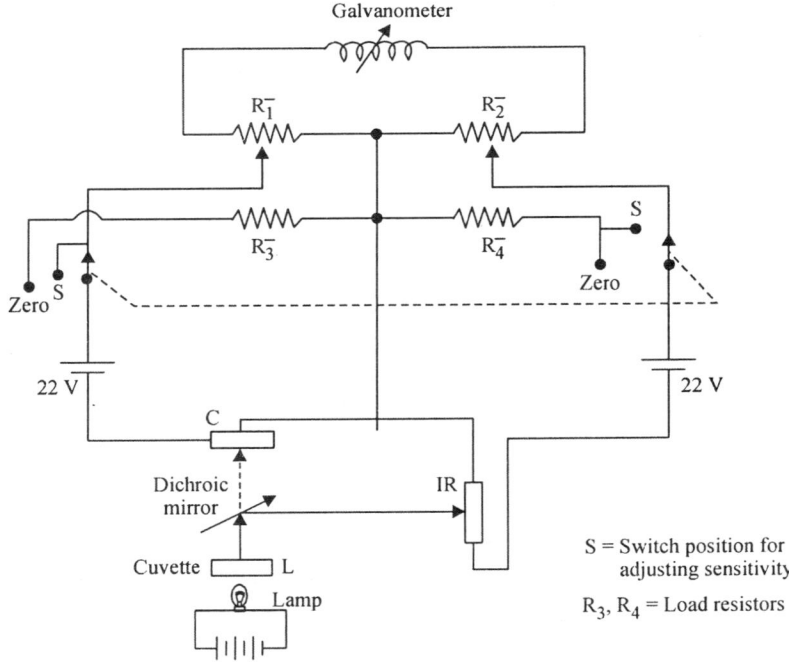

Fig. 6.2. Optical arrangement of a two-wavelength densitometer.

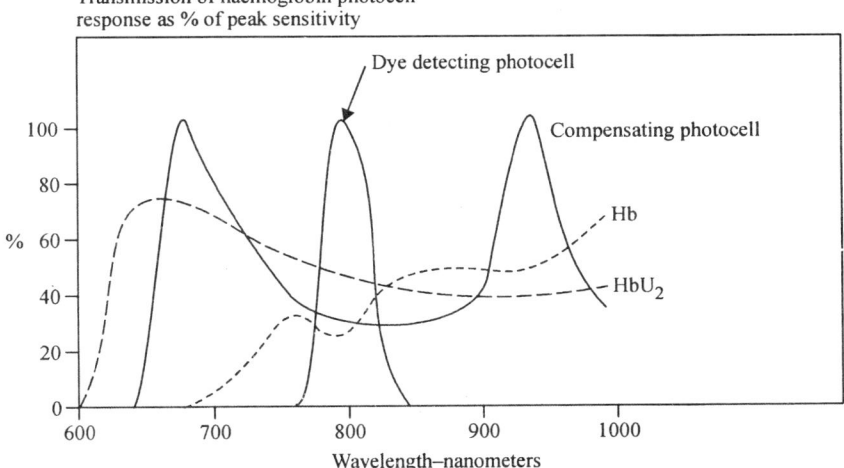

Fig. 6.3. Spectral response of the photocells used in the two-wavelength densitometer.

The sensitivity of the photocells can be adjusted by potentiometers R_1 and R_2. These are 10-turn helical potentiometers in the galvanometer circuit. The load resistors R_3 and R_4 keep the load on the photocells constant and hence minimise drift. When a dye dilution curve is to be recorded, the control switch is first placed in position 0 and the zero reading of the galvanometer is adjusted to a convenient baseline position towards the bottom of the associated recorder's chart using the recorder shift control. Whilst blood is being drawn through the cuvette, R_1 is used to adjust the sensitivity of the compensating photocell to bring the recorder pack to the baseline. With the switch in the S-operate position and blood still flowing, R_2 is adjusted to again return the recorder pen to the baseline. The outputs from the pair of photocells are then nearly equal and opposite. The sensitivity of the densitometer is proportional to the difference in the galvanometer or recorder readings with the switch in the S and 0 positions. The pair of photocells, the lamp and the cuvette are all mounted in a cylindrical housing 25 mm in diameter by 70 mm long. The volume of the cuvette and its inlet tube is only 0.05 ml in total thus ensuring that the instrument has a good dynamic response.

A venous catheter is placed in the right atrium and a bolus of dye injected through it. For adults the dose of dye would typically be 5 mg in 1 ml, for children it would be 2.5 mg. Meanwhile a constant flow of blood, typically 0.4 ml per second is withdrawn from an artery such as the radial through the cuvette by means of a motor driven syringe, (Fig. 6.4). A suitable speed for the chart recorder used to display the output signal from the densitometer would be 5 mm per second. Some operators prefer to chase the bolus of dye immediately with an injection of saline to wash it into the circulation.

The most accurate method for the estimation of cardiac output by the dye dilution technique is invasive and require the drawing of arterial blood through the densitometer cuvette. This imposes a rigid requirement for sterility and also the need to ensure that there are no leaks in the line through which air might be entrained to form air bubbles which can spoil the baseline of the recording. The presence of the dye in the circulation can also be detected by shining a beam of light through the pinna of the ear onto a pair of photocells each covered with an optical filter. When the recorder tracing is constant following the dye curve, it is assumed that the dye concentration in the circulation is constant and a venous blood sample is drawn and pulled through a cuvette which has been substituted for the earpiece. The cuvette is calibrated with blood samples containing known dye concentrations and in this way the concentration of the equilibrium blood sample is determined and this is then used to calibrate the dilution curve obtained from the earpiece. This method is applicable to dyes as Evans blue which remain in the circulation sufficiently long for a stable equilibrium blood level to occur.

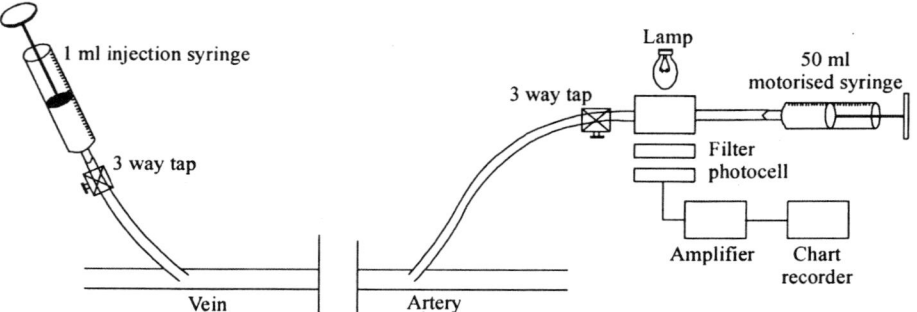

Fig. 6.4. Schematic diagram of the arrangement used for recording a dye curve.

Manual calculation of the area under the dye curve without recirculation

The first procedure is to extrapolate the exponential downslope of the dye dilution curve to a dye concentration equivalent to one per cent of the peak concentration. This is done by re-plotting the exponential portion of the downslope on semi-logarithmic graph paper to yield a straight line. This is extended to take in a concentration which is one per cent of the peak value and points read off from the line are re-plotted on the original dye curve to extend the downslope without recirculation, (Fig. 6.5). The area under the re-plotted curve can now be measured in arbitary units by counting squares or more usually by the use of a planimeter. For use in the calculation of the cardiac output the area under the curve must be expressed in mg per litre × seconds. The cardiac output in litres per minute is then given by

$$Q \text{ litres/minutes} = \frac{\text{mg of dye injected} \times 60}{\text{area under curve in mg/litre} \times \text{seconds}}$$

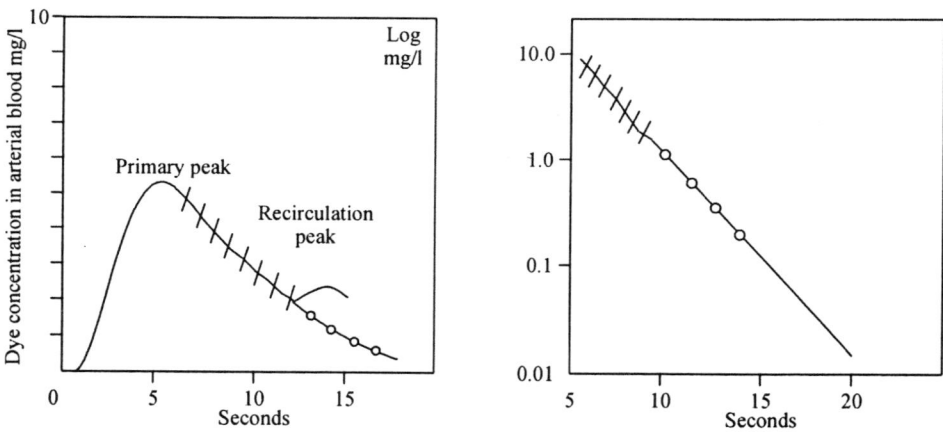

Fig. 6.5. The re-plotting of the downslope of a dye dilution curve on semi-logarithmic graph paper.

The densitometer recorder chart is calibrated by drawing blood through the cuvette which contains a known concentration of dye. Suppose that the recorder deflects by 50 mm when the dye concentration is 5 mg per litre and that the chart speed is 5 mm per second. A rectangle 50 × 25 mm drawn on the chart is equivalent to 25 mg per litre × seconds. A calibration factor can be found to give the area under the dye curve in mg per litre × seconds by running the planimeter round this known area. An approximation to the area under the curve can be found by summing the dye concentrations occurring at one second intervals from the start to the finish of the curve.

Use of a radioactive indicator

The use of indocyanine green dye is well-established but requires access to arterial blood for the best accuracy. The fact that the dye is cleared rapidly from the blood makes it difficult to obtain an equilibrium level for use in calibrating an earpiece. The dye method has been checked against the Fick method.

Another approach which is of value in an intensive care unit is to make use of a gamma-emitting radio-isotope as the indicator. Only a venous blood sample is needed and if a double peaked dilution curve is generated much additional information on the state of the patient's circulation can be obtained. Due to the rise in the background radioactivity level of the patient's blood it is usual to make only two cardiac output determinations within the space of a few hours. Veall and Vetter have described the use of human serum albumin (RISA) labelled with gamma ray emitting isotope iodine–131, as a suitable indicator. A typical concentration would be 100 micro-curies in a volume of 1 ml. The protein concentration should be approximately 2 per cent v/v to prevent errors due to absorption on the glassware.

The passage of the radioactivity through the heart is detected by means of a collimated 2 in diameter scintillation counter using a thallium-activated sodium iodide crystal. Veall and Vetter recommend the use of a collimator having a cylindrical aperture 25 mm in diameter and 50 mm deep. The shielded counter and collimator assembly is mounted on an adjustable stand so that it can be positioned over the heart of a supine patient. The counter stand forms part of a mobile trolley which carries the e.h.t supply, pulse amplifier, discriminator and linear ratemeter. This should have a range of 1000 counts per second full-scale with a time constant of 0.4 seconds and the possibility of increasing this to 5 seconds. A zero control should be provided so that the baseline of the ratemeter can be set to zero in order for the background activity arising from previous injections to be offset during serial determinations. The output signal from the ratemeter is fed to a potentiometric recorder having a balancing time of 0.5 seconds for full-scale deflection and a chart speed of 10 mm per second.

Before the injection is made, a standard calibration solution is prepared by injecting approximately 0.1 ml of the RISA solution into 100 ml of water in a volumetric flask. The actual value of the dilution produced is found by weighing the syringe before and after making the dilution. A 5 ml syringe full of the diluant is counted for radioactivity by placing it in a jig at a convenient distance from the face of the scintillation counter. Next it is necessary to check that the dilution curve recorded from the patient will not exceed the range of the counting equipment. This is done by placing the standard solution in the aperture of the collimator and adjusting the value of the e.h.t voltage or the discriminator setting to produce a deflection which is about 75 per cent of full scale on the recorder. The maximum amount of information concerning the state of patient's circulation can be extracted from a dilution curve which is double peaked, (Fig. 6.6), so that the collimator should be positioned in the region of the apex of the heart and directed to view both halves of the heart. With the ratemeter time constant set at 0.4 seconds an accurately known volume of the RISA (0.1 ml, 10 micro-curies) is injected as smoothly and rapidly as possible into an arm vein and followed with a bolus of physiological saline solution.

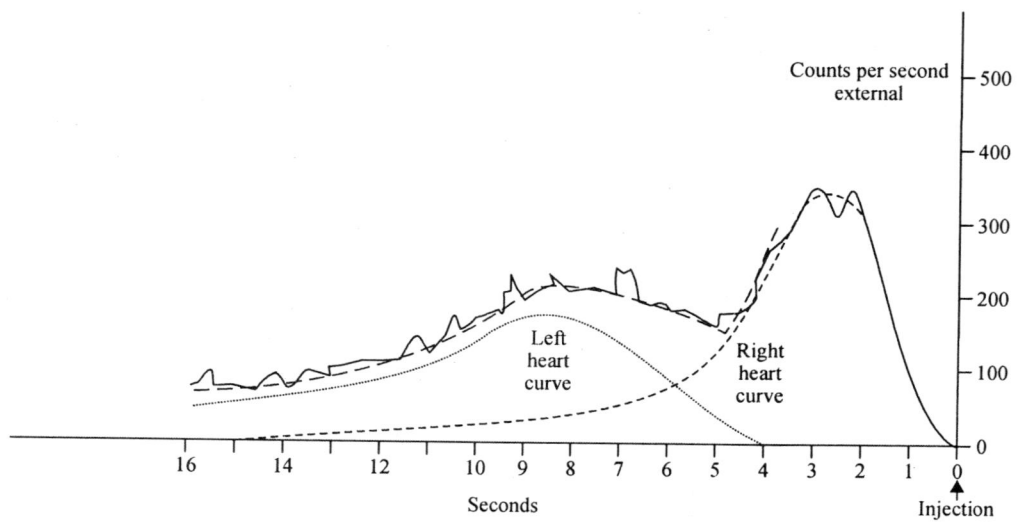

Fig. 6.6. The right and left heart components of a normal radiocardiogram.

A mark is make at the time of the injection on the recorder chart. After waiting for about ten minutes in order for a steady blood level of activity to be obtained, a recording is made with the ratemeter time constant increased to 5 seconds and at this time a 5 ml blood sample is drawn. For some patients, such as those with mitral valve incompetence or a low cardiac output, more time will have to be allowed for mixing of the indicator to occur. The blood sample is then counted in the jig used for counting the standard solution. In order to reduce the uptake of the RISA by the thyroid gland, potassium iodide may be administered orally. Uhrenholdt gave 750 mg of potassium iodide orally before and then four days after a radiocardiogram for which the dose was 45-55 micro-curies of I-131 RISA. If V = the volume of RISA injected in ml

D = the dilution of injectate to produce the standard solution.

S = activity of the standard in counts per minute per 5 ml.

Then the counts per minute of I-131 injected = V × D × S/5, let E = the activity in counts per minute recorded over the heart at the time of drawing the blood sample.

B = activity of the blood sample in counts per minute per 5 ml.

Define a known area on the chart record bounded by a rectangle with sides of X seconds and Y counts per second over the heart. This area is equal to A = (X · Y) × 60 × 200 × B/E expressed in (counts per minute per litre of blood) × seconds. Using a planimeter it is found that the area under the total dilution curve with the left heart downslope extrapolated to eliminate the effects of recirculation is f × A. The factor 200 converts from the counts measured for a blood sample of 5 ml to counts per litre and the factor 60 converts from the measured counts per second to counts per minute.

For the patient whose curve is shown in Fig. 6.6, V = 0.396 ml, S = 17618, E = 10902, D = 773; B = 1729; X = 5 seconds, Y = 400 counts per second; and f = 3.34.

$$\text{Cardiac output in litres per minute} = \frac{(Vxx\ D \times S/5) \times 60}{f \times X \times Y \times 60 \times 200 \times B/E}$$

The dose injected (V × D × S/5) = 0.396 × 773 × 17618/5 = 1.078602 × 10^6 counts per minute.

Area under the curve $= 3.34 \times 5 \times 400 \times 60 \times 200 \times 1729/10902$
$$= 12.712955 \times 10^6 \text{ counts per minute per litre of blood x seconds.}$$
Cardiac output in litres per minute
$$= 60 \text{ x dose/area}$$
$$= 60 \text{ x } 1.078602/12.712955 = 5.1 \text{ litres per minute.}$$

Analysis of double-peaked radiocardiograms

When calculating the cardiac output from a radiocardiogram, the total area under the curve corrected for recirculation must be used, i.e., the area under both peaks if left and right heart peaks are present. Some authors only mention single peaked radiocardiograms and whether one peak or two is seen depends on both the shape of the collimator used and the positioning of the detector. The boundary of the area used in the cardiac output calculation is defined by the projection of the exponential down-slope of the single peak or the left peak in a double peaked curve to a value equal to one per cent of the peak activity. When the dilution curve is double peaked, the total area must be employed since the height of the final equilibrium plateau is derived from activity emanating from both the right and left halves of the heart.

The contribution of the right heart curve to the total area is first found by extrapolating the exponential down-slope of the right heart peak (Fig. 6.6). Subtracting the amplitudes of the right heart curve from that of the total curve gives the curve due to the left heart only. For both the right and left heart curves the mean transit time 't' is calculated from the expression $t = \Sigma C_n t_n dt/\Sigma C_n dt$. In practice dt is made one second so that commencing at the start of each curve the count rate is noted at 1, 2, 3 ... seconds up to the end of the curve. The calculation of the mean transit time is discussed by Hamilton and Zierler. Let t_L and t_R be the values of the mean transit times for the right and left heart curves, then $(t_L - t_R)$ is the central mean transit time (CMTT). The central blood volume (CBV) is given by the product of the cardiac output in litres per minute and the CMTT in minutes. When a distinct dip occurs between the right and left heart peaks of the radiocardiogram, the dip is likely to coincide with the peak of radioactivity in the lungs. A more accurate approach is to inject a mixture of RISA labelled with I-131 and I-125 and to obtain a lung curve with a second scintillation counter mounted over the lungs and the associated pulse height analyser set to pick up the weaker gamma radiation emitted by I-125. The CMTT can now be divided into arterial (right-heart peak-to-lung peak) and venous (lung peak-to-left heart peak) portions. In patients with severe heart disease and whose radiocardiograms are flattened in appearance (Fig. 6.7) this technique can only be performed if a separate I-125 lung curve is available. The ratio A/H is a useful parameter where 'H' is the activity expressed in counts per minute per litre of blood recorded by the counter over the heart and 'A' is the area of the total dilution curve, expressed in counts per minute per litre of blood × seconds. Another useful parameter is the ratio CMTT/cardiac output. Johnson showed that in patients with normal hearts this has a value of less than unity.

A compartmental analysis should be performed on the radiocardiogram, as described by Valentinuzzi and Hill. The build-up time t_{pR} and peak concentration C_{pR} are noted. The circulation lying between the sites of injection and detection is assumed to consist of N identical compartments connected in series. Each is assumed to have the same time constant and to be perfused with the same volume flow. The conventional Stewart-Hamilton formula for cardiac output is modified to give $\dot{Q} = (m \times 60 \times \alpha)/(C_{pR} \times t_{pR})$ where C_{pR} is the peak activity of the right heart curve and t_{pR} is the build-up time for that curve. A knowledge of the other terms in that equation allows α to be calculated and a value for N found. Figure 6.8 shows the relationship between N and α_N. The value of α for N = 1 was extrapolated by iteration based upon successive ratios of N and the assumption that these ratios tend towards a constant value. The expression for the calculation of N is $\alpha_N = [1/(N-2)!] \, (N-1) \, (N^{-1}) \, \exp[-(N-1)]$. Since this expression only has meaning for integer values of N, adjacent points were joined by straight lines to allow for interpolation. A similar procedure is adopted for the left heart, but now the build-up time for the left heart peak is taken as (t_{PL} −CMTT).

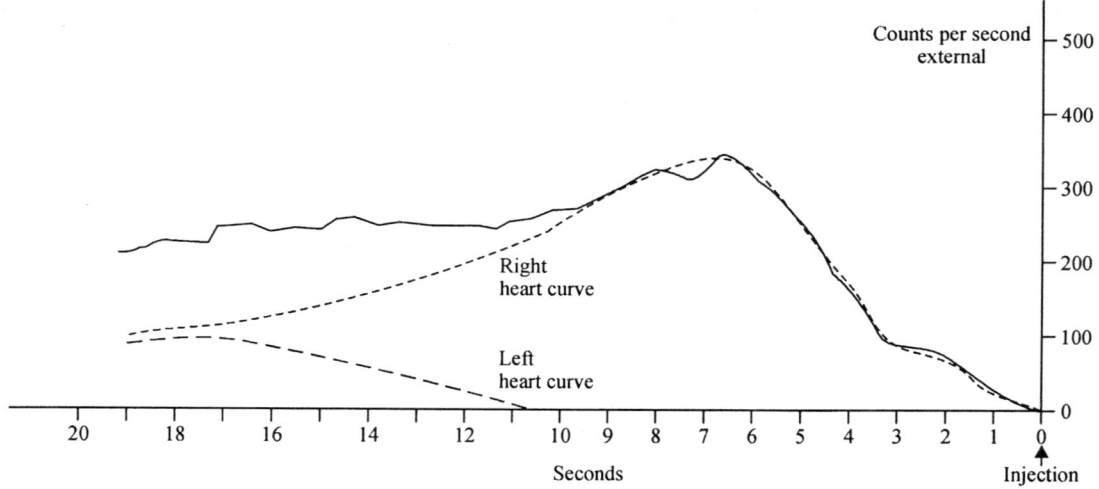

Fig. 6.7. The radiocardiogram of a patient in partially compensated left ventricular failure.

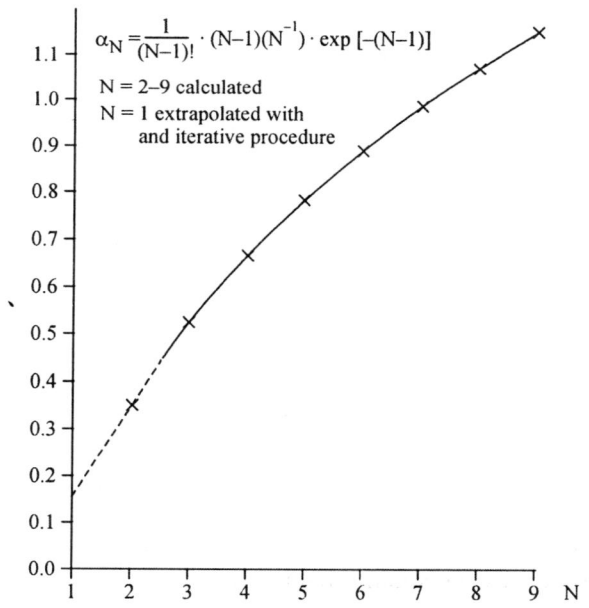

Fig. 6.8. The variation of αN with N for integer values of N

$$\alpha_N = \frac{1}{(N-2)!}(N-1)(N^{-1})\exp[-(N-1)]$$

N = 2 to 9 calculated, N = 1 extrapolated with an iterative procedure.

Preferably, a two channel recorder should be used, one channel recording the radiocardiogram and the other giving an indication of each heart beat from an ECG or peripheral pulse recording. From a knowledge of time of occurrence of each contraction of the heart it is possible to calculate a better estimate of the pulmonary blood volume (PBV) rather than only the CBV. The CBV includes contributions from both the right and left heart as well as lungs. Assuming that the right heart curve has an exponential downslope, a constant fraction R of the blood volume in the right ventricle will be expelled per beat as the stroke volume. Knowing this fraction from the right heart curve and the stroke volume SV enables the volume which filled the ventricle to be calculated, i.e., the right ventricular end-diastolic volume (VDV). Thus VDV = SV/R. The ventricular residual volume remaining after injection (VRV) is given by VRV = VDV – SV.

The patient whose radiocardiogram is shown in Fig. 6.6 had a cardiac output of 5.1 litres per minute, a CMTT of 5.2 seconds, a CBV of 439 ml, CMTT/$\dot{Q}$ = 1.01, a venous fraction of 49 per cent, 3.5 compartments for the right heart and 2.7 for the left heart, an A/H of 37.1, a body surface area of 1.61 m^2, a heart rate of 74.1 beats per minute, a stroke volume of 69 ml, a blood pressure of 130/75, a total peripheral resistance of 0.018 PRU, a pulmonary blood volume of 268 ml, an ejection fraction of 0.19, a ventricular diastolic volume of 370 ml and a ventricular residual volume of 301 ml.

If absolute values of cardiac output are required, rather than changes in output, it is desirable that the values obtained from the particular apparatus be compared with simultaneous measurements obtained using the Fick method or indocyanine green dye. The evidence in the literature is conflicting. For example, Uhrenholdt found that the radio-isotope method always read higher than the dye dilution method (mean difference 18.3 per cent range +6.6 to +35.2 per cent). The correlation coefficient was 0.877 and the regression equation $\dot{Q}_{RISA} = \dot{Q}_{dye} \times 0.986 + 1.280$. In contrast, Lorimer found identical means, a correlation coefficient of 0.94 and a regression equation of $\dot{Q}_{RISA} = \dot{Q}_{dye} + 0.89 \times 0.42$.

Use of cool saline as the indicator

In the thermal dilution method, a bolus of cool saline is used as an indicator. In this case the indicator is colloquially known as 'coolth' (negative heat). Lowe showed that when a bolus of cooled indocyanine green dye was injected there was no systematic difference between the area under the curves of dye concentration and blood temperature against time as recorded in the aorta of a dog, the injection being made into the right atrium. The dye curve reached its peak earlier and its down-slope was steeper than that of the thermal dilution curve. These findings arise from the fact that the thermal indicator does in practice leave the circulation and is initially distributed in an unknown proportion to the heart blood vessels and lung parenchyma. It returns from these structures to the blood when the temperature gradient which has been established becomes reversed as blood at normal temperatures flows past again. The advantages of the thermal dilution techniques are that the cool saline is inexpensive and no re-circulation peak occurs since during the second pass through the circulation the indicator warms up to body temperature.

Lowe states that the major problem in the determination of cardiac output by thermal dilution is due to uncertainty over how much of the coolth injected takes part in the dilution curve. As much as one-half can be lost to the atrial catheter and its surrounding blood. The loss can be reduced to less than two per cent by making a rapid injection through a catheter which has low thermal capacity and thermal conductivity together with a small dead space. Lowe recommends for use in man a concentric tube catheter with each polythene tube separated by an air space. With an inner tube diameter of 1 mm, Lowe could inject 10 ml of cooled saline by hand through a 40 cm long catheter in less than two seconds. Another major advantage of the thermal dilution techniques lies in its application to serial cardiac output determinations since five to ten serial measurements can be made.

Adequate mixing can be obtained by interposing just one heart chamber between the sites of injection and detection. For example, the coolth can be injected into the right ventricle and detected in the pulmonary artery, the two catheters being passed via the neck. One design of injection catheter for adults is thin-walled and 80 cm long with an internal diameter of 2.24 mm and an external diameter of 3.33 mm. The tip is closed but there are six side openings at the end which ensures an almost complete mixing of the coolth with the blood. It has been shown that with this arrangement the temperature achieved at the catheter tip is virtually independent of the volume of coolth injected. Detection is by means of a thermistor bead located at the tip of a catheter placed in the pulmonary artery. Prior to the injection, blood is drawn through this detection catheter for four seconds in order to warm up to body temperature the portion of the catheter situated outside the body. After this, saline at 0.5°C is injected as rapidly as possible. A 4 ml injectate is usual for normal hearts and this is increased to 8 ml for hearts which are substantially dilated. Following the injection, if another is to be made soon after, 4 ml of blood is drawn through the sampling catheter to re-warm it. Once the cooled blood has returned to body temperature which takes about 5 to 8 seconds, a further injection of coolth may be made.

In one commercial arrangement, the detection thermistor has a resistance of approximately 1100 ohms at 37°C and a sensitivity of about 30 ohms per °C. It forms one arm of a Wheatstone bridge, the output of which is taken via a DC amplifier to the chart recorder, whose speed is normally 10 mm per second. A typical sensitivity would be 1 cm for a 0.1°C change from body temperature.

The cardiac output measured by thermal dilution is given by:

$$\dot{Q} = \frac{V(t_1 - t_2)d_1 s_1 \times 60}{A \times K \times S \times d_2 \times s_2} \text{ litres per minute,}$$

where,

V	is the volume in ml of the cool saline injected
t_1	is the temperature of the blood in the pulmonary artery measured on the recorder
C_2	is the temperature of the saline at the tip of the injection catheter (7.4°C for a Lehman No.10 catheter and a saline volume of 4.13 ml with a body temperature of 37°C)
d_1	the density of the saline solution (1.005 gram per ml)
d_2	is the density of the blood in gram per ml
s_1	is the specific heat of the saline solution (0.997 cal per gram)
s_2	is the specific heat of the blood (cal per gram)
A	is the area under the thermal dilution curve in mm^2
K	is the temperature calibration factor of the recorder (°C per mm)
S	is the chart speed in mm per second

Both the specific heat and the density of blood are haematocrit dependent as follows:

Haematocrit %	Specific heat calories per gram	Density grams per ml
30	0.89	1.049
35	0.88	1.053
40	0.87	1.058
45	0.865	1.061
50	0.86	1.064
55	0.85	1.068
60	0.84	1.073

A critical account of the factors which affect the accuracy of the thermal dilution technique is given by Wilson, particularly in regard to serial determinations performed over prolonged periods. Because there is no re-circulation peak, the measurement of the area under the curve by integration is easy and this lends itself to analogue computation.

Estimation of Cardiac Output from Thoracic Electrical Impedance Changes

Kubicek showed how, in patients with normal chests and hearts, it was possible to estimate the stroke volume and hence cardiac output indirectly from observations of the diminution in the thoracic electrical impedance accompanying each systole. In Kubicek's technique, two current and two voltage strip electrodes are applied to the patient's thorax as shown in Fig. 6.9. The electrodes are disposable, each consisting of a 0.25 inch (6.4 mm) wide aluminium band backed by an adhesive plastic strip.

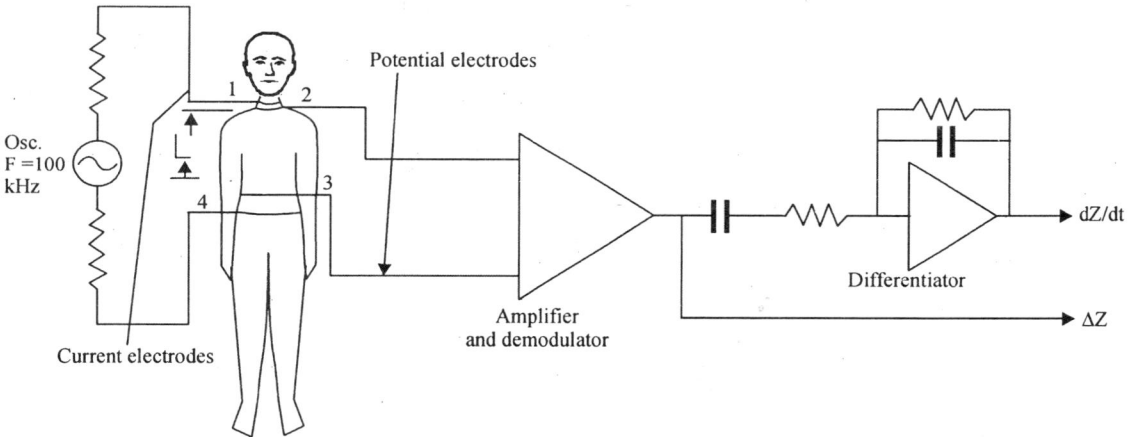

Fig. 6.9. Four electrode arrangement for the non-invasive measurement of cardiac output by the electrical impedance technique.

The upper two electrodes are placed around the neck with a spacing of not less than 20 mm. Electrode No. 3 is located at the level of the xiphisternal joint with electrode No. 420 mm below. Electrodes 1 and 4 are supplied with approximately 4 mA rms at 100 kHz from a constant current source. The voltage variations accompanying each systole are picked-up at electrodes 2 and 3 amplified and demodulated. The standing voltages arising from the thoracic electrical impedance Z_0 is backed-off and the impedance change ΔZ occurring with each systole is displayed on a chart recorder. A differentiating circuit is provided to give a voltage proportional to dZ/dt. It is also very convenient to have another channel on the recorder available to show the patient's phonocardiogram. A fourth channel can display the electrocardiogram. If only a two channel recorder is available, dZ/dt would be recorded on one channel and the other used to record alternatively the phonocardiogram and ECG. A typical recording is shown in Fig. 6.10. The impedance change ΔZ is somewhat similar in form to an arterial blood pressure recording. Kubicek base his calculation for stroke volume upon the well-known formula for specific resistance (resistivity) $p = RA/L$ or $R = pL/A$ where R is the resistance in ohms of the material having a resistivity of p ohm-cm, a length of L cm and a cross-sectional area of A cm^2. Thus $R = pL/A = (pL/A) \times (L/L) = pL^2/AL$, but $AL = V$ the volume of a cylinder if the volume is taken as a cylindrical conductor of homogeneous material and uniform current density distribution. Differentiating R with respect to V, $dR/dV = pL^2/V^2$ or $dR = -p(L^2/V^2)dV$.

Since $R = pL^2/V$, $dR = p(R^2/L^2)dV$ and $dV = -p(L^2/R^2)dR$. For a specified material and size of cylinder, $-p(L^2R^2)$ is a constant $= K$ so that $dV = KdR$, i.e., the change in resistance is directly proportional to the change in volume. So far the discussion has centred around resistance which implies DC conditions. In the general case, the modulus of the impedance is substituted for R so that $dV = p(L^2/Z^2)dZ$. In order to use this expression for the calculation of stroke volume the various terms are expressed as follows:

- dV   is the stroke volume in ml
- p   is the haematocrit of the patient's blood. If the haematocrit is unknown but can be taken as normal, a typical value is 150 ohm-cm.
- L   is the distance between the two potential electrodes (2 and 3 in Fig. 6.9) in cm.
- Z   is taken as Z_0 the impedance in ohms existing between the potential electrodes immediately prior to the rapid decrease in impedance which accompanies ventricular systole.
- dZ   is the diminution in impedance in ohms associated with the stroke volume.

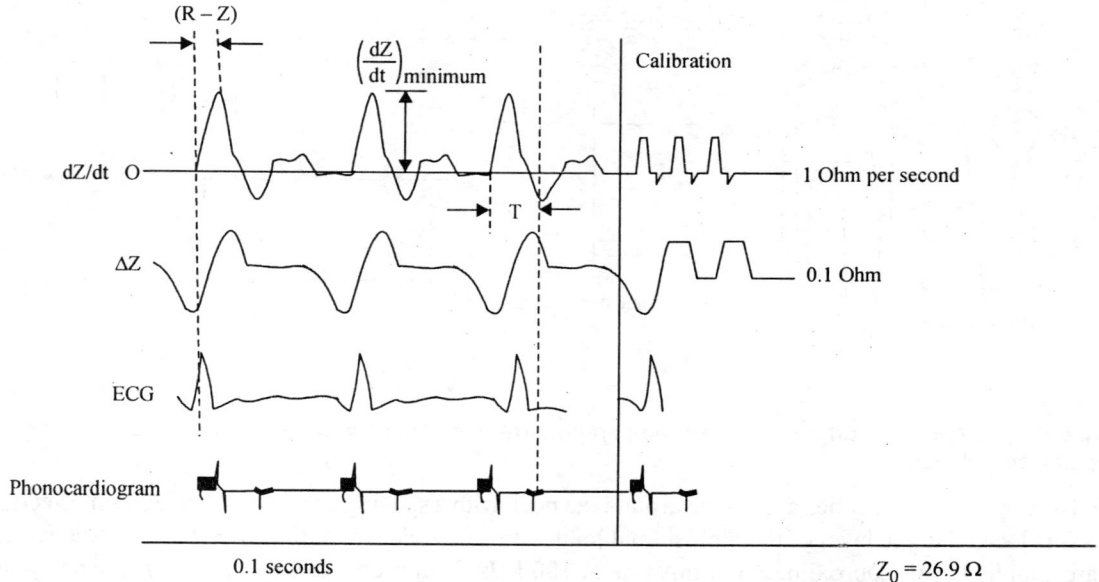

Fig. 6.10. The use of the second heart sound to locate the end of ventricular ejection in the calculation of stroke volume by the electrical impedance method.

The interpretation of dZ requires some consideration. Dealing with peripheral arteries, Nyboer showed that the impedance change observed was related to a change in blood volume in the segment of artery considered. Thus the impedance changes observed across the thorax with each heart beat are taken as corresponding with the difference in blood flow into and out of the thorax. It is also assumed that when ventricular contraction occurs and the aortic and pulmonic valves open, blood is ejected into the aorta so rapidly that the rate of ejection is established before any significant degree of arterial run-off has occurred (loss of blood from the thorax). In this case, multiplication of the initial rate of change of the impedance with time by the time interval during which the two output valves are open should represent the impedance change which would have occurred if there had been no arterial run-off. This change would be proportional to the stroke volume. The maximum rate of the change of the impedance waveform can simply be located by observing the output of the differentiating circuit calibrated in ohms per second and fed with the impedance waveform from the pick-up electrodes. The maximum rate of the change (dz/dt_{max}) of the impedance waveform in ohms per second in then multiplied by a time interval 'T' derived from the impedance rate of the change waveform and a phonocardiogram. The start of the interval 'T' is taken from when the up-slope of the main dZ/dt peak crosses the baseline $(dZ/dt = 0)$ to the onset of the second heart sound. In many patients, but not all, the occurrence of the second heart sound coincides with the appearance of the distinct notch in the dZ/dt waveform. The formula for stroke volume is $SV = (- pL^2/Z_0^2) T (dZ/dt)_{max}$. During systole, Z_0 decreases so that $(dZ/dt)_{max}$ has a negative value thus making the stroke volume SV positive.

An alternative derivation of the stroke volume equation can be obtained by considering that at end-diastole the blood in the thorax has a resistance R_0. Consequent upon systole an additional resistance r due to the stroke volume expelled from the heart is placed in parallel with R_0. The rapid ejection of the stroke volume gives rise to the sudden fall seen in R_0 with each systole. If R_{min} is the equivalent resistance of R_0 and r in parallel then $1/R_{min} = 1/R_0 + 1/r$ so that $r = (R_0 R_{min})/(R_0 - R_{min})$. Since R_0 and R_{min} will differ by only about 0.4 per cent we can take R_0 and R_{min} as being approximately equal. Hence $r = R_0^2/(R_0 - R_{min})$ $= R_0^2/\Delta R$. Assuming that both the volumes of blood corresponding with R_0 and r can be represented as uniform conductors having a length L and cross-sectional areas 'A' and 'a' respectively, then $r = pL/a$ where p is the resistivity of blood, so that the volume change accompanying systole is $L \cdot a = pL^2/r$. This volume change is the stroke volume so that $SV = pL^2/r = pL^2 \Delta R/R_0^2$. In the general case Z_0 is substituted for R_0 and $(T \times dZ/dt_{max})$ for ΔR where T is the ejection time and dZ/dt_{max} is the maximum value of dZ/dt. As before the expression for stroke volume becomes $SV = (- pL^2/Z_0^2)T(dZ/dt)_{max}$.

The ΔZ waveform is markedly affected by respiratory thoracic movements and hence it is simpler to work from the dZ/dt waveform. Because of the circuitry's shorter time constant it is frequently feasible to measure $(dZ/dt)_{max}$ in the presence of spontaneous or assisted respiration which is not very vigorous. The best reproducibility is obtainable by measuring $(dZ/dt)_{max}$ close to the end of the expiration. It may be required in an intensive care unit to follow changes in a patient's cardiac output consequent upon increments of exercise, perhaps a two-step test. After the required number of steps, the patient should be asked to hold his breath for about 5 heart beats whilst a recording is made. If a two-channel recorder is available, the dZ/dt waveform should be recorded with the ECG and then with the phonocardiogram. The record should also contain a one ohm per second dZ/dt calibration signal. If the patient is anaesthetised but making excessively vigorous spontaneous respiratory movements, the anaesthetist can render the patient apnoeic for a short period by squeezing the re-breathing bag to over-ventilate the patient and reduce his arterial carbon dioxide tension. On the other hand, if the patient is connected to an automatic lung ventilator, this can usually be turned off for about one minute whilst the recording is made.

Accuracy of cardiac output determinations by the electrical impedance technique

The impedance method for cardiac output measurement is essentially a beat-by-beat method and for this reason a comparison with methods such as the Fick and dye dilution is not easy as these give a cardiac output averaged over perhaps 20 beats. In 20 children without shunts or valvular insufficiency, Lababidi found a 5.5 per cent mean difference between impedance and dye dilution cardiac output values with the impedance mean being greater than the dye dilution mean. Sova found a correlation of 0.78 for 20 comparisons of the impedance and dye dilution methods in normal patients. He found a correlation of 0.80 in 9 heart disease patients at rest and this increased to 0.95 in these patients after exercise.

Patients with pulmonary oedema or who have inhaled vomit will have values of the thoracic impedance Z_0 markedly less than 20 ohms and the cardiac output values obtained from the impedance traces are likely to be in error. In patients with normal values of Z_0 (20 to 30 ohms in adults) and without valvular incompetance or marked degrees of arrhythmia, the impedance method is very reproducible and is of great use in indicating trends in a patient's condition. It can, for example, be valuable in guiding the adjustment of an isoprenaline drip. In many situations, within limits, a knowledge of the absolute value of the cardiac output can be of smaller significance than a knowledge of changes occurring in the cardiac output.

The value of the stroke volume in ml calculated using the impedance method is directly proportional to the patient's haematocrit. Geddes and Sadler have found a best-fit equation relating the specific resistance in ohm-cm of human blood to the percentage haematocrit H. This is $p = 53.2 \exp(0.022H)$. On this basis the value of $p = 150$ ohm-cm which is often used corresponds with a 47 per cent haematocrit. The values for 40, 30 and 20 per cent are respectively 128, 103 and 83. This represents a very significant correction, for example, in the case of renal dialysis patients who often have haematocrit values of 20 and 30 per cent. The following tables shows the magnitude of the change found when using the calculated resistivity instead of a nominal 150 ohm-cm:

Radioisotope cardiac output	Impedance cardiac output	Impedance cardiac output
4.68 L/minute	7.23 (p = 150) L/minute	4.22 (p = 90.2, Hct = 24 per cent) L/minute
4.51	7.95	4.38 (p = 90.2, Hct = 24 per cent)
6.95	8.06	7.36 (p = 137, Hct = 43 per cent)
8.90	14.6	8.0 (p = 83.6, Hct = 20 per cent)

It should be remembered, that whilst the non-invasive nature and convenience of use makes the impedance method attractive for monitoring cardiac output changes, the method is indirect and cannot be specific in regard to cardiac action. The basic formula is unlikely to apply to patients with pathology of the heart and thorax. A more complicated equation would be required which took into account possible redistributions of blood within the thorax. Under some circumstances, the dZ/dt peak at systole may not be well pronounced or may become bifurcated. The usual calculation for stroke volume cannot then be used.

Use of the electrical impedance technique to monitor changes in myocardial contractility

Siegel found a correlation of 0.88 between the time interval from the preceding R-wave of the ECG and the occurrence of $(dZ/dt)_{max}$ and the interval from the preceding R-wave to the maximum rate of change of left ventricular pressure $(dP_{LV})_{max}$. The reciprocal of the latter is known to be a function of the state of contractility of the myocardium.

Denote the time from the R-wave to $(dZ/dt)_{max}$ by T_{R-Z}. Dr. Loren Heather of Minneapolis has suggested that a more sensitive index of the contractility would be $(dZ/dt)_{max}/T_{R-Z}$ where $(dZ/dt)_{max}$ is in ohms per second and T_{R-Z} in seconds. Thus for a patient whose myocardium is in a good contractile state $(dZ/dt)_{max}$ might be 3.5 and T_{R-Z} 0.108 giving a Heather index of 32.4. Whereas for a patient with some degree of heart failure and a poorly contracting myocardium, the Heather index might be of the order of 16 to 19.

Use of transthoracic impedance measurement to monitor for the detection of pulmonary oedema

Pomerantz has shown that the monitoring of Z_0 provides a useful guide to intrathoracic fluid volumes. In one patient with a pleural effusion, the value of Z_0 rose by 1 ohm for each 200 ml of fluid removed. In two cases of respiratory distress syndrome Z_0 was less than 19–20 ohms. In dogs Pomerantz showed that

Z_0 changed by as much as 45 minutes before changes were detected in the central venous pressure, pulmonary complicance, arterial blood pressure or blood-gas values. They also found in cardiac by-pass patients that the post-operative value of Z_0 was lower than the pre-operative value. Over the subsequent 7 to 10 days Z_0 rose to above its pre-operative level as the patient's cardiopulmonary dynamics improved. Van de Water also found the monitoring of Z_0 to be of value in the management of thoracic surgery patients. Hill has measured a Z_0 of 4.5 ohms in a patient who had inhaled vomit. After automatic lung ventilation with a positive end-expiratory pressure for some days, Z_0 attained a value of 30 ohms and the patient's chest radiograph was clear. The simple measurement of Z_0 may well be a useful technique in the management of patients with the 'shocked lung' syndrome. Luepker has shown a quantitative relationship in dogs between Z_0 and thoracic fluid volume.

Estimation of Left Ventricular Work and Total Systemic Resistance

If the cardiac output and mean arterial blood pressure are known, it is possible to derive a value for the left ventricular work. Strictly speaking, the mean aortic pressure should be used, but for patient monitoring purposes it is only the systemic peripheral arterial pressure which is available.

Work is expressed as the product of force × distance and the unit of work on the SI system is the Joule or meter-Newton. It is the work done when the force of 1 Newton moves its point of application through a distance of 1 meter, (1 Newton will give a mass of k kg an acceleration of 1 m per second per second). Power is the rate of doing work and 1 Watt equals one joule per second. In order to be able to link the work done by the heart with the cardiac output it is convenient to calculate the power developed by the left heart in watts. Taking the density of mercury as 13.6 gram per cc., the power in watts is given by $0.0022 \times P \times \dot{Q}$ where P is the mean arterial pressure in mm Hg and $\dot{Q}$ is the cardiac output in litres per minute. If P = 100 mm Hg and Q = 5 litres per minute then the power developed by the left heart = 1.1 watts.

Using a hydraulic version of Ohm's law the ratio (Pressure drop across the heart)/cardiac output = total systemic resistance. This is often called the total peripheral resistance since the bulk of the resistance to blood flow resides in the periphery. The pressure used in the calculation is strictly (mean aortic pressure– –right atrial pressure) but for monitoring purposes if the patient is not markedly hypotensive it is taken simply as the mean arterial blood pressure. By expressing the cardiac output in ml per minute and the pressure in mm Hg the result is given in PRU (peripheral resistance units). For a cardiac output of 5000 ml per minute and a mean arterial blood pressure of 100 mm Hg, the total peripheral resistance would be 100/5000 = 0.02 PRU.

In the intensive care situation, it is convenient to have a set of nomograms which will give the patient's body surface area in order to be able to calculate the cardiac index (Q/body surface area), the left ventricular stroke work and the total peripheral resistance. Body surface area is usually calculated from the formula of Dubois which relates body surface area to the patient's height and weight, i.e., BSA = $W^{0.425} + H^{0.725} \times 71.84$ where BSA is in m^2, W is in Kg and H is in cm. Mitchell have shown that using a photometric technique to measure body surface area directly, the measured results showed a good correlation (0.97) with the values calculated from the Dubois formula, but the Dubois values were systematically lower than the measured values. Their regression equation was: measured body surface area in m^2 = +0.945 Dubois area (m^2) + 0.208 for predicted areas within the range 1.3 to 2.1 m^2.

Origins of the Impedance Changes Associated with Cardiac Activity

The sudden diminution in thoracic impedance which occurs with each systole has been related by Karnegis and Kubieck to other events in the cardiac cycle by comparing the dZ/dt waveform with a lead 2 ECG and the left ventricular pressure waveform. Lababidi have correlated the dZ/dt waveform with the phonocardiogram. The origin of the impedance changes is complicated and cannot be ascribed to a single event such as ejection from the left ventricle, this has been confirmed in a comprehensive investigation in dogs by Kubicek. The contribution to the signal from the right heart, pulmonary circulation and volume changes in the aorta have yet to be clarified. Geddes and Baker showed that in dogs the impedance method over-estimated because of a significant contribution from the right heart, but this is not necessarily the case in man. Comparison of the impedance method in patients with the radio-cardiogram technique has revealed that the impedance results are consistently lower than the isotope results which are likely to over-estimate because of the contribution from paracardiac tissues.

Pulse contour methods for monitoring stroke volume changes

Many attempts have been made to be able to deduce changes in the stroke volume from accompanying changes in the arterial blood pressure waveform. At its simplest, many physicians feel happy when they observe a good pulse pressure (systolic-diastolic pressure). Herd showed that the difference between the mean pressure and the end-diastolic pressure measured in the ascending aorta of dogs provided a useful index of stroke volume over the range 50 to 150 per cent of the control cardiac output. A calibration factor was obtained by using dye dilution to measure the cardiac output. Although a peripheral arterial pressure can be used, the greatest accuracy will be obtainable with a central pressure. Herd found that the scatter of their data points was about twice as much using the femoral artery pressure as was found when using the aortic pressure close to the heart.

Warner proposed an index of stroke volume based upon measurement of the central aortic pressure. The equation is $SV = K \cdot P_{md} (1 + S_a/D_a)$ where SV is the stroke volume in ml, K is a constant, S_a is the systolic pressure area (the mean pressure which acts at the periphery of the arterial bed during systole multiplied by the duration of systole) and D_A is the diastolic pressure area (the mean pressure at the periphery during diastole multiplied by the duration of diastole). Let U be the total volume of blood in all arteries extending from the aortic arch to the arterioles at the end of systole minus the volume of this arterial bed at the end of the previous diastole. As no blood will enter the aorta from the left ventricle during diastole, the diastolic drainage will equal this volume increment of the arterial bed which is present at the end of systole. The corresponding increment in mean pressure between the end of diastole and the end of systole, multiplied by a constant, will be equal to the volume increment, i.e., $U = K \cdot P_{md}$.

In order to estimate P_{md} from the central aortic pressure, the time of transmission of the pulse wave from the aorta to the periphery of the arterial tree must be taken into account. As it is impossible to measure the transmission times from the aorta to each point in the periphery and calculate their mean, the time is measured between two sites such as aorta to femoral artery or brachial to radial arteries and multiplying this by a constant chosen to give a reasonable value for the mean time of transmission in the resting, supine, position (100 to 110 ms). The ratio S_a/D_a and P_{md} can now be determined from the central aortic pressure waveform. A calibration constant can be found by performing a dye dilution cardiac output.

Warner has used the method for following stroke volume changes with an on-line digital computer patient monitoring system. However, Kouchoukos has shown that the constant of proportionality relating stroke volume to the contour of the aortic pressure pulse is dependent on both the pulse wave velocity and the radii of the proximal large arteries. Hence Warner's method will be affected by interventions or drugs which give rise to pulse wave reflections in the aorta or changes in the tone of the vessels. Kouchoukos used the formula $SV = K \cdot P_{sa}(1 + T_s/T_d)$ where K is a constant, P_{sa} is the area lying under the systolic portion of the aortic pressure curve above end-diastole, T_s is the duration of systole and T_d is the duration of diastole. Nicholls deduced that the constant of proportionality between the stroke volume and the systolic area of the aortic pressure curve would depend on the of value of the total peripheral resistance, i.e., $SV = K(P_{sa}/R)$ where R is determined from a dye cardiac output and the mean aortic pressure. Another stroke volume formula is that of Guier which is claimed to be valid also for ectopic beats. Baker compared the stroke volume changes in dogs having a sinus rhythm with the P_{sa} alone and the formulae of Kouchoukos, Nicholls and Guier. There was little to choose between them, all producing a correlation coefficient of about 0.89. All these approximations are liable to give erroneous result if the patient is receiving catecholamines and other sympathomimetic drugs which might be conducive to the formation of reflected waves in the aorta. From the viewpoint of implementing the simplest version of on-line computer monitoring, it would seem to be worthwhile just monitoring the systolic area changes.

Direct monitoring of stroke volume and cardiac output by means of an extractable blood flow probe

The development of a flexible electromagnetic blood flow probe which can be fixed in place around the aorta with a snare during thoracic surgery and subsequently left in place for several days has opened up the possibility of the direct measurement of stroke volume on a beat-by-beat basis. The electromagnet, soft iron core and collecting electrodes are located inside a silicone rubber housing of uniform cross-sectional area. This can be sterilised in ethylene oxide gas. The housing is sufficiently flexible that it will assume an almost straight configuration under traction. The snare is brought outside the chest alongside the probe cable. Fixation of both is achieved with ordinary skin sutures. Removal of the fixing snare allows the probe to straighten and it can then be withdrawn from the patient by gentle traction upon the cable. In use the probe coil is fed with a sinewave current at a frequency of several hundred hertz. The interaction of the magnetic field from the coil with the flowing blood stream generates an electrical signal in a plane which is mutually perpendicular to the planes of the field and the direction of blood flow. The signal is picked up from a pair of electrodes in contact with the vessel wall. Its amplitude is proportional to the blood velocity and its sign corresponds the direction of blood flow. By integrating the flow signal, the stroke volume is obtained. Multiplication by the heart rate gives the cardiac output.

BEDSIDE AND PORTABLE MONITORS

Bedside monitors are electronic instrument packages used to keep track of certain patient parameters and to sound alarms or take other action should one of these parameters go outside certain pre-determined limits. Their purpose is to provide—on a continuous basis—medical data that is normally difficult to obtain. They also free the nursing staff for more pressing duties.

Bedside monitors are usually found in intensive care units, coronary care units, operating rooms, emergency rooms and certain other special or critical care areas of the hospital. Portable monitors are found in all of these places as well as in crash carts, ambulances and other places where critical care may have to be render in an emergency but where there is no convenient source of AC power.

These units are manufactured by the medical division of Hewlett-Packard and are good examples of the modular approach. On this model the user can select a channel (channel 1, channel 2 or both at the same time) and position its beam vertically on the CRT screen.

One interesting feature on this instrument is that each channel is provided with two parallel-connected input jacks so that signals can be simultaneously fed to the oscilloscope and routed to other instruments, such as a strip chart recorder, in a 'daisy chain' manner. If the oscilloscope is used for ECG, as is frequently the case, the alternate jack on the oscilloscope's ECG channel might also be sent to a defibrillator's synchronisation input for use in cardioversion procedures. Both modules of this instrument can be unlocked and easily removed for servicing or re-configuring the mainframe with another instrument or pair of instruments. The ECG pre-amplifier is a three-lead design and has a built-in heart rate meter and alarm capability. The alarms can be set to certain high and low limits, using the slide scale located immediately below the digital readout of the heart rate meter (also called a cardiotachometer by some people). If the patient's heart rate, which is electronically derived from the ECG signal, exceeds the preset limits, then the alarm will trip. On this particular instrument, high or low panel lights will come on and a terminal connector on the rear panel will be grounded. In this manner, remote alarms can also be triggered easily.

The criterium for triggering the alarms is the heart rate. This is determined by either counting the patient's R-waves over a certain period of time and then multiplying by a factor to obtain beats per minute or by determining the R-to-R time interval, taking the reciprocal and multiplying by the appropriate scale factor to obtain the heart rate in beats per minute. In both systems, artifacts can affect the cardiotach and erroneously push the counted rate over the limit to sound a false alarm. Some electronic pacemakers occasionally used on patient's with certain heart diseases can create a pulse or spike on the ECG waveform. This pulse is often interpreted by the cardiotach as an additional R-wave. In such cases, the heart rate meter reading will be almost precisely twice the normal or correct reading taken by the manual methods.

It is sometimes possible to eliminate 'falsing' by lowering the gain of the ECG pre-amplifier. Whenever you examine a false alarm situation, look first to the ECG display and determine if it is of excessive amplitude. If it is high, then back-off on the pre-amplifier gain and note whether or not the 'falsing' ceases or lessens in severity. Some patients have ECG waveforms that are responsible for fooling the cardiotach and these cannot be helped in any substantial manner. If one of the other wave features is the same height as the R-wave, then some falsing might occur. If the monitor uses a lead selector switch, try going to another lead; if none is used, reposition the electrodes on the patient. There are certain electronic circuit defects that can also cause this problem and these will be covered later in this chapter.

The bedside monitor of Fig. 6.11 is an arterial pressures module. This unit is equipped to calculate the diastolic and systolic arterial pressures, the mean pressure as derived from the arterial pressures and the venous pressure. A switch on the front panel selects which of these is to be displayed on the single digital readout. The arterial waveform developed in the carrier amplifier is available for display on the oscilloscope. Note that the pressures module is also equipped with limit alarms below the readout display.

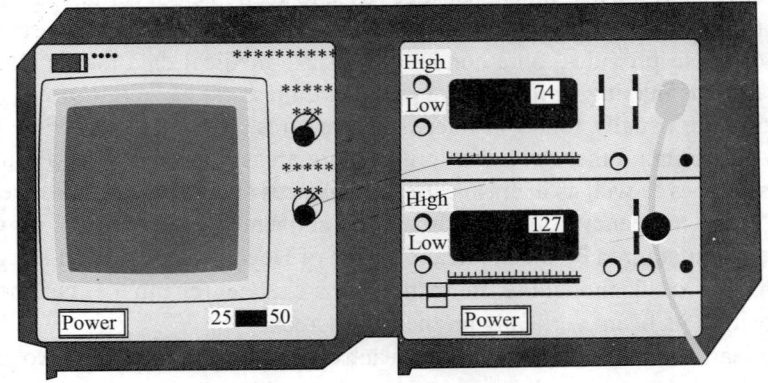

Fig. 6.11. Two-channel bedside patient monitor.

The bedside monitor (Fig. 6.12) represents an example of the 'integrated mainframe' approach to monitor system design. The ECG and pressures modules in this instrument are actually sub-assemblies (as was true in the Hewlett-Packard design) and they can be removed easily for servicing. In this case, however, they are in a common mainframe with the non-fade display medical oscilloscope and share a common AC on/off switch (lower right). The ECG pre-amplifier in this model is a full 12-lead type and also uses a digital readout for the heart rate meter.

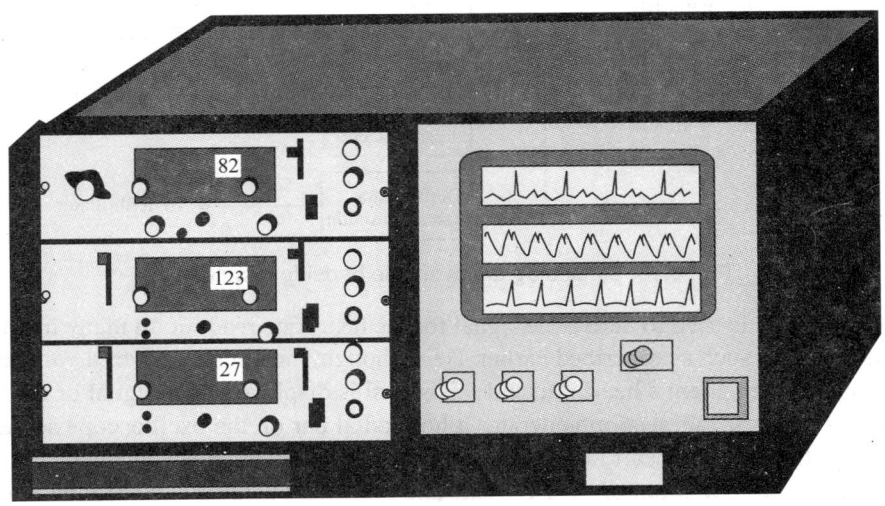

Fig. 6.12. Three-channel bedside patient monitor.

The PC boards are arranged by function (e.g., high-voltage power supply, low-voltage power supply, alarms, oscilloscope deflection amplifiers, etc.) so that even relatively inexperienced technicians with limited diagnostic acumen can return the instrument to service with only minimum down time. The approach even lends itself to repair by unskilled persons—on a limited basis, of course—through the use of step-by-step 'cookbook' troubleshooting procedures.

Typical Bedside Monitor Systems

A block diagram of a simple bedside monitor is shown in Fig. 6.13. Only ECG can be monitored in this example, but other monitors frequently include are arterial blood pressure amplifier or some other form of instrument along with the standard ECG. We have already discussed ECG pre-amplifiers to some extent and will expand on the theme in due course.

The purpose of the ECG pre-amplifier is to amplify or build up the 1.0 millivolt ECG signal acquired from the patient to a level around 1.0 volt (peak), which is compatible with the oscilloscope input requirements. It is the oscilloscope that is normally used for moment-to-moment monitoring, but if certain waveform features begin to appear or certain changes take place, the staff can easily make permanent records using the strip chart recorder. The defibrillator synchronisation block in the figure may or may not exist in any particular model. Its function is to supply an ECG signal to the defibrillator. In some cases, a monostable multivibrator (one-shot) is triggered by the R-wave and its output is fed to the defibrillator synchronisation circuit. In most cases, though, the defibrillator synchronisation signal is just the regular ECG signal buffered by some amplifier stage or resistor network.

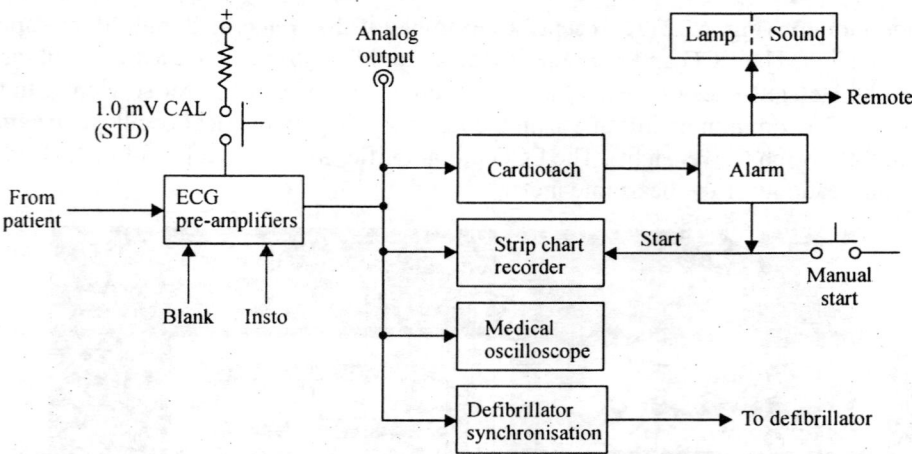

Fig. 6.13. Block diagram of simple bedside monitor.

The cardiotachometer is used to derive the signal for the heart rate readout. In many instruments this might be a special circuit such as described earlier. Here, though, the circuit derives a voltage or current that is proportional to the patient's heart rate and this signal is displayed on a digital or analog readout meter. In some instruments, this section generates a horizontal bar on the oscilloscope screen having a length that is proportional to the heart rate.

An alarm section is used to monitor the ECG rate and to let the operator know if it exceeds an upper limit or drops below a lower limit, both indications of potential trouble. Locally, the alarms generally turn on a lamp or possibly sound a tone. At the remote output connector there will be either a voltage level or more commonly, a grounded condition whenever an alarm situation is present. This output is used to turn on the alarm at the nurse's station or monitor desk. Alarms are also used to automatically start the strip chart recorder so that a permanent record can be made, latch an alarm light or possibly put a halt command into the control circuits of a tape recorder cardiac memory. Many bedside monitors use a non-latching alarm at bedside and a latching type at the central monitoring station. Others, such as the H-P, use a latching circuit in the bedside monitor but provide a special re-set line on the remote connector so that it is not necessary to go into the patient's room to re-set a false alarm. Most alarms will have a manual re-set.

ECG Pre-amplifiers

ECG pre-amplifiers used in bedside monitoring equipment, as well as in ECG machines, have changed quite a bit over the past few years. This metamorphosis was given a certain impetus by the advancing technology of electronics and by increased concerns over matters of patient safety. In the earliest instruments, such amplifiers were single ended, so the operators had to tolerate a large amount of 60 Hz interference. Once the differential amplifiers became known, its advantages soon became apparent and it was incorporated into ECG equipment design. In both cases, however, the common connection (patient's right leg) was made to the machine's chassis ground and this was connected to AC powerline ground. Obviously, this could open the patient to danger from 60 Hz leakage currents that always exist on the chassis of AC operated electrical equipment, especially if a ground fault occurred. In later designs, some of which are still seen in older but now obsolete systems, a 5 mA (1/200 ampere) fuse is connected in series with the right leg, common connection.

In newer ECG designs, a common-mode amplifier (called the right leg amplifier in ECG terminology) sums the signals from each of the two inputs of the differential pair and uses them to derive a common 'ground' line—actually the right-leg signal. This common-mode amplifier produced two extremely useful results. First, it improved the common-mode rejection characteristics of the differential amplifier enough to greatly improve rejection of 60 Hz power line interference. Secondly, it lifted the patient off chassis ground, thereby reducing the possibility of danger from stray leakage currents or catastrophic component failures within the amplifier itself. Make no mistake—those leakage currents, although small enough to seem harmless, can present a very large danger in certain medical contexts.

An intermediate step, before the use of common-mode amplifiers, used a resistor network to sum the common-mode signals, rather than an amplifier and such equipment is still in use at some places.

It is often the case that ECG cables are double shielded. The outer shield is terminated only at the machine end (the other end is left floating) where it is connected to chassis ground. The inner shield is concentric to the outer shield and is connected to the output of the common-mode amplifier and to the wire from the patient's right-leg electrode. This inner shield, whether used in ECG work or some other small signal application, is usually called the guard shield. Modern low-level and medium-level pre-amplifiers are usually fitted with input connectors designed to accommodate the guard shield.

The most recent style of ECG pre-amplifier design and the one still favoured for modern use, is the so-called isolated pre-amplifier.

In order to achieve this level of isolation, it is necessary that the DC power supply for the input stages of the pre-amplifier be completely separated from the normal DC power supplies used to power the remainder of the circuit. In the circuit this is accomplished by the use of an inverter/rectifier circuit. A two-transistor, 100 kHz, power oscillator obtains its DC power from the instrument's main power supply. The 100 kHz AC signal developed in this oscillator is fed via oscillator transformer T1 to the isolated portion of the pre-amplifier circuit, where DC power for those few stages in the isolated section is derived by rectifying this 100 kHz signal. The 100 kHz signal is also used to chop the ECG signal so that it can pass through modulation transformer T2 back to the main portion of the pre-amplifier. Both transformers, incidentally, are specially designed to pass ultrasonic AC signals in the 100 kHz range but to be very inefficient at 60 Hz. This is done to assist in the improvement of isolation to 60 Hz power line.

The insto circuit creates a short across the amplifier input in order to keep it from latching up during excessive input voltage conditions, such as will exist when a defibrillator is used on the patient. As a result, this keeps the baseline of the display constant so that the ECG waveform will return to view on the screen of the oscilloscope or on the strip chart recorder rapidly after the defibrillator is fired. In some cases, an insto switch is provided that must be manually pushed, but in other pre-amplifier designs, provision is made for an insto input pulse from the defibrillator. In either event, the insto circuit stabilises the baseline and prevents amplifier latch-up under high input-voltage conditions.

Cardiotachometers

A block diagram of cardiotach logic is shown in Fig. 6.14. ECG signals from the pre-amplifier output having a maximum amplitude of about 1 volt are fed to an absolute-value amplifier. This is a stage that produces a positive-going output signal, regardless of input signal polarity. If the input signal is already positive going, this transistor stage will pass the signal appearing at its emitter. (In the emitter-follower configuration, a transistor has an output that is in phase with its input.) If, on the other hand, the input signal is negative going, the circuit automatically passes the inverted version appearing normally at the collector of the transistor. Diodes in the collector and emitter circuits are used to prevent signals of incorrect polarity from appearing at the input of the stage following the absolute-value amplifier.

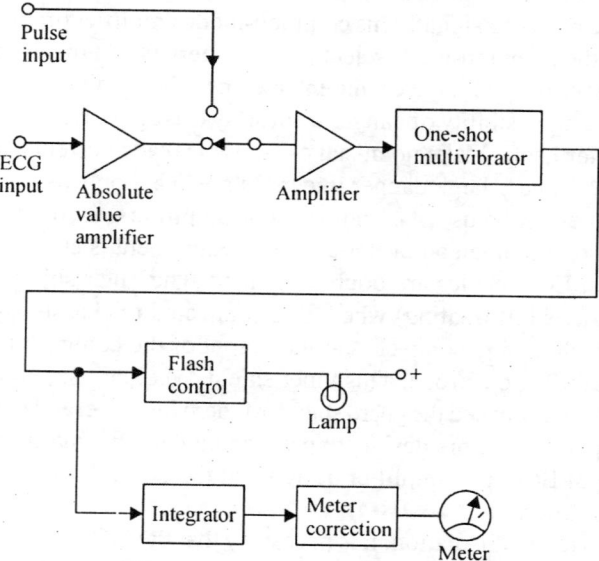

Fig. 6.14. Cardiotachometer block diagram.

A manual switch, in the line following this stage, allows the user to select, from the front panel of the instrument, whether an ECG signal or an alternate pulse input from a photoplethysmograph is to be used as the trigger signal for the cardiotachometer. The stage following the manual selector switch provides further amplification and its output is fed to the trigger point in a monostable multivibrator or one-shot.

The purpose of the one-shot is to generate one pulse of constant amplitude and duration (period) for each and every R-wave received from the ECG pre-amplifier. This, incidentally, is a very common technique that is used in many different types of medical and scientific instruments, since it permits the next stage, an integrator, to produce a DC level that is proportional to the frequency of the incoming signal. Some service manuals will call this integrator stage a low-pass filter, but that is substantially the samething.

If the one-shot was not used, if we merely integrated the incoming R-waves, we would just get erroneous values. The integrator's output is actually dependent upon the area underneath the patient's R-wave complex curve and this can vary considerably from one patient to the next and with the settings of the amplifier gain control. The one-shot is used to normalise the signal for a wide range of input conditions.

The one-shot is also used to trigger a transistor lamp switch so that a flash can be generated for every R-wave. This lamp, located on the front panel, is usually referred to as either a systole lamp or pulsometer by the nurses using the equipment. If the readout device is a digital readout, such as a digital panel meter (DPM), we can use the integrator's output directly. Only level scaling and perhaps some buffering need be provided and even that might be redundant. Where analog panel meters are used, however, Hewlett-Packard uses a meter correction circuit that is designed to expand the middle range of 50–120 beats per minute, the normal range for human heart rates.

Monitor Alarms

Most bedside monitoring equipment provides alarms to alert medical personnel if certain pre-set limits are exceeded. Figure 6.15 shows a typical alarm circuit. The two integrated circuits used (U1 and U2) are voltage comparators, which issue an output whenever one input voltage exceeds the other. These comparators can be either special integrated circuits such as the LM311 or operational amplifiers connected as comparators.

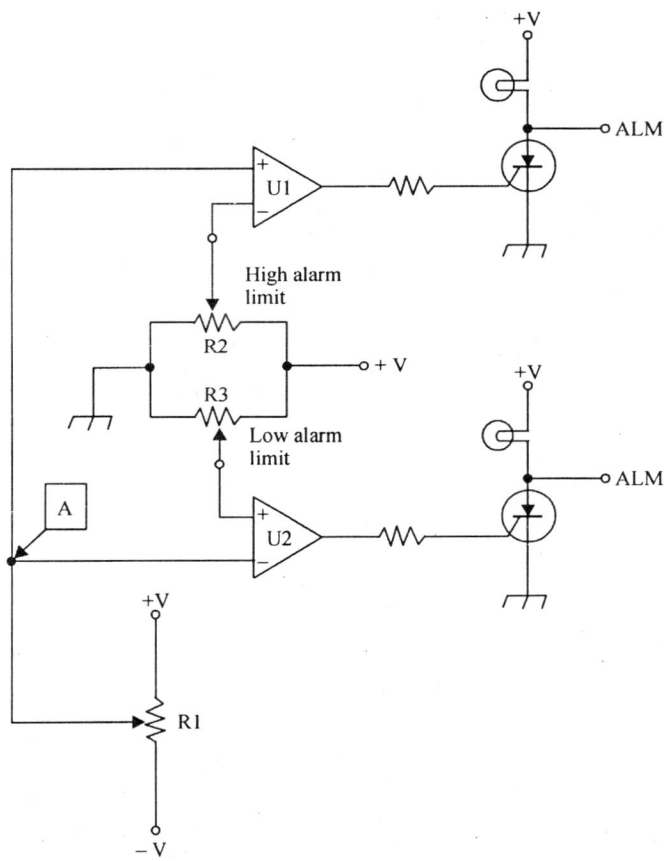

Fig. 6.15. Alarm circuit for bedside monitor.

In this example, the circuits are merely operational amplifiers connected without the normal feedback resistors. This means the gain of the circuit approximates the open-loop gain of the op-amp and that is typically 50000 to 10,00,000. Obviously, then, even a small differential voltage at the op-amp's inputs will saturate the output. In the circuit shown, the comparator output will snap to a positive DC level whenever the plus input exceeds the minus input. This DC level is used to turn on the gate of a silicon controlled rectifier (SCR).

One input to the two comparators, the voltage at point A, is proportional to the patient's heart rate and is generated by potentiometer R1. This variable resistor is located inside of the meter housing and its wiper is gauged to and operated by the meter pointer. The reference voltage to each comparator comes from the appropriate limit potentiometer—R2 for the high alarm limit or R3 for the low alarm limit.

These potentiometers may be either separately mounted on the front panel, with scales calibrated in the same units as the meter face or they may be located inside the meter housing. When inside the meter housing, 'set', tabs ganged to the potentiometer wipers would be available to the user outside of the meter housing. The actual meter scale is then used as the alarm scale and the set tabs positioned to coincide with the desired limit points.

BLOOD PRESSURE AND OTHER PHYSIOLOGICAL PRESSURES

The systemic arterial blood pressure is virtually always measured, commonly by a non-invasive indirect (bloodless) method, in patients whose condition is being monitored. In patients who are seriously ill, a direct arterial puncture method will be used in the interests of greater accuracy and it is also very likely that the central venous pressure will be monitored. It can be argued that a knowledge of regional blood flow rates would be even more useful than a knowledge of the systemic arterial pressure alone but in man it is generally easier to measure the pressure. The widespread interest in the measurement of blood pressure and particularly in its monitoring over periods of many hours, has led to the development of a variety of techniques and equipment for this purpose. The indirect methods are based upon the use of an inflating cuff and techniques such as detection of the Korotkoff sounds, cuff pressure oscillation or vessel wall movement in a suitable blood vessel and the direct methods required some form of transducer to transform the blood pressure into a visual and/or electrical signal. Whilst simple, mechanical systems, for either the direct or indirect approach are valuable at the bedside or in the operating room, the use of electrical systems has the great advantage of allowing the pressure to be observed or recorded at other locations in addition to providing this facility close to the patient.

Pressure is defined as force per unit area. In English and American engineering practice, the unit of force was taken as the pound weight—the force due to gravity acting on a mass of one pound and the unit of area was the square inch. Thus the gas pressure inside the cylinders connected to an anaesthetic machine is measured in pounds per square inch (psi). However, force due to gravity varies by about 0.5 per cent over the earth's surface, it is now customary to use an absolute (gravity independent) unit of force. On the centimetre-gram-second (cgs) system this is the dyne, where one dyne is that force which will give one gram an acceleration of one centimetre per second per second. Currently, in Europe, a change is being made to the SI (Système International d'Unités) system of units. Here, the unit of length is the metre, the unit of mass is the kilogram and the unit of force is the Newton. This is the force which will give a mass of one kilogram an acceleration of one metre per second per second. The SI unit of pressure is the Pascal (Pa) which is one newton per square metre. In the physiological literature, pressures are quoted in dynes per cm^2 or newtons per m^2 when it is required to use these in conjunction with the calculation of cardiac work or total systemic resistance.

In clinical practice, blood pressure are quoted in terms of the height of a column of mercury which the pressure can support. For example, a typical systolic pressure would be capable of supporting a vertical column of mercury 120 mm high. From Newton's law of motion, force = mass × acceleration. Consider a vertical column of mercury 120 mm high and having a 1 cm^2 cross-section. Taking the density of mercury as 13.6 grams per cm^3 at room temperature, the mass of the column is $12 \times 1 \times 1 \times 13.6$ grams. The acceleration due to gravity is 981 cm per second per second so that the force on the 1 cm^2 area due to the column is $12 \times 13.6 \times 981 = 1,60,099$ dynes per $cm^2 = 16010$ newtons per m^2. This is equal to 16.01 kilo-Pascals (kPa). On this basis 1 mm Hg = 133.4 Pascals. Using an accurate figure for the density of mercury, the official relationship is that 1 mm Hg = 133.32 Pascals. In the United Kingdom, it is being recommended that the Pascal replace the mm of Hg for blood-gas tensions, but it has not been recommended for blood pressure measurements. Incidently, the torr which is numerically equal to 1 mm Hg and is the unit used in vacuum measurements is not an SI unit.

Pressure Transducer Cuvette and Diaphragm

Pressure transducer commonly used to record blood pressures, the transducer is placed outside the patient's body and a physical connection made with the blood vessel concerned via a saline filled needle or cannula when a systemic arterial or venous pressure is to be measured. A suitable catheter will be substituted when central aortic, atrial or ventricular pressures or central venous pressure have to be measured. The needle, cannula or catheter is joined to the entry point of the transducer's cuvette via a 3-way tap and Luer taper connections which are usually of the locking type. The cuvette is made from a transparent plastic material to facilitate the observation of bubbles.

In many models, the complete cuvette can be unscrewed from the transducer housing thus exposing the diaphragm for cleaning and the removal of air bubbles. The exit from the cuvette is via a second Luer connection. The inlet and outlet connections are normally joined to 3-way stopcocks. These are often made of stainless steel and can be sterilised by autoclaving.

BLOOD PRESSURE MEASUREMENT

Determining an individual's blood pressure is a standard clinical measurement, whether taken in a physician's office or in the hospital during a specialised surgical procedure. Blood-pressure values in the various chambers of the heart and in the peripheral vascular system help the physician determine the functional integrity of the cardiovascular system. A number of direct (invasive) and indirect (non-invasive) techniques are being used to measure blood pressure in the human. The accuracy of each should be established, as well as its suitability for a particular clinical situation.

Fluctuations in pressure recorded over the frequency range of hearing are called sounds. The sources of heart sounds are the vibration set up by the accelerations of blood.

The function of the blood circulation is to transport oxygen and other nutrients to the tissues of the body and to carry metabolic waste products away from the cells. The heart serves as a four-chambered. pump for the circulatory system. The heart is divided into two pumping systems, the right side of the heart and left side of the heart. These two pumps and their associated valves are separated by the pulmonary circulation and the systemic circulation. Each pump has a filling chamber, the atrium, which helps to fill the ventricle, the stronger pump.

Figure 6.16 is a schematic diagram of the circulatory system. The left ventricle ejects blood through the aortic valve into the aorta and the blood is then distributed through the branching network of arteries, arterioles and capillaries. The resistance to blood flow is regulated by the arterioles, which are under local, neural and endocrine control. The exchange of the nutrient material takes place at the capillary level. The blood then returns to the right side of the heart via the venous system. Blood fills the right atrium, the filling chamber of the right heart and flows through the tricuspid valve into the right ventricle. The blood is pumped from the right ventricle into the pulmonary artery through the pulmonary valve. It next flows through the pulmonary arteries, arterioles, capillaries and veins to the left atrium. At the pulmonary capillaries, O_2 diffuses from the lung alveoli to the blood and CO_2 diffuses from the blood to the alveoli. The blood flows from the left atrium, the filling chamber of the left heart, through the mitral valve into the left ventricle. When the left ventricle contracts in response to the electric stimulation of the myocardium, blood is pumped through the aortic valve into the aorta.

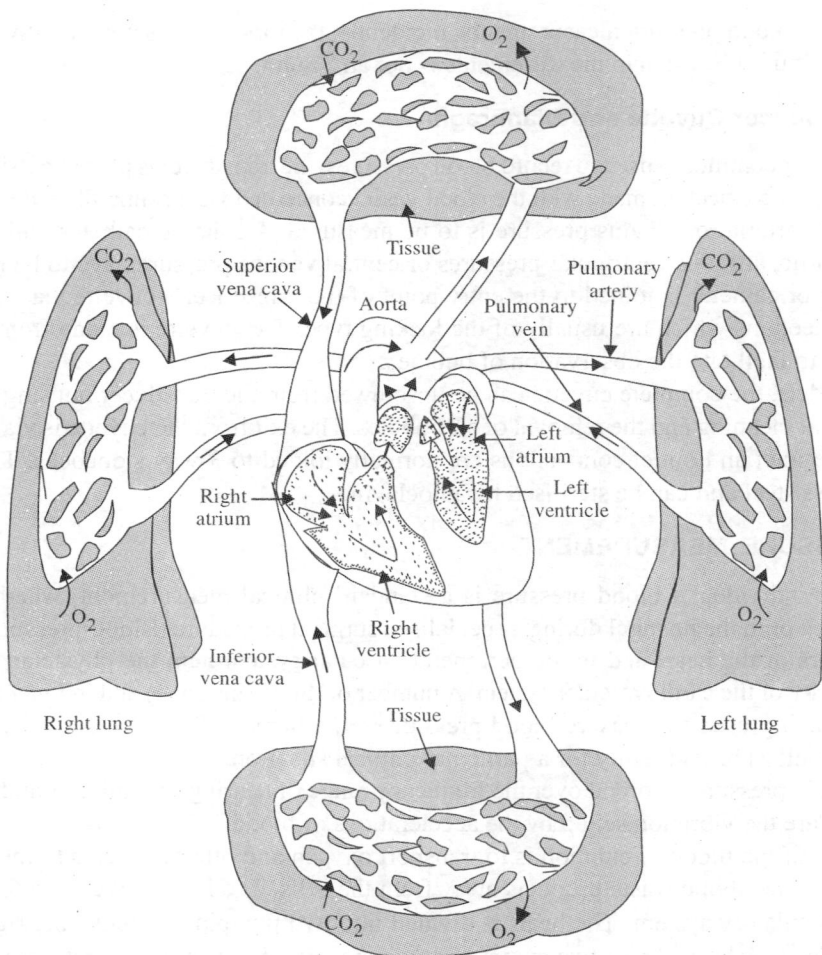

Fig. 6.16. The left ventricle ejects blood into the systemic circulatory system. The right ventricle ejects blood into the pulmonary circulatory system.

The pressures generated by the right and left sides of the heart differ somewhat in shape and in amplitude (Fig. 6.17). As already discussed, cardiac contraction is caused by electric stimulation of the cardiac muscle. An electric impulse is generated by specialised cells located in the sinoatrial node of the right atrium. This electric impulse quickly spreads over both atria. At the junction of the atria and ventricles, the electric impulse is conducted after a short delay at the atrial-ventricular node. Conduction quickly spreads over the interior of both ventricles by means of a specialised conduction throughout both ventricles. This impulse causes mechanical contraction of both ventricles. Mechanical contraction of the ventricular muscle generates ventricular pressures that force blood through the pulmonary and aortic valves into the pulmonary circulation and the systemic circulation, causing pressures in each. The heart sounds are associated with the movement of blood during the cardiac cycle. Murmurs are vibrations caused by the turbulence in the blood moving rapidly through the heart.

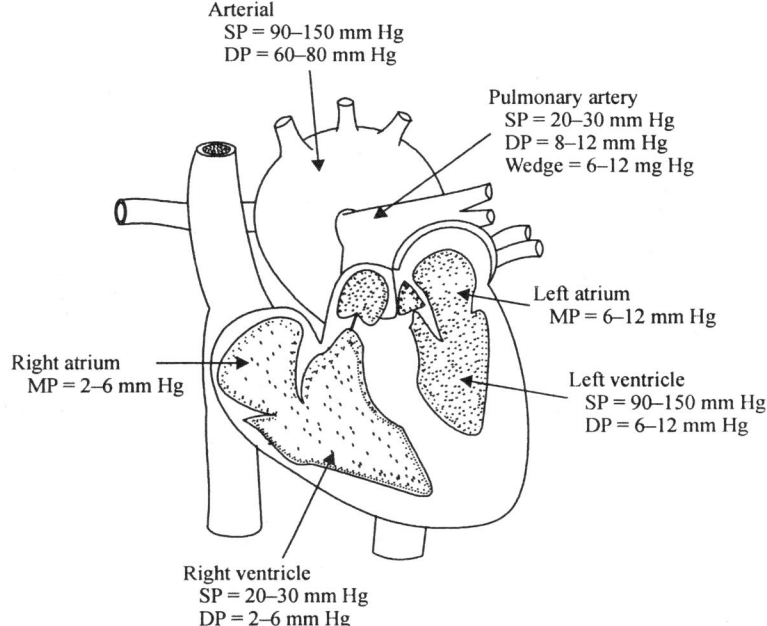

Arterial
SP = 90–150 mm Hg
DP = 60–80 mm Hg

Pulmonary artery
SP = 20–30 mm Hg
DP = 8–12 mm Hg
Wedge = 6–12 mg Hg

Left atrium
MP = 6–12 mm Hg

Right atrium
MP = 2–6 mm Hg

Left ventricle
SP = 90–150 mm Hg
DP = 6–12 mm Hg

Right ventricle
SP = 20–30 mm Hg
DP = 2–6 mm Hg

Fig. 6.17. Typical values of circulatory pressures SP is the systolic pressure, DP the diastolic pressure and MP the mean pressure.

Direct Measurements

Blood-pressure sensor systems can be divided into two general categories according to the location of the sensor element. The most common clinical method for directly measuring pressure is to couple the vascular pressure to an external sensor element via a liquid-filled catheter. In the second general category, the liquid coupling is eliminated by incorporating the sensor into the tip of a catheter that is placed in the vascular system. This device is known as an intravascular pressure sensor.

A number of different kinds of sensor elements may be used; they include strain gauge, linear-variable differential transformer, variable inductance, variable capacitance, optoelectronic, piezoelectric and semiconductor devices.

Extravascular sensors

The extravascular sensor system is made up of a catheter connected to a three-way stopcock and then to the pressure sensor (Fig. 6.18). The catheter-sensors system, which is filled with a saline-heparin solution, must be flushed with the solution every few minutes to prevent blood from clotting at the tip.

The physician inserts the catheter either by means of a surgical cut-down, which exposes the artery or vein or by means of percutaneous insertion, which involves the use of a special needle or guide-wire technique. Blood pressure is transmitted via the catheter liquid column to the sensor and finally, to the diaphragm, which is deflected. Figure 6.18 highlights modern disposable blood-pressure sensors.

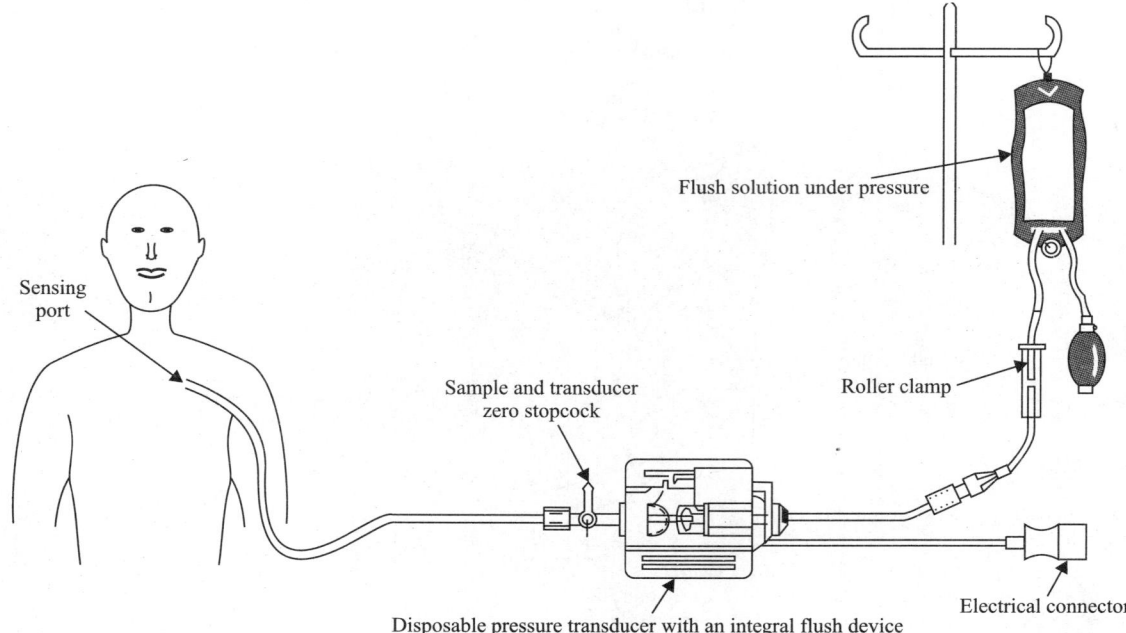

Fig. 6.18. Extravascular pressure-sensor system. A catheter couples a flush solution (heparinised saline) through a disposable pressure sensor with an integral flush device to the sensing port. The three-way stopcock is used to take blood samples and zero the pressure sensor.

Intravascular sensors

Catheter-tip sensors have the advantage that the hydraulic connection via the catheter, between the source of pressure and the sensor element, is eliminated. The frequency response of the catheter-sensor system is limited by the hydraulic properties of the system. Detection of pressures at the tip of the catheter without the use of a liquid-coupling system can thus enable the physician to obtain a high frequency response and eliminate the time delay encountered when the pressure pulse is transmitted in a catheter-sensor system.

A number of basic types of sensors are being used commercially for the detection of pressure in the catheter tip. These include various types of straingauge systems bonded onto a flexible diaphragm at the catheter tip. Gauges of this type are available in the F5 catheter (1.67 mm OD) size. In the French scale (F), used to denote the diameter catheters, each unit is approximately equal to 0.33 mm. Smaller-sized catheters may become available as the technology improves and the problems of temperature and electric drift, fragility and non-destructive sterilisation are solved more satisfactorily. A disadvantage of the catheter-tip pressure sensor is that it is more expensive than others and may break after only a few uses, further increasing its cost per use.

The fibre-optic intravascular pressure sensor can be made in sizes comparable to those described above, but at a lower cost. The fibre-optic device measures the displacement of the diaphragm optically by the varying reflection of light from the back of the deflecting diaphragm. These devices are inherently safer electrically, but unfortunately they lack a convenient way to measure relative pressure without an additional lumen either connected to a second pressure sensor or vented to the atmosphere.

A fibre-optic microtip sensor for *in vivo* measurements inside the human body is shown in Fig. 6.19a in which one leg of the bifurcated fibre bundle is connected to a light-emitting diode (LED) source and the other to a photodetector. The pressure-sensor tip consists of a thin metal membrane mounted at the common end of the mixed fibre bundle. External pressure causes membrane deflection, varying the coupling between the LED source and the photodetector. Figure 6.19b shows the output signal versus membrane deflection. Optical fibres have the property of emitting and accepting light within a cone defined by the acceptance angle θ_A, which is equal to the fibre numerical aperture, N_A. The coupling between LED source and detector is a function of the overlap of the two acceptance angles on the pressure-sensor membrane. The operating portion of the curve is the left slope region where the characteristic is steepest.

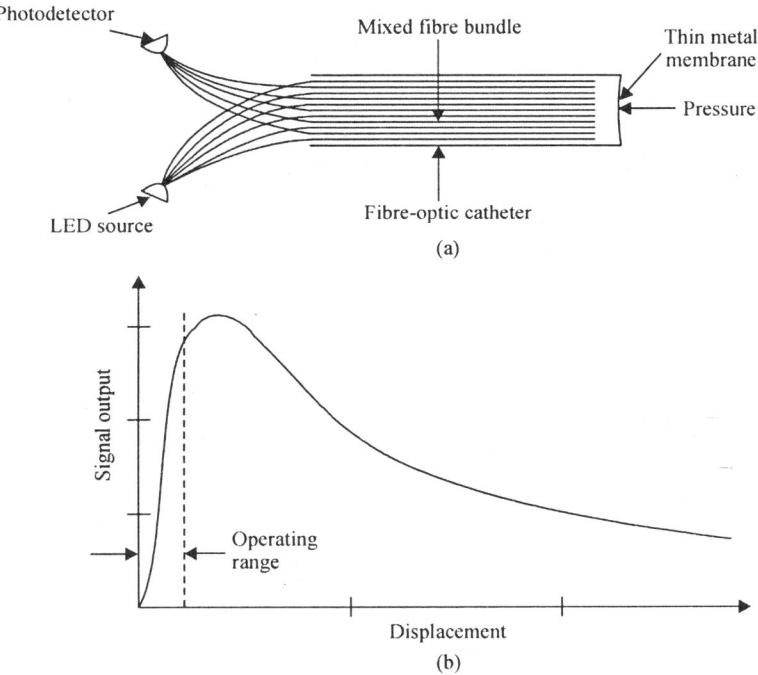

Fig. 6.19. (a) Schematic diagram of an intravascular fibre-optic pressure sensor. Pressure causes deflection in a thin metal membrane that modulates the coupling between the source and detector fibres. (b) Characteristic curve for the fibre-optic pressure sensor.

Roos and Carroll describes a fibre-optic pressure sensor for use in magnetic resonance imaging (MRI) fields in which a plastic shutter assembly modulates the light transversing a channel between source and detector. Neuman has described a fibre-optic pressure sensor for intracranial pressure measurements in the newborn. Figure 6.20 shows a schematic of the device, which is applied to the anterior fontanel. Pressure is applied with the sensor such that the curvature of the skin surface is flattened. When this applanation occurs, equal pressure exists on both sides of the membrane, which consists of soft tissue between the scalp surface and the dura. Monitoring of the probe pressure determines the dura pressure. The membrane position is determined by a reflector that is attached to the membrane and varies the amount of light coupling between the source and detector fibres.

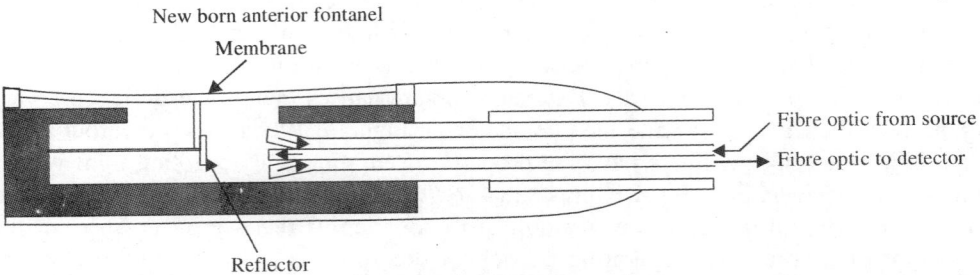

Fig. 6.20. Fibre-optic pressure sensor for intracranial pressure measurements in the new born. The sensor membrane is placed in contact with the anterior fontanel of the new born.

Air pressure from a pneumatic servo system controls the air pressure within the pressure sensor, which is adjusted such that diaphragm—and thus the fontanel tissue—is flat, indicating that the sensor air pressure and the fontanel or intracranial pressure are equal.

Similar pressure-unloading techniques are used in thin, compliant sensors that measure interface pressures between the skin and support structures such as seat cushions.

Silicon fusion bonding is used to fabricate micro silicon pressure-sensor chips. A wedge-shaped cavity is etched in a silicon wafer to form a diaphragm. Piezoresistive strain gauges are implanted and a metal connection is made in order to create a sensor for a catheter tip micropressure sensor.

Disposable pressure sensors

Traditionally, physiological pressure sensors have been re-usable devices, but most modern hospitals have adopted inexpensive, disposable pressure sensors in order to lower the risk of patient cross-contamination and reduce the amount of handling of pressure sensors by hospital personnel. Because re-usable pressure sensors are subject to the abuses of re-processing and repeated user handling, they tend to be less reliable than disposable sensors.

By micromachining silicon, a pressure diaphragm is etched and piezoresistive strain gauges are diffused into the diaphragm for measuring its displacement. This process results in a small, integrated, sensitive and relatively inexpensive pressure sensor. This silicon chip is incorporated into a disposable pressure-monitoring tubing system. The disposable pressure sensor system also contains a thick-film resistor network that is laser-trimmed to remove offset voltages and set the same sensitivity for similar disposable sensors. In addition, a thick-film thermistor network is usually incorporated for temperature compensation. The resistance of the bridge elements is usually high in order to reduce self-heating, which may cause erroneous results. This results in a high output impedance for the device. Thus, a high-input impedance monitor must be used with disposable pressure sensors.

Pressure sensors can monitor blood pressure in post-surgical patients as part of a closed-loop feedback system. Such a system injects controlled amounts of the drug nitroprusside to stabilise the blood pressure.

Harmonic Analysis of Blood-Pressure Waveforms

The basic sine-wave components of any complex time-varying periodic waveform can be dissected into an infinite sum of properly weighted sine and cosine functions of the proper frequency that, when added, reproduce the original complex waveform. It has been shown that researchers can apply techniques of Fourier analysis when they want to characterise the oscillatory components of the circulatory and respiratory systems, because two basic postulates for Fourier analysis—periodicity and linearity—are usually satisfied.

Cardiovascular physiologists and some clinicians have been employing Fourier-analysis techniques in the quantification of pressure and flow. Fourier analysis used bandpass filters. More recent analysts have used computer technique to obviate the need for special hardware. The advantage of the technique is that it allows for a quantitative representation of a physiological waveform; thus it is quite easy to compare corresponding harmonic components of pulses.

The blood-pressure pulse can be divided into its fundamental component (of the same frequency as the blood-pressure wave) and its significant harmonics. Figure 6.21 shows the first six harmonic components of the blood-pressure wave and the resultant sum. When we compare they original waveform and the waveform re-constructed from the Fourier components, we find that they agree quite well, indicating that the first six harmonics give a fairly good reproduction. Note that the amplitude of the sixth harmonic is approximately 12 per cent of the fundamental. We can achieve more faithful reproduction of the original waveform by adding higher harmonic components.

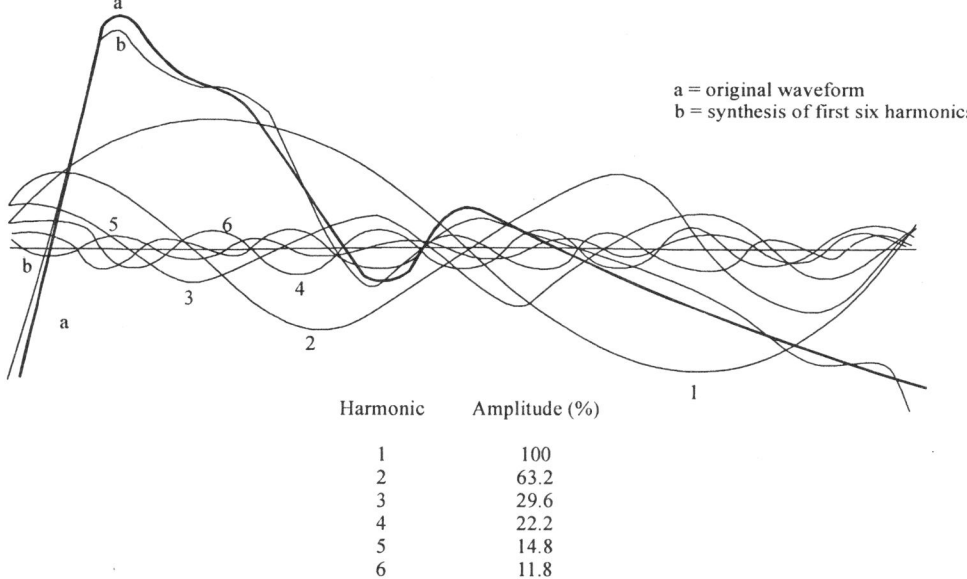

a = original waveform
b = synthesis of first six harmonics

Harmonic	Amplitude (%)
1	100
2	63.2
3	29.6
4	22.2
5	14.8
6	11.8

Fig. 6.21. The first six harmonics of the blood-pressure waveform. The table gives relative values for amplitudes.

Dynamic properties of pressure-measurement systems

An understanding of the dynamic properties of a pressure-measurement system is important if we wish to preserve the dynamic accuracy of the measured pressure. Errors in measurement of dynamic pressure can have serious consequences in the clinical situation. For instance, an underdamped system can lead to overestimation of pressure gradients across stenotic (narrowed) heart valves. The liquid-filled catheter sensor is a hydraulic system that can be represented by either distributed or lumped-parameter models. Distributed parameter models gives an accurate description of the dynamic behaviour of the catheter-sensor system. However, distributed-parameter models are not normally employed, because the single-degree-of-freedom (lumped-parameter) model is easier to work with and the accuracy of the results obtained by using these models is acceptable for the clinical situation.

Bandwidth Requirements for Measuring Blood Pressure

When we know the representative harmonic components of the blood-pressure waveform—or for that matter, any periodic waveform—we can specify the bandwidth requirements for the instrumentation system. As with all biomedical measurements, bandwidth requirements are a function of the investigation.

For example, if the mean blood pressure is the only parameter of interest, it is of little value to try to achieve a wide bandwidth system. It is generally accepted that harmonics of the blood-pressure waveform higher than the tenth may be ignored. As an example, the bandwidth requirements for a heart rate of 120 beats/minute (or 2 Hz) would be 20 Hz.

For a perfect reproduction of the original waveform, there should be no distortion in the amplitude or phase characteristics. The waveshape can be preserved, however, even if the phase characteristics are not ideal. This is the case if the relative amplitudes of the frequency components are preserved but their phases are displaced in proportion to their frequency. Then the synthesised waveform gives the original waveshape, except that it is delayed in time, depending on the phase shift.

Measurements of the derivative of the pressure signal increase the bandwidth requirements, because the differentiation of a sinusoidal harmonic increases the amplitude of that component by a factor proportional to its frequency. As with the original blood-pressure waveform, the bandwidth requirements for the derivative of the blood pressure can be estimated by a Fourier analysis of the derivative signal. The amplitude-versus-frequency characteristics of any catheter-manometer system used for the measurement of ventricular pressures that are subsequently differentiated must remain flat to within 5 per cent, up to the twentieth harmonic.

Typical Pressure-Waveform Distortion

Accurate measurements of blood pressure are important in both clinical and physiological research. This section gives examples of typical types of distortion of blood-pressure waveform that are due to an inadequate frequency response of the catheter–sensor system.

There may be serious consequences when an underdamped system leads to overestimation of the pressure gradients across a stenotic (narrowed) heart valve.

Figure 6.22 shows examples of distortion of pressure waveform. The actual blood-pressure waveform [Fig. 6.22a] was recorded with a high-quality pressure sensor with a bandwidth from DC to 100 Hz. Note that in the underdamped case, the amplitude of the higher-frequency components of the pressure wave are amplified, whereas for the overdamped case these higher-frequency components are attenuated. The actual peak pressure [Fig. 6.22a] is approximately 130 mm Hg (17.3 kPa). The underdamped response [Fig. 6.22b] has a peak pressure of about 165 mm Hg (22 kPa), which may lead to a serious clinical error if this peak pressure is used to asses the severity of aortic-valve stenosis. The minimal pressure is in error, too; it is –15 mm Hg (–2 kPa) and the actual value is 5 mm Hg (0.7 kPa). There is also a time delay of approximately 30 ms in the underdamped case.

The overdamped case [Fig. 6.22c] shows a significant time delay of approximately 150 ms and an attenuated amplitude of 120 mm Hg (16 kPa); the actual value is 130 mm Hg (17.3 kPa). This type of response can occur in the presence of a large air bubble or a blood clot at the tip of the catheter.

An underdamped catheter-sensor system can be transformed to an overdamped system by pinching the catheter. This procedure increases the damping ratio ζ and has little effect on the natural frequency.

Another example of distortion in blood-pressure measurements is known as catheter whip. Figure 6.23 shows these low-frequency oscillations that appear in the blood-pressure recording. This may occur when an aortic ventricular catheter, in a region of high pulsatile flow, is bent and whipped about by the accelerating blood. This type of distortion can be minimised by the use of stiff catheters or by careful placement of catheters in regions of low flow velocity.

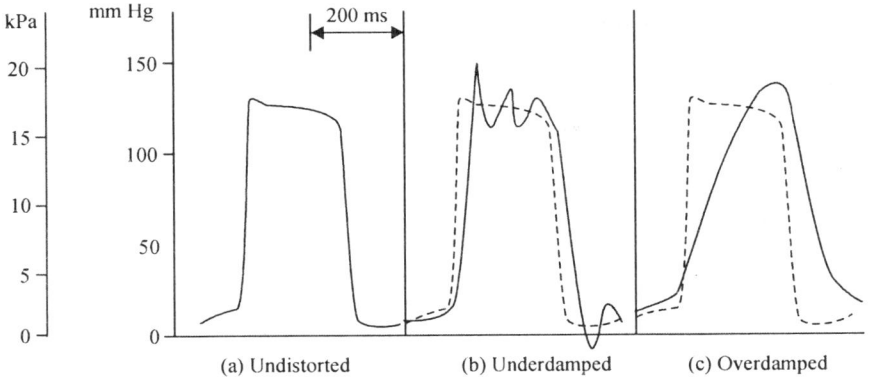

Fig. 6.22. Pressure-waveform distortion. (a) Recording of an undistorted left-ventricular pressure waveform via a pressure sensor with bandwidth DC to 100 Hz. (b) Underdamped response, where peak value is increased. A time delay is also evident in this recording. (c) Overdamped response that shows a significant time delay and an attenuated amplitude response.

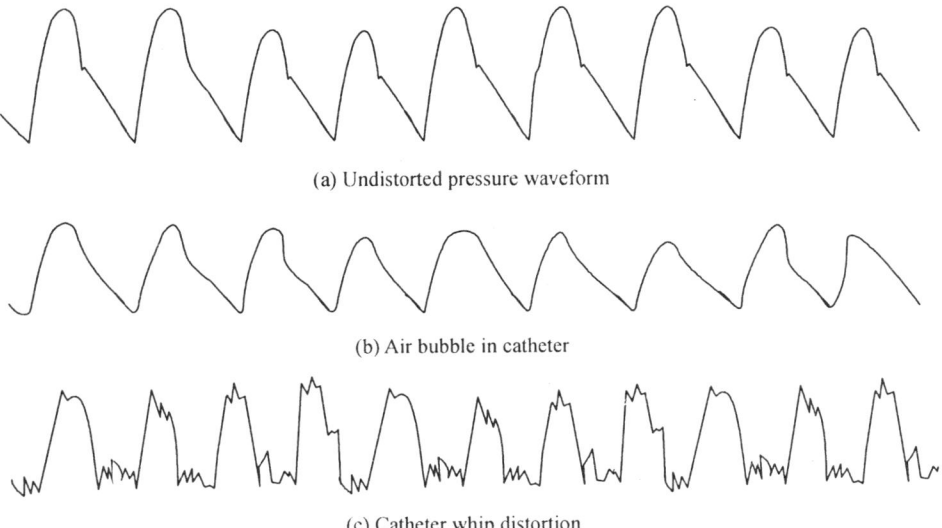

Fig. 6.23. Distortion during the recording of arterial pressure. The bottom trace is the response when the pressure catheter is bent and whipped by accelerating blood in regions of high pulsatile flow.

Systems for Measuring Venous Pressure

Measurements of venous pressure are an important aid to the physician for determining the function of the capillary bed and the right side of the heart. The pressure in the small veins is lower than the capillary pressure and reflects the value of the capillary pressure. The intrathoracic venous pressure determines the diastolic filling pressure of the right ventricle. The central venous pressure is measured in a central vein or in the right atrium. It fluctuates above and below atmospheric pressure as the subject breathes, whereas the extrathoracic venous pressure is 2 to 5 cm H_2O (0.2 to 0.5 kPa) above atmospheric. The reference level for venous pressure is at the right atrium.

Central venous pressure is an important indicator of myocardial performance. It is normally monitored on surgical and medical patients to assess proper therapy in cases of heart dysfunction, shock, hypervolemic or hypovolemic states or circulatory failure. It is used as a guide to determine the amount of liquid a patient should receive.

Physicians usually measure steady-state or mean venous pressure by making a percutaneous venous puncture with a large-bore needle, inserting a catheter through the needle into the vein and advancing it to the desired position. The needle is then removed. A plastic tube is attached to the intravenous catheter by means of a stopcock, which enables clinicians to administer drugs or fluids as necessary. Continuous dynamic measurements of venous pressure can be made by connecting to the venous catheter a high-sensitivity pressure sensor with a lower dynamic range than that necessary for arterial measurements.

Problems in maintaining a steady baseline occur when the patient changes position. Errors may arise in the measurements if the catheter is misplaced or if it becomes blocked by a clot or is impacted against a vein wall. It is normal practice to accept venous-pressure values only when respiratory swings are evident. Normal central venous pressures range widely from 0 to 12 cm H_2O (0 to 1.2 kPa), with a mean pressure of 5 cm H_2O (0.5 kPa).

Oesophageal manometry uses a similar low-pressure catheter system. A hydraulic capillary infusion system infuses 0.6 ml/min to prevent sealing of the catheter orifice in the Oesophagus.

Table 6.1 demonstrate the relative importance of the kinetic-energy term in different parts of the circulation. As Table 6.1 shows, there are situations in the aorta, venae cavae and pulmonary artery in which the kinetic energy term is a substantial part of the total pressure. For the laminar-flow case, this error decreases as the catheter pressure port is moved from the centre of the vessel to the vessel wall, where the average velocity of flow is less. The kinetic energy term could also be important in a disease situation in which an artery becomes narrowed.

Table 6.1. Relative importance of the kinetic energy term in different parts of the circulation.

Vessel	Vel (cm/s)	KE (mm Hg)	Systolic (mm Hg)	(kPa)	% KE of total
Aorta (systolic)					
At rest	100	4	120	(16)	3
Cardiac output at 3 × rest	300	36	180	(24)	17
Brachial artery					
At rest	30	0.35	110	(14.7)	0.3
Cardiac output at 3 × rest	90	4	120	(16)	3
Venae cavae					
At rest	30	0.35	2	(0.3)	12
Cardiac output at 3 × rest	90	3.2	3	(0.4)	52
Pulmonary artery					
At rest	90	3	20	(2.7)	13
Cardiac output at 3 × rest	270	27	25	(3.3)	52

Indirect Measurements of Blood Pressure

Indirect measurement of blood pressure is an attempt to measure intra-arterial pressures non-invasively. The most standard manual techniques employ either the palpation or the auditory detection of the pulse distal to an occlusive cuff. Figure 6.24 shows a typical system for indirect measurement of blood pressure. It employs a sphygmomanometer consisting of an inflatable cuff for occlusion of the blood vessel, a rubber bulb for inflation of the cuff and either a mercury or an aneroid manometer for detection of pressure.

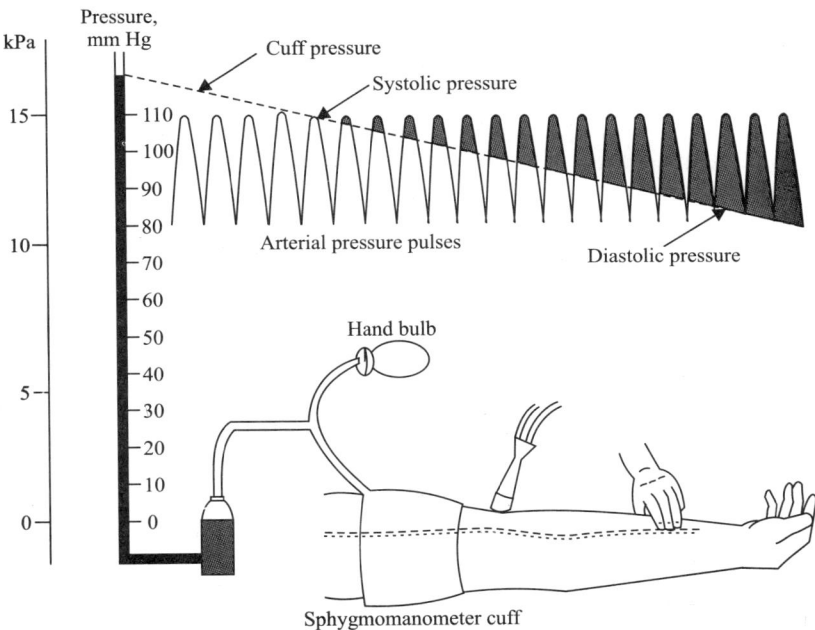

Fig. 6.24. Typical indirect blood-pressure measurement system. The sphygmomanometer cuff is inflated by a hand bulb to pressures above the systolic level. Pressure is then slowly released and blood flow under the cuff is monitored by a microphone or stethoscope placed over a downstream artery. The first Korotkoff sound detected indicates systolic pressure, whereas the transition from muffling silence brackets diastolic pressure.

Blood pressure is measured in the following way. The occlusive cuff is inflated until the pressure is above systolic pressure and then is slowly bled off (2–3 mm Hg/s) (0.3–0.4 kPa/s). When the systolic peaks are higher than the occlusive pressure, the blood spurts under the cuff and causes a palpable pulse in the wrist (Riva-Rocci method). Audible sounds generated by the flow of blood and vibrations of the vessel under the cuff are heard through a stethoscope. The manometer pressure at the first detection of the pulse indicates the systolic pressure. As the pressure in the cuff is decreased, the audible Korotkoff sounds pass through five phases. The period of transition from muffling (phase IV) to silence (phase V) brackets the diastolic pressure.

In employing the palpation and auscultatory techniques, you should take several measurements, because normal respiration and vasomotor waves modulate the normal blood-pressure levels. These techniques also suffer from the disadvantage of failing to give accurate pressures for infants and hypotensive patients.

Using an occlusive cuff of the correct size is important if the clinician is to obtain accurate results. The pressure applied to the artery wall is assumed to be equal to that of the external cuff. However, the cuff pressure is transmitted via interposed tissue. With a cuff of sufficient width and length, the cuff pressure is evenly transmitted to the underlying artery. It is generally accepted that the width of the cuff should be about 0.40 times the circumference of the extremity. However, no general agreement appears to exist about the length of the pneumatic cuff. If a short cuff is used, it is important that it be positioned over the artery of interest. A longer cuff reduces the problem of misalignment. The cuff should be placed at heart level to avoid hydrostatic effects.

The auscultatory technique is simple and requires a minimum of equipment. However, it cannot be used in a noisy environment, whereas the palpation technique can. The hearing acuity of the user must be good for low frequencies from 20 to 300 Hz, the bandwidth required for these measurements. Bellville and Weaver have determined the energy distribution of the Korotkoff sounds for normal patients and for patients in shock. When there is a fall in blood pressure, the sound spectrum shifts to lower frequencies. The failure of the auscultation technique for hypotensive patients may be due to low sensitivity of the human ear to these low-frequency vibrations.

There is a common misconception that normal blood pressure is 120/80, meaning that the systolic value is 120 mm Hg (16 kPa) and that the diastolic value is 80 mm Hg (10.7 kPa). This is not the case. A careful study showed that the age and sex of an individual determine the 'normal value' of blood pressure.

A number of techniques have been proposed to measure automatically indirectly the systolic and diastolic blood pressure in human. The basic technique involves an automatic sphygmomanometer that inflates and deflates an occlusive cuff at a pre-determined rate. A sensitive detector is used to measure the distal pulse or cuff pressure. A number of kinds of detectors have been employed, including ultrasonic, piezoelectric, photoelectric, electroacoustic, thermometric, electrocardiographic, rheographic and tissue-impedance devices. Three of the commonly used automatic techniques are described in the following paragraphs.

The first technique employs an automated auscultatory device wherein a microphone replaces the stethoscope. The cycle of events that takes place begins with a rapid (20–30 mm Hg/s) (2.7–4 kPa/s) inflation of the occlusive cuff to a preset pressure about 30 mm Hg higher than the suspected systolic level. The flow of blood beneath the cuff is stopped by the collapse of the vessel. Cuff pressure is then reduced slowly (2–3 mm Hg/s) (0.3–0.4 kPa/s). The first Korotkoff sound is detected by the microphone, at which time the level of the cuff pressure is stored. The muffling and silent period of the Korotkoff sounds is detected and the value of the diastolic pressure is also stored. After a few minutes, the instrument displays the systolic and diastolic pressures and recycles the operation.

The ultrasonic determination of blood pressure employs a transcutaneous Doppler sensor that detects the motion of the blood-vessel walls in various states of occlusion. Figure 6.25 shows the placement of the compression cuff over two small transmitting and receiving ultrasound crystals (8 MHz) on the arm. The Doppler ultrasonic transmitted signal is focused on the vessel wall and the blood. The reflected signal (shifted in frequency) is detected by the receiving crystal and decoded. The difference in frequency, in the range of 40 to 500 Hz, between the transmitted and received signals is proportional to the velocity of the wall motion and the blood velocity. As the cuff pressure is increased above diastolic but below systolic, the vessel opens and closes with each heartbeat, because the pressure in the artery oscillates above and below the applied external pressure in the cuff. The opening and closing of the vessel are detected by the ultrasonic system.

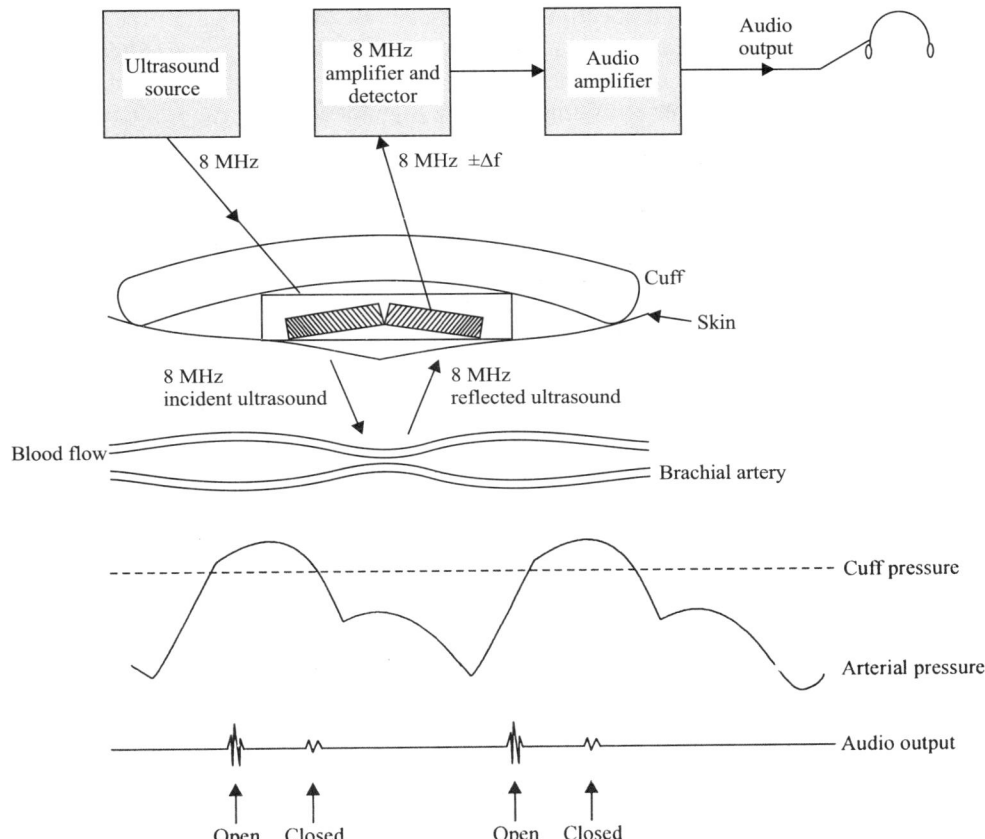

Fig. 6.25. Ultrasonic determination of blood pressure. A compression cuff is placed over the transmitting (8 MHz) and receiving (8 MHz ± Δf) crystals. The opening and closing of the blood vessel are detected as the applied cuff pressure is varied.

As the applied pressure is further increased, the time between the opening and closing decreases until they coincide. The reading at this point is the systolic pressure. Conversely, when the pressure in the cuff is reduced, the time between opening and closing increases until the closing signal from one pulse coincides with the opening signal from the next. The reading at this point is the diastolic pressure, which prevails when the vessel is open for the complete pulse.

The advantages of the ultrasonic technique are that it can be used with infants and hypotensive individuals and in high-noise environment. A disadvantage is that movements of the subject's body cause changes in the ultrasonic path between the sensor and the blood vessel. Complete re-construction of the arterial-pulse waveform is also possible via the ultrasonic method. A timing pulse from the ECG signal is used as a reference. The clinician uses the pressure in the cuff when the artery opens versus the time from the ECG R wave to plot the rising portion of the arterial pulse. Conversely, the clinician uses the cuff pressure when the artery closes versus the time from the ECG R-wave to plot the falling portion of the arterial pulse. The oscillometric method, a non-invasive blood pressure techniques, measures the amplitude of oscillations that appear in the cuff pressure signal which are created by expansion of the arterial wall each time blood is forced through the artery. The uniqueness of the oscillometric method, a blood-pressure cuff technique, is that specific characteristics of the compression cuff's entrained air volume are used to identify and sense blood-pressure values. The cuff-pressure signal increases in strength in the systolic pressure region; reaching a maximum when the cuff pressure is equal to mean arterial pressure. As the cuff pressure drops below this point, the signal strength decreases proportionally to the cuff air pressure bled rate. There is no clear transition in cuff pressure oscillations to identify diastolic pressure since arterial wall expansion continues to happen below diastolic pressure while blood is forced through the artery. Thus, oscillometric monitors employ proprietary algorithms to estimate the diastolic pressure.

Ramsey has indicated that, using the oscillometric method, the mean arterial pressure is the single blood-pressure parameter which is the most robust measurement, as compared with systolic and diastolic pressure, because it is measured when the oscillations of cuff pressure reach the greatest amplitude. This property usually allows mean arterial pressure to be measured reliably even in case of hypotension with vasoconstriction and diminished pulse pressure.

When the cuff pressure is raised quickly to pressures higher than systolic pressure it is observed that the radial pulse disappears. Cuff pressures above systolic cause the underlying artery to be completely occluded. However, at suprasystolic cuff pressures, small amplitude pressure oscillations occur in the cuff pressure due to artery pulsations under the upper edge of the cuff, which are communicated to the cuff through the adjacent tissues. With slow cuff-pressure reductions, when the cuff pressure is just below systolic pressure, blood spurts through the artery and the cuff-pressure oscillations become larger. Figure 6.26 illustrates the ideal case in which the cuff pressure is monitored by a pressure sensor connected to a strip chart recorder. A pressure slightly above systolic pressure is detected by determining the shift from small-amplitude oscillations at cuff pressure slightly above systolic pressure and when the cuff pressure begins to increase amplitude (Point 1). As the cuff continues to deflate, the amplitude of the oscillations increases reaching a maximum and then decreases as the cuff pressure is decreased to zero. Point 2 in Fig. 6.26 is the maximum cuff pressure oscillation which is essentially true mean arterial pressure. Since there is no apparent transition in the oscillation amplitude as cuff pressure passes diastolic pressure, algorithmic methods are used to predict diastolic pressure.

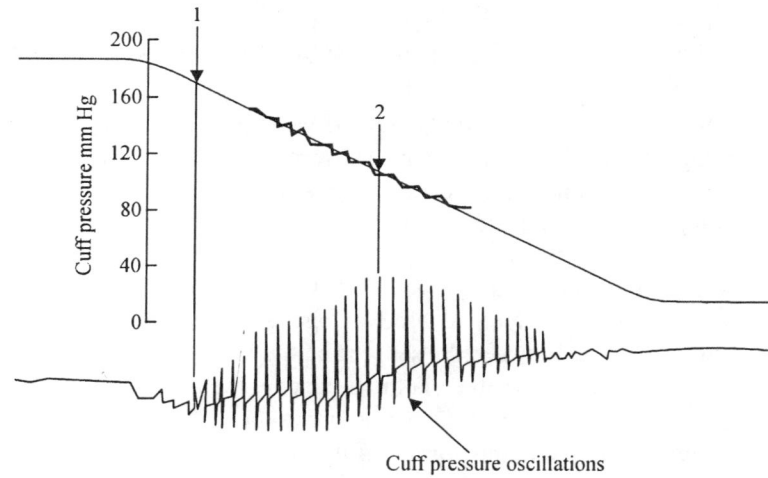

Cuff pressure oscillations

Fig. 6.26. The oscillometric method. A compression cuff is inflated above systolic and slowly deflated. Systolic pressure is detected (Point 1) where there is a transition from small amplitude oscillations (above systolic pressure) to increasing cuff-pressure amplitude. The cuff-pressure oscillations increase to a maximum (Point 2) at the mean arterial pressure.

The system description begins with the blood-pressure cuff which compresses a limb and its vasculature by the encircling inflatable compression cuff pressures. The cuff is connected to a pneumatic system (Fig. 6.27). A solid-state pressure sensor senses cuff pressure and the electric signal proportional to pressure is processed in two different circuits. One circuit amplifies and corrects the zero offset of the cuff-pressure signal before the analog-to-digital digitisation. The other circuit high-pass filters and amplifies the cuff-pressure signal. Cuff pressure is controlled by a microcomputer which activates the cuff inflation and deflation systems during the measurement cycle.

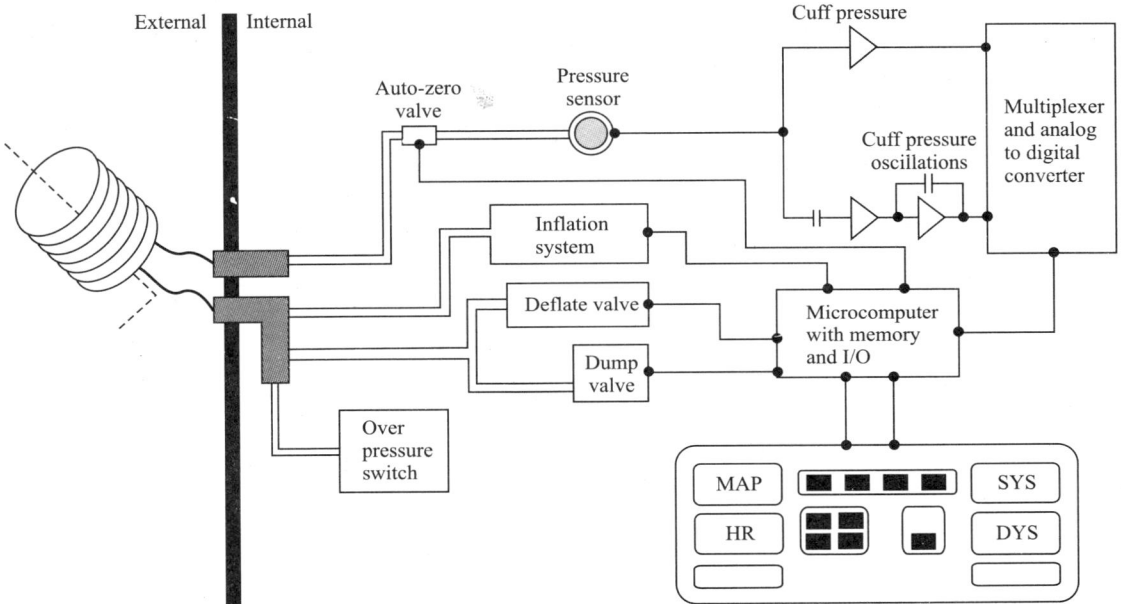

Fig. 6.27. Block diagram of the major components and sub-systems of an oscillometric blood-pressure monitoring device, based on the Dinamap unit, I/O = input/output; MAP = mean arterial pressure; HR = heart rate; SYS = systolic pressure; and DYS = diastolic pressure.

HEART RATES

The auscultation of the heart gives the clinician valuable information about the functional integrity of the heart. More information becomes available when clinicians compare the temporal relationships between the heart sounds and the mechanical and electric events of the cardiac cycle. This latter approach is know as phonocardiography.

There is a wide diversity of opinion concerning the theories that attempt to explain the origin of heart sounds and murmurs. More than 40 different mechanisms have been proposed to explain the first heart sound. A basic definition shows the difference between heart sounds and murmurs. Heart sounds are vibrations or sounds due to the acceleration or deceleration of blood, whereas murmurs are vibrations or sounds due to blood turbulence.

Mechanism and Origin

Figure 6.28 shows how the four heart sounds are related to the electric and mechanical events of the cardiac cycle. The first heart sound is associated with the movement of blood during ventricular systole.

As the ventricles contract, blood shifts toward the atria, closing the atrioventricular valves with a consequential oscillation of blood. The first heart sound further originates from oscillations of blood between the descending root of the aorta and ventricle and from vibrations due to blood turbulence at the aortic and pulmonary valves. Splitting of the first heart sound is defined as an asynchronous closure of the tricuspid and mitral valves. The second heart sound is low-frequency vibration associated with the deceleration and reversal of flow in the aorta and pulmonary artery and with the closure of the semi-lunar valves (the valves situated between the ventricles and the aorta or the pulmonary trunk). This second heart sound is coincident with the completion of the T-wave of the ECG.

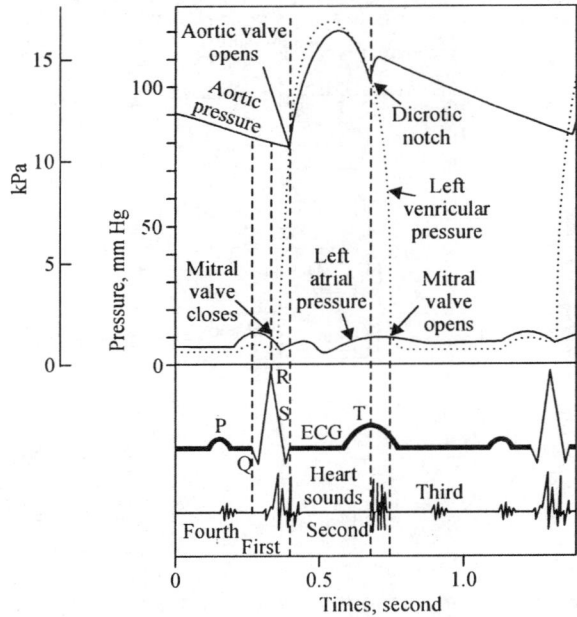

Fig. 6.28. Correlation of the four heart sounds with electric and mechanical events of the cardiac cycle.

The third heart sound is attributed to the sudden termination of the rapid-filling phase of the ventricles from the atria and the associated vibration of the ventricular muscle walls, which are relaxed. This low-amplitude, low-frequency vibration is audible in children and in some adults.

The fourth or atrial heart sound—which is not audible but can be recorded by the phonocardiogram—occurs when the atria contract and propel blood into the ventricles.

The sources of most murmurs, developed by turbulence in rapidly moving blood, are known. Murmurs during the early systolic phase are common in children and they are normally heard in nearly all adults after exercise. Abnormal murmurs may be caused by stenoses and insufficiencies (leaks) at the aortic, pulmonary and mitral valves. They are detected by noting the time of their occurrence in the cardiac cycle and their location at the time of measurement.

Auscultation Techniques

Heart sounds travel through the body from the heart and major blood vessels to the body surface. Because of the acoustical properties of the transmission path, sound waves are attenuated and not reflected. The largest attenuation of the wave-like motion occurs in the most compressible tissues, such as the lungs and fat layers. There are optimal recording sites for the various heart sounds, sites at which the intensity of sound is the highest because the sound is being transmitted through solid tissues or through a minimal thickness of inflated lung. There are four basic chest locations at which the intensity of sound from the four valves is maximised (Fig. 6.29).

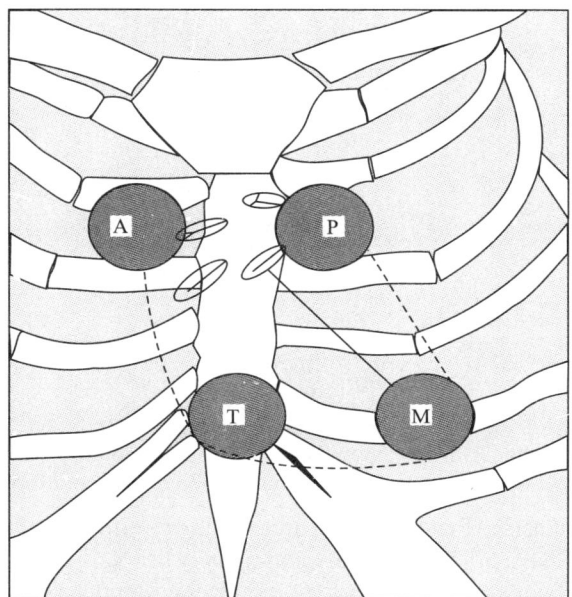

Fig. 6.29. Auscultatory areas on the chest. A, aortic; P, pulmonary; T, tricuspid; and M, mitral areas.

Heart sounds and murmurs have extremely small amplitudes, with frequencies from 0.1 to 2000 Hz. Two difficulties may result. At the low end of the spectrum (below about 20 Hz), the amplitude of heart sounds is below the threshold of audibility. The high-frequency end is normally quite perceptible to the human ear, because this is the region of maximal sensitivity. However, if a phonocardiogram is desired, the recording device must be carefully selected for high frequency-response characteristics. That is, a light-beam, ink-jet or digital-array recorder would be adequate, whereas a standard pen strip-chart recorder would not.

Because heart sounds and murmurs are of low amplitude, extraneous noises must be minimised in the vicinity of the patient. It is standard procedure to record the phonocardiogram for non-bedridden patients in a specially designed, acoustically quiet room. Artifacts from movements of the patient appear as baseline wandering.

Stethoscopes

Stethoscopes are used to transmit heart sounds from the chest wall to the human ear. Some variability in interpretation of the sounds stems from the user's auditory acuity and training. Moreover, the technique used to apply the stethoscope can greatly affect the sound perceived.

Ertel has investigated the acoustics of stethoscope transmission and the acoustical interactions of human ears with stethoscopes. He found that stethoscope acoustics reflected the acoustics of the human ear.

Younger individuals revealed slightly better responses to a stethoscope than their elders. The mechanical stethoscope amplifies sound because of a standing-wave phenomenon that occurs at quarter-wavelengths of the sound. Figure 6.30 is a typical frequency-response curve for a stethoscope; it shows that the mechanical stethoscope has an uneven frequency response, with many resonance peaks.

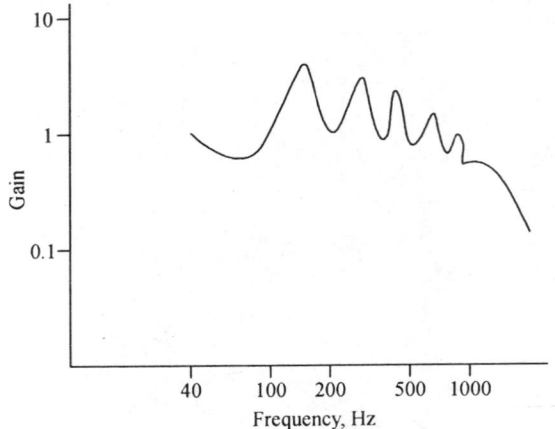

Fig. 6.30. The typical frequency-response curve for a stethoscope can be found by applying a known audiofrequency signal to the bell of a stethoscope by means of a headphone-coupler arrangement. The audio output of the stethoscope earpiece was monitored by means of a coupler microphone system.

These investigators emphasised that the critical area of the performance of a stethoscope (the clinically significant sounds near the listener's threshold of hearing) may be totally lost if the stethoscope attenuates them as little as 3 dB. A physician may miss, with one instrument, sounds that can be heard with another.

When the stethoscope chest piece is firmly applied, low frequencies are attenuated more than high frequencies. The stethoscope housing is in the shape of a bell. It makes contact with the skin, which serves as the diaphragm at the bell rim. The diaphragm becomes taut with pressure, thereby causing an attenuation of low frequencies.

Loose-fitting earpieces cause additional problems, because the leak that develops reduces the coupling between the chest wall and the ear, with a consequent decrease in the listener's perception of heart sounds and murmurs.

Many types of electronic stethoscopes have been proposed by engineers. These devices have selectable frequency-response characteristics ranging from the 'ideal' flat-response case and selected bandpasses to typical mechanical-stethoscope responses. Physicians, however, have not generally accepted these electronic stethoscopes, mainly because they are unfamiliar with the sounds heard with them. Their size, portability, convenience and resemblance to the mechanical stethoscope are other important considerations.

Phonocardiography

A phonocardiogram is a recording of the heart sounds and murmurs. It eliminates the subjective interpretation of these sounds and also makes possible an evaluation of the heart sound and murmurs with respect to the electric and mechanical events in the cardiac cycle. In the clinical evaluation of a patient, a number of other heart-related variables may be recorded simultaneously with the phonocardiogram. These include the ECG, carotid arterial pulse, jugular venous pulse and apex cardiogram. The indirect carotid, jugular and apex-cardiogram pulses are recorded by using a microphone system with a frequency response from 0.1 to 100 Hz. The cardiologist evaluates the results of phonocardiograph on the basis of changes in waveshape and in a number of timing parameters.

CARDIAC CATHETERISATION

The cardiac-catheterisation procedure is a combination of several techniques that are used to assess hemodynamic function and cardiovascular structure. Cardiac catheterisation is performed in virtually all patients in whom heart surgery is contemplated. This procedure yields information that may be crucial in defining the timing, risks and anticipated benefit for a given patient. Catheterisation procedures are performed in specialised laboratories outfitted with X-ray equipment for visualising heart structures and the position of various pressure catheters. In addition, measurements are made of cardiac output, blood and respiratory gases, blood-oxygen saturation and metabolic products. The injection of radiopaque dyes into the ventricles or aorta makes it possible for the clinician to assess ventricular or aortic function. In a similar fashion, injection of radiopaque dyes into the coronary arteries makes possible a clinical evaluation of coronary-artery disease. In the following paragraphs, we shall discuss a number of specific procedures carried out in a catheter laboratory.

Clinicians can measure pressures in all four chambers of the heart and in the great vessels by positioning catheters, during fluoroscopy, in such a way that they can recognise the characteristic pressure waveforms. They measure pressures across the four valves to determine the valve's pressure gradients.

An example of a patient with aortic stenosis will help illustrate the procedure. Figure 6.31a shows the pressure of the stenotic patient before the operation: Note the pressures in the left ventricle and in the aorta and the systolic pressure gradient. Figure 6.31b reflects the situation after the operation: Note the marked decrease in the pressure gradient brought about by the insertion of a ball-valve aortic prosthesis. These pressures may be measured by using a two-lumen catheter positioned such that the valve is located between the two catheter openings. The clinician can find the various time indices that describe the injection and filling periods of the heart directly from the recordings of blood pressure in the heart.

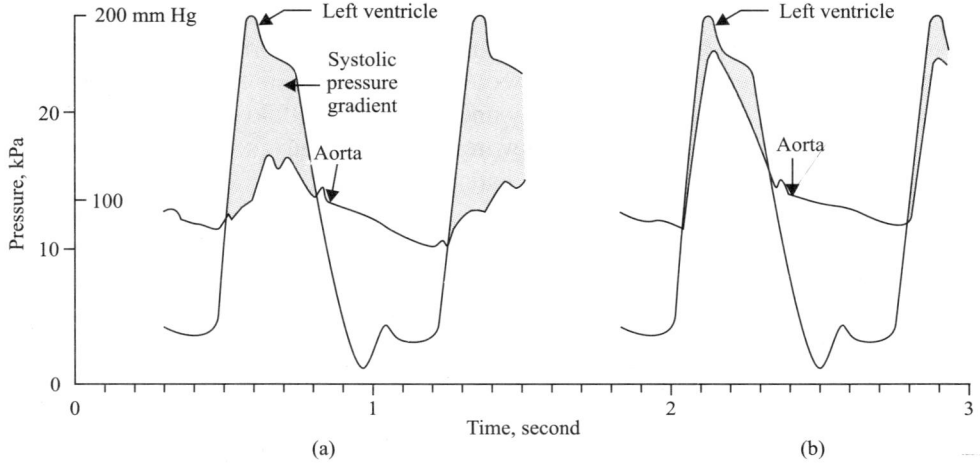

Fig. 6.31. (a) Systolic pressure gradient (left ventricular-aortic pressure) across a stenotic aortic valve. (b) Marked decrease in systolic pressure gradient with insertion of an aortic ball valve.

Clinicians can also use balloon-tipped, flow-directed catheters without fluoroscopy. An inflated balloon at the catheter tip is carried by the bloodstream from the intrathoracic veins through the right atrium, ventricle and pulmonary artery and into a small pulmonary artery—where it is wedged, blocking the local flow. The wedge pressure in this pulmonary artery reflects the mean pressure in the left atrium, because a column of stagnant blood on the right side of the heart joins the free-flowing blood beyond the capillary bed.

This catheter is also commonly used to measure cardiac output using the principle of the thermodilution. Cardiac output is valuable for assessing the pumping function of the heart and can also be measured using dye dilution, the Fick method and impedance cardiography.

Blood samples can be drawn from within the various heart chambers and vessels where the catheter tip is positioned. These blood samples are important in determining the presence of shunts between the heart chambers or great vessels. For example, a shunt from the left to the right side of the heart is indicated by a higher-than-normal O_2 content in the blood in the right heart in the vicinity of the shunt. The O_2 content is normally determined by an oximeter. Cardiac blood samples are also used to assess such metabolic end products as lactate, pyruvate, CO_2 and such injected substances are radioactive materials and coloured dyes.

Angiographic visualisation is an essential tool used to evaluate cardiac structure. Radiopaque dye is injected rapidly into a cardiac chamber or blood vessel and the hemodynamics are viewed and recorded on X-ray film, movie film or videotape. Specially designed catheters and power injectors are used in order that a bolus of contrast material can be delivered rapidly into the appropriate vessel or heart chamber. Standard angiographic techniques are employed, where indicated, in the evaluation of the left and right ventricles (ventriculography), the coronary arteries (coronary arteriography), the pulmonary artery (pulmonary angiography) and the aorta (aortography). During heart catheterisation, ectopic beats and/or cardiac fibrillation frequently occur. These are usually caused by a mechanical stimulus from the catheter or from a jet of contrast material. For this reason, clinicians must have a functional defibrillator readily available in the catheterisation laboratory.

The percutaneous translumenal coronary angioplasty (PTCA) catheter is used to enlarge the lumen of stenotic coronary arteries, thereby improving distal flow and relieving symptoms of ischemia and signs of myocardial hypoperfusion. After initial coronary angiography is performed and the coronary lesions are adequately visualised, a guiding catheter is introduced and passed around the aortic arch. The PTCA catheter is then placed over the guidewire and connected to a manifold (for pressure recording and injections) and to the inflation device. The guidewire is generally advanced into the coronary artery, across from and distal to the lesion to be dilated. A balloon catheter is advanced over the wire and placed across the stenosis. The pressure gradient across the stenosis is measured by using the pressure lumens on the PTCA catheter. This measurement is done to determine the severity of the stenosis. The balloon is repeatedly inflated—usually for 30 to 60 seconds each time—until the stenosis is fully expanded. Test injections are performed to determine whether the coronary artery flow has been improved.

A successful PTCA is an alternative to coronary by-pass surgery for a large proportion of patients with coronary artery disease. It avoids the morbidity associated with thoracotomy, cardiopulmonary by-pass and general anaesthesia. In addition, the hospital stay is much shorter. The patient can be discharged about two days after the procedure. Re-stenosis following coronary angioplasty has been shown to recur in 15 to 35 per cent of cases. Areas of a valve orifice can be calculated from basic fluid-mechanics equations. Physicians can assess valvular stenosis by measuring the pressure gradient across the valve of interest and the flow through it.

PERIPHERAL PULSE TRANSDUCERS

In patient monitoring systems there is a requirement for transducers capable of producing an electrical output signal corresponding to the peripheral arterial pulse contour picked up, for example, from a digit or thumb, the pinna of the ear or from the forehead. Normally only the pulsatile component of the waveform is required so that an AC coupled arrangement is appropriate. The pulsatile signal can be used to trigger a heart rate meter and this may be an arrangement which is less susceptible to electrical artefacts than one triggered from an ECG. In the presence of a low blood pressure or a marked degree of vasoconstriction the pulse signal may diminish or vanish, thus causing heart rate recording to cease. However, if an alarm condition is activated it may be of value in any case for the staff to investigate which factors have led to the loss of the pulse signal.

The commonest form of sensing the peripheral pulse is based upon the technique of photoplethysmography which is a non-invasive method of monitoring changes in peripheral blood volume. The skin at the point where the pulse is to be detected is illuminated with light from a low power bulb or a light-emitting diode. A photosensor is then used to detect light which is either transmitted through or reflected from the vascular bed. Fine and Weinman have given a detailed account of the use of photoconductive cells as detectors in photoplethysmography. These authors point out that physiological events recorded by a photoplethysmographic sensor are the periodic blood-volume pulse and also blood volume variations due to vasomotor activity. The latter are much slower but they can give rise to light variations which are several times greater in intensity than those due to the blood volume pulse. This occurs because of changes in blood volume caused by the pulsatile blood pressure and its profile will thus depend upon the elastic nature of the particular vessel's wall. For an ideally elastic vessel it would be identical with the blood pressure waveform, whereas for an ideally still vessel the blood volume pulse would be zero. Fine and Weinman have investigated the drift and small-signal dynamic properties of a cadmium sellenide photoconductive cell in regard to its suitability for this application. Van Nie has described an improved ear-clip for use with photoplethysmography. The design of the clip is aimed at eliminating artefacts produced when the patient moves without requiring an excessive clamping force on the pinna of the ear. The 37.5 mW infra-red gallium arsenide light emitting diode and the silicon photodiode are each mounted in a cup which can turn slightly with respect to the relevant arm of the clip. When the clip is attached to the ear the cup turns until its flat side is in good contact with the ear. Subsequent loosening of the clip leaves the position of the cup fixed by friction even when the patient moves. Pollard has described a reflected light photoplethysmograph.

When a peripheral pulse waveform is present further information may be obtained from its amplitude. This can be affected by factors such as the blood pressure, degree of vasoconstriction and the occurrence of vascular spasms. In order to be able to operate alarms from physiological changes occurring in the peripheral pulse amplitude it is clearly necessary to have removed possible artefacts. Those due to movement of the patient's head have been eliminated in the pick-up of Van Nie whilst the use of a light-emitting diode enables a modulated light to be employed, thus preventing interference from fluorescent or other light sources present in the room. The small power consumption, typically 38 mW, of the diode also prevents the patient from receiving a burn.

Carotid Pulse Transducers

The monitoring of the carotid pulse waveform can provide a non-invasive substitute for the aortic pulse waveform in the calculation of the left ventricular ejection time. A convenient way of obtaining this is with a light-weight crystal pick-up mounted over the area of the carotid pulse in the neck and feeding into a high input impedance amplifier. It is also possible to place a suction cup over the carotid pulse and detect the pulse by a sensitive air pressure transducer coupled to the cup via a length of rubber tubing. However, movement of the tubing can generate troublesome artefacts. A more faithful pulse waveform can be obtained with an applanation transducer such as the Hewlett Packard which produces a DC output signal when energised with a 6V DC supply. It can be used for either the carotid or jugular pulses or the apex beat. The transducer's frequency range is DC to 300 Hz and its pressure range is 0 to 180 mm Hg. With an excitation of 6 V at 20 mA the sensitivity is 1.5 mV per mm Hg. The operating principle of the applanation transducer is based upon the fact that a solid guard ring on the base of the transducer flattens the body surface upon which it is placed and the internal pressure from the body at the location displaces a spring-retained metal core relative to the surface of the guard ring by an amount proportional to the pressure to be measured. The transducer provides a DC output voltage which is proportional to the core movement. It is a differential transformer arrangement energised with an audio frequency carrier.

Although crystal microphones do not have a frequency response which extends down to DC, the response of a microphone such as the Hewlett Packard Model 21050 is 3 dB down at 0.05 Hz relative to its response at 0.1 Hz when used with a cut-off filter which gives a flat response from 1 to 10 Hz with a 10 dB drop at 100 Hz. A second filter can be used to give a response which is flat from approximately 80 to 1000 Hz with a −10 dB level at 10 Hz. By means of such a splitting network it is possible to separate the low frequency pulse displacement signals from the higher frequency sounds of the phonocardiogram. This facility can be most useful when it is required to monitor both the mechanical motion of the apex beat and the phonocardiogram.

Measurement of Other Physiological Pressures

Transducers which are capable of measuring both venous and arterial blood pressure are also suitable for the measurement of pressure such as airway, oesophageal, urethral, bladder and rectal pressure which might lie in the range 10–100 cm H_2O (73.5 mm Hg). A more sensitive transducer is likely to be required for use with pneumotachograph head for recording respiratory flow rates.

The application technique has been widely applied to the measurement of intra-occular and intra-uterine pressures. Here the applied pressure acts on the pressure sensitive element of the transducer to make it co-planar with a surrounding flat guard ring. When this occurs the force exerted by the transducer balances the pressure to be measured. This system is known as a tonometer.

In neurosurgical intensive care units, the monitoring of intra-cranial pressure may be of considerable value in the detection of post-operative haemorrhage. Various technique have been developed including the use of a pressure transducer mounted in a burr hole drilled through the skull and the use of a radio telemetry link to avoid infection arising when a physical connection has to be made through the skull.

RESPIRATORY MEASUREMENT

Respiration is the process by which gas is exchanged across cell membranes in all living systems. At the cellular level, oxygen enters the cell and carbon dioxide is excreted. This process occurs even in dormant systems such as seeds. In human beings, the lung transfers O_2 from the ambient air to the blood and exhausts CO_2 into the atmosphere. The blood in turn carries O_2 and CO_2 from the cells. To control the rate at which this transfer occurs, an elaborate control system has evolved, as illustrated in Fig. 6.32.

In this process, contraction of respiratory muscles such as the diaphragm and intercostal muscles between the ribs expands the thorax, creating a negative pressure in the lung and drawing in oxygen-rich air. The alveoli exchange O_2 for CO_2 in the blood flowing into the lung. The output blood then stimulates

CO_2-sensitive cells called CO_2 receptors in the arteries near the carotid sinus. These cells, along with stretch receptors in the respiratory muscles, send out nerve impulses the medulla oblongata region of the brain stem. The output from the brain stem is fed back to the respiratory muscles. This controls the breathing rate. Measurements of blood partial pressure of CO_2, called $^P CO_2$ or partial pressure of O_2, called $^P O_2$, show that the respiration rate is controlled by these factors. An increase in $^P CO_2$ increases the breathing rate, as illustrated in Fig. 6.33. CO_2 is a waste product of respiration that must be swept away as it builds up in the lung. On the other hand, as $^P CO_2$ increases, the breathing rate slows down, as indicated in the figure. In this case, the demand for oxygen-rich fresh air decreases.

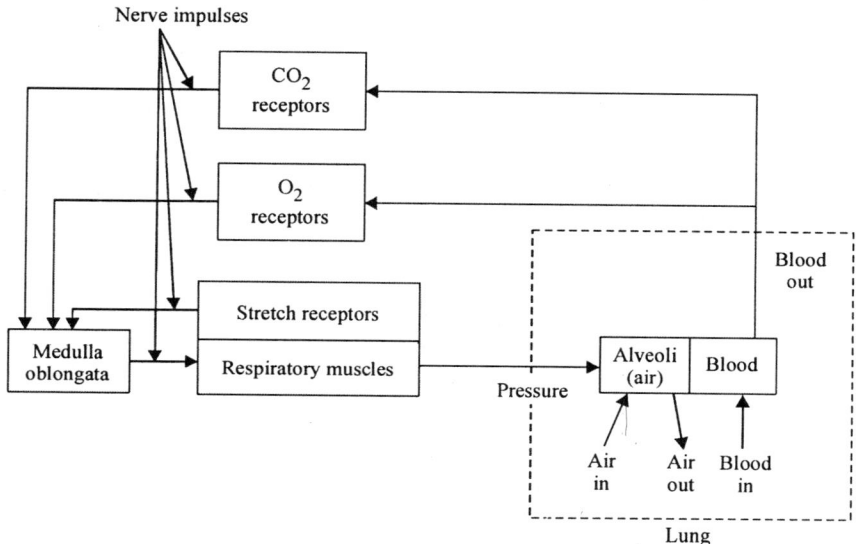

Fig. 6.32. A simplified block diagram of respiratory control.

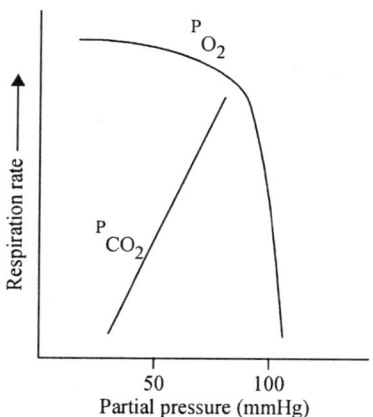

Fig. 6.33. The effect of blood $^P CO_2$ and $^P O_2$ on the respiration rate.

In order to diagnose disease of the lung such as emphysema or bronchitis, clinicians need to measure air volumes and flow rates. The nominal volumes are measured by spirometers and plethysmographs, such as are described further in this chapter.

Measurement of Gas Volumes and Flow Rates

In intensive care situations it is commonplace to monitor the patient's body temperature, ECG and blood pressure and it is increasingly possible to quickly check blood gas tensions and blood pH. Many commercial patient monitor systems make provision for monitoring the respiratory rate, but few can measure the minute volume and respired gas composition. Of course, when the patient is connected to an automatic lung ventilator or respirator there is much more control over the ventilatory volume and regular checks can be made of the blood gases. A knowledge of the tidal volumes and airway pressures can give a valuable insight into the patient's respiratory mechanics and in the case of spontaneously breathing patients a recording of the minute volume changes can be valuable.

Tidal and minute volume meters

A number of turbine-type meters are available for the indication of the tidal volume and in some cases a timer is added to give the minute volume. The mechanism is a miniature air turbine having a very low inertia. The revolutions of the two-bladed rotor can be recorded, in the mechanical version, by means of a gear train and a dial similar to that used in a watch. The dial shows the number of litres of the gas which have traversed the respirometer between two successive readings. Gas entering the respirometer emerges from a series of fixed tangential slots to strike the rotor so that the meter responds to gas flows in one direction only and does not require valves. The ratio of the indicated volume to that actually passed through the meter is flow-rate dependent since slip of gas past the rotor will occur to a greater degree at high flow rates. At very low flows there will be insufficient force to turn the rotor, whilst at high flows the reading tends towards a constant value. Nunn and Ezi-Ashi reported that the Wright respirometer under-read at low flows and over-read at the high flows. During anaesthesia, they found that the combination of the respiratory waveform and the gas mixtures used combined to minimise the small error which would normally arise with hypoventilation. With hyperventilation they always expected over-reading and found that it exaggerated any departure from normality.

Whilst spot checks can readily be made with the purely mechanical Wright's respirometer of a patient's tidal and minute volume, for patient monitoring purposes a need exists for a version with a meter display and electrical outlets for a recorder. Figure 6.34 shows an electronic version of the Wright respiration monitor. The same turbine principle is used as in the original mechanical version, but now the gear train and 'clock type' dial have been replaced by lamp and phototransistor which sense the rotation of the turbine rotor. The resulting electric pulses are counted to give an indication of the tidal volume and totalled over a minute to give the minute volume. The tidal volume range is between 200 and 1500 cc's and the minute volume range from 4 to 30 litres per minute.

The device is claimed to respond to gas flows as low as 2 litres per minute and the accuracy is quoted as being of the order of plus or minus two per cent of the indicated reading. A push button permits a changeover from tidal to minute volume readings. The meter can be powered from the mains supply or from a self-contained rechargeable battery which can operate for 10 hours. The flow head can be sterilised by autoclaving at a maximum temperature of $121°C$ or by the use of ethylene oxide gas. The flow head weighs only 200 gram which makes it convenient to mount on an endotracheal tube or tracheotomy tube, but care must be taken not to drop the respirometer on the floor as false readings may subsequently be obtained. The need to routinely check the calibration of respirometer is brought out by Lunn and Hillard. They found that an individual respirometer performance could differ from the mean of a group by up to plus or minus 15 per cent.

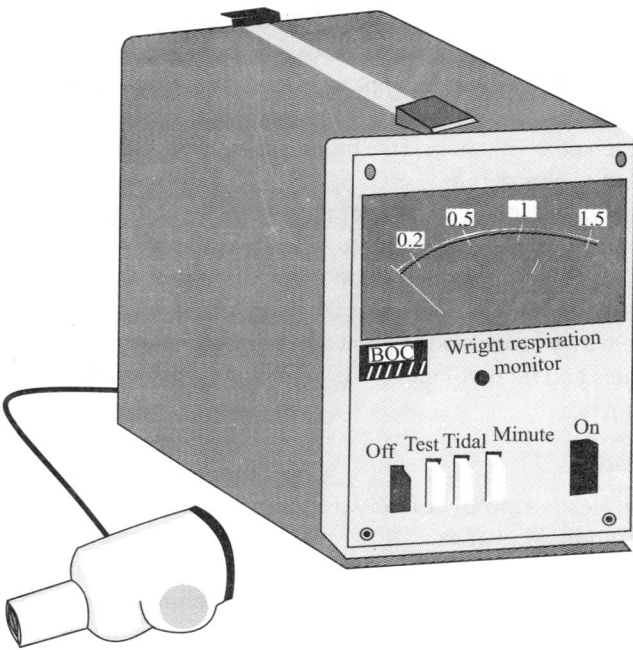

Fig. 6.34. Electronic Wright respiration monitor.

Respirometers can be calibrated for particular flow patterns using a large capacity spirometer or a dry gas meter. Reynolds described the addition of a chopper-disc to a dry gas meter in order to drive a chart recorder or a motor and electromagnetic counter when a chart record is not required. Re-set switches are required to allow the instrument to be used for single breath studies. Cooper discusses the estimation of minute volume during anaesthesia.

Particularly when an automatic lung ventilator is being used to ventilate a patient via an endotracheal tube, it is advisable to place the respirometer so that it measures expiratory and not inspiratory minute volume. The reasoning for this becomes obvious if the cuff of the tube becomes deflated. In this case a constant volume ventilator would supply the pre-set tidal volume but the majority of this might be lost through the leak around the cuff. If the expired minute volume was adequate then at least this much would be recorded as the inspired minute volume. In long-term applications of a ventilator when a humidifier is used, a considerable problem may arise from a condensation of expired water vapour in the respirometer. An electrically heated (low voltage) version of the Dräger volumeter is available to overcome this problem. When a circle anaesthetic system is in use, the carbon dioxide absorber is usually placed in front of the respirometer and traps the majority of the water vapour.

The availability of respirometers having an electrical output enables an alarm to be given if the minute volume should drop below a pre-set value.

Pneumotachograph

A pneumotachograph is essentially a device for the measurement of gas volume flow rates and like the Wright respirometer it is attractive in that the pneumotachograph can conveniently be mounted on a facemask or endotracheal tube. In principle, the head offers a small resistance, typically a few mm of water pressure, to the inspiratory and expiratory tidal flow of gas. The flow through the head is laminar over a stated flow range so that the pressure drop across the head is a linear function of the volume flow rate through the head. The pressure difference appearing across the head is sensed by a sensitive transducer whose output signal is then the time variation of the flow rate. By integrating the flow rate signal an indication is obtained of each tidal volume and the minute volume is obtainable by summing the inspiratory or expiratory tidal volumes over a minute.

In practice, the accurate operation of an integrating pneumotachograph is complicated by the fact that the sensitivity may not be the same for inspiratory and expiratory flows, it will be affected by the composition of the gas flows and the condensation of water vapour and upset by baseline shifts which are not uncommon with sensitive transducers. For these reasons, pneumotachographs tend to be used in research applications where they can provide a great deal of information and not for the routine monitoring of patient's respiratory rates and tidal volumes. They are being used as part of computer systems for the analysis of pulmonary function.

Pneumotachograph heads

Many pneumotachograph heads employ a fine wire mesh gauge as the resistance to flow (Fig. 6.35). This arrangement is commonly known as a 'flow can' and consists of a sheet of 400 mesh wire gauge supported between two metal cones. Provision is usually made to heat the gauge from a low voltage source to prevent the condensation of water vapour from occluding the holes of the gauge. Adjacent to each side of the gauge is a series of small holes around the periphery of the cones. Each set communicates with an annular chamber fitted with a side-arm. A pair of plastic or rubber tubes connect the sidearms to a sensitive pressure transducer. The holes together with the pressure take-off chambers minimise negative pressure effects which may arise at a single orifice due to interaction with the gas stream. Fry evaluated the performance of three types of pneumotachograph head. Gregory and Kitterman have described a pneumotachograph head suitable for use with infants during spontaneous or assisted ventilation. It is constructed from plastic endotracheal tube connectors having an internal diameter of 11 mm and a 400 mesh stainless steel gauge. The output is said to be linear for volume flow rates of 0.05 to 20 litres per minute at respiratory rates from 30 to 120 per minutes. The internal volume of the head is 3.4 ml and the resistance to flow 0.9 mm H_2O per litre per minute. It is desirable to have a range of pneumotachograph heads available to cater for children and adults at rest or exercising. Typical characteristics would be:

Subject	Maximum flow rate	Area	Pressure drop
Children	90 l/min	645 mm^2	8.5 mm H_2O
Adult (resting)	180	1290	6.1
Adult (working)	600	4515	8.5

It is possible to mount the gauge and one cone on to a facemask, but the system is then not symmetrical and difficulty may be experienced in measuring both inspiratory and expiratory flows with the same calibration. Capacitance, unbounded strain gauge, differential transformer and photoelectrical pressure transducers have all been used in conjunction with pneumotachograph heads. An unbounded strain gauge transducer for this purpose has a pressure range of 0 to plus or minus 25 mm H_2O with an output of 5 mV full scale per volt of excitation. The Hewlett Packard Model 270 differential transformer gas pressure transducer has a full scale range of –500 to +400 mm H_2O with a volume displacement of 1.5 mm^3 per mm H_2O and thermal zero drift of 0.07 mm H_2O per degree centigrade.

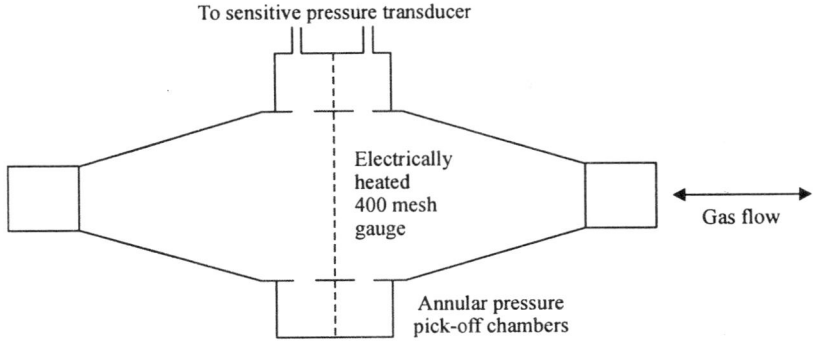

To sensitive pressure transducer

Electrically
heated
400 mesh
gauge

Gas flow

Annular pressure
pick-off chambers

Fig. 6.35. Wire gauge pneumotachograph head.

Another form of pneumotachograph head which is popular is that due to Fleisch. In effect it consists of a large number of small lumen parallel metal tubes. This construction helps to maintain a laminar flow pattern over a wider range of flow rates than is possible with a gauge. Four sizes of head are available to cover the flow range from 0 to 60 and 0 to 1000 litres per minute. For each head the maximum pressure drop developed is approximately 7 mm H_2O. The heads can be electrically heated.

For a given flow rate the pressure drop developed across the head will depend upon the viscosity of the gas mixture. Hobbes showed that the pressure drop increases linearly with an increasing nitrous oxide concentration and that the effect of saturating air at 37°C with water vapour was to reduce the output from the head by 1.2 per cent in comparison with dry air at 37°C. He also reported that raising the temperature of a Fleisch head from ambient to 37°C increased the output from the head by 1 per cent for each degree C rise.

The sudden inspiratory flow rates produced by some forms of automatic lung ventilator can give rise to artefacts in the flow signal produced by a pneumotachograph. Unless care is taken, there is a possibility of a pressure pulse reaching one side of the pressure transducer's diaphragm before it arrives at the other. As a result, a transient pressure difference appears across the diaphragm which is recorded as a high peak of flow. It follows that the pneumatic capacities must be accurately balanced on either side of the flow head. Thick walled rubber tubes, which are tied together, should connect the pneumotachograph head to the transducer. A Fleisch-type head or one consisting of a rigid bundle of parallel metal tubes is preferable to a gauge-type head for use with a ventilator. The cross-section area of the holes may not be the same for inspiratory and expiratory flows and the gauge is likely to be deflected by a pressure pulse.

Use of a pneumotachograph with an integrator

A simple pneumotachograph tracing is useful for measuring the respiratory rate and for indicating inspiration and expiration. However, the addition of an integrator can give the same information plus an indication of the tidal volumes. In Fig. 6.36, the pneumotachograph tracing of volume flow rate against time has been divided into a number of strips each of width dt minutes. Thus the inspiratory and expiratory tidal volumes are given by:

$$\int_{t=t_1}^{t=t_2} f dt \quad \text{and} \quad \int_{t=t_2}^{t=t_3} f dt$$

where f is the instantaneous volume flow rate in litres per minute. Figure 6.37 shows a pneumotachogram together with its integral. The amplitude of the pneumotachogram is proportional to the instantaneous volume flow rate whilst the peak amplitude of the integral trace is proportional to the tidal volume. If the inspired and expired tidal volumes are equal (unity respiratory quotient) the mean level of the integral tracing will be horizontal. With a normal respiratory quotient of say 0.8, the trace will drift and this is arranged to be offset by introducing an equal and opposite signal into the integrator.

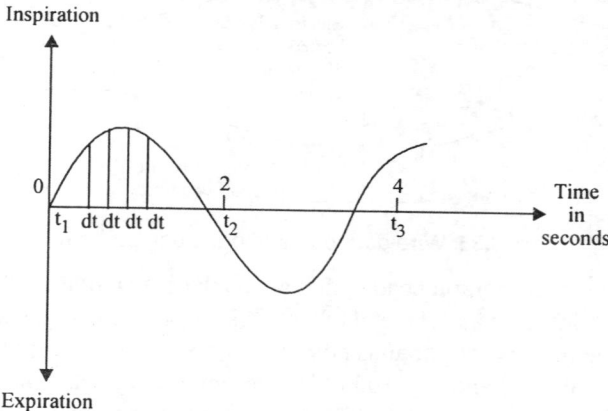

Fig. 6.36. Summation technique for the estimation of the area under a curve of respiratory volume flow rate against time to give the tidal volume.

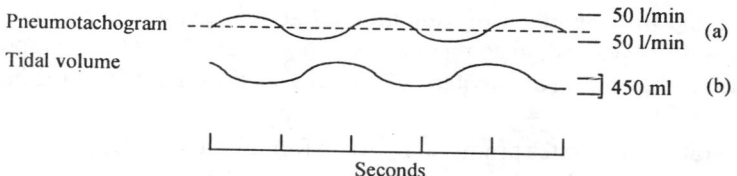

Fig. 6.37. A pneumotachogram (a) and its integral (b).

The tidal volume trace is 90° out of phase with the pneumotachogram since the integral of a sinewave is a cosine wave. For patient monitoring purposes it is convenient to use an integrating circuit which is re-set whenever the respiratory flow rate falls to zero, i.e., twice per respiratory cycle. In this way any baseline drift of the integrator is cancelled at the end of each inspirator and expiration and the trace is kept on the chart paper. This system is described by Whelpton and Watson. Provision is often made to be able to select either the inspiratory or the expiratory tidal volumes and to sum these over an interval of a minute to obtain the minute volume.

Calibration of pneumotachographs

The calibration of a pneumotachograph in terms of volume flow rate is accomplished by passing known flow rates through the flow head. For steady flows a good quality vacuum cleaner is often employed in conjunction with a suitable rotameter-type flowmeter. When it is required to investigate the frequency performance of a pneumotachograph, for example, in relation to hyperventilating patients, then a variable speed sine wave pump is used. For a true sine wave flow pattern, Fry showed that the peak volume flow rate is equal to π times the minute volume. For a minute volume of 10 litres per minute the peak flow would be 31.42 litres per minute. For routine patient monitoring purposes a large plastic syringe, typically of 400 ml capacity, is used to calibrate an integrating pneumotachograph in terms of tidal volume. The plunger is moved in and out at approximately the patient's respiratory rate.

As has been previously mentioned, the task of accurately calibrating a pneumotachograph under conditions of varying gas mixture composition is not easy.

Monitoring of Respiratory Rate

The majority of modular patient monitoring systems make provision for the monitoring of respiratory rate. The rate is usually displayed on a panel meter and provision made to give an alarm if a respiration has not been detected for 15 seconds. Several methods are available, some of which respond to the tidal flow of respiratory gases and some to chest movements only. This can be an important distinction in cases of respiratory obstruction.

Use of a thermistor probe

A thermistor (thermally sensitive resistor) is a small bead of semi-conductor material which posses a marked negative temperature coefficient of resistance. In use, the thermistor probe is taped to the upper lip so that it is bathed by the respiratory gas flow. During expiration, the warm expired air reduces the resistance of the thermistor relative to that obtaining during inspiration. The thermistor is connected as one arm of the Wheatstone bridge network and the out-of-balance voltage from the bridge which occurs with each respiratory cycle is fed to a ratemeter circuit which has a time constant of several seconds. If the length of the rigid probe is excessive it will tend to move away from the lip and out of the airstream. The technique usually works well unless the patient is restless and objects to having anything attached to his face. When oxygen is being administered via a facemask, it is convenient to mount the thermistor in a disposable mask so that it projects into the stream of tidal air.

With patients who have a tracheotomy or who are intubated, the thermistor can be mounted so that its sensitive tip projects into the airway. Gelbrich described the use of a thermistor probe in conjunction with an EEG recorder to measure respiratory rate.

Use of twin thermocouples

Gundersen has reported the use of a pair of thermocouples to monitor the respiratory rate. The two thermocouples are connected in series and one junction is situated 5 mm from the lips and the other 5 mm below one of the nostrils. The reference junctions are located inside a metal tube which is suspended from the subject's forehead. During inspiration all the junctions are at the same temperature and the output signal from the pair of thermocouples is zero. During expiration, on the other hand, the temperature of the external junctions is raised by the warm breath and an output signal results. A curve is still obtained whether the subject breathes through his nose or mouth or both.

Use of a spring-loaded switch

The thermistor technique has the distinct advantage that it does respond to the tidal flow of respiratory gases. If this approach is not possible then it is usual to monitor an indirect variable such as thoracic motion or thoracic electric impedance changes. Chest expansions and contractions as small as 0.5 mm can be detected by means of a sensitive spring-loaded switch which is actuated by means of a light strap or cord placed around the thorax. Expansion of the chest during inspiration causes the switch contacts to close and operate a trigger circuit which produces a pulse for feeding to a respiratory ratemeter. The method is simple, but finding the optimum tension for the strap may require care. Triggering may fail should the patient's mode of respiration change significantly, e.g., if the main respiratory movement changes from the thorax to the abdomen.

Use of a pneumograph

The pneumograph consists of about nine inches (230 mm) of narrow corrugated rubber tube sealed at one end and with the other connected via a flexible tube to a sensitive pressure transducer. A tape joining the two ends of the tube holds it in position around the chest. Respiratory movements cause a fluctuating pressure change in the corrugated tube which is sensed by the transducer and can be displayed on a meter or recorder. The method is simple and reliable but it does require a transducer. It is open to the same criticism as the switch arrangement if the mode of respiratory movement alters and should only be used for the monitoring of respiratory rate and not tidal volume. An alternative approach is to use a mercury-in-rubber strain gauge at the umbilical level.

Monitoring of respiratory rate from the ECG or central venous pressure recording

Many signals such as the ECG, the arterial blood pressure and the external anal sphincter EMG show a more or less marked modulation arising from the effect of respiration. Since many seriously ill patients will have their central venous pressure monitored and the tip of the catheter will lie within the thorax it is feasible to extract the respiratory component from the electrical output of the central venous pressure transducer and use this to monitor respiratory rate. Meagher employed a low-pass filter to extract the respiratory signal from the central venous signal.

The amplitude of the R-waves of an ECG is also subject to respiratory modulation. In practice, Whitlock placed a pair of electrodes one on either side of the chest and a few inches below the armpit. A band-pass filter with 3 dB points at 8 and 12 Hz was used to select the R-waves whilst removing the P and T-waves. Each R-wave is caused to operate a peak follower the output of which is fed into a low-pass filter having a 3 dB point variable from 0.5 to 1 Hz. Whitlock showed that the output waveform from this filter is very similar to a pneumotachogram. The method is suitable for monitoring respiratory rates but cannot be correlated reliably with the tidal volume. Figure 6.38 illustrates an ECG tracing with the electrodes placed for the optimum respiratory modulation of the R-wave amplitudes, but a correlation of only 0.74 was found using an on-line digital computer to correlate the tidal volumes obtained from an integrating pneumotachograph with the R-wave amplitudes.

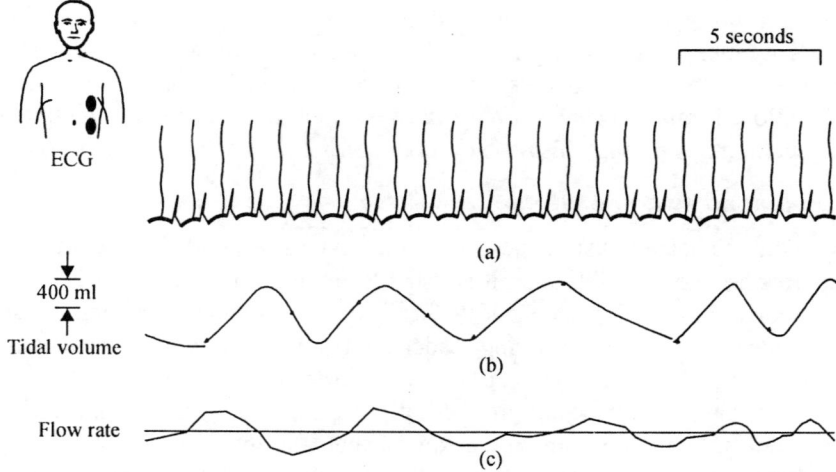

Fig. 6.38. Electrocardiogram (a) obtained from the electrodes placed vertically on the left side of the chest; (b) the corresponding pneumotachogram; and (c) its integral—the tidal volume tracing.

Use of an Impedance Pneumograph for the Measurement of Respiratory Rate and Volume

It has been shown by a number of investigators, that a quantitative relationship exists between the tidal volume and the transthoracic electrical impedance change. Pacela has examined various techniques for measuring the impedance changes. Baker showed that over the frequency range 50–100 kHz the changes found in the transthoracic impedance which accompanied respiration were essentially due to changes of the resistive component only and were independent of the frequency over this range.

Figure 6.39 shows the block diagram of a two-terminal impedance pneumograph, the pair of disk electrodes being placed bilaterally along the mid-axillary lines. The impedance measured across the thorax is given by $(Z_0 + \Delta Z)$ where Z_0 is the standing impedance and ΔZ is the impedance change which accompanies respiration. The output impedance of the oscillator supplying the signal current to the patient is higher than $(Z_0 + \Delta Z)$ so that the circuit is essentially a constant current arrangement. The voltage developed across the two electrodes is given by $(V_0 + V_1) = i(Z_0 + \Delta Z)$. Z_0 is usually of the order of 200 ohms whilst ΔZ will be a few ohms per litre tidal volume. After amplification, the output voltage is rectified and smoothed to give DC components V_{0DC} and V_{1DC}. With this system it is possible to monitor both the respiratory changes of the impedance and also any variations which may occur in the standing impedance. However, for respiratory monitoring it is usual to employ an AC coupled amplifier and to display only the ΔZ signal on a recorder. For silver disk electrodes 10 mm in diameter, the contact impedance is about 250 ohms and the potential drop at each electrode is 0.25 V giving a total power dissipation of about 0.5 mW at the electrodes with a further 0.25 mW in the thorax. One commercial patient monitoring system passes 5 mA rms at 500 kHz across the patient's thorax. The detection system after demodulation of the radio frequency signal has a frequency response of 0.05–1 Hz (–3 dB) and is scaled 0–50 breaths per minute.

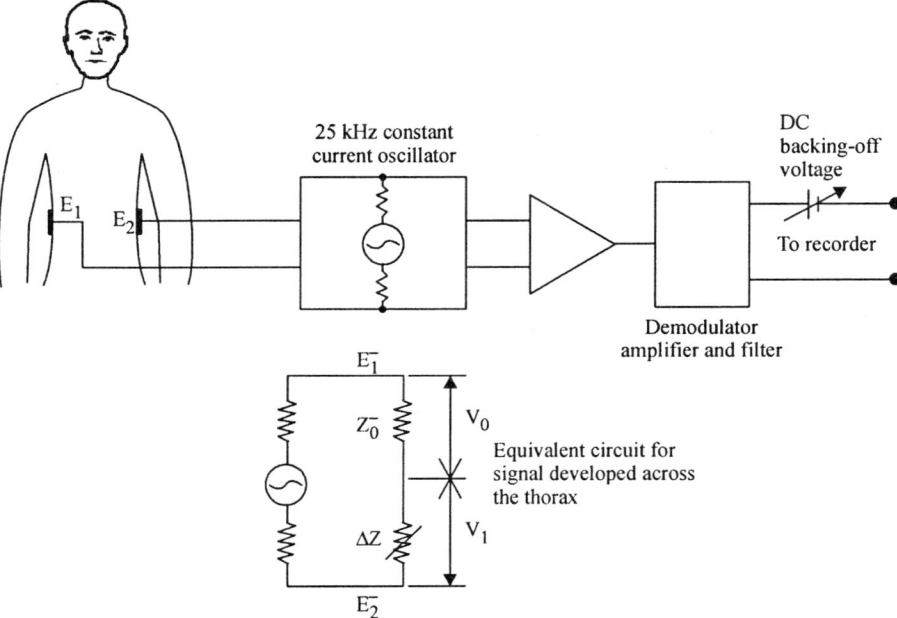

Fig. 6.39. Block diagram of a 2-terminal impedance pneumograph.

The impedance electrodes will also pick-up an ECG signal if the lead 1 input of an electrocardiograph is connected to them. This is a non-standard ECG signal, but it is useful for monitoring heart rate changes. Because of the low transthoracic impedance hum pick-up is small and Colline has obtained clean respiration and ECG recordings from a patient connected to the impedance pneumograph by twenty feet (6.1 m) of cable. The simple two-terminal pneumograph is convenient to use with resting or anaesthetised patients. Since the electrode contact impedance is of the same order as the resting transthoracic impedance, artefact signals will arise if movement of the electrodes significantly alters the contact impedance. Movement artefacts can be reduced by the use of a four-terminal system (Fig. 6.40). The two outer electrodes 1 and 4 act as a feed for the constant current, whilst the potential variations are detected at electrodes 2 and 3. These only carry the small input current of the amplifier and not the oscillator current. With the four-terminal arrangement only ΔZ is measured.

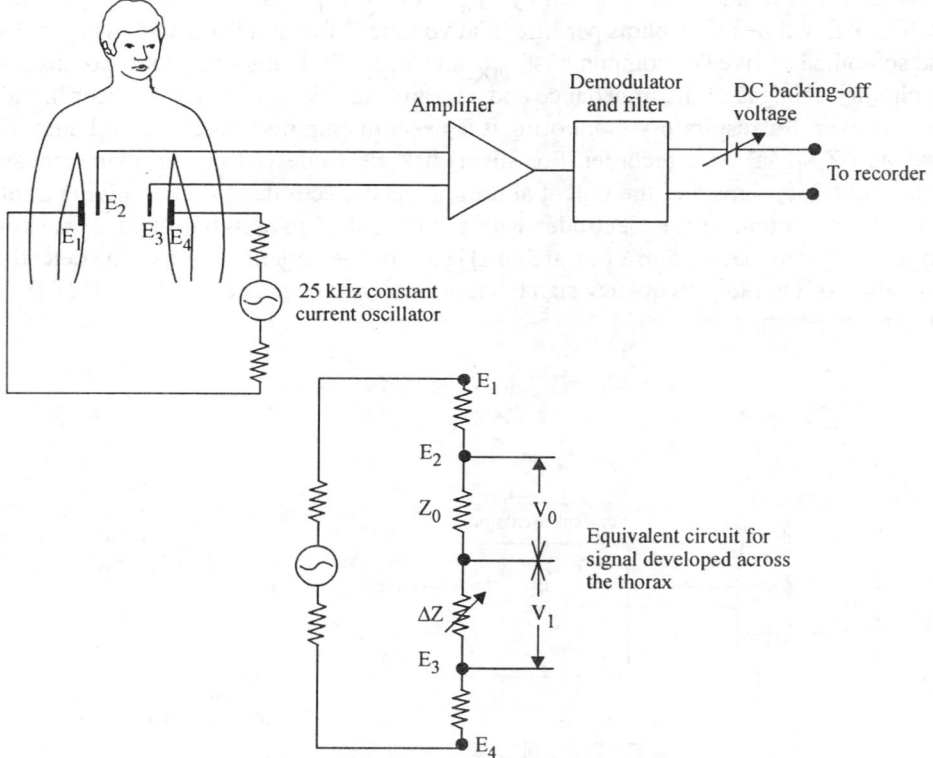

Fig. 6.40. Block diagram of a 4-terminal impedance pneumograph.

Barker and Brown have described a simple two-terminal impedance pneumograph and an associated integrator to give an output proportional to the minute volume. In order to generate an output signal proportional to the minute volume, the demodulated respiratory signal is further amplified, full-wave rectified and the peak voltage excursions stored. As the demodulated signal passes through zero, successive positive and negative voltage changes are produced at the output of the first operational amplifier. These voltages are used to gate the peak voltages at P via Tr_3 and Tr_4. The resulting pulses are integrated to give an output which is proportional to the minute volume. This output is quoted as being linear within plus or minus 5 per cent of full-scale over the respiratory rate range of 12–60 breaths per minute and an impedance range of 0.2 to 2 ohms.

Calibration of an impedance pneumograph

The Z_0 reading of a two-terminal impedance pneumograph can be calibrated by connecting the leads to a decade resistance box whose resistance can be altered in 1 ohm steps and adjusting the box until the recorder baseline for the pneumograph is the same as it was with the patient connected. The respired volume for a given ΔZ will vary for each patient and must be determined for the individual concerned. For spontaneously breathing patients the pneumograph can be calibrated against a device such as the Wright respirometer or an electrically recording fast response spirometer. For anaesthetised patients who have received a muscle relaxant drug the calibration factor of the pneumograph in ohms per litre can be found from the known stroke volume of the automatic lung ventilator or by inflating the patient's lungs with a large (400 ml) volume syringe.

Application of impedance pneumographs

Geddes used the method with conscious patients and Pallett and Scopes have used it with newborn infants. Gougerot and Kitterman found the method accurate if the calibration was performed at the start of the monitoring but errors up to 20 per cent in the tidal volume were found if a calibration was not performed and an average value assumed for $\Delta V/\Delta Z$. Lewis found the respiratory rate could be monitored indefinitely with the technique, but the tidal volume calibration could not be relied upon to stay the same after periods of an hour or more. Baker found the method convenient to use with anaesthetised, paralysed, patients. Figure 6.41 shows the straight-line calibration they obtained for ΔZ against tidal volume for a 54 years old woman undergoing surgery for the removal of a bladder stone. The slope of the line was 2.27 ohms per litre. Superimposed recordings are shown in Fig. 6.42 of ΔZ for this patient when the time periods of inspiration and expiration were varied but their sum was fixed at 5 seconds. The recordings show that the peak amplitude of ΔZ is independent of the ratio of inspiratory to expiratory times and that the pneumograph faithfully indicates tidal volume over this pattern of ventilation. Using two 4-terminal impedance pneumographs operating respectively at 20 and 50 kHz, Baker has shown that it is possible to monitor the ventilation of the right and left lungs in patients with a previously diagnosed pulmonary pathology. Farman and Juett found the impedance technique of a value in the monitoring of post-operative patients. However, it must be pointed out that the technique monitors thoracic movements and not respired gas flow directly. Thus if a patient suffers a respiratory obstruction, perhaps due to the kinking of an endotracheal tube, an alarm will only be given when chest movements cease or previously to this when they have become markedly abnormal.

Geddes showed that the high frequency currents used in impedance pneumographs do not constitute a ventricular fibrillation hazard, whilst Cooley showed that unless the electrodes were large in area, two-terminal impedance pneumographs measure predominantly localised changes in the impedance of the thoracic wall at their point of placement.

Gundersen make the point that with the high respiratory rates of infants difficulty may be experienced from cardiac pulsations which are difficult to filter out under these circumstances without affecting the respiratory signal.

A number of commercially available impedance pneumograph respiration modules are offered for use in patient monitoring systems. It is claimed that tidal volumes as small as 10 ml can be measured with a 4-terminal 50 kHz system. An alarm can be given if the tidal volume diminishes by a pre-set percentage. An apnoea alarm can be set to operate if no respiratory excursion is detected after 5, 10 or 20 seconds. With some apnoea alarms a valid breath has to be detected within 20 seconds and this is defined in adults as a tidal volume of at least 200 cc's and a flow rate of at least 200 cc's per second.

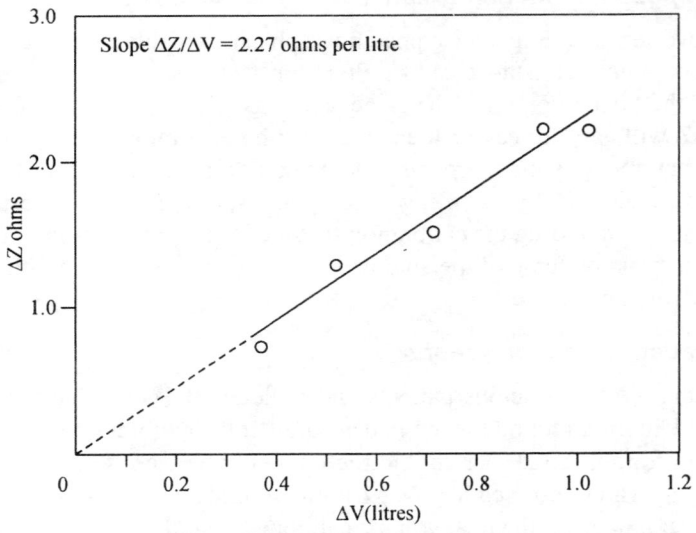

Fig. 6.41. Straight line calibration obtained for a 2-terminal impedance pneumograph..

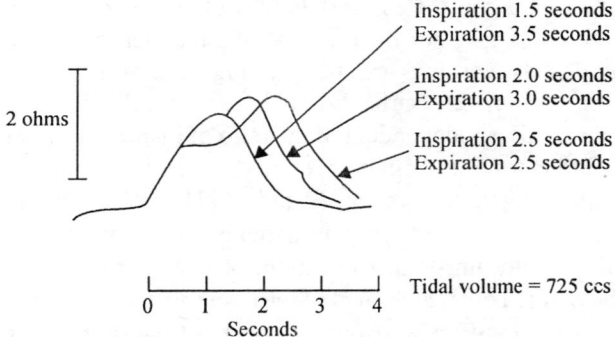

Fig. 6.42. The effect of changing the ratio inspiratory time/expiratory time for a constant tidal volume on the output from a 2-terminal impedance pneumograph.

Ultrasonic spirometer

An interesting method for the continuous monitoring of a patient's respiratory rate, tidal and minute volume operates by measuring the velocity of a beam of ultrasound when it is travelling with and against the tidal flow of respired gas. It is similar in principle to that of Franklin for the measurement of arterial blood flows. The breathing tube of the spirometer is 100 mm long and weighs 85 gram. It is connected to the patient's airway or facemask so that the tidal flow of gas passes through the tube. A pair of piezoelectric crystals C_1 and C_2 are placed at the ends of a cross-tube whose axis makes an angle of approximately 45° with the axis of gas flow. The crystals transmit bursts of ultrasound alternately upstream and downstream, each crystal alternating at 2.5 ms intervals as the transmitter and receiver. The velocity of the gas flow parallel to the axis of the ultrasound transmission adds to the velocity of the ultrasound when the two are in the same direction and subtracts from it when they are opposed. The difference in the transit times is then proportional to the gas velocity and hence to the tidal volume if the flow signal is integrated. The ultrasonic frequency is approximately 100 kHz. Small ports in the breathing tube allow for the simultaneous recording of airway pressure, carbon dioxide concentration and oxygen content breath-by-breath. The ultrasonic crystals can be removed to allow the breathing tube to be sterilised. The respiration rate range is 0–50 breaths per minute, the tidal volume range 0–1.5 litres and the minute volume range 0 to 25 litres. The respiratory flow rate range is 0 to plus or minus 2 litres per second. A linearity of plus or minus 1 per cent is claimed for flow rate and respiratory rate, plus or minus 3 per cent for tidal volume and plus or minus 5 per cent for minute volume. The performance of the ultrasonic spirometer has been analysed by Blumenfeld. It was shown that corrections must be made for the effects of temperature, moisture and gas composition otherwise significant errors in the readings can be expected. For example, calibration with dry air at 30°C and measurement of air at 40°C having a 44 mm Hg partial pressure of water vapour will give a reading which is 5.3 per cent too high (3.5 per cent due to the temperature increase and 1.8 per cent due to the water vapour). Similarly, changing from air to 100 per cent oxygen alters the velocity of the ultrasound and produced a 9 per cent error. Blumenfeld point out that under clinical conditions a 5 per cent error in the measurement of the respiratory flow can give rise to a 25 per cent error in the calculation of oxygen consumption.

Detection of Apnoea in Infants

The monitoring of respiration in infants is complicated by the high respiratory rate encountered and the need not to encumber the infant with wires. Pallet and Scopes used an electrical impedance arrangement, whilst Caro and Bloice used the Doppler shift obtained by reflecting a beam of microwave (10 GHz) radiation from the infant's chest.

The wavelength involved was about 3 cm resulting in a marked frequency shift due to respiratory movements. Lewin placed the baby upon a segmental air filled mattress. The segments were connected by tubes arranged to puff air over a thermistor as long as there was a respiratory motion. The performance of the device has been validated by Blake and Gundersen and Dahlin. Figure 6.43 shows how, for various sensitivity settings, the indication from the mattress of respiration agreed with that obtained using a mercury-in-rubber strain gauge placed around the infant's body at the umbilical level. Gundersen and Dahlin found that in this position the mercury strain gauge pneumograph worked well whether the child was breathing with its thorax or abdomen.

A number of commercial apnoea alarms for neonates are based upon impedance pneumography. Some, such as the Backman Vital Signs Monitor utilise a three stage alarm logic in order to minimise false alarms in babies who are breathing irregularly without sacrificing an early detection of distress. In the first stage a breath pause light is activated if a breath does not occur within a pre-set interval in the range 5 to 15 seconds. A second stage alarm consisting of a visible and an intermittent audible signal is activated if a breath does not occur within the interval 15 to 25 seconds. Both first and second stage alarms are cancelled if the infant overcomes his difficulties and achieves 24 breaths per minute. If this is not achieved a red 'apnoea' light is turned on and a continuous audio alarm is sounded. The third stage alarms must be silenced by the intervention of a nurse. Some systems such as the Air-Shields neonatal intensive care system incorporate a check on the contact impedance of the electrodes. This arrangement minimises the possibility of false alarms due to loose or detached electrodes.

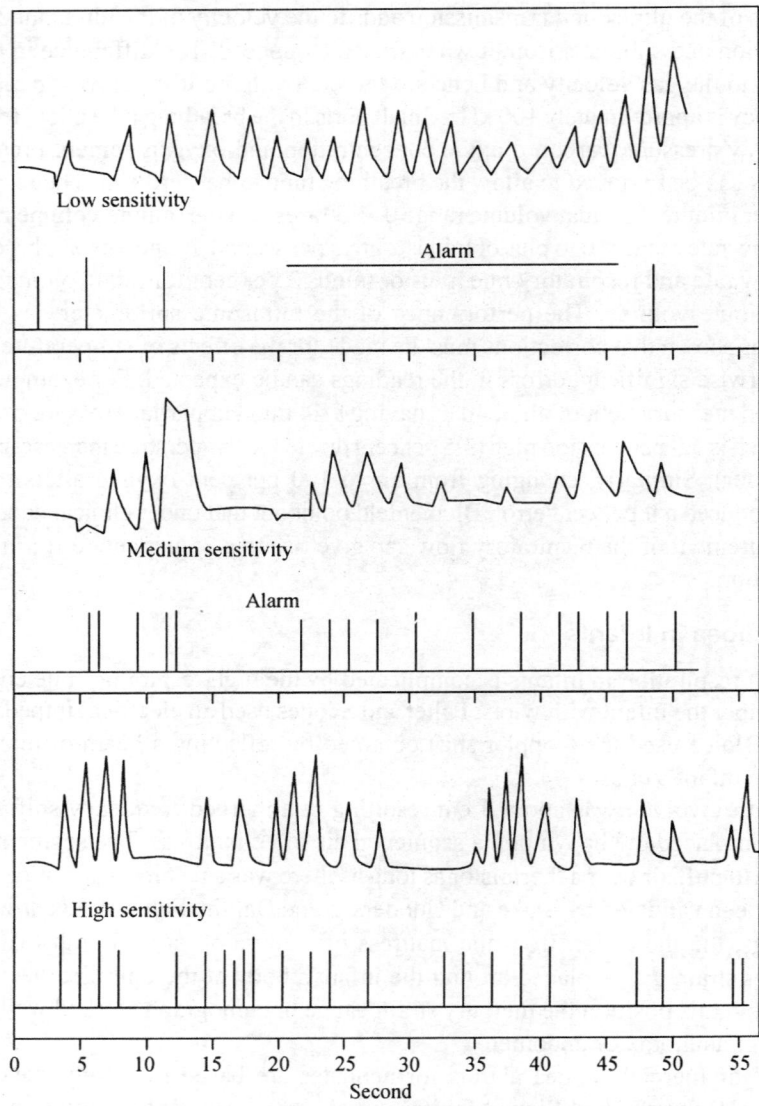

Fig. 6.43. The effect of adjusting the sensitivity of the segmental mattress system in comparison with the respiratory indications from a mercury-in-rubber strain gauge.

Peak flow meter

Wright and McKerrow showed that the maximum forced expiratory flow rate ('peak flow rate') was a convenient and reliable index of a patient's ventilatory capacity. They describe a portable peak flow meter which is often found in intensive care units. The principle of the meter is shown in Fig. 6.44. A cylindrical cavity about 127 mm in diameter and 36 mm deep has a radial inlet nozzle (1) and contains a moveable vane (2) pivoted in the centre of the cylinder and fitting closely without touching. A fixed partition (3) extends from one side of the inlet orifice to within a short distance of the boss of the vane but also does not touch it. A spiral spring (4) attached to one end of the vane's spindle tends to rotate it towards the inlet orifice, a stop (5) prevents it from passing the orifice. A pointer (6) on the other end of the spindle counterbalances the vane and indicates its position on a scale. An annular orifice (7) extends around the periphery of the cylinder at the back from one side of the inlet orifice to the other. The subject takes a deep breath and then blows as hard as possible into the instrument.

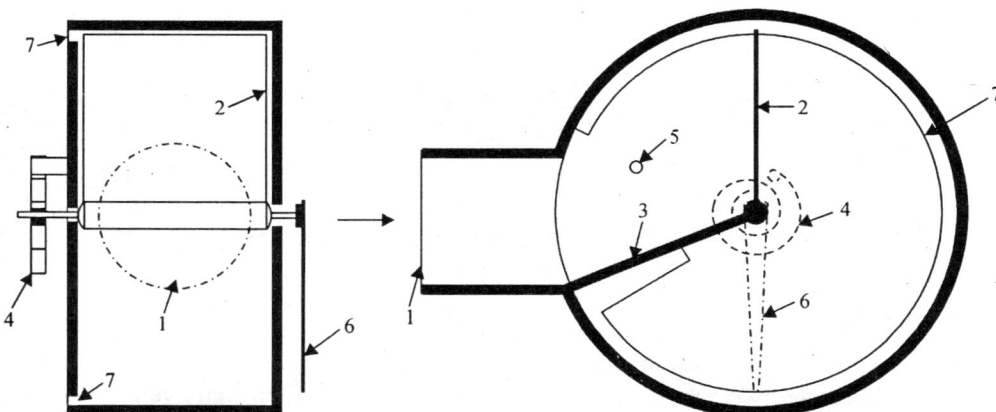

Fig. 6.44. Constructional details of the peak flowmeter.

The air cannot escape (except for a small amount which leaks past the vane) until the vane has moved and uncovered part of the annular orifice. When the area uncovered is such that the pressure behind the vane is just sufficient to balance the force of the spring, the vane will come to rest in a position dependent upon the peak flow rate. The spring tension increases with deflection so that the deflection is less for high flows than for low flows. A ratchet holds the vane in its position of maximum deflection until released manually. Flows in the range 50 to 1000 litres per minute can be measured. The average of three successive attempts is taken. Disposeable cardboard mouthpieces can be used or a plastic mouthpiece which can be washed and sterilised.

Chapter 7

Biotelemetry

INTRODUCTION

Telemetry systems are special cases of patient monitor systems in which the monitoring is done from a remote location. There are two basic forms of telemetry system: radio telemetry and landline telemetry. The radio form uses a small radio transmitter attached to the patient that picks up electrocardiograph (ECG) or some other electrophysical parameter and transmits it via radio waves to a central monitoring point. The landline form of telemetry uses an audio tone to represent the analog ECG or other signal and then transmits over telephone lines.

Telemetric transmission of functional and physiological information offers many advantages in medical diagnostics and patient surveillance. The telemetric data link avoids direct connections to the recording or monitoring equipment, which are sometimes embarrassing and re-straining, thus leaving the patients freely movable. They can be monitored in their natural environment and during work. Accordingly, the measurement does not influence the physiological system under study, thus avoiding severe artifacts. This advantage is especially important in behavioural studies involving both human and animals. Implantable telemetry systems transmit internal physiological signals or serve to control and programme implanted devices, such as stimulators and drug infusion systems, without the need of transcutaneous wire connections which always carry the risk of infection.

CLASSIFICATION AND PRINCIPLES OF BIOTELEMETRY

Biotelemetry is defined as the transmission of biomedical signals and parameters to a remote recorder by means that do not cause substantial disturbances and restraints to the animal or human being monitored. The classification of systems is based on the technical principles of transmission (i.e., wireless or by wire, radio wave, ultrasonic wave or light wave). Further classification is according to the range of transmission, number of simultaneous data channels, modulation techniques and application (implanted, ingestible or portable), as show in Table 7.1.

Depending on the distance between patient and remote recorder, on-wire transmission is realised either as a direct connection between transducer and recorder or uses interference-reducing pre-amplifiers-driven cable connections or even interference-proof signal modulation (Fig. 7.1). Wireless telemetry transmits the signals by modulation of a carrier wave that serves as a transmission link (Fig. 7.2). Besides the commonly used battery-operated systems, passive telemetry transmitters, which do not require any power supply, exist for applications in long-term implantable devices, offering unlimited operation times.

Table 7.1. Application of various biotelemetry techniques and devices.

Application	Wire telemetry	Radio telemetry	Ultrasonic telemetry	Light telemetry	Telephonic telemetry	Implanted devices	Ingestible devices	Portable devices	Fixed devices
Animal application									
Remote measurements		x	x	x		x	x	x	
Tracking		x	x					x	
Human application									
Patient monitoring	x	x	x	x	x	(x)		x	
Function tests		x	x	x	x	x	x	x	
Rehabilitation		x	x	x	x			x	
Remote diagnosis	x				x			x	
Mobile clinical emergency systems		x						(x)	
Work and sport		x	x	x			x	x	
Research		x	x	x			(x)	x	

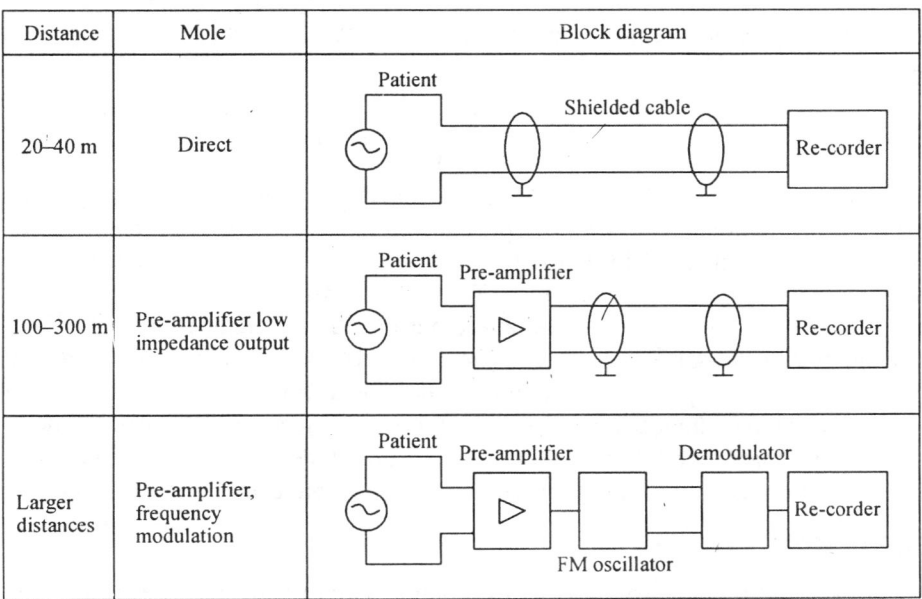

Fig. 7.1. Block diagrams of wire telemetry for different transmission ranges.

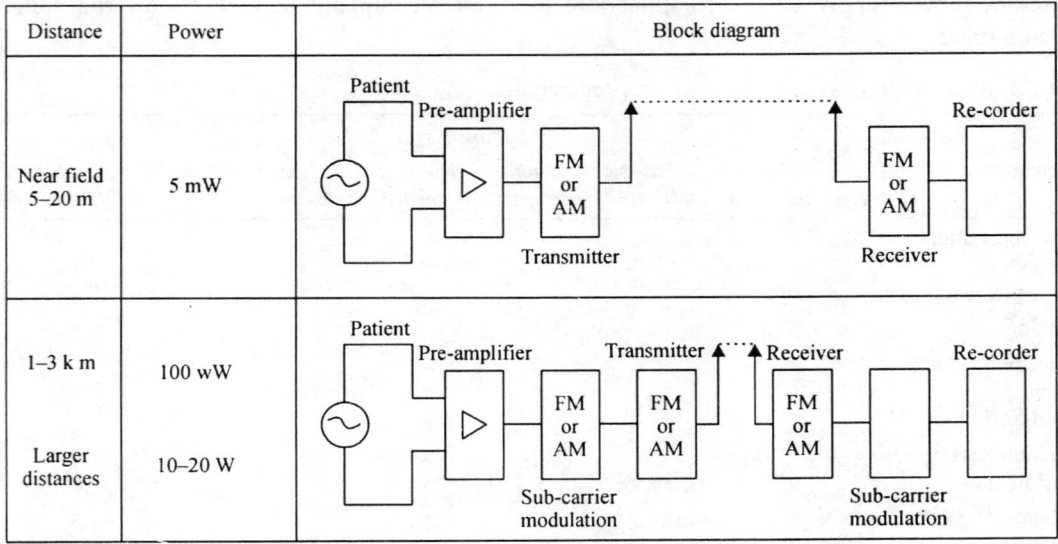

Fig. 7.2. Block diagrams of wireless telemetry for different transmission ranges.

CABLE TRANSMISSION

The easiest way to transmit data from the patient to the recorder is to use a shielded cable link. Transmission is limited in range and bandwidth because the cable reactance causes frequency-dependent attenuation of the signal. Within the bandwidth range of physiological signals, cable capacitance is the most important limiting factor. The bandwidth of a shielded cable, driven from a voltage source with an output resistance R, is given by

$$f_{3dB} = \frac{0.16 \times 10^{12}}{RCl} \text{(Hz)} \qquad \qquad ... (7.1)$$

where C is the capacitance of the shielded cable in picofarads per metre and l the length of the cable in metres. Thus a 300 m shielded cable with a capacitance of 100 pF/m, driven from a source resistance of 100 Ω, provides a bandwidth of 50 kHz. Additional parameters, such as cable inductance and resistance, further reduce bandwidth or transmission range. Thus wire transmission in excess of about 50 m uses signal pre-amplifiers offering signal gain and an output impedance matched to that of the cable. The cable is terminated with the same impedance. The signal receiver is usually a differential amplifier, avoiding ground loops and suppressing common mode interference signals. Transmission over very long distances, where signal attenuation, noise and interference are severe problems, is done by using a high-frequency carrier that is modulated by the signal in amplitude or frequency. Thus, by modulation, the attainable signal-to-noise ratio (SNR) for the transmitted signal can be increased substantially.

RADIO-TELEMETRY SYSTEMS

Many hospitals used radio-telemetry systems to monitor certain patients. The most common use of radio-telemetry is to keep track of improving cardiac patients while at the same time keeping them ambulatory. These units are sometimes called post-coronary care units (PCCU), step-down CCU or some other name that indicates a less rigorous monitoring and care regime than the full coronary care unit where new heart patients are treated. The telemetry unit is sort of a 'half-way house' between the full-up CCU and either the general medical floor patient population or discharge to home care.

The telemetry unit uses a tiny cigarette pack-sized VHF or UHF radio transmitter that is attached to the patient either by a belt clip or in a small sack hung around the patient's neck. The transmitter contains an analog ECG section that acquires the signal and uses it to frequency modulate (FM) the radio transmitter. The nurse's station is equipped with a bank of radio receivers tuned to the same frequencies as the various transmitters. The receiver demodulates the FM signal to recover the analog ECG waveform. The waveform is then displayed on an oscilloscope and/or strip-chart recorded as in any other patient monitoring systems. The signal may also be input to a computerised monitoring system (indeed, today it probably will be so processed).

It is common practice to use either specialised frequencies set aside by the Federal Communications Commission (FCC) for medical telemetry use or television channel frequencies. It is not unusual for a telemetry transmitter to operate in the quietest 'guard band' between the video carrier and sound carrier to TV channels. These VHF and UHF frequency selections allow the telemetry system designer to use hardware that was originally designed for the master antenna TV (MATV) or cable TV industries to process signals for the medical system.

Many different types of radio-telemetry systems are being used. Their basic construction, however, is always the same. Transducers provide the signal to be transmitted and a radio-frequency (rf) carrier is modulated by the signal and fed to the radiating antenna. For short-range transmission, the antenna is often omitted, radiation being emitted by the oscillator coil as in the simple radio transmitter shown in Fig. 7.3a. The antimony/silver chloride (Sb/AgCl) electrodes that are in contact with the gastric acid represent a galvanic element that provides pH-dependent voltage modulation of the transistor. The magnesium/antimony (Mg/Sb) electrodes together with the physiologic sodium chloride (NaCl) solution form a battery providing the operating power. The capsule is swallowed and then transmits a frequency according to the sensed pH.

In most applications, however, batteries are required as well as a distinct modulator. Figure 7.3b shows an ultrahigh-frequency (UHF) tunnel-diode (TD) transmitter. Frequency modulation is achieved by the two variable capacitance diodes (CD) that are controlled by the signal voltage U_s. The frequency range of this transmitter is about 100–250 MHz, the mass without battery is less than 0.5 gram, the volume is a disk of about 5 mm diameter and 2 mm height and the range of transmission is up to about 20 m. Longer ranges are achieved by additional rf amplifiers and/or antennas, increasing the emitted power. A two-stage circuit for accomplishing this is shown in Fig. 7.4.

The need for short-range telemetry with an operating range of only a few feet might seem questionable. However, wireless transmission is required from totally implanted devices to eliminate any transcutaneous wires with their healing and infection problems. Transmission from the implanted system to the body surface is all that is required to solve this problem.

The range of radiotelemetry systems is affected mainly by power, frequency bandwidth and antenna gain. Environmental conditions, such as shielding by steel-concrete buildings, also influence transmission characteristics. Steel-concrete is penetrated easily only by carrier frequencies above 100 MHz.

Two principles of electromagnetic energy transmission are possible: inductions and rf radiation. Inductive coupling is effective only over very short range of several feet, whereas rf waves enable far-reaching transmission links. Inductive transmission is based on the electromagnetic coupling of two transmission coils, where the information is transferred from the primary coil to the secondary coil induction flow. Long-range transmission is based on the emission of radio waves from the transmitter antenna and the sensing of the high-frequency electromagnetic field by the receiving antenna. As induction and radio-wave systems base on dissimilar principles of transmission, optimum carrier frequencies differ greatly.

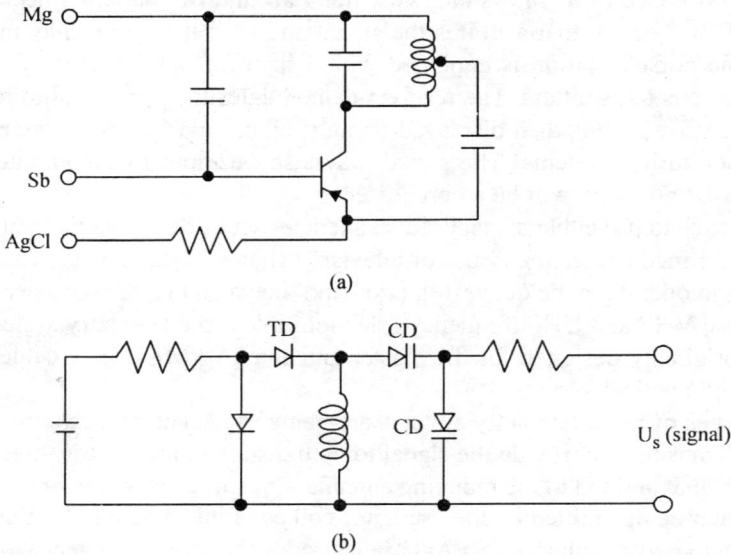

(a)

(b)

Fig. 7.3. Circuits of simple radio transmitters. (a) Single-stage electrode powered pH-transmitted; and (b) tunnel-diode battery-operated modulation stage.

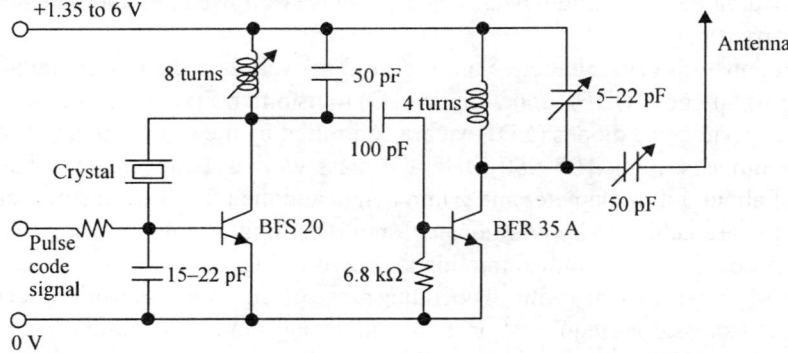

Fig. 7.4. Circuit diagram of a two-stage transmitter for pulse code telemetry. Frequency range is 100–150 MHz.

CARRIER FREQUENCY

Inductive systems typically use frequencies in the range of 1 kHz to 1 MHz, much lower than radio-wave transmitters which have frequencies between 20 and 500 MHz. This has several advantages: simple construction, adequate frequency stability without employing crystal oscillators, negligible generation of rf radiation and thus, usually no regulatory control to impose severe restrictions on radiation transmitters. Disadvantages include the fact that the low carrier frequency of inductive systems, which are sometimes subject to invincible limitations (e.g., in metallic encapsulated implants where the frequency cannot surpass 20 kHz for reasons of eddy currents) also limits the maximum possible rate of data flow within the telemetry system.

High transmission frequencies are chosen for radio-wave transmitters for several reasons: Passive components such as capacitors and coils have very small sizes to facilite miniaturisation, high data transfer capacity is enabled, the small wavelengths do not need large antennas and in-house transmission is possible over longer distances in spite of metallic constructions.

MULTIPLEXING

Many applications require the transmission of various signals at the same time. For this purpose multichannel telemetry systems provide simultaneous data transfer by either frequency-division or time-division multiplexing procedures. Frequency multiplexing uses sub-carriers with various frequencies that are frequency-modulated by the measuring signal. Figure 7.5 shows a two-channel frequency-division multiplex radiotelemetry system. The sub-carriers are linearly mixed and the resulting signal modulates the main carrier. The sub-carrier frequencies must be chosen such that no overlapping of the signal-modulated spectra occurs. The receiver first demodulates the carrier signal and then separates the modulated sub-carriers by appropriate band-pass filters. Subsequent sub-carrier demodulation yields the single signals.

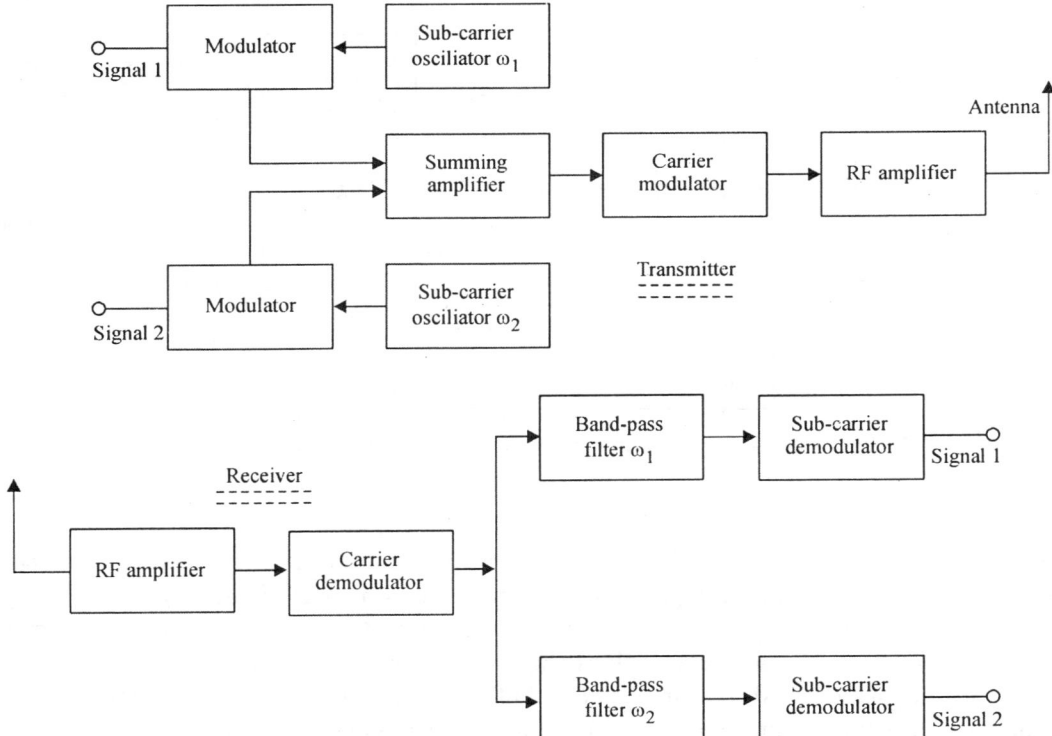

Fig. 7.5. Block diagram of two-channel frequency-division multiplex radiotelemetry system.

In a time-division multiplexing system, as shown in Fig. 7.6, the single channel are sampled periodically. If the sampling theorem is satisfied (i.e., the sampling frequency is at least twice the highest signal frequency), no information is lost. The sampling values of the different channels are then arranged side by side by a commutator that opens the transfer channel successively for the various signal channels, which results in a pulse train representing each of the channels for a certain time interval. In the receiver, another commutator demultiplexes the signal samples, which are first fed to a sample-and-hold circuit and then reconstructed by low-pass filters. To identify the single channels in the receiver, an additional channel, the frame reference signal, is transmitted to indicate the beginning of a new cycle. The reference signal is marked by some characteristics property, for example, a longer duration or a special amplitude. The bandwidth of the signals is determined by the sampling rate.

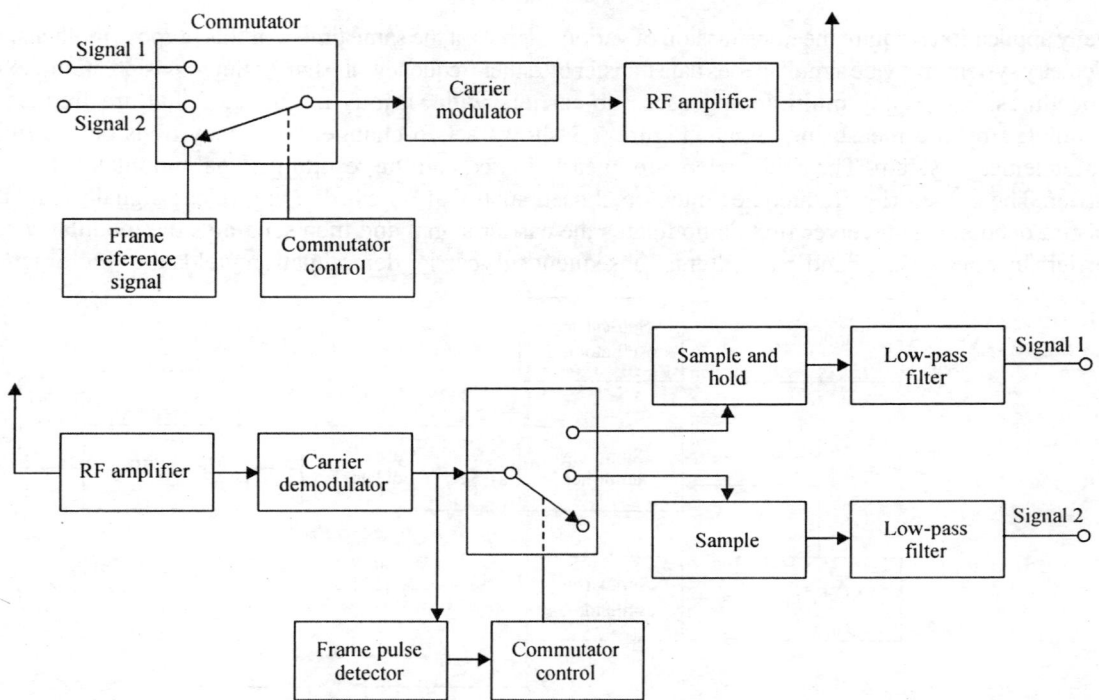

Fig. 7.6. Block diagram of two-channel time-division multiplex radiotelemetry system.

Modulation

The physiological signal alone cannot be transmitted with reasonable efficiency as a radio wave because of its low frequency. Therefore a high-frequency carrier wave is used as transmitting vehicle. The signal information is forced upon the carrier by modulation, that is, by a signal-dependent (and thus time-variant) characteristics parameter such as amplitude, frequency or phase.

Amplitude modulation (AM) is a simple method of signal transmission; its applications, however, is rather limited. Since the amplitude of the received signal depends on many parameters, such as distance between transmitter and receiver or orientation of the antennas, absolute signal amplitudes can only be determined in the receiver if a calibration signal is included in the transmission. Moreover, AM signals are more adversely affected by sources of interference that additively superimpose the carrier than are the signals modulated by other procedures. Demodulation of an AM signal is simply done by rectifying and low-pass filtering the carrier, which corresponds to envelope detection.

Frequency modulation (FM) provides absolute values for the signal amplitudes. Fading (i.e., amplitude variations in the received FM signal due to time-variant transfer conditions such as changing antenna orientations) is compensated by an automatic gains control (AGC), thus always ensuring the same conditions for the demodulator. Noise interferes much less with the reception that in AM systems, since the addition of a disturbing signal up to a certain limit does not influence demodulation which determines only the momentary frequency of the carrier, independent from amplitude (Fig. 7.7).

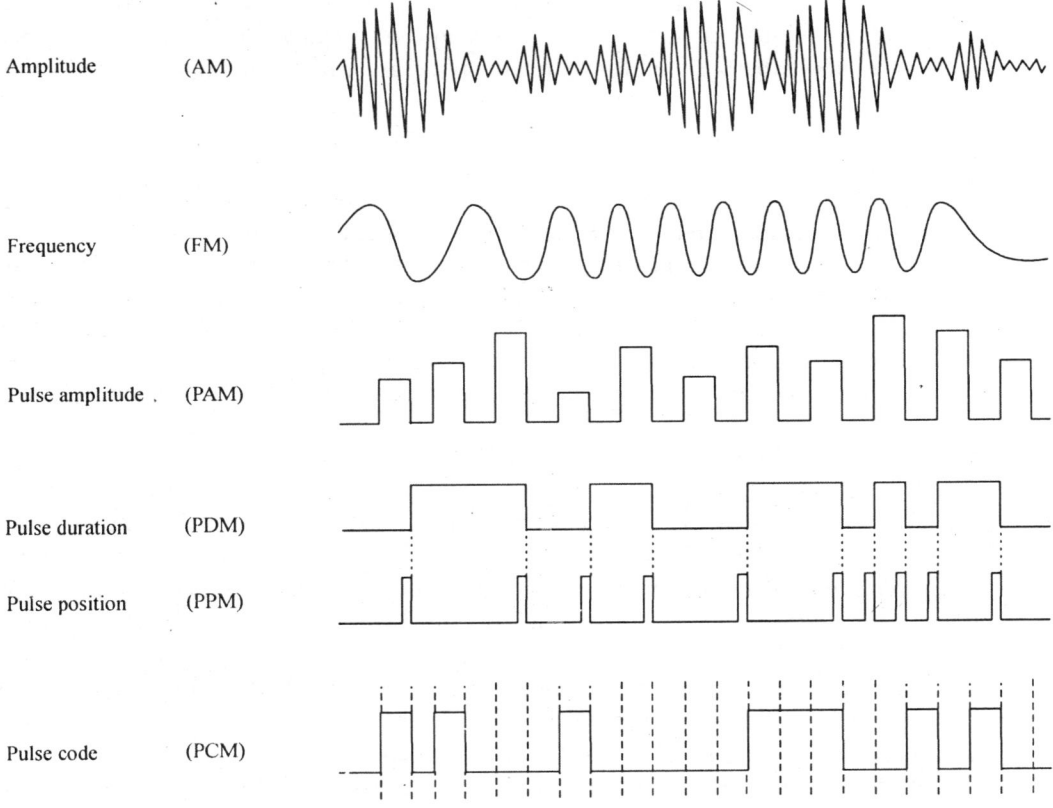

Amplitude	(AM)
Frequency	(FM)
Pulse amplitude	(PAM)
Pulse duration	(PDM)
Pulse position	(PPM)
Pulse code	(PCM)

Fig. 7.7. Modulation and coding techniques.

Many different methods of FM demodulation are known. Direct demodulation converts the FM signal to an AM signal by differentiation. Succeeding envelope detection provides the signal. Indirect demodulation uses a phase-locked loop (PLL) that is especially efficient in the presence of noise.

Multichannel telemetry systems use double modulation. Both the sub-carriers and the radio-wave carrier have to be modulated. Modulation principles must not be identical but are chosen according to the best realisation for the special application. Four different combinations are possible: AM/AM, AM/FM, FM/AM and FM/FM.

Pulse Modulation

In pulse modulation techniques, only discrete samples representing the signal are used to modulate the carrier. The advantage of signal sampling can already be seen in the realisation of the time-division multiplexing telemetry system. In pulse modulation these discrete samples are used to vary a parameter of a pulse waveform. Such parameters are the amplitude (pulse amplitude modulation, PAM), duration (PDM) or position (PPM) of the pulse. Representative waveforms for the different modulation techniques are shown in Fig. 7.7. Another coding system is pulse code modulation (PCM), in which the analog signal is converted to digital sample points and the series of binary digits is transmitted.

Using the described basic modulation procedures, one can develop arbitrary complex combined coding and modulation techniques. Digital modulation techniques especially offer a variety of possibilities, each optimised for a special purpose, as for optimum speed, information content or minimum error probability.

Passive Telemetry Systems

For control of medical implants and surveillance of patients, continuous data flow of physiological signals and functional parameters is required. Simple inductive telemetry systems are best suited for this application. However, power consumption by telemetry shortens the operating time of the implant substantially, because the battery capacity is very limited and the necessary radio-wave power is often higher than the power consumption by the intrinsic implant electronics. In this situation one can use a passive telemetry system, which does not need its own power supply, thus avoiding both lifetime reduction and problems, resulting from an inductive energy transmission into the implant (i.e., reduced reliability and additional components).

The function of passive telemetry systems is based on the coupling of two components, either by induction or by electromagnetic or ultrasonic wave fields, so that the extracorporeal component, the information receiver, changes a characteristics parameter (e.g., its impedance) according to variations of the second, implanted component's conditions. In this situation, the data transmitter operates as a modulated energy receiver. The two components can be two induction coils in which the load impedance of the secondary coil is reflected back to the primary coil, two piezoelectric crystals in which the impedance of an ultrasound-emitting transducer changes according to the load of the implanted receiver or two antennas, in which the radio-wave emission is influenced by the load of the receiving antenna. No matter what type of transmitters are used, load modulation of the implanted device can be achieved with neglible power consumption if a field-effect transistor is used as a modulation component (Fig. 7.8). This of course presumes an electric signal to be transmitted. In the case of non-electric biological signals other possible variable-load components are piezoelectric crystals with pressure or temperature-dependent capacitance.

Depending on the type of oscillator used in the primary circuit, variations of the load impedance provide either amplitude or frequency modulation of the carrier. The highest efficiency of the telemetry system is obtained when the secondary circuit is tuned to resonance.

The application of passive telemetry in an implantable pacemaker system uses inductive coupling of coils. The implanted coil alternatively serves as a secondary coil for the passive telemetry system, transmitting the intracardiac ECG as well as pacer parameters to an extracorporeal receiver or as a secondary coil in a conventional active telemetry system, by which the extracorporeal control system or programmer transmits commands to the implanted device.

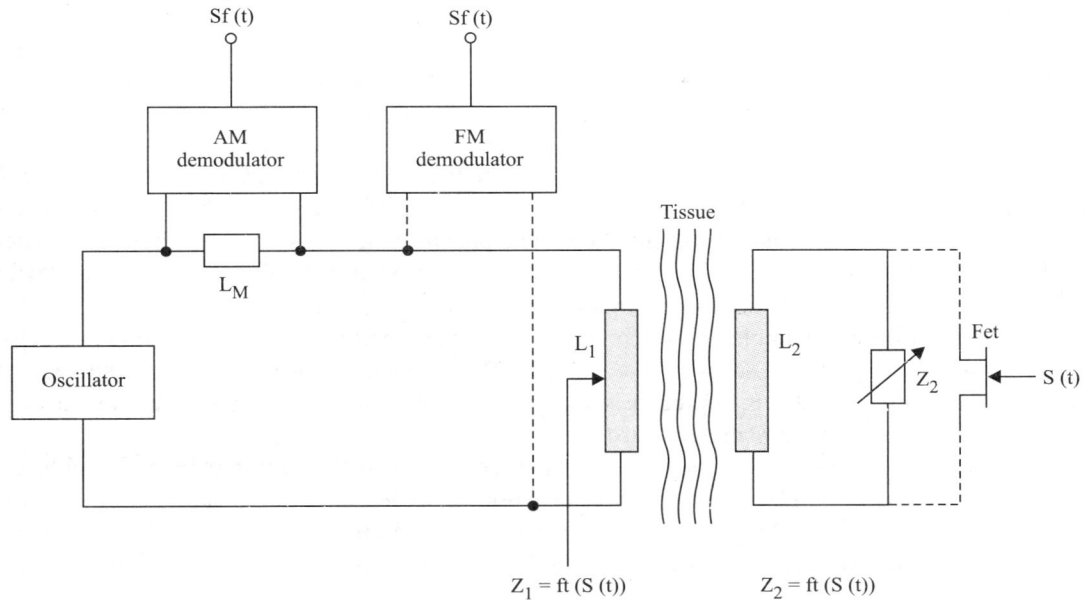

Fig. 7.8. Block diagram of passive telemetry system.

ULTRASOUND AND LIGHT TELEMETRY

The limitations of radio-wave telemetry—such as legal regulations that prevent the availability of sufficient radio frequencies with adequate bandwidths, interference problems, with other radio-wave transmitters, or even physical shortcomings such as the impossibility or radio-wave transmission in underwater telemetry—recommend the use of ultrasound or infrared light as information carriers in some special applications. In underwater animal tracking, ultrasonic telemetry is the most common technique. Infrared light telemetry has proved its value in clinical environment for in-room transmission of data, especially within surgical units, thus avoiding inconvenient cable connection between patient and remote recorders. Technically, there are not major differences from radio-wave telemetry except for the use of different signal transducers.

TROUBLESHOOTING TELEMETRY SYSTEMS

ECG telemetry systems are like all other hardware, so from time to time they will malfunction. Some of the faults can be handled directly by the user, while others must be referred to various grades or levels of service shop.

Nurses, EMTs and other medical personnel can perform several minor trouble shooting tests. First, the patient electrodes and the wires that connect them to the transmitter are usually replaceable by the user, so can be checked before taking a unit out of service. Second, the battery (which is the usual fault) can be replaced on most units by the user. Finally, it is permissible for users to swap telemetry transmitters and receivers on most systems and therefore restore operation (if on a different channel) by a simple process of elimination. The problem on single-channel systems is that this process does not reveal whether it is the receiver or transmitter that is at fault.

For routine troubleshooting of the telemetry system by a service technician, much can be said for owning either a television field strength meter (which can also be used in making site surveys) or a continuously tunable VHF/UHF receiver that covers all the operating frequencies that might normally be expected to be covered. The receiver or FSM can be used to monitor the output of the transmitter to determine whether or not the transmitter is putting out a signal.

Receiver troubleshooting requires a signal generator that covers the frequency of operation. The selected instrument should be an FM generator that is capable of external modulation so that a low-frequency square wave, simulated ECG from a 'chicken heart' generator or other source can be used to modulate the FM output of the signal generator. The FM signal generator should be capable of deviating at least 25 KHz and preferably the entire range of the deviation expected in the system.

If no FM generator is available, then a common CW (i.e., unmodulated) signal generator can also be used by the technician who knows what she is doing. The telemetry transmitter can also sometimes be used as a signal source, but this approach is fraught with difficulty when there is an ambiguity over whether the receiver or the transmitter is at fault.

Also useful in this type of servicing are the usual collection of DC multimeters and oscilloscopes needed for all forms of complex electronic service work. However, be aware that most of the faults are 'trauma' items like broken battery connectors, open switches and other components that are subject to abuse in normal use. Then there is always the unit that got drenched in saline IV solution.

Portable Telemetry Units

The rise of emergency medical technicians in the rescue services of local communities gives us an immensely useful tool in dealing with trauma and coronary victims outside of the hospital. Although very highly trained, the EMT is not a physician, so some means is often required to communicate physiological data to the local hospital where they are interpreted by a physician. In addition, two-way voice communications must be established for the EMT team to converse with and receive instructions from the physician at the hospital. Specialised communications equipment is often used to meet these requirements.

Figure 7.9 shows a portable telemetry system that has the range and power needed for the EMT/ambulance crew to establish a data link to the hospital. The transmitter might be a special unit or most often, it is a modified version of the standard walkie-talkie that is commonly used by police, fire and rescue units. The modulating signal, however, is an analog signal such as the ECG, the output of a blood pressure transducer or other physiological source. The signal is transmitted over the airwaves to a base station transceiver (transmitter and receiver in the same cabinet) at the hospital. From there, the demodulation and display is similar to that of other telemetry systems. Because the size of handheld transceivers used for telemetry and voice communications is necessarily small, the available power output is low. As a result, the range is short for these units. Where the require range is greater, however, a repeater system can be used. At critical locations around the city receiver sites can pick up the small signal from the handheld units. Another method, shown in Fig. 7.10, is to install the repeater on the ambulance itself. The handheld unit only has to transmit on frequency F1 as far as the vehicle, where the signal is picked up and re-radiated at higher power on a different frequency (F2) to the hospital site.

Telephonic Telemetry

Telemetry by public telephone can improve clinical surveillance of non-hospitalised patients. The main application fields are the surveillance of pregnancy, the post-operative monitoring of patients with cardiac diseases and the control of cardiac pacemakers (Fig. 7.11).

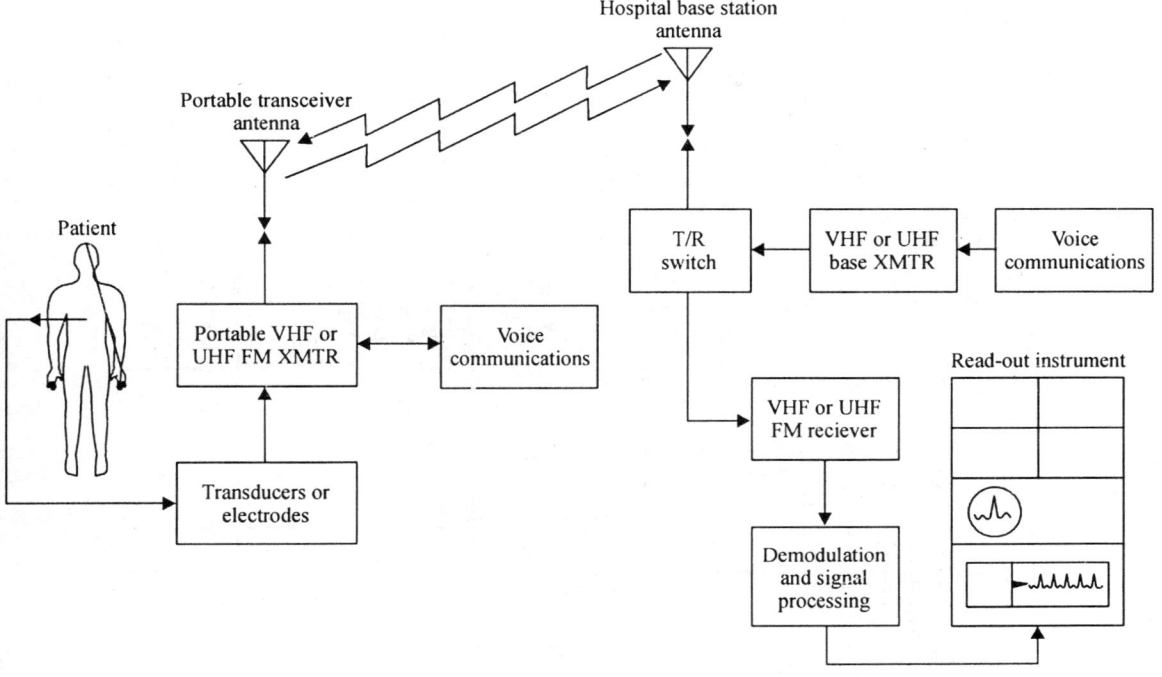

Fig. 7.9. Portable telemetry system.

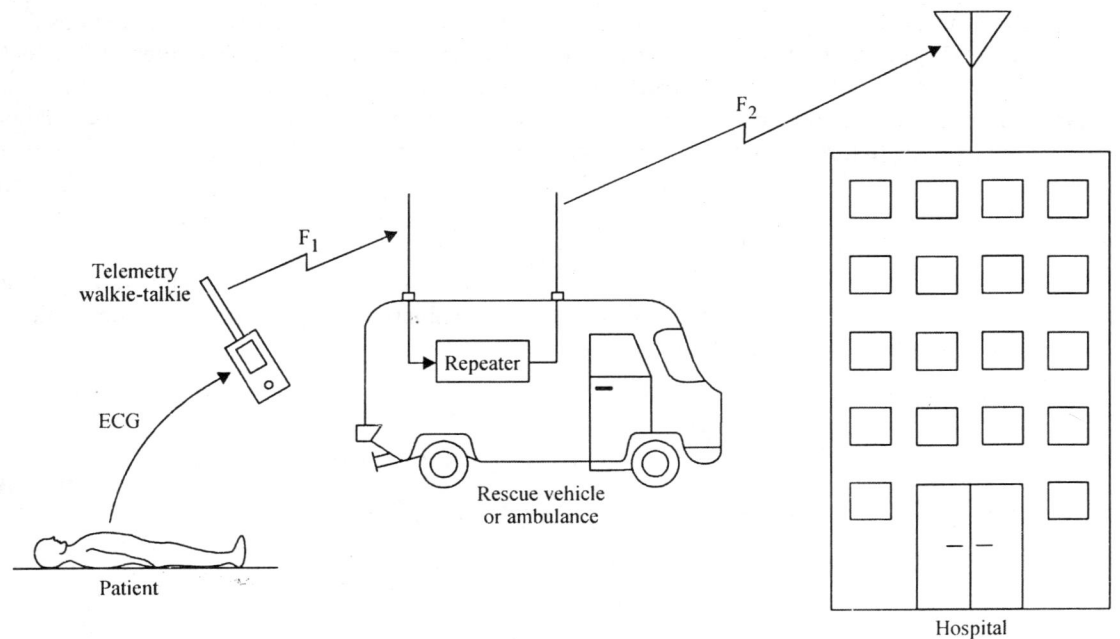

Fig. 7.10. Installation of the repeater on ambulance.

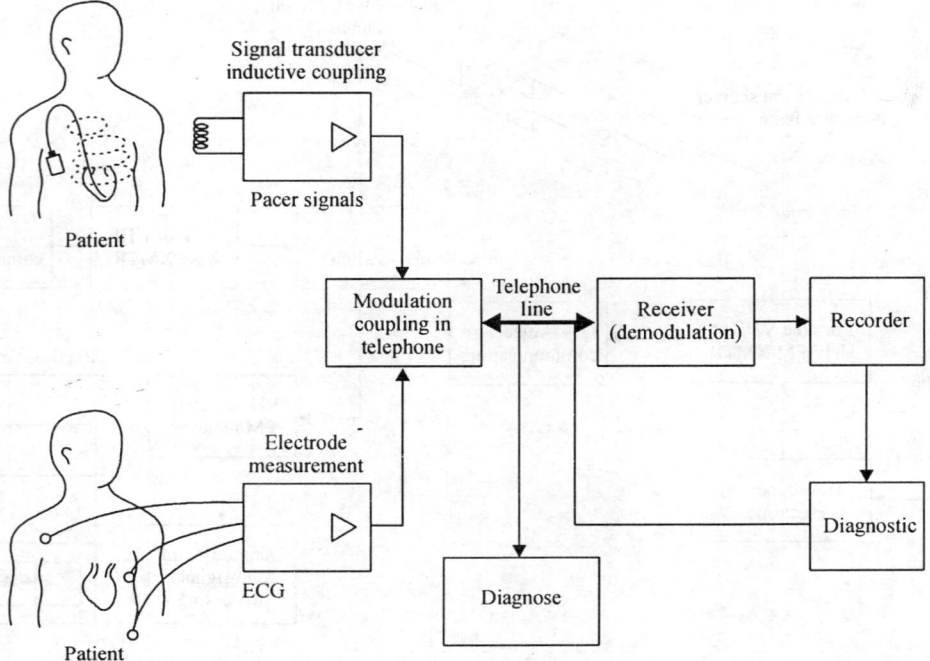

Fig. 7.11. Block diagram of telephonic telemetry system.

Providing the patient with simple measuring equipment enables him either to contact the hospital at regular intervals or to have immediate access to examination if he suspects an emergency. Telemetric monitoring of pregnancy has especially proven its value in rural areas, where the alternatives without telemetry often are hospitalisation or the complete absence of surveillance. Besides the psychological aspects of pregnancy that recommend limiting hospitalisation to the absolutely necessary minimum and the augmented risk of unmonitored pregnancy, telephone telemetry also offers strong financial arguments.

The basic principle of telephonic telemetry is shown in Fig. 7.11. The patient system consists of an ECG amplifier, a modulator, usually FM and an adapter or converter that translates the signal to a form corresponding to the regulations of telephonic data transfer. The receiver demodulates the signal and feeds it to normal registration equipment. Computerised evaluation of the signals provide immediate 24 hours control without any restrictions of patient mobility.

Chapter 8

Cardiac Output Measurement

INTRODUCTION

Cardiac output is the amount of blood pumped by the right or left ventricular per unit of time. It is expressed in litres per minute (l/min) and normalised by division by body surface area in square meters (m^2). The resulting quantity is called the cardiac index. Cardiac output is sometimes normalised to body weight, being expressed as ml/min per kilogram. A typical resting value for a wide variety of mammals is 70 ml/min per kg. With exercise, cardiac output increases. In well-trained athletes, cardiac output can increase five-fold with maximum exercise. During exercise, heart rate increases, venous return increases and the ejection fraction increases. Parenthetically, physically fit subjects have a low resting heart rate and the time for the heart rate to return to the resting value after exercise is less than that for subjects who are not physically fit.

There are many direct and indirect (non-invasive) methods of measuring cardiac output. Of equal importance to the number that represents cardiac output is the left-ventricular ejection fraction (stroke volume divided by diastolic volume), which indicates the ability of the left ventricle to pump blood.

INDICATOR-DILUTION METHOD

The principle underlying the indicator-dilution method is based on the upstream injection of a detectable indicator and on measuring the downstream concentration-time curve, which is called a dilution curve. The essential requirement is that the indicator mixes with all the blood flowing through the central mixing pool. Although the dilution curves in the outlet branches may be slightly different in shape, they all have the same area.

Figure 8.1a illustrates the injection of m g of indicator into an idealised flowing stream having the same velocity across the diameter of the tube. Figure 8.1b shows the dilution curve recorded downstream. Because of the flow-velocity profile, the cylinder of indicator and fluid becomes teardrop in shape, as shown in Fig. 8.1c. The resulting dilution curve has a rapid rise and an exponential fall, as shown in Fig. 8.1d. However, the area of the dilution curve is the same as that shown in Fig. 8.1a. Derivation of the flow equation is shown in Fig. 8.1 and the flow is simply the amount of indicator (m gm) divided by the area of the dilution curve (gm/ml × s), which provides the flow in ml/s.

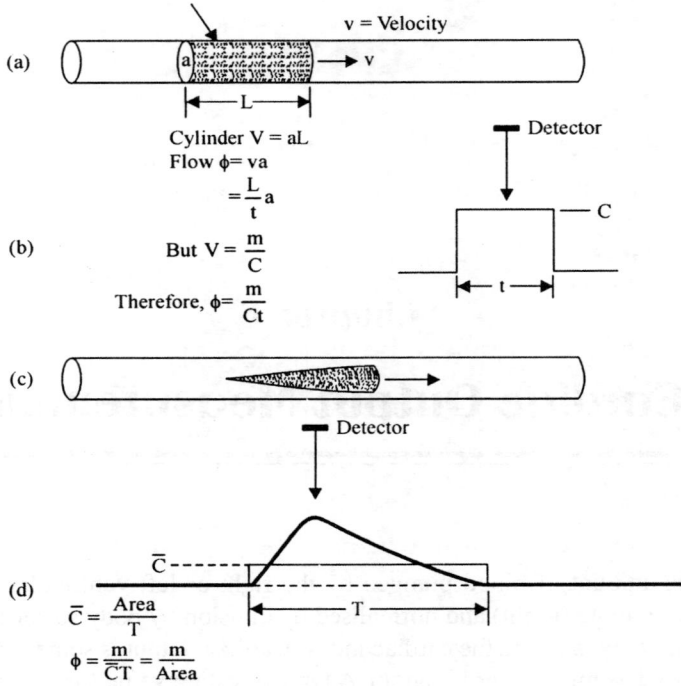

Fig. 8.1. Genesis of the indicator-dilution curve.

Indicators

Before describing the various indicator-dilution methods, it is useful to recognise that there are two types of indicator, diffusible and non-diffusible. A diffusible indicator will leak out of the capillaries. A non-diffusible indicator is retained in the vascular system for a time that depends on the type of indicator. Whether cardiac output is overestimated with a diffusible indicator depends on the location of the injection and measuring sites. Table 8.1 lists many of the indicators that have been used for measuring cardiac output and the types of detectors used to obtain the dilution curve. It is obvious that the indicator selected must be detectable and not alter the flow being measured. Importantly, the indicator must be non-toxic and sterile.

Table 8.1. Indicators.

Material	Detector	Retention data
Evans blue	Photoelectric 640 mu.	50 per cent loss in 5 days
Indocyanine green	Photoelectric 800 mu.	50 per cent loss in 10 minutes
Coomassie blue	Photoelectric 585-600 mu.	50 per cent loss in 15–20 minutes
Saline (5 per cent)	Conductivity cell	Diffusible*
Albumin l^{131}	Radioactive	50 per cent loss in 8 days
Na^{24}, K^{42}, D_2O, DHO	Radioactive	Diffusible*
Hot-cold solutions	Thermodetector	Diffusible*

* It is estimated that there is about 15 per cent loss of diffusible indicators during the first pass through the lungs.

When a diffusible indicator is injected into the right heart, the dilution curve can be detected in the pulmonary artery and there is no loss of indicator because there is no capillary bed between these sites; therefore the cardiac output value will be accurate.

Thermal Dilution Method

Chilled 5 per cent dextrose in water or 0.9 per cent NaCl can be used as indicators. The dilution curve represents a transient reduction in pulmonary artery blood temperature following injection of the indicator into the right atrium. Figure 8.2 illustrates the method and a typical thermodilution curve. Note that the indicator is really negative calories. The thermodilution method is based on heat exchange measured in calories and the flow equation contains terms for the specific heat (C) and the specific gravity (S) of the indicator (i) and blood (b). The expression employed when a #7F thermistor-tipped catheter is used and chilled D5W is injected into the right atrium is as follows:

$$CO = \left[\frac{V(T_b - T_i)60}{A} \right] \left[\frac{S_i C_i}{S_b C_b} \right] F$$

where
V = volume of indicator injected in ml
T_b = temperature (average of pulmonary artery blood in (°C)
T_i = temperature of the indicator (°C)
60 = multiplier required to convert ml/s into ml/min
A = area under the dilution curve in (seconds × °C)
S = specific gravity of indicator (i) and blood (b)
C = specific heat of indicator (i) and blood (b)

$\left(\dfrac{S_i C_i}{S_b C_b} = 1.08 \text{ for 5 per cent dextrose and blood of 40 per cent packed-cell volume} \right)$

F = empiric factor employed to correct for heat transfer through the injection catheter (for a #7F catheter, F = 0.825 [2])

Entering these factors into the expression gives

$$CO = \frac{V(T_b - T_i)53.46}{A}$$

where
CO = cardiac output in ml/min
53.46 = $60 \times 1.08 \times 0.825$

To illustrate how a thermodilution curve is processed, cardiac output is calculated below using the dilution curve shown in Fig. 8.2.

V = 5 ml of 5 per cent dextrose in water
T_b = 37°C
T_i = 0°C
A = 1.59°C second

$$CO = \frac{5(37 - 0)53.46}{1.59} = 6220 \text{ ml/min}$$

Although the thermodilution method is the standard in clinical medicine, it has a few disadvantages. Because of the heat loss through the catheter wall, several series 5 ml injections of indicator are needed to obtain a consistent value for cardiac output. If cardiac output is low, i.e., the dilution curve is very broad, it is difficult to obtain an accurate value for cardiac output. There are respiratory-induced variations in PA blood temperature that confound the dilution curve when it is of low amplitude. Although room-temperature D5W can be used, chilled D5W provides a better dilution curve and a more reliable cardiac output value. Furthermore, it should be obvious that if the temperature of the indicator is the same as that of blood, there will be no dilution curve.

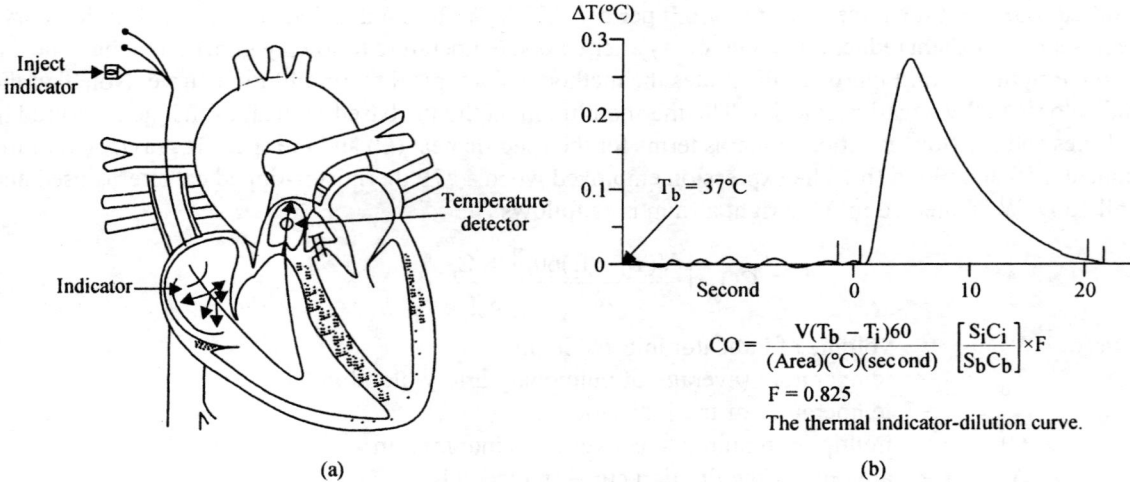

$$CO = \frac{V(T_b - T_i)60}{(Area)(°C)(second)} \left[\frac{S_i C_i}{S_b C_b}\right] \times F$$

$$F = 0.825$$

The thermal indicator-dilution curve.

(a)　　　　　　　　　　　　　　(b)

Fig. 8.2. (a) the thermodilution method; and (b) a typical thermal indicator dilution curve

Indicator Recirculation

An ideal dilution curve shown in Fig. 8.2 consists of a steep rise and an exponential decrease in indicator concentration. Algorithms that measure the dilution-curve area have no difficulty with such a curve. However, when cardiac output is low, the dilution curve is typically low in amplitude and very broad. Often the descending limb of the curve is obscured by recirculation of the indicator or by low-amplitude artifacts. Figure 8.3a is a dilution curve in which the descending limb is obscured by recirculation of the indicator. Obviously it is difficult to determine the practical end of the curve, which is often specified as the time when the indicator concentration has fallen to a chosen percentage (e.g., 1 per cent) of the maximum amplitude (C_{max}). Because the descending limb represents a good approximation of a decaying exponential curve (e^{-kt}), fitting the descending limb to an exponential allows reconstruction of the curve without a recirculation error, thereby providing a means for identifying the end for what is called the first pass of the indicator.

In Fig. 8.3b, the amplitude of the descending limb of the curve in Fig. 8.3a has been ploted on semilogarithmic paper and the exponential part represents a straight line. When recirculation appears, the data points deviate from the straight line and therefore can be ignored and the linear part (representing the exponential) can be extrapolated to the desired percentage of the maximum concentration, say 1 per cent of C_{max}. The data points representing the extrapolated part were replotted on Fig. 8.3a to reveal the dilution curve undistorted by recirculation.

Commercially available indicator-dilution instruments employ digitisation of the dilution curve. Often the data beyond about 30 per cent of C_{max} are ignored and the exponential is computed on digitally extrapolated data.

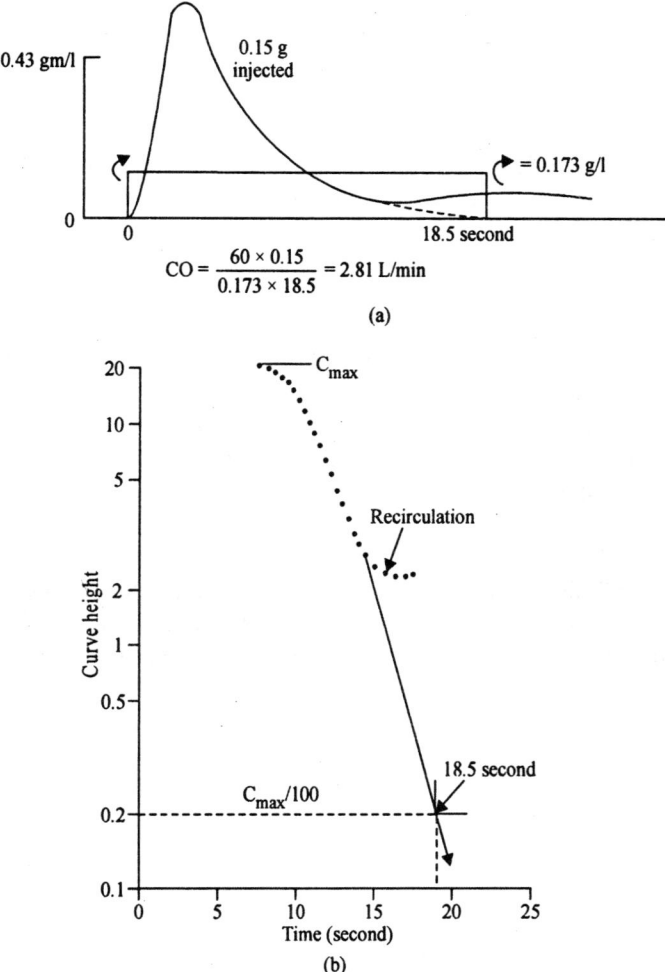

Fig. 8.3. (a) dilution curve obscured by recirculation; and (b) a semi-logarithmic plot of the descending limb.

FICK METHOD

The Fick method employs oxygen as the indicator and the increase in oxygen content of venous blood as it passes through the lungs, along with the respiratory oxygen uptake, as the quantities that are needed to determine cardiac output, $CO = O_2$ uptake/$(A - VO_2$ difference). Oxygen uptake (ml/min) is measured at the airway, usually with an oxygen-filled spirometer containing a CO_2 absorber. The $A - VO_2$ difference is determined from the oxygen content (ml/100 ml blood) from any arterial sample and the oxygen content (ml/100 ml) of pulmonary arterial blood. The oxygen content of the blood used to be difficult to measure. However, the new blood-gas analysers that measure, pH, pO_2, pCO_2, hematocrit and haemoglobin provide a value for O_2 content by computation using the oxygen-dissociation curve.

There is a slight technicality involved in determining the oxygen uptake because oxygen is consumed at body temperature but measured at room temperature in the spirometer. Consequently, the volume of

O_2 consumed per minute displayed by the spirometer must be multiplied by a factor, F. Therefore the Fick equation is

$$CO = \frac{O_2 \text{ uptake/min (F)}}{A - VO_2 \text{ difference}}$$

The Fick method does not require the addition of a fluid to the circulation and may have value in such a circumstance. However, its use requires stable conditions because an average oxygen uptake takes many minutes to obtain.

EJECTION FRACTION

The ejection fraction (EF) is one of the most convenient indicators of the ability of the left (or right) ventricle to pump the blood that is presented to it. Let v be the stroke volume (SV) and V be the end-diastolic volume (EDV); the ejection fraction is v/V or SV/EDV.

Measurement of ventricular diastolic and systolic volumes can be achieved radiographically, ultrasonically and by the use of an indicator that is injected into the left ventricle where the indicator concentration is measured in the aorta on a beat-by-beat basis.

Indicator-Dilution Method for Ejection Fraction

Holt described the method of injecting an indicator into the left ventricular during diastole and measuring the stepwise decrease in aortic concentration with successive beats (Fig. 8.4). From this concentration-time record, end-diastolic volume, stroke volume and ejection fraction can be calculated. No assumption need be made about the geometric shape of the ventricle.

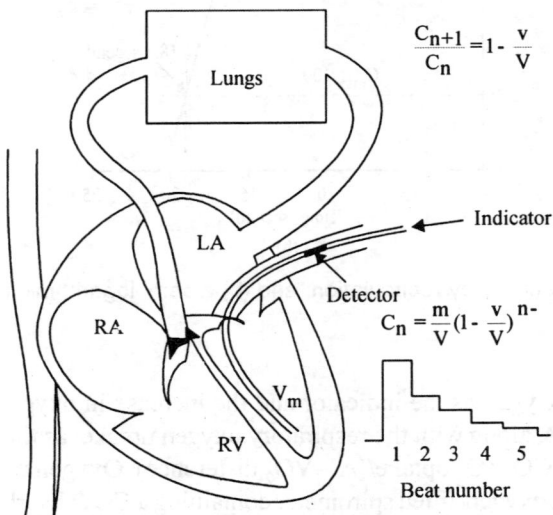

$$\frac{C_{n+1}}{C_n} = 1 - \frac{v}{V}$$

$$C_n = \frac{m}{V}\left(1 - \frac{v}{V}\right)^{n-}$$

Fig. 8.4. The saline method of measuring ejection fraction, involving injection of m gm of NaCl into the left ventricle and detecting the aortic concentration (C) on a beat-by-beat basis.

Chapter 9

Noninvasive Optical Monitoring

INTRODUCTION

Optical measures of physiologic status are attractive because they can provide a simple, non-invasive, yet real-time assessment of medical condition. Non-invasive optical monitoring is taken here to mean the use of visible or near-infrared light to directly assess the internal physiologic status of a person without the need of extracting a blood of tissue sample or using a catheter. Liquid water strongly absorbs ultraviolet and infrared radiation and thus these spectral regions are useful only for analysing thin surface layers or respiratory gases, neither of which will be the subject of this review. Instead, it is the visible and near-infrared portions of the electromagnetic spectrum that provide a unique 'optical window' into the human body, opening new vistas for non-invasive monitoring technologies.

Various molecules in the human body possess distinctive spectral absorption characteristics in the visible or near-infrared spectral regions and therefore make optical monitoring possible. The most strongly absorbing molecules at physiologic concentrations are the haemoglobins, myoglobins, cytochromes, melanins, carotenes and bilirubin (Fig. 9.1). Perhaps less appreciated are the less distinctive and weakly absorbing yet ubiquitous materials possessing spectral characteristics in the near-infrared: water, fat, proteins and sugars. Simple optical methods are now available to quantitatively and non-invasively measure some of these compounds directly in intact tissue. The most successful methods to date have used haemoglobins to assess the oxygen content of blood, cytochromes to assess the respiratory status of cells and possibly near-infrared to assess endogenous concentrations of metabolites, including glucose.

OXIMETRY AND PULSE OXIMETRY

Failure to provide adequate oxygen to tissues—hypoxia—can in a matter of minutes result in reduced work capacity of muscles, depressed mental activity and ultimately cell death. It is therefore of considerable interest to reliably and accurately determine the amount of oxygen in blood or tissues. Oximetry is the determination of the oxygen content of blood of tissues, normally by optical means. In the clinical laboratory the oxygen content of whole blood can be determined by a bench-top co-oximeter or blood gas analyser. But the need for timely clinical information and the desire to minimise the inconvenience and cost of extracting a blood sample and later analyse it in the laboratory has led to the search for alternative non-invasive optical methods. Since the 1930s, attempts have been made to use multiple wavelengths of light to arrive at a complete spectral characterisation of a tissue. These approaches, although somewhat successful, have remained of limited utility owing to the awkward instrumentation and unreliable results.

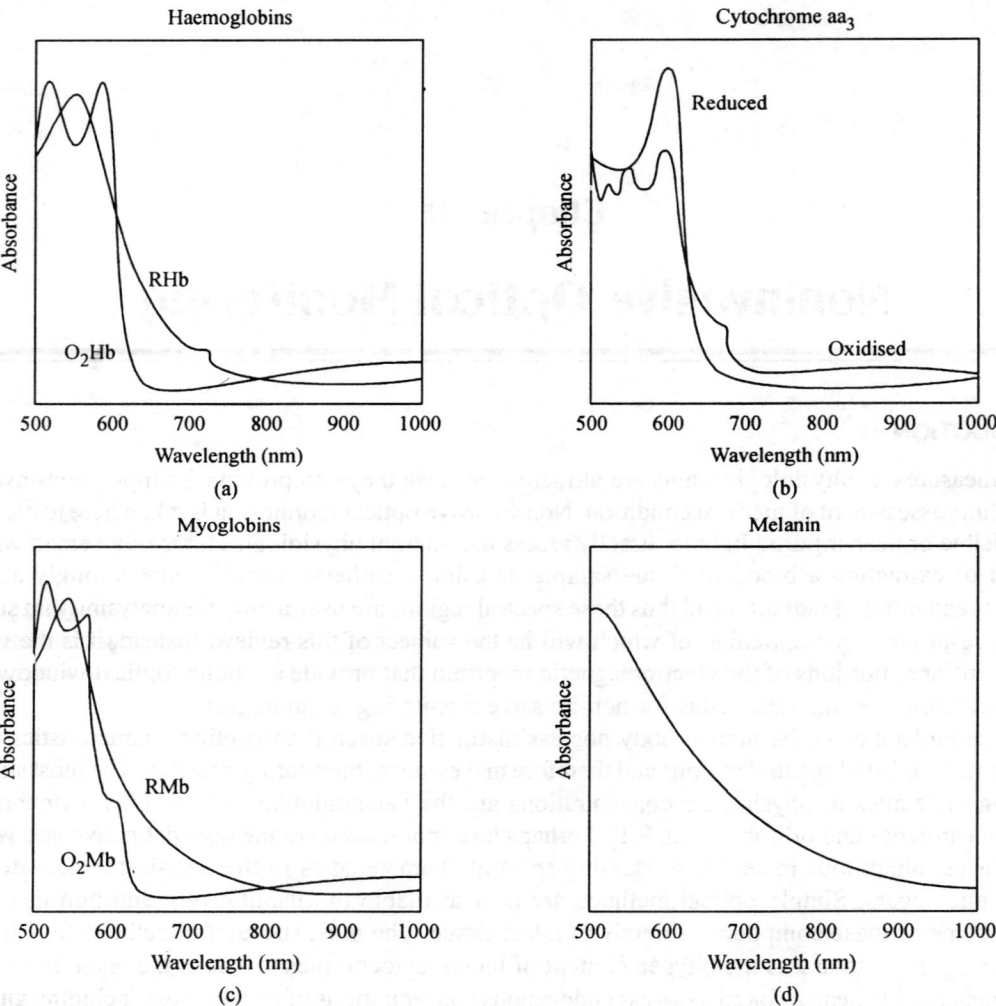

Fig. 9.1. Absorption spectra of some endogenous biologic materials (a) haemoglobins; (b) cytochrome aa$_3$; (c) myoglobins; and (d) melanin.

It was not until the invention of pulse oximetry in the 1970s and its commercial development and application in the 1980s that non-invasive oximetry became practical. Pulse oximetry is an extremely easy-to-use, non-invasive and accurate measurement of real-time arterial oxygen saturation. Pulse oximetry is now used routinely in clinical practice, has become a standard of care in all US operating rooms and is increasingly used wherever critical patients are found. The pulse oximetry is the most significant technological advance ever made in monitoring the well-being and safety of patients during anaesthesia, recovery and critical care.

The remarkable success of pulse oximetry has established non-invasive optical monitoring of vital physiologic functions as a modality of considerable value. Hardware and algorithm advances in pulse oximetry are beginning to broaden its use outside the traditional operating room and critical care areas. Other promising applications of non-invasive optical monitoring are emerging, such as for measuring deep tissue oxygen levels, determining cellular metabolic status or for quantitative determination of other important physiologic parameters such as blood glucose. Although these latter applications are not yet practical, they may ultimately impact non-invasive clinical monitoring just as dramatically as pulse oximetry.

The partial pressure of oxygen (pO_2) in tissues need only be about 3 mmHg to support basic metabolic demands. This tissue level, however, requires capillary pO_2 to be near 40 mmHg, with a corresponding arterial pO_2 of about 95 mmHg. Most of the oxygen carried by blood is stored in red blood cells reversibly bound to haemoglobin molecules. Oxygen saturation (SaO_2) is defined as the percentage of haemoglobin-bound oxygen compared to the total amount of haemoglobin available for reversible oxygen binding. The relationship between the oxygen partial pressure in blood and the oxygen saturation of blood is given by haemoglobin oxygen dissociation curve as shown in Fig. 9.2. The higher the pO_2 in blood, the higher the SaO_2. But due to the highly co-operative binding of four oxygen molecules to each haemoglobin molecule, the oxygen binding curve is sigmoidal and consequently the SaO_2 value is particularly sensitive to dangerously low pO_2 levels. With a normal arterial blood pO_2 above 90 mmHg, the oxygen saturation should be at least 95 per cent and a pulse oximeter can readily verify a safe oxygen level. If oxygen content falls, say to a pO_2 below 40 mmHg, metabolic needs may not be met and the corresponding oxygen saturation will drop below 80 per cent. Pulse oximetry therefore provides a direct measure of oxygen sufficiency and will alert the clinician to any danger of imminent hypoxia in a patient.

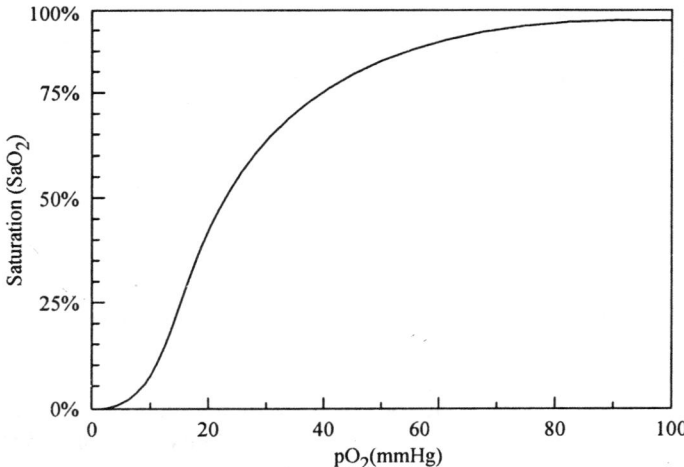

Fig. 9.2. Haemoglobin oxygen dissociation curve showing the sigmoidal relationship between the partial pressure of oxygen and the oxygen saturation of blood. The curve is given approximately by per cent $SaO_2 = 100\%/[1 + P_{50}/pO_2^n]$, with $n = 2.8$ and $P_{50} = 26$ mmHg.

Although endogenous molecular oxygen is not optically observable, haemoglobin serves as an oxygen-sensitive 'dye' such that when oxygen reversibly binds to the iron atom in the large heme prosthetic group, the electron distribution of the heme is shifted, producing a significant colour change. The optical absorption of haemoglobin in its oxygenated and deoxygenated states is shown in Fig. 9.1. Fully oxygenated blood absorbs strongly in the blue and appears bright red; deoxygenated blood absorbs through the visible region and is very dark (appearing blue when observed through tissue due to light scattering effects). Thus the optical absorption spectra of oxyhaemaglobin (O_2Hb) and 'reduced' deoxyhaemoglobin (RHb) differ substantially and this difference provides the basis for spectroscopic determinations of the proportion of the two haemoglobin states. In addition to these two normal functional haemoglobins, there are also dysfunctional hemoglobins—carboxyhaemoglobin, methemoglobin and sulhaemoglobin—which are spectroscopically distinct but do not bind oxygen reversibly. Oxygen saturation is therefore defined in Eq. (9.1) only in terms of the functional saturation with respect to O_2Hb and RHb:

$$S_aO_2 = \frac{O_2Hb}{RHb + O_2Hb} \times 100 \text{ per cent}$$

... (9.1)

Co-oximeters are bench-top analysers that accept whole blood samples and utilise four or more wavelengths of monochromatic light, typically between 500 and 650 nm, to spectroscopically determine the various individual haemoglobins in the sample. If a blood sample can be provided, this spectroscopic method is accurate and reliable. Attempts to make an equivalent quantitative analysis non-invasively through intact tissue have been fraught with difficulty. The problem has been to contend with the wide variation in scattering and non-specific absorption properties of very complex heterogeneous tissue. One of the more successful approaches, marketed by Hewlett-Packard, used eight optical wavelengths transmitted through the pinna of the ear. In this approach a 'bloodless' measurement is first obtained by squeezing as much blood as possible from an area of tissue; the arterial blood is then allowed to flow back and the oxygen saturation is determined by analysing the change in the spectral absorbance characteristics of the tissue. While this method works fairly well, it is cumbersome, operator dependent and does not always work well on poorly perfused or highly pigmented subjects.

It has been proved that most of the interfering non-specific tissue effects could be eliminated by utilising only the change in the signal during an arterial pulse. Although an early prototype was built in Japan, it was not until the refinements in implementation and application by Biox (now Ohmeda) and Nellcor Incorporated in the 1980s that the technology became widely adopted as a safety monitor for critical care use.

Theory

Pulse oximetry is based on the fractional change in light transmission during an arterial pulse at two different wavelengths. In this method the fractional change in the signal is due only to the arterial blood itself and therefore the complicated non-pulsatile and highly variable optical characteristics of tissue are eliminated. In a typical configuration, light at two different wavelengths illuminating one side of a finger will be detected on the other side, after having traversed the intervening vascular tissues (Fig. 9.3). The transmission of light at each wavelength is a function of the thickness, colour and structure of the skin, tissue, bone, blood and other materials through which the light passes. The absorbance of light by a sample is defined as the negative logarithm of the ratio of the light intensity in the presence of the sample (I) to that without (I_0): $A = -\log(I/I_0)$. According to the Beer-Lambert law, the absorbance of a sample at a given wavelength with a molar absorptivity (ε) is directly proportional to both the concentration (c) and pathlength (l) of the absorbing material: $A = \varepsilon cl$. (In actuality, biologic tissue is highly scattering and the Beer-Lambert law is only approximately correct). Visible or near-infrared light passing through about one centimeter of tissue (e.g., a finger) will be attenuated by about one or two orders of magnitude for a typical emitter-detector geometry, corresponding to an effective optical density (OD) of 1–2 OD (the detected light intensity is decreased by one order of magnitude for each OD unit).

Although haemoglobin in the blood is the single strongest absorbing molecule, most of the total attenuation is due to the scattering of light away from the detector by the highly heterogeneous tissue. Since human tissue contains about 7 per cent blood and since blood contains typically about 14 g/dl haemoglobin, the effective haemoglobin concentration in tissue is about 1 g/dl (~150 uM). At the wavelengths used for pulse oximetry (650–950 nm); the oxy and deoxyhaemoglobin molar absorptivities fall in the range of 100–1000 $M^{-1}cm^{-1}$ and consequently haemoglobin accounts for less than 0.2 OD of the total observed optical density. Of this amount, perhaps only 10 per cent is pulsatile and consequently pulse signals of only a few per cent are ultimately measured, at times even one-tenth of this.

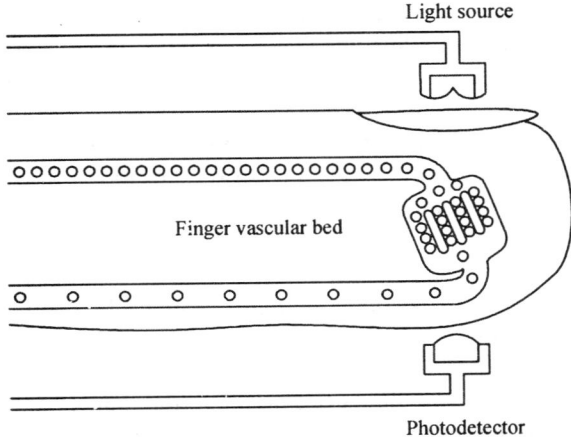

Fig. 9.3. Typical pulse oximeter sensing configuration on a finger. Light at two different wavelengths is emitted by the source, diffusely scattered through the finger and detected on the opposite side by a photodetector.

Application and Future Directions

Pulse oximetry is now routinely used in nearly all operating rooms and critical care areas in the United States and increasingly throughout the world. It has become so pervasive and useful that it is now being called the 'fifth' vital sign (for an excellent review of practical aspects and clinical applications of the technology). The principal advantages of pulse oximetry are that it provides continuous, accurate and reliable monitoring of arterial oxygen saturation on nearly all patients, utilising a variety of convenient sensors, re-usable as well as disposable. Single-patient-use adhesive sensors can easily be applied to fingers for adults and children and to arms for legs or neonates. Surface reflectance sensors have also been developed based on the same principles and offer a wider choice for sensor location, though they tend to be less accurate and prone to more types of interference.

Limitations of pulse oximetry include sensitivity to high levels of optical or electric interference, errors due to high concentrations of dysfunctional haemoglobins (methemoglobin or carboxyhaemoglobin) or interference from physiologic dyes (such as methylene blue). Other important factors, such as total haemoglobin content, fetal haemoglobin or sickle cell trait, have little or no effect on the measurement except under extreme conditions. Performance can also be compromised by poor signal quality, as may occur for poorly perfused tissues with weak pulse amplitudes or by motion artifact.

Hardware and software advances continue to provide more sensitive signal detection and filtering capabilities, allowing pulse oximeters to work better on more ambulatory patients. Already some pulse oximeters incorporate ECG synchronisation for improved signal processing. A pulse oximeter for use in labour and delivery is currently under active development by several research groups and companies. A likely implementation may include use of a reflectance surface sensor for the fetal head to monitor the adequacy of fetal oxygenation. This application is still in active development and clinical utility remains to be demonstrated.

NON-PULSATILE SPECTROSCOPY

Non-pulsatile optical spectroscopy has been used for more than half a century for non-invasive medical assessment, such as in the use of multiwavelength tissue analysis for oximetry and skin reflectance measurement for bilirubin assessment in jaundiced neonates. These early applications have found some limited use, but with modest impact. Recent investigations into new non-pulsatile spectroscopy methods for assessment of deep-tissue oxygenation (e.g., cerebral oxygen monitoring), for evaluation of respiratory status at the cellular level and for the detection of other critical analytes, such as glucose, may yet prove more fruitful. The former applications have led to spectroscopic studies of cytochromes in tissues and the latter has led to considerable work into new approaches in near-infrared analysis of intact tissues.

Cytochrome Spectroscopy

Cytochromes are electron-transporting, heme-containing proteins found in the inner membranes of mitochondria and are required in the process of oxidative phosphorylation to convert metabolytes and oxygen into CO_2 and high-energy phosphates. In this metabolic process the cytochromes are reversibly oxidised and reduced and consequently the oxidation-reduction states of cytochromes c and aa_3 in particular are direct measures of the respiratory condition of the cell. Changes in the absorption spectra of these molecules, particularly near 600 nm and 830 nm for cytochrome aa_3, accompany this shift. By monitoring these spectral changes, the cytochrome oxidation state in the tissues can be determined. As with all non-pulsatile approaches, the difficulty is to remove the dependence of the measurements on the various non-specific absorbing materials and highly variable scattering effects of the tissue. To date, instruments designed to measure cytochrome spectral changes can successfully track relative changes in brain oxygenation, but absolute quantitation has not yet been demonstrated.

Near-Infrared Spectroscopy and Glucose Monitoring

Near-infrared (NIR), the spectral region between 780 nm and 3000 nm, is characterised by broad and overlapping spectral peaks produced by the overtones and combinations of infrared vibrational modes. Figure 9.4 shows typical NIR absorption spectra of fat, water and starch. Exploitation of this spectral region for *in vivo* analysis has been hindered by the same complexities of non-pulsatile tissue spectroscopy described above and is further confounded by the very broad and indistinct spectral feature characteristic of the NIR. Despite these difficulties, NIR spectroscopy has garnered considerable attention, since it may enable the analysis of common analytes.

Karl Norris and co-workers pioneered the practical application of NIR spectroscopy, using it to evaluate water, fat and sugar content of agricultural products. The further development of sophisticated multivariate analysis techniques, together with new scattering models (e.g., Kubelka-Munk theory) and high-performance instrumentation, further extended the application of NIR methods. Over the past decade, many research groups and companies have touted the use of NIR techniques for medical monitoring, such as for determining the relative fat, protein and water content of tissue and more recently for non-invasive glucose measurement. The body composition analyses are useful but crude and are mainly limited to applications in nutrition and sports medicine. Non-invasive glucose monitoring, however, is of considerable interest.

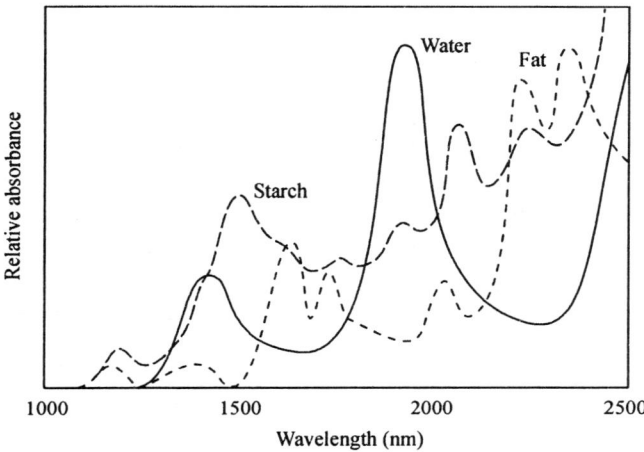

Fig. 9.4. Typical near-infrared absorption spectra of several biologic materials.

More than two million diabetics in the United States lance their fingers three to six times a day to obtain a drop of blood for chemical glucose determination. The ability of these individuals to control their glucose levels and the quality of their life generally, would dramatically improve if a simple, non-invasive method for determining blood glucose levels could be developed. Among the non-invasive optical methods proposed for this purpose are optical rotation, NIR analysis and Raman spectroscopy. The first two have received the most attention. Optical rotation methods aim to exploit the small optical rotation of polarised light by glucose. To measure physiologic glucose levels in a 1cm thick sample to an accuracy of 25 mg/dl would require instrumentation that can reliably detect an optical rotation of at least 1 millidegree. Finding an appropriate *in vivo* optical path for such measurements has proved most difficult, with most approaches looking to use either the aqueous humour or the anterior chamber of the eye. Although several groups have developed laboratory analysers that can measure such a small effect, so far *in vivo* measurement has not been demonstrated, due both to unwanted scattering and optical activity of biomaterials in the optical path and to the inherent difficulty in developing a practical instrument with the required sensitivity.

NIR methods for non-invasive glucose determination are particularly attractive, although the task is formidable. Glucose has spectral characteristics near 1500 nm and in the 2000–2500 nm band where many other compounds also absorb and the magnitude of the glucose absorbance in biologic samples is typically two orders of magnitude lower than those of water, fat or protein. The normal detection limit for NIR spectroscopy is on the order of one part in 10^3, whereas a change of 25 mg/dl in glucose concentration corresponds to an absorbance change of 10^{-4} to 10^{-5}. In fact, the temperature dependence of the NIR absorption of water alone is at least an order of magnitude greater than the signal from glucose in solution. Indeed, some have suggested that the apparent glucose signature in complex NIR spectra may actually be the secondary effect of glucose on the water.

Sophisticated chemometric (particularly multivariate analysis) methods have been employed to try to extract the glucose signal out of the noise. Several groups have reported using multivariate techniques to quantitate glucose in whole blood samples, with encouraging results. And despite all theoretical disputations to the contrary, some groups claim the successful application of these multivariate analysis methods to non-invasive *in vivo* glucose determination in patients.

Time-Resolved Spectroscopy

The fundamental problem in making quantitative optical measurements through intact tissue is dealing with the complex scattering phenomena. This scattering makes it difficult to determine the effective pathlength for the light and therefore attempts to use the Beer-Lambert law or even to determine a consistent empirical calibration, continue to be thwarted. Application of new techniques in time-resolved spectroscopy may be able to tackle this problem. Thinking of light as a packet of photons, if a single packet from a light source is sent through tissue, then a distant receiver will detected a photon distribution over time—the photons least scattered arriving first and the photons most scattered arriving later. In principle, the first photons arriving at the detector passed directly through the tissue. For these first photons the distance between the emitter and the detector is fixed and known and the Beer-Lambert law should apply, permitting determination of an absolute concentration for an absorbing component. The difficulty in this is, first, that the measurement time scale must be on the order of the photon transit time (sub-nanosecond) and second, that the number of photons getting through without scattering will be extremely small and therefore the detector must be exquisitely sensitive. Although these considerable technical problems have been overcome in the laboratory, their implementation in a practical instrument applied to a real subject remains to be demonstrated. This same approach is also being investigated for non-invasive optical imaging, since the unscattered photons should produce sharp images.

Chapter 10

Clinical Laboratory Instruments

INTRODUCTION

Most hospitals have a laboratory area separate from patient areas that is used solely for chemical analyses and measurements of body fluids and tissues. Typically, analysis is done on blood and urine and on body tissue. These measurements are made to aid physicians in the diagnosis of disease states and to help them monitor the effects of therapy. For example, when oxygen therapy is given to a patient it is necessary to frequently monitor the partial pressure of oxygen and carbon dioxide in the patient's blood. Accuracy of measurement is critical in the laboratory. And because the chemical parameters are sensitive to environmental factors such as temperature, light and humidity, equipment calibration must constantly be monitored. The chemical solutions are often active and cause ageing and wearing effects that may impair accuracy. These effects are most clearly evident in the chemical electrode.

OPERATION OF THE CLINICAL LABORATORY

In the typical hospital, the clinical laboratory performs tests on a variety of specimens of diverse origin. These may be samples of normal body fluids (blood, cerebrospinal fluid, etc.), abnormal body fluids (pleural or peritoneal effusions, cyst contents, etc.), abnormal products (purulent secretions, exudates, etc.), products of normal excretory functions (feces, urine, etc.) and others. Such specimens and samples may be obtained directly by laboratory personnel (phlebotomists) from inpatients or outpatients or may be brought from the patient's ward to the laboratory by nursing personnel.

The timing of a test may be mandated by the condition of the patient. A medical emergency may require that certain determinations be performed STAT (a term that means, in hospital parlance, that the specimen must by obtained immediately, the test performed and the result reported back to the requesting patient care area as soon as it becomes available). Other tests may be performed on samples obtained under specific conditions, such as blood cultures during periods of spiking fever. Some must be obtained at a certain time of day (e.g., plasma cortisol) or over a period of time (urinary catecholamines during a 24 hour period). However, most routine determinations are scheduled so that samples are obtained the morning after the day of the request and tests are performed in batches, in many cases using automated laboratory equipment.

After the samples are obtained, the specimens are routed to the corresponding section of the clinical laboratory where the pertinent tests are routinely performed. In certain selected cases, however, a sample may be sent to a reference laboratory which may be located in another city or even another state. Figure 10.1 illustrates the general flow of information to and from the clinical laboratory.

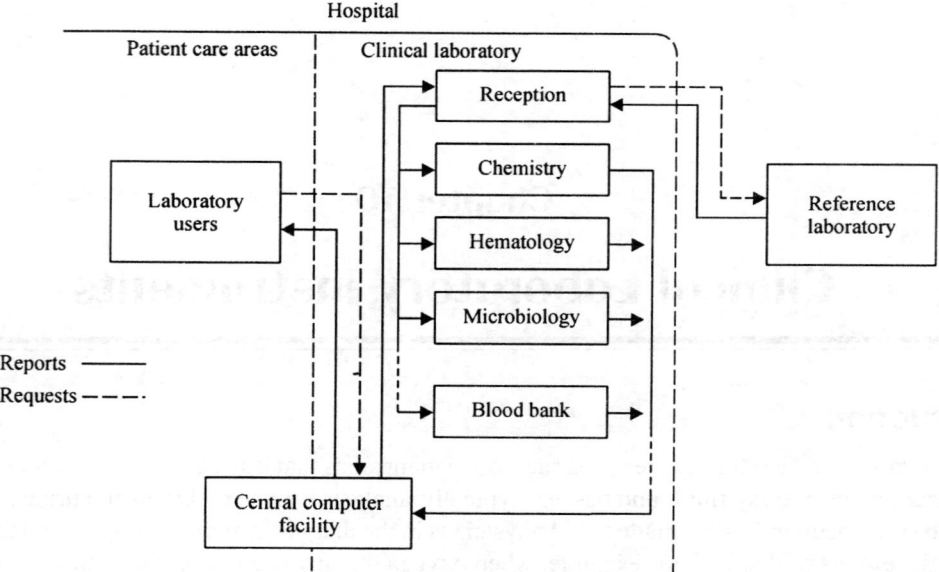

Fig. 10.1. Flow of information to and from the clinical laboratory. Requests arrive via computer in the reception area and are distributed to various laboratory sections. Results are reported via computer to requesting sites.

The results of a test may be expressed in one or more of the following ways:

1. Quantitatively, as a value followed by a unit of measure, such as 'serum cholesterol, 150 mg per cent'.
2. Qualitatively, as an indication of the presence or absence of a particular substance or element in a specimen, such as albumin in a urinalysis as 'trace,' occult blood in stools as ' 3 +,' platelets in a blood sample as 'adequate,' or a blood culture as 'negative'.
3. In narrative form, such as 'no malignant tells were found' in a report of a biopsy specimen (cytology).
4. In interpretive form, such as 'further laboratory evidence of myocardial damage' in one of a series of daily sequential reports of a cardiac profile.

If the result is a number, it may fall within the range of normal values for that particular test or it may be abnormally elevated or abnormally lowered. Extreme deviations from the normal range, which pose an immediate threat to the life or well-being of a patient, are called critical or panic values. Table 10.1 depicts some frequently made determinations in the key laboratory areas of chemistry and hematology, including test names, range of normal values, units of measure and critical limits.

All test results that fall in the critical or panic category, as well as those that are requested STAT, should be reported to the attending staff at once after adequate validation. Other normal and noncritical abnormal results can be reported in batches at least once daily or more often if possible, at preestablished time(s) of day. The time elapsed between the initiation of the request for the test until the result becomes available to the attending staff is sometimes referred to as the test turnaround time.

Table 10.1. Some common laboratory tests, with normal value ranges adjusted by sex, units of measure and critical care limits where applicable.

Test name	Sex	Low	High	Units	Critical low	Critical high
Chemistry						
Random serum glucose	M-F	70	120	mg/dl	50	300
Serum sodium	M-F	135	145	mEq/l	120	150
Serum potassium	M-F	3.5	5.0	mEq/l	3	5.9
Serum calcium	M-F	8.5	10.5	mg/dl	7	13
Cholesterol	M-F	150	300	mg/dl	–	–
Uric acid	M-F	2.5	8.0	mg/dl	–	–
Triglycerides	M-F	30	150	mg/dl	–	–
Haematology						
Haemoglobin	M	14	18	gm %	10	–
	F	12	16	gm %	10	–
Haematocrit	M	42	52	%	–	–
	F	37	47	%	–	–
White blood cell count	M-F	4800	10800	cells/mm^3	–	–
Reticulocyte count	M-F	0.5	1.5	%	–	–
Platelet count	M-F	1,50,000	3,50,000	cell/mm^3	50000	

CHEMICAL ELECTRODES

Chemical electrodes produce a potential that depends on the ionic concentration of fluids under test. These potentials are determined by the Goldman equation or the Nernst equation. These equations show that these potentials are directly proportional to temperature. Ions that are of particular interest in body fluid analysis include calcium, potassium, sodium, lithium and the chlorides.

Chemical electrodes range in complexity from a simple solid in contact with the solution under test to multiple-element structures. A chloride membrane electrode, for example, consists of silver chloride membrane on the tip of a glass tube. A wire from one side of the membrane connects to a high-impedance voltmeter. The membrane potential is a function of the chloride content of perspiration of the skin in contact with the electrode.

pH Electrode

The pH of normal blood must be maintained within a narrow range in human beings. Therefore, electrodes for accurate and convenient measurement of pH are essential. Furthermore, the pH electrode is a component from which more complex electrodes may be constructed.

The Goldman equation, shows that electrolyte membrane potentials are proportional to the logarithm of the ion concentration. In a solution containing the hydrogen ion, a membrane separating two solutions has a potential proportional to the hydrogen $[H^+]$ ion concentration. For example, at 25°C,

$$V_m = -60 \log [H^+] + C \text{ (in mV)}$$

where C is a constant. Usually, pH meters are calibrated so that the effect of this constant is cancelled.

The pH is a measure of the hydrogen ion concentration and is defined as

$$pH = - \log [H^+]$$

Therefore,

$$V_m = 60 \text{ pH} + C$$

In a pH meter, illustrated in Fig. 10.3, the constant C is compensated for by calibration so that the meter scale is proportional to pH. V_m is also proportional to the absolute temperature, T and ranges from zero to several tenths of a volt. The pH electrode consists of a reference terminal and an active terminal. The reference terminal uses a metal, in this case silver-silver chloride (Ag-AgCl), in a potassium chloride electrolyte. A salt bridge consisting of a fibre wick saturated with KCl is inert to the solution under test. However, it maintains the KCl at the potential of the solution and keeps the reference terminal potentials essentially the same regardless of the solution under test. The active terminal is sealed with common glass except for a tip made of pH-sensitive glass. The pH-sensitive glass consists of a hydrated gelatinous glass layer. Its membrane potential is proportional to the log [H$^+$] and therefore is proportional to the pH of the solution under test. The pH-sensitive glass very slowly dissolves in solution, taking as long as several years to become ineffective. In general, all boundary potentials in the electrode except those across the pH-sensitive glass are independent of the solution, so long as the temperature remains constant. The temperature is held constant in a pH meter by thermal compensation circuits that control the temperature of the sample chamber, as shown in Fig. 10.2.

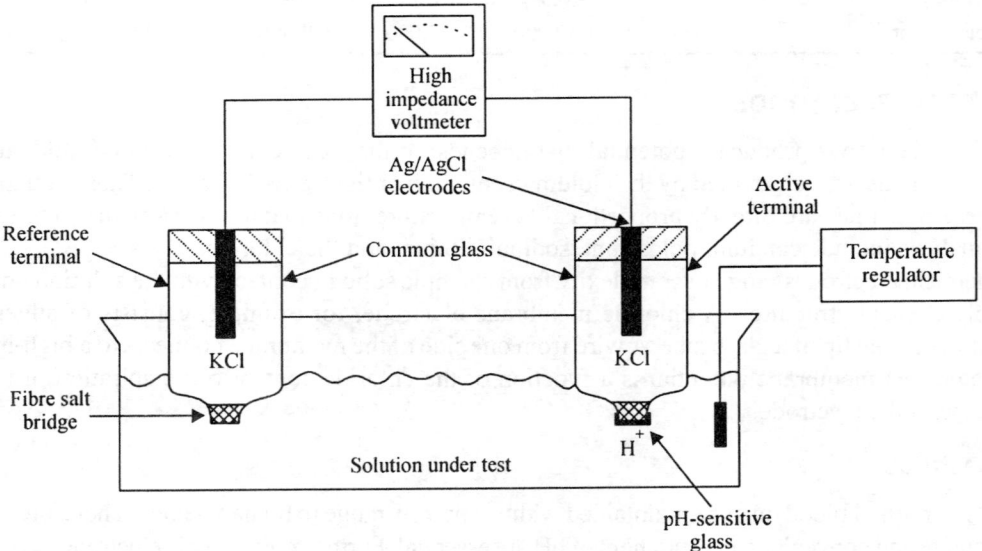

Fig. 10.2. A pH meter.

The care of pH electrodes include cleaning to avoid contamination by the sample solution. They must be replaced periodically because they are a wearing element. To compensate for unknown variables, the meter is calibrated with a solution of known pH when used for tests in the clinical setting. pH electrodes are wearing elements that may fail because of ageing. The pH electrode is also a building block of other chemical electrodes. In particular, it is a component of blood gas analyser electrodes.

BLOOD GAS ANALYSER

A major function of blood is to carry oxygen to the cells and carbon dioxide to the lungs for expiration. These gases mix with the blood to form a partial pressure in the blood.

A blood gas analyser is used to measure the partial pressure of oxygen, $^{P}O_2$, the partial pressure of carbon dioxide, $^{P}CO_2$ and the blood pH. The fundamental measurement from which the others are derived is the pH measurement. In normal blood this must be maintained between 7.34 and 7.44, slightly basic. pH readings from 0 to 7 are acidic and readings from 7 to 14 are basic. Since pH measurements are very much dependent on temperature, that parameter is carefully regulated to normal body temperature, 37°C. A pH electrode, as illustrated in Fig. 10.2, may be used in a blood gas analyser. Again, because errors in measurement can cause a dangerous misdiagnosis of disease, careful calibration procedures are followed.

$^{P}CO_2$ Electrode

The pH electrode is used as a component of a $^{P}CO_2$ electrode to measure the partial pressure of CO_2 by the arrangement shown in Fig. 10.3. Blood or another fluid to be measured enters a sample chamber and comes in contact with a teflon or silicon rubber membrane. This membrane separates the fluid from a sodium solution but is permeable to the CO_2 in the solution. The CO_2 combines with water so as to produce free hydrogen ions in the sodium solution. This changes the solution pH in proportion to the partial pressure of CO_2 in the blood.

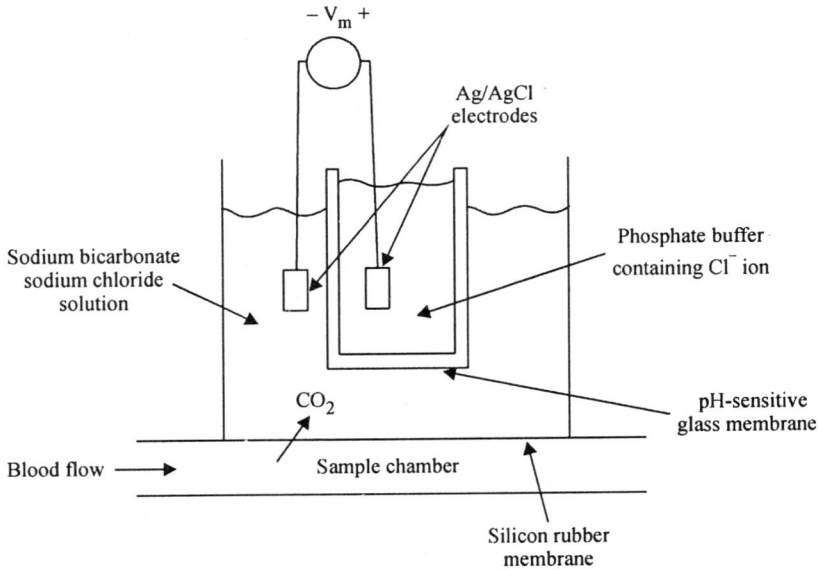

Fig. 10.3. A cell for measuring $^{P}CO_2$.

A chemical reaction in the electrode is

$$H_2O + CO_2 \rightleftharpoons H_2CO_3 \longrightarrow H^+ + HCO_3^-$$

Notice here that the CO_2 is proportional to the hydrogen ion, H^+. The pH meter then measures pH-sensitive membrane voltage, Vm, which in turn is proportional to the pH. The voltmeter is calibrated in units of $^{P}CO_2$. The electrode is maintained at body temperature with temperature-regulating circuits. The input impedance of the electrode ranges from 50 to 1000 MΩ; therefore a high-input-impedance voltmeter is required. One form of the $^PCO_2$ electrode is called a Severinghaus electrode, named for its developer.

$^PO_2$ Electrode

The $^PO_2$ electrode known as a Clark electrode, in honour of its inventor, is an oxygen sensor for blood. It consists of two chambers separated by a polypropylene membrane that is permeable to oxygen. The blood sample is injected into the lower sample chamber, as illustrated in Fig. 10.4. The upper chamber contains the electrode. The O_2 in the blood permeates the polypropylene membrane and reacts chemically with a phosphate buffer contained in the upper chamber. The buffer maintains the solution pH at a constant level. The O_2 combines with water in the buffer, producing electrons in proportion to the number of oxygen molecules according to the formula:

$$O_2 + 2H_2O + 4e^- \longrightarrow 4OH^-$$

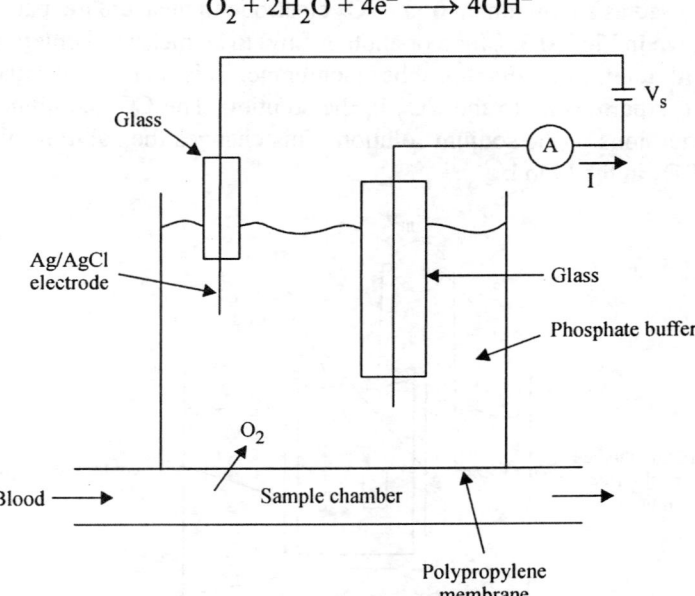

Fig. 10.4. The Clark electrode for $^PO_2$.

The electron current I is measured by the ammeter A in Fig. 10.4. The electron current is proportional to the $^PO_2$. The electrons on the left side of the equation that drive the reaction are provided by a source voltage, V_s, that polarises the electrode and has a value between 0.4 and 0.8 V. The need for this polarising voltage gives rise to the name polarographic electrode for the Clark electrode. The meter scale is then calibrated in units of partial pressure of oxygen ($^PO_2$) in the blood.

This electrode depends on current flow rather than membrane potential, as was the case with the pH-electrode-based devices. As with the other electrodes, procedures for calibration for environmental effects, electrode ageing, corrosion and contamination must be developed and followed.

A blood gas analyser that measures blood serum pH, $^PCO_2$ and $^PO_2$. The sample is drawn into the instrument through a capillary. The measured quantities appear on a front panel display and are printed on paper to provide hard copy. In order to calibrate the instrument, two known solutions of pH 7.384 and

6.840 are used. After each sample, a flushing solution cleans the tubing and sample chambers and ejects the waste into the container shown.

Non-invasive Blood Gas Monitoring

The blood gas analyser described in the previous section makes measurements on blood samples drawn from a patient and carried to the instrumentation. The process has the disadvantages of discomfort to the patient in drawing the blood and a time delay in obtaining the data. Real-time, immediately available measurement of $^PO_2$ and $^PCO_2$, as well as oxyhaemoglobin saturation SaO_2, can be achieved by use of non-invasive transducers applied directly to the surface of the skin. Such monitoring instrumentation is especially valuable in the OR, where immediate knowledge of the patient's oxygen and carbon dioxide is of critical importance.

It has long been known that both O_2 and CO_2 diffuse through the skin, as well as through the alveoli of the lung. Although the diffusion is minimal, it can be increased significantly by heating the skin. Therefore, to measure the $^PO_2$, the Clark electrode in Fig. 10.2 can be modified by placing it in a heating coil that heats the skin. The polypropylene membrane is placed against the skin and O_2 passes through it into the electrode, where it can be measured as described earlier.

In a similar manner the $^PCO_2$ electrode may also be modified. Its silicon rubber membrane is then placed against the patient's skin so that real-time $^PCO_2$ measurement can be made.

The $^PO_2$ can also be measured optically by using the fact that oxygenated blood tends to be red and low-oxygen blood tends to be blue. About 98 per cent of oxygen in the blood combines with haemoglobin (Hb) to form oxyhaemoglobin (HbO_2). The ratio of HbO_2 to Hb in the blood is called the percentage oxyhaemoglobin saturation (SaO_2). SaO_2 also is related in a known manner to $^PO_2$ for given values of blood pH and temperature. To measure SaO_2 optically, two light-emitting diodes are used side by side to illuminate the tissue, such as a finger tip. One light is red and the other is near infrared. The absorption of the red light is very dependent on the SaO_2 and the infrared light is independent of this value. Therefore the ratio of the light intensity as detected on corresponding photodetector diodes can be used to drive an output display calibrated to give the SaO_2 value. A finger transducer for monitoring blood gas is shown in Fig. 10.5. In addition to measuring the SaO_2, the instrument shown in Fig. 10.6 measures the end tidal CO_2 ($ETCO_2$). This instrument is called a pulse oximeter, end tidal (POET).

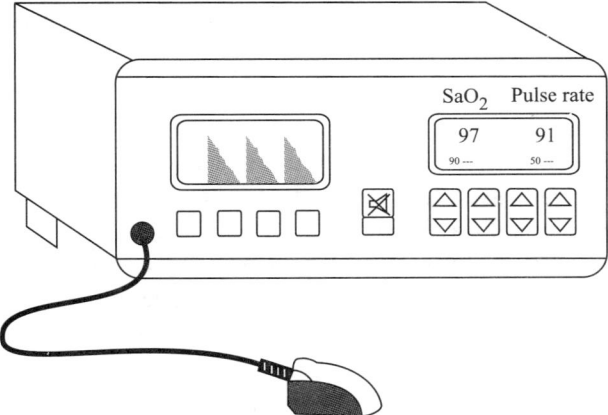

Fig. 10.5. The saturated blood oxygen (SaO_2) and pulse rate are measured non-invasively through a finger.

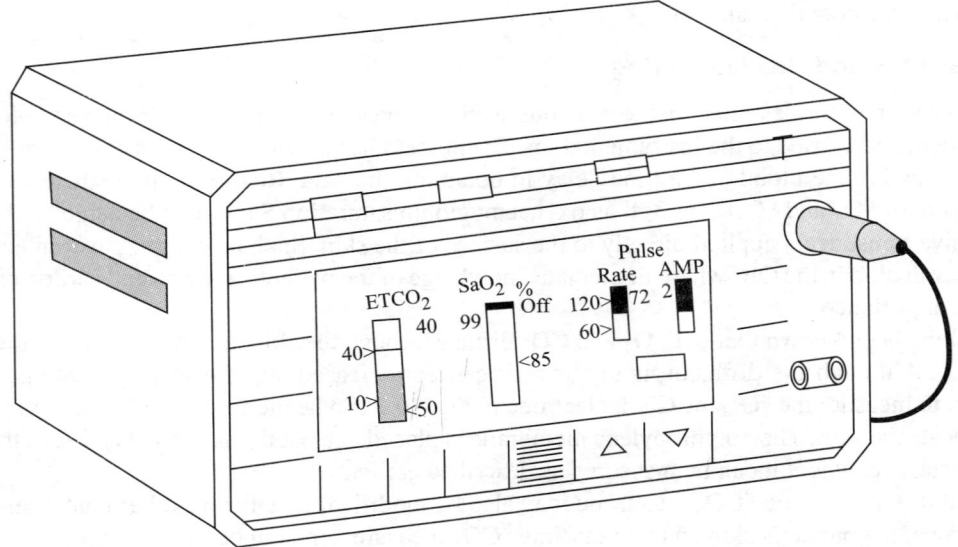

Fig. 10.6. A device for monitoring O_2 and CO_2.

PHOTOMETERS AND COLORIMETERS

The chemical content of biological substances can be determined by measuring how they either absorb or emit visible light. The colorimeter uses light absorption to determine blood proteins and iron levels. In order to enhance the colour of these substances in blood serum, it is necessary to mix it with reagents. Measurements of light emitted by ions, such as sodium or potassium in serum or urine, excited by heat are made with a flame photometer.

A colorimeter consists of a light source broken into its spectrum of colours by a prism or diffraction grating. The individual colours are then passed through the sample. The amount of each colour absorbed is measured to determine the type and concentration of substances in the sample. Since these measurements are highly temperature dependent, control of this parameter is necessary.

Diffraction Gratings

Colorimeters and spectrophotometers, which are used to measure the light transmitted and absorbed as it passes through a sample, typically use diffraction gratings to break the light source into individual colours, as defined by their frequencies and wavelengths.

A diffraction grating consists of slits or openings, on an opaque plate, as illustrated in Fig. 10.7. The slits are spaced D meter apart. For each colour there is an angle, ϕ, with respect to the plane of the grating, in the direction of which path lengths from adjacent slits differ by integer numbers of wavelengths. Therefore the colour experiences constructive interference along that path, which makes it visible to an observer. In Fig. 10.7, white light containing all colours is incident on the left side of the plate. An observer moving around a circle as indicated on the right side of the plate would see violet, yellow or red depending on his or her position. A flame photometer may be constructed with photodetectors at each of those positions. They are interconnected to the potassium, sodium and lithium channels of the flame photometer.

To find the directional angle ϕ, observe that the difference in path length to an observation point from adjacent slits in Fig. 10.8 may be defined as $M\lambda$, where M is an integer 1, 2, 3, ... etc.

Thus,

$$M\lambda = D \cos\phi \qquad \qquad ... (10.1)$$

for values of λ for which there is constructive interference at the observation point. In other words, the angle ϕ at which an observer sees the colour having a wavelength λ may be computed from Equation (10.1).

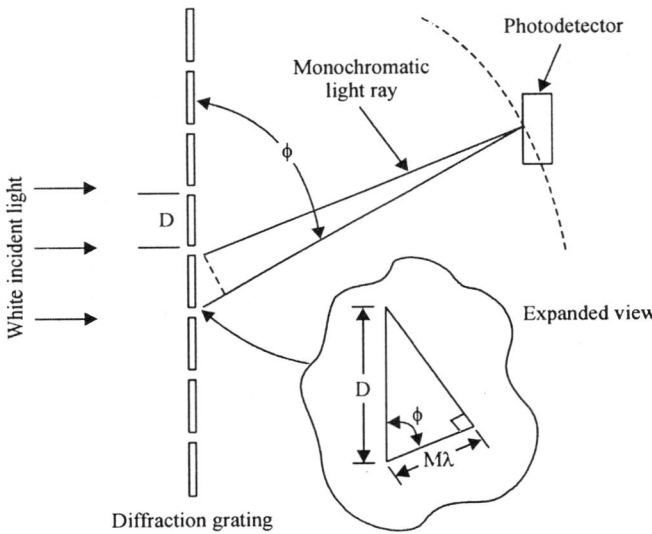

Fig. 10.7. A diffraction grating showing an incident beam of white light and a ray of monochromatic light emerging.

In order to cause light of different wavelengths to take a path through the sample under test to the photodetector, it is possible to rotate the diffraction grating on its axis, while holding the detector in one position. By measuring the detector output versus its angle of rotation, it is then possible to record the sample absorption versus light wavelength or colour. This data then leads to the identity of these substances and their concentration.

Flame Photometers

A flame photometer is used to analyse urine or blood in order to determine the concentration of potassium (K), sodium (Na) and lithium (Li). Sodium and potassium are present in normal urine. Lithium is used as a calibrating substance, unless it appears in the serum or urine because of medication.

A flame photometer operates on the same principle as that used for chemical analysis with a Bunsen burner. A liquid sample, as shown in Fig. 10.8, is aspirated into the flame by the gas and air mixture. Depending upon the chemical content of the sample, the flame has different colours resulting from high-temperature thermal collisions that force atoms into excited states. For medical analysis, the commonly analysed ions and the respective colours they make in the flame as the excited atoms return to the ground state are as follows:

Element	Colour	Wavelength (A)
Potassium, K	Violet	4047
Sodium, Na	Yellow	5890
Lithium, Li	Red	6708

The actual intensity of the colour is quite variable because of changes in the flow rate of the gas that draws the sample into the flame. Electronic circuitry is used to compensate for the variations.

The light from the flame in the flame photometer is filtered, then directed along individual channels for the three major substances, Li, Na and K. The simplest filter consists of coloured glass. Violet glass, for example, passes violet colour in the flame but rejects the other colours. It may be considered an optical filter. Glass filters generally cause relatively high attenuation of the light and tend to get hot. Flame photometers typically use diffraction gratings to filter the light, as described earlier.

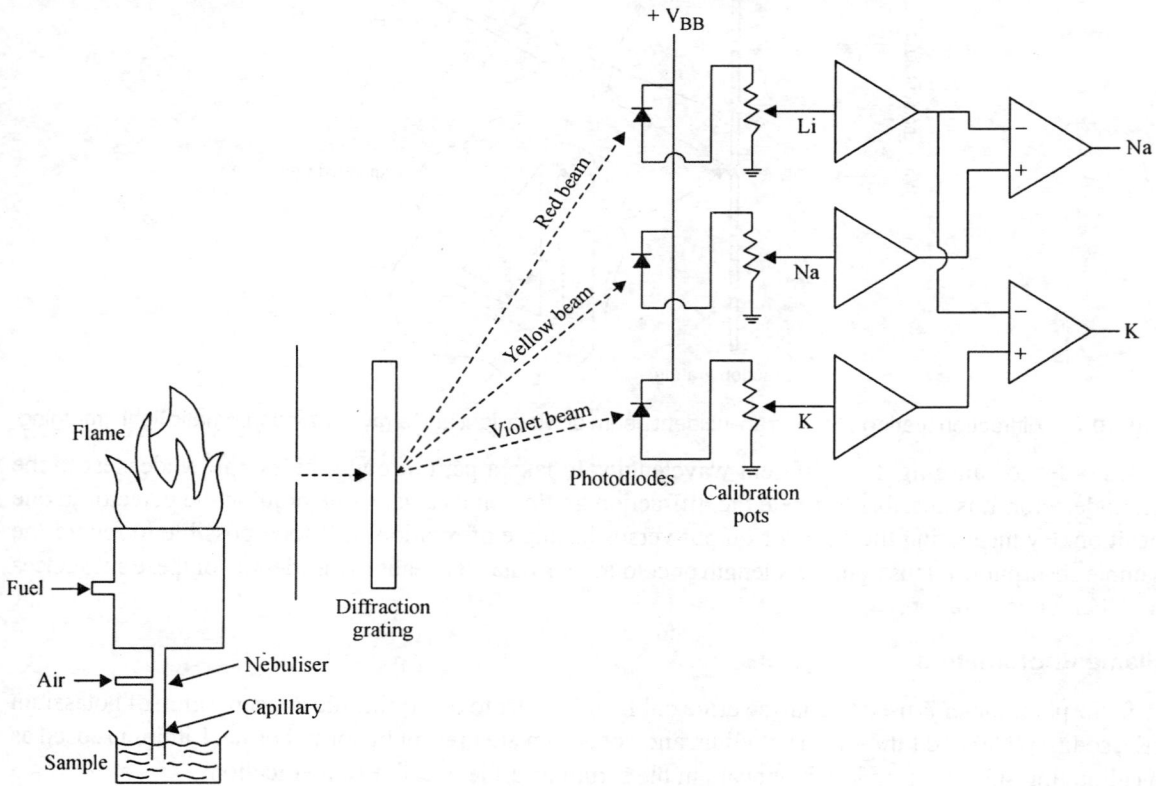

Fig. 10.8. Flame photometer functional diagram.

The flame photometer illustrated in Fig. 10.8 has a separate photodetector for each channel. The photodetector is a reverse-biased diode for which current increases as intensity of light incident upon it increases. Calibration potentiometers in each channel are used to calibrate the instrument with known, standard solutions. The output of the Na and K channel is compared with that of the Li channel. In normal use the sample to be tested in this instrument should not contain an unknown amount of Li. Rather, a known, standard amount of Li is added to the sample. The output Na and K concentrations are calibrated in terms of differences with the known Li, called a stock standard. This procedure compensates for variations in the flame that are common to all channels.

BLOOD CELL COUNTER

Knowledge about the number of particles in blood is important data from which a physician can diagnose disease. These particles are commonly known as red blood cells (RBCs), white blood cells (WBCs) and platelets (PLTs). They can be distinguished from each other by virtue of their size and density, as Table 10.2 shows. Because of these distinguishing features it is possible to use a microscope to count the particles or to use electronic circuitry to do the task automatically. Notice in the table that the RBCs are more numerous but smaller than the WBCs. Table 10.2 shows that most of the particles in blood are RBCs. To determine relative proportion of blood volume made up by cell particles, known as the hematocrit (ht), a centrifuge is used (the centrifuge is sometimes called a hematocrit also). The blood sample is placed on a test tube, which is spun so that the cells are packed on the bottom under centrifugal force.

The ht value equals the height of the packed cells divided by the height of the blood in the tube. This is typically 45 per cent.

Table 10.2. Blood particles.

Type	Density (millions/μl)	Individual size (μm)
RBC	4.26–6.2	6.8–7.5
PLT	0.15–0.40	2–4
WBC	0.004–0.011	6–18

The function of the red blood cell is to carry haemoglobin to the cells of the body. It is important to know the mean volume of each red blood cell (MCV) in litres. MCV is defined as:

$$MCV = \frac{ht}{RBC} \text{ (in litres/cell)}$$

where RBC represents the density of red blood cells in cells per litre. A measure of haemoglobin is made by destroying the red blood cells with an acid and releasing the red colour haemoglobin into solution 1 in a process called lysing. The haemoglobin is then separated and weighed. A measure of the mean cell haemoglobin (MCH) is then computed by the definition

$$MCH = \frac{\text{Haemoglobin (g/litre)}}{\text{RBC (litre}^{-1})}$$

The units of MCH are grams per cell. The concentration of haemoglobin in the blood is then given by the mean cell haemoglobin concentration (MCHC) in grams per litre:

$$MCHC = \frac{\text{Haemoglobin (g/litre)}}{ht}$$

A circuit for electronic measurement of the number of cell particles in the blood is shown in Fig. 10.10. The transducer consists of an orifice through which the sample is drawn by a vacuum.

Since the blood cells have high-resistance membranes, the cells in the orifice increase its resistance R_{OUT}. That is,

$$R_{OUT} = R + \Delta R \qquad \text{... (10.3)}$$

where ΔR is the change in resistance due to a cell in the orifice and the value of the orifice resistance clear of cells is R. ΔR produced by each white blood cell is larger than that of a red blood cell or a platelet because its size is greater. The Wheatstone bridge in Fig 10.9 produces a voltage V_{OUT} due to changes in R_{OUT} as follows:

$$V_{OUT} = \left(\frac{R_{OUT}}{R_{OUT} + R} - \frac{1}{2} \right) V_{BB} = \left(\frac{R_{OUT} - R}{2(R_{OUT} + R)} \right) V_{BB} \qquad \text{... (10.4)}$$

Where V_{BB} is the bias voltage on the bridge. Inserting Equation (10.3) into (10.4) gives

$$V_{OUT} = \frac{\Delta R}{4R + 2\Delta R} V_{BB}$$

$$\approx \frac{\Delta R}{4R} V_{BB} \qquad \text{... (10.5)}$$

where $\Delta R \ll R$. Therefore V_{OUT} is proportional to ΔR, which is in turn proportional to the size of the blood cell in the orifice. In Fig. 10.10, V_{OUT} is amplified by a differential amplifier of gain A. An oscilloscope trace of the output is illustrated in Fig. 10.11. Notice that the highest peaks are fewest in number.

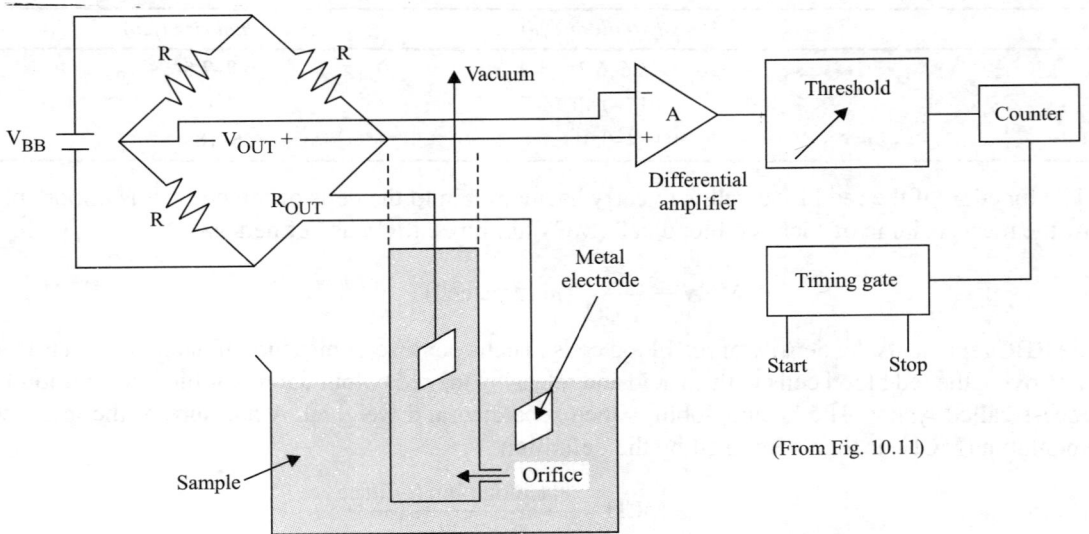

Fig. 10.9. A circuit for electronic measurement of blood cell count.

These are due to the WBCs, which are correspondingly largest in size and fewest in number according to Table 10.1. The RBCs are represented by the peaks between threshold T_2 and T_1. They are much greater in number than the WBCs but make less resistance change in the orifice. In the operation of the instrument, the threshold is first set to zero and the counter will read N_0, the total number of particles per litre,

$$WBC + RBC + PLT = N_0 \qquad \text{... (10.6)}$$

where WBC is the number of white blood cells per litre, RBC the number of red blood cells per litre and PLT the number of platelets per litre. The threshold is then set to T_1 and the counter will read those signals that exceed the threshold and give the number N_1:

$$RBC + WBC = N_1 \qquad\qquad ... (10.7)$$

Then the threshold is set to T_2 and the counter will read just WBC. The RBC is then computed from Equation (10.7) and the PLT from Equation (10.6).

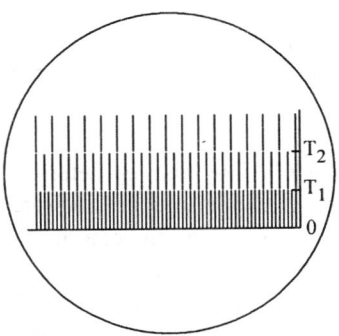

Fig. 10.10. A blood cell counter display.

The counter must be started and stopped over well-timed periods. A vacuum fluid arrangement for doing this timing is shown in Fig. 10.11. To operate the mechanism, valves V and F are both initially opened. This draws a flushing solution through glass tubing into the waste to get rid of any bubbles.

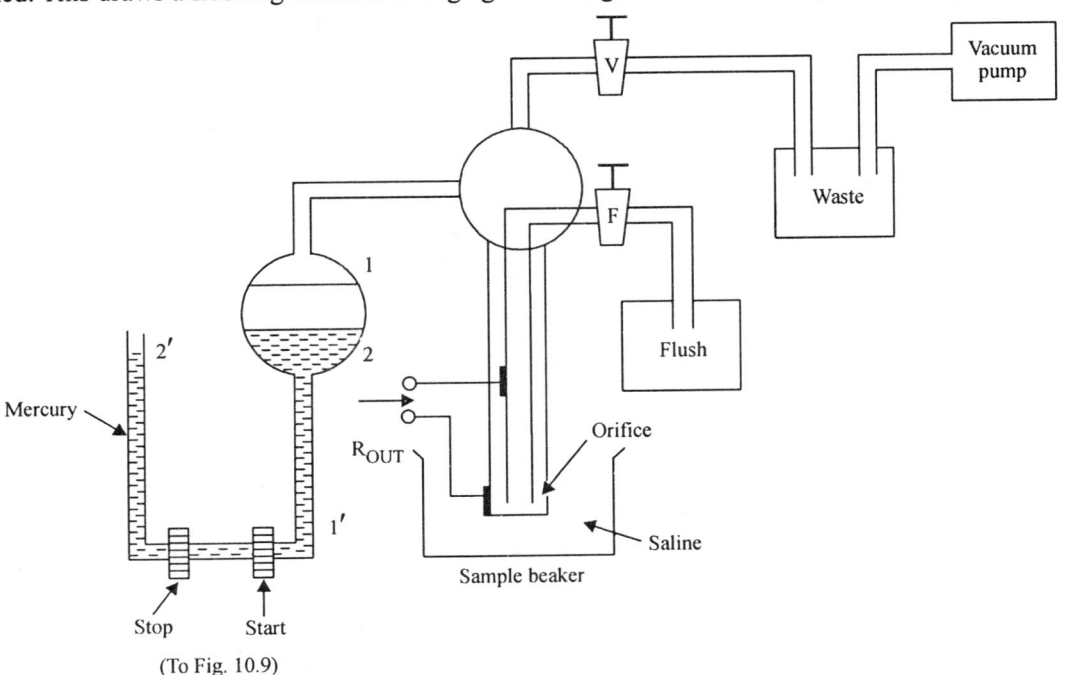

Fig. 10.11. Glass tubing for a blood cell counter using a mercury timer.

Valves F and V are then closed. A sample of dilute blood is then placed in the beaker and valve V is opened. The vacuum thus created will cause the sample to enter the orifice. Simultaneously the mercury will be drawn up into the bulb so that it is confined between the levels 1 and 1′. Valve V is then closed, cutting off the vacuum pump from the sample and mercury. The mercury surface then moves from the levels 1 and 1′ to become confined between the levels marked 2 and 2′ in the figure as it seeks its own level because of the atmospheric pressure at both ends. As the mercury surface travels from position 1–1′ to position 2–2′, it activates first the start switch to begin the counter. When it arrives at the stop switch the counter stops. As the mercury falls it also draws a fixed volume of the sample through the orifice. The counter therefore reads the number of particles per unit volume. This mechanism controls the rate of flow through the orifice so the digital display can be calibrated in units of cells per microlitre.

Optical Methods of Cell Counting

The cell counts RBC, WBC, PLT and MCV may also be determined by measuring the light scattered from each cell particle as it passes through an aperture, as illustrated in Fig. 10.12. The blood is heavily diluted to reduce the number of particles counted to one at a time. A sheath fluid is directed around the blood stream to confine it to the centre of the aperture. The cell is illuminated by a light source such as a laser. The angle of scattered light is different for different-size cells. The scattering angles of platelets and red blood cells are sufficiently separate that these two types of cells can be distinguished by directing the scattered light to different detectors. To separate white blood cells from red blood cells, it is necessary to destroy the red blood cells with a lysing agent. This also frees the haemoglobin so that it can be measured. Instrumentation based on this principle presents a display of RBC, WBC, PLT, ht, MCV, MCH and MCHC.

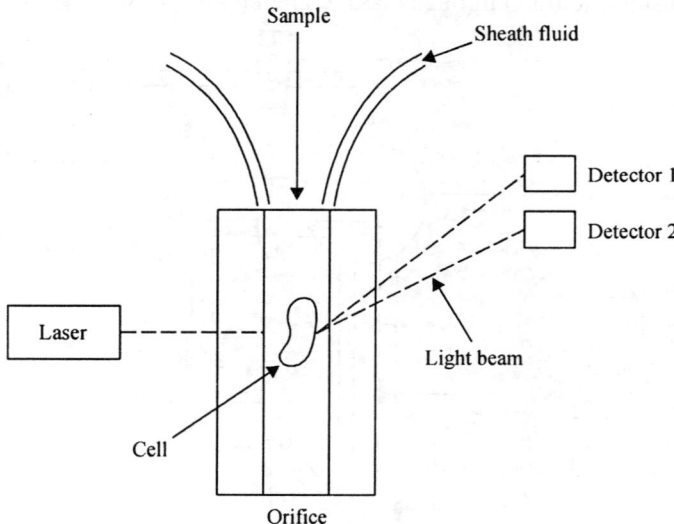

Fig. 10.12. Optical cell counting.

RADIATION DETECTORS

The gas-filled tube is probably the most popular type of radiation detector. Such tubes can be operated in any of three modes: ionisation chamber, proportional counter and Geiger counter. The main difference between these three is the voltage level applied to the gas-filled tube. A schematic of a typical gas-filled tube is shown in Fig. 10.13 with its operating curve.

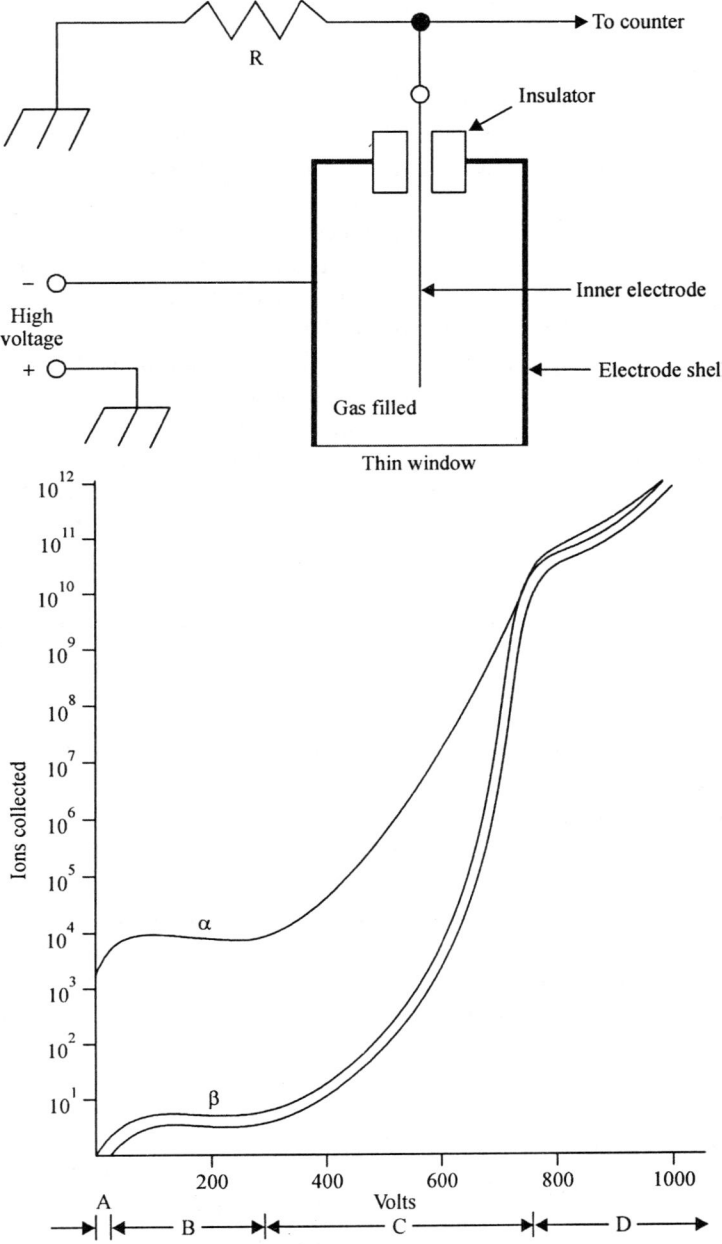

Fig. 10.13. The mechanical construction of a gas-filled radiation detector. The characteristic curve shows the properties and operating conditions of the gas-filled tube.

Regardless of the mode, the operation of this tube is dependent upon an internal electric field set up through the application of a high potential difference across the two electrodes. Radiation particles, which enter mostly through the thin window on the end of the tube, ionise some of the gas molecules. The electric field can then operate on these particles and pull some of them toward the inner electrode, where they form a current that flows out through the external resistance. This current has an impulse character and so produces a spike-like pulse across the resistor. This pulse is the signal fed to the counter.

The gas-filled radiation detector is most popularly associated with the hand-held Geiger counter. In some laboratory instruments, on the other hand, the gas-filled 'tube' is actually a dome and the inner electrode is a small loop of wire. In these instruments there is a little compartment, accessible through a trap door, that accepts samples for radioactive testing.

Figure 10.14 shows the operating curve of a typical gas-filled tube. Two curves are given here, one for alpha (α) particles and the other for beta (β) particles (high-speed electrons). A low-voltage bias (region A of the graph) creates only a weak electric field inside the tube. This field is too weak to attract many of the particles formed when radiation ionises the gas.

The second zone, however, presents a somewhat different situation. In region B, which extends from approximately 100 to 240 volts, the tube operates as an ionisation chamber. Nearly all of the ions produced in this region of operation appear as a current flow in external resistance R. The voltage drop across R is proportional to the level of radiation intensity. We can, therefore, use a gas-filled tube as an ionisation chamber to measure the intensity of gamma-ray sources such as X-ray generators.

The third region on the characteristic curve, region C, extends from around 240 volts up to just under 800 volts. In this part of its curve, the gas-filled tube operates as a proportional counter. In this type of operation it is found that the electric field is strong enough to impart sufficient kinetic energy to the ionised gas particles that they create additional ions through the mechanism of collision. Because of this, the ionic current in the external resistor producing the voltage spike is magnified proportionally to the applied voltage. The proportional counter is thus capable of counting ions in the chamber on a one-by-one basis.

The name proportional counter is derived from the fact that the amplitude of the output pulse is proportional to the kinetic energy of the incident ionising radiation particle. A particle with higher levels of energy will ionise more gas molecules than low-energy particles. This current can be multiplied by as much as a million times through the creation of new ions by the collision of the original ions with un-ionised gas particles.

The last region of the curve, region D, is where the gas-filled tube becomes a Geiger counter—the name erroneously applied to instruments of all three classes. At voltage levels from around 800 to well over 2000 volts, the gas-filled tube operates in a somewhat different manner than described previously. The ion multiplication effect of the proportional counter becomes so intense in this region that the tube can be said to abruptly discharge or avalanche. This produces as single pulse across the external resistor with pretty much the same amplitude every time it occurs, which implies that Geiger counter output pulses are totally independent of the kinetic energy of the impinging radiation.

Gas-filled tube specifications vary somewhat from one manufacturer to another. Most tubes use argon, at a gauge pressure of approximately 100 torr, as the internal gas. A small amount of impurity (usually bromine) is added to quench the discharge; otherwise, the tube would remain ionised and would behave more like an argon glow lamp than a radiation detector. Typical output pulses from these tubes are on the order of a few microseconds, so the amplifier circuitry must be able to follow moderate to fast rise-time pulses.

SCINTILLATION COUNTERS

Scintillation is a word used to denote a process similar to that which generates light on the screen of a cathode ray tube. When a radiation particle strikes an atom of certain phosphorous materials, its kinetic energy may be added to the energy of the orbital electrons. When an electron is thus excited, it jumps to a higher energy level. It is, however, unstable in this high-energy state and will soon fall back to its normal or ground state. But energy must be conserved and just as it attained extra energy from the radiation, it must lose energy as it returns to its normal state. This energy is released in the form of light energy called photons. Quite simply then, a scintillator is a device that allows the counting of the light flashes produced by scintillation.

A stylised scintillator tube is shown in Fig. 10.14. In this instrument, the scintillation crystal is attached to a photomultiplier tube—a specialised vacuum tube capable of making a very large output current for even very dim light inputs. The cathode of the photomultiplier is a photoemitter material that produces an electron for every impinging photon.

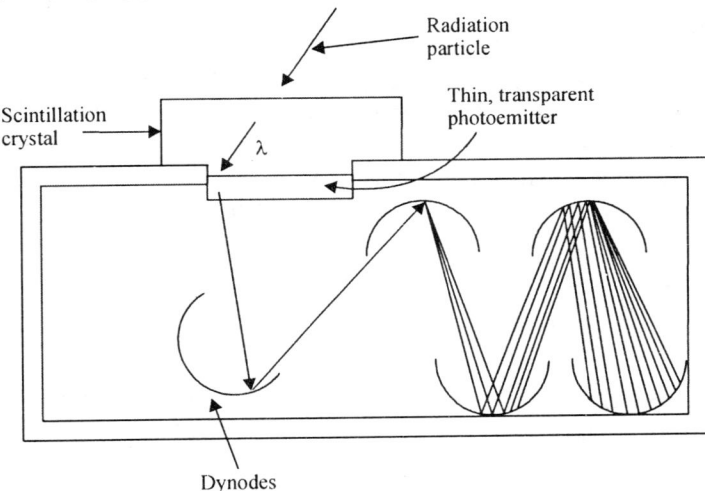

Fig. 10.14. A scintillation radiation detector uses a photomultiplier tube to increase its output current levels.

The typical photomultipler tube has 10 anodes or dynodes arranged so that electrons reflected from the first will strike the second, those from the second strike the third and so forth. Each dynode has a potential with respect to the cathode that is approximately 100 volts higher than that of the preceding dynode. This is usually implemented by connecting each successive dynode to an appropriate tap on a resistive voltage divider.

Each electron emitted by the cathode surface is therefore accelerated by a potential of approximately 100 electron volts (eV). This means that each electron will have a 100 eV kinetic energy when it strikes the next dynode. And when it does strike the next dynode, its kinetic energy will knock loose several more electrons from the metallic dynode material; these are sometimes called secondary electrons. This process continues, the electron count increasing at each dynode, until the tenth dynode, where it is collected and delivered to the external circuit.

The scintillator/photomultiplier produces a current that is proportional to the kinetic energy of the indicent radiation. Such tubes, then are used to measure the energy of the radiation. Most of the better scintillation assemblies can generate nanosecond duration pulses up to a very high counting rate, making them more sensitive than the gas-filled tubes. The scintillation assembly is often associated with a cathode ray tube that displays the pulse count along the vertical axis and the kinetic energy along the horizontal axis; this comprises a radiation spectrometer. Many of these instruments use a computer-like memory and an add-to-memory circuit for accumulating pulse counts.

SEMI-CONDUCTOR RADIATION DETECTORS

The elements of semi-conductor theory form the basis for the operation of diodes and transistors and this should be somewhat familiar to you. If a radiation particle strikes the semi-conductor crystal, its kinetic energy can dislodge an electron and through the normal semi-conductor mechanism, a current is generated. This current can be accelerated by an external electric field applied across the crystal, creating an even greater current pulse. The pulse amplitude from this type of detector is substantial and it is nearly linear for a wide range of particle kinetic energy (usually 20 keV to 200 MeV). Pulse durations down to the nanosecond range can be achieved.

COMPUTER IN THE CLINICAL LABORATORY

The advent of the computer allowed speeding up of communications between the area of the hospital requesting a test and the laboratory. In cases in which the laboratory is a subset of a larger overall computer-based hospital information system, requests for tests can be initiated and results received using remote computer stations located in nursing units, special care facilities, outpatient department, surgery, physicians' offices and other places where patient care is provided (Fig. 10.15).

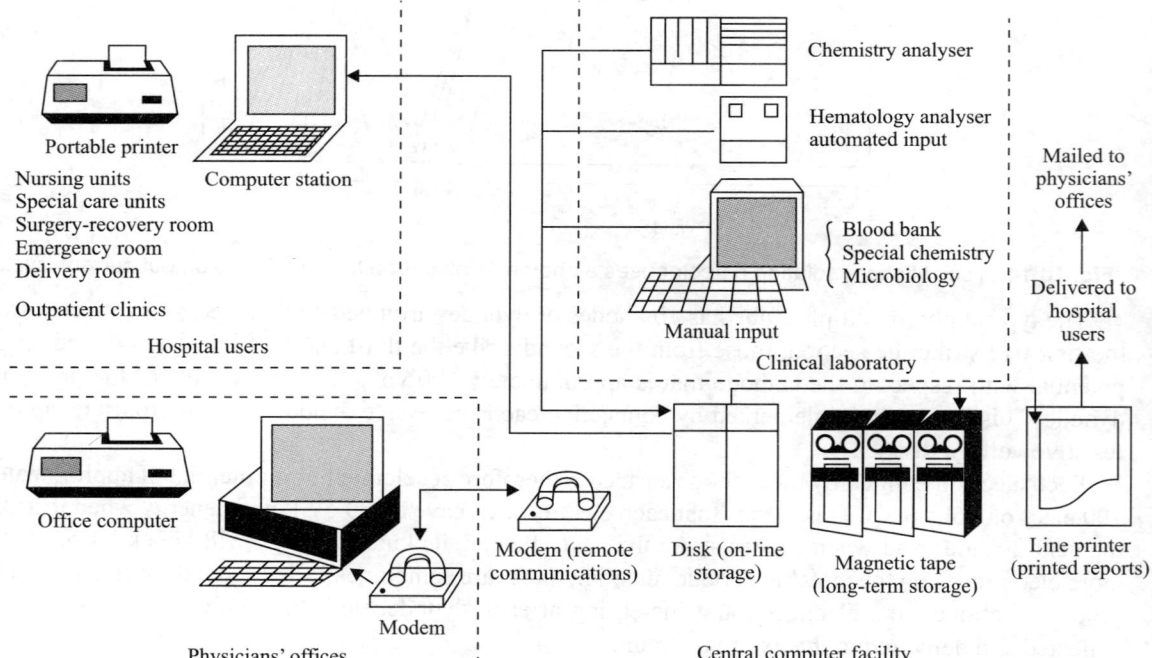

Fig. 10.15. Clinical laboratory information is transmitted to remote computer stations via hardwire and to office computers via modem. Printed reports may be hand-carried to hospital users or mailed to physicians' offices.

Currently, video display terminals (VDT) are the most commonly used stations. Requests arriving in the laboratory may be printed on portable or desktop printers and/or may be held in storage in order to generate a collection list for the following morning. This list facilitates sequential collection of samples and provides specimen labels and other information. Work lists for the pertinent laboratory sections may also be printed, detailing sequentially the various steps required for the completion of the tests.

In some cases, the arrival in the laboratory of a STAT test request or a request for a test that needs to be done at a time prior to the printing of the next collection list is signaled to laboratory personnel by devices that incorporate visible or audible (or both) alarms. Similar devices are used in patient areas to alert the staff that the result of a test requested as STAT or a routine request that produced a critical or panic result, is now available for review on the VDT screen.

If a link between a laboratory computer and a central installation computer exists or if the laboratory is an integral part of a hospital-wide information system, it is possible to make available to the laboratory the demographic or background information on the patient for whom a test has been requested, thus avoiding repetitive entry of information. However, regardless of where the information is entered into the system, the software should (i) provide for logical error checks; (ii) produce adequate audit trails for tracking human or system failures; and (iii) facilitate obtaining derived or secondary data when possible without human intervention. The laboratory, in turn, may report the results of the tests performed, as soon as they become available, directly to the remote stations in patient care areas. Then the results are reported on a VDT screen, including abnormal result flags (H = high, L = low and ALERT = critical value) and units of measure.

Test results that are produced by automated laboratory equipment, such as multiple chemistry and hematology analysers, can be transferred to a central (hospital-wide) computer system or to a local (laboratory) computer.

Bar-code self-adhesive labels are, in some cases, affixed to specimen tubes to provide the automated laboratory analysers or the laboratory blood bank with patient identification data and test types requested. These machine readable labels can be generated by central computer or a laboratory computer using information entered by other departments.

In all cases in which information is exchanged automatically between laboratory equipment and a computer system, it is advisable to ensure that a manual override mechanism exists. This override can be used by a technologist to monitor the exchange process and detect and delete invalid results produced by technical problems before they are reported to the attending staff. Typically, if a test result produced by automated laboratory equipment (such as a multiple chemistry analyser or a hematology counter) falls in the critical ranges or consists of values not logically compatible with the output of the instrument, manual override procedures come into effect. The result in question, usually presented to laboratory personnel and flagged as abnormal on a VDT screen or a hard-copy device, is not allowed to be reported to the requesting patient care area. The test is then repeated, using another instrument or a different reagent or methodology, until laboratory personnel are satisfied as to the validity of the result. In some cases it may be necessary to obtain a new specimen from the patient. The manual override procedure then allows laboratory personnel to enter the correct result in the patient's result report file using a VDT or other input device. Test results that are produced by non-automated laboratory equipment or by equipment that has not been interfaced can be entered manually through a VDT into the central or laboratory computer. It should be kept in mind that this transcription process can be a frequent source of human error.

Procedure descriptions and specimen collection instructions for nursing personnel can be made available on-line to the nursing units if the clinical laboratory is tied into a hospital-wide information system. This information can be maintained current at all times through updates entered in the system by laboratory personnel. Finally instructions are displayed to nursing personnel on a VDT screen for a fasting blood glucose determination.

The secondary gains that can be obtained from the use of a central or dedicated computer in the clinical laboratory are:

1. Automatic generation and maintenance of a database containing test descriptions, normal values and ranges, units of measure, adjustments for age, sex, height and weight and so on.
2. Laboratory census and statistics on daily, monthly and yearly basis by laboratory section and patient type.
3. Historical data on patients with multiple hospitalisations.
4. Quality control procedures.

SELECTION OF A COMPUTER SYSTEM

There are two main approaches to the automation of a hospital clinical laboratory.

Turnkey Systems

Turnkey systems, which are available for purchase or lease from a number of vendors, can be either software/hardware combination packages or just software that is designed to run on one or more popular computers. In most cases, these packages operate satisfactorily shortly after their installation, providing the laboratory with a tried-and-tested system, usually at an attractive initial cost. This obviates the time and expense needed to develop software and to rent, lease or purchase hardware. However, modification to these turnkey systems can be expensive and frequently they have an inherent inflexibility that, in many cases, requires that the laboratory modify its operational procedures to accommodate the system. Additionally, the system can be more expensive in the long run because of the cost of hardware maintenance, software upgrades and escalating rental or lease fees. Should this type of system be considered, the long-term viability of the vender, the size of the vendor's customer base, the user satisfaction and the quantity and quality of support offered by the company should all be carefully investigated.

In-House Systems

In-house systems may consist of a hardware-software combination that serves exclusively the needs of the clinical laboratory and perhaps interfaces in on-line or off-line mode with other computers used in the hospital for accounting and billing or for patient registration. In other cases, the laboratory is an integral part of a hospital-wide information system using a mainframe computer with or without satellite systems. In general, the hardware for these systems is more expensive and the software may require extended periods of development time before it becomes fully operational. However, in-house systems can be custom-tailored to the user's needs, are less expensive to maintain and may be less costly over the long run than turnkey systems. Other advantages include the interchangeability of peripheral equipment such as VDTs and desktop or portable printers with other users or areas of application. Ordering and reporting software can be shared with other hospital departments, using single remote stations in nursing units or other patient care areas, which avoids proliferation of peripheral hardware and overlapping of software. The system described earlier in Figs. 10.1 and 10.3 are examples of in-house development.

The increasing popularity of small personal and business computers has brought a new dimension to the clinical laboratory. These devices, which continue to increase in performance, storage capacity and range of available peripherals as their cost decreases, can be used as stand-alone tools in specific applications, as satellite units of a larger system or as part of a network. Numerous programmes are commercially available and many laboratory professionals have learned to programme their personal computers using available high-level languages.

Particular attention should be paid to the test result reports printed by the laboratory, since they become a permanent part of the patient's record. They should be easy to read, clearly indicate which laboratory section originated them: and help in spotting trends at a glance if any are present. The cumulative-type reports that are offered by many vendors may not be acceptable to physicians or nurses and may be misplaced or lost. Overlapping printed reports, on which the pertinent laboratory sections are identified by colour or labels and which allow review of one week of group-related tests on one page may be preferable.

Whatever approach is chosen, it is imperative (to avoid costly failures) to involve upper-level management in both the laboratory and the hospital administration in the early stages of the development of an in-house system or in the procurement of a turnkey system. Experience has shown that the delegation of these responsibilities to lower-level clerical or technical personnel is generally not helpful although their input and eventual feedback should not be neglected.

Chapter 11

Hearing Aids

INTRODUCTION

This chapter presents hearing fundamentals, symptoms and causes of hearing disorders, hearing aid fundamentals, design, systems and fitting procedures.

The human auditory system is one of the most remarkable biological information processing systems known. As such, it has been the focus of intensive scientific study. Consequently, much is known concerning the function of various parts of the ear as they relate to the hearing process.

From an acoustical point of view, the external ear is the least important component of the auditory system (Fig. 11.1). Unlike the external ear of several other members of the animal kingdom, the human pinna or auricle does not prevent dirt and fluid from entering the ear canal, nor does it move independently of the head to facilitate judgement of the direction of sound waves. It does, however, exhibit a transfer function that emphasises high frequencies and it offers an irregular three-dimensional (3-D) shape that promotes the acoustic seal of custom-made hearing aid moulds.

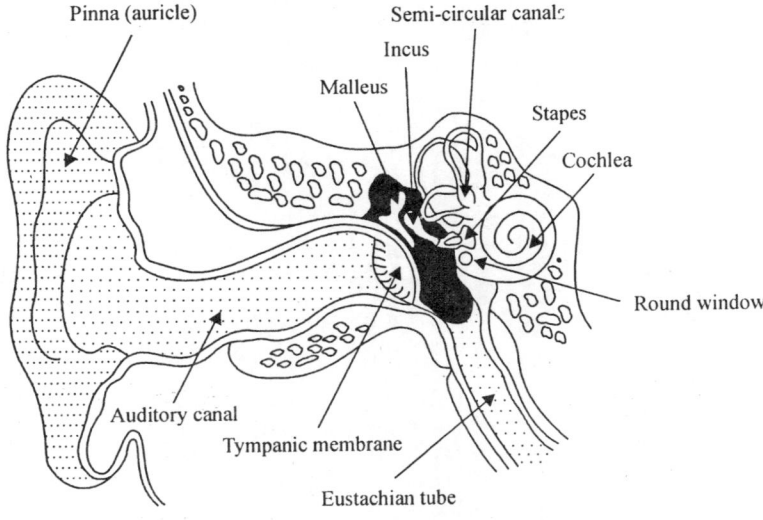

Fig. 11.1. Anatomical view of the ear.

The cross-section of the ear canal is approximately oval and extends a distance of nearly an inch from the pinna to the tympanic membrane or ear drum. The size and shape of the ear canal varies greatly from one individual to another. This variation causes a variation in the acoustic impedance of the ear canal and is a major factor creating difficulty in accurately fitting a hearing aid to a patient, as discussed later.

The middle ear is comprised of the tympanic membrane, the air-filled cavity behind it and the group of bones (malleus, incus and stapes) known as the ossicles. Sound waves are conducted through the external ear canal to the ear drum, causing it to vibrate. These vibrations are coupled mechanically by the ossicles to the inner ear at the oval window. The eustachian tube connects the middle ear to the rear of the nasal cavity to allow the air pressures on both sides of the ear drum to be equalised. The middle ear effects an impedance match between the air of the outer ear and the fluid of the inner ear. Hence it increases the sensitivity of the ear.

The inner ear, which includes the snail-shaped, bony structure known as the cochlea and the three semi-circular canals, is the most complex chamber of the ear. The semi-circular canals are associated with our sense of balance and are not directly related to the sense of hearing. The cochlea is a very complex organ, whose detailed function is not yet fully understood. Consequently, it continues to be the subject of intensive scientific research at numerous institutions worldwide. The macroscopic function of the cochlea is to convert mechanical vibrations, coupled via the stapes of the middle ear through the oval window, into nerve impulses on the auditory nerve.

Pressure exerted on the incompressible fluid in the cochlea by the vibrations at the oval window is relieved at the round window, which is a second opening to the bone that encloses the cochlea. The cochlea is partitioned into three fluid-filled regions (i.e., the vestibular and tympanic canals and the cochlear duct) by two membranes that run the length (3.5 cm) of the cochlea from the oval window to near the apex. These are the basilar membrane and Reissner's membrane. At the apex there is a small gap between the membranes and the end of the bony cochlear coil to allow for equalisation of fluid pressure in the vestibular and tympanic canals. Hair cells are distributed along the entire length of the basilar membrane. When they are disturbed by vibrations traveling down the basilar membrane, they initiate neural activity in the structures connected to them and cause a flow of electrical impulses through the auditory nerve to the central nervous system. There are approximately 2500 hair cells in the inner ear, which are encoded by 30000 neurons.

SYMPTOMS AND CAUSES OF HEARING DISORDERS

Hearing impairments are classified by cause and severity. There are three general categories of hearing impairment: (i) poor conduction of the sounds from the outer to the inner ear; (ii) abnormal transformation of inner ear waves to nerve pulses or abnormal transmission of nerve pulses to the central nervous system via the auditory nerve; and (iii) dysfunction of the central nervous system. These are known as conduction, excitation/transmission and interaction/perception disorders, respectively. The common form for excitation/transmission disorders is sensorineural hearing loss. A combination of conductive and sensorineural hearing loss is called a mixed loss. A person may have normal hearing, in that he has a normal threshold curve, but also have poor speech intelligibility due to an abnormality of the central nervous system. These disorders are called dysacusis.

An outstanding feature of the human ear is its extraordinary dynamic range of operation. In fact, at 4 kHz the ear has a dynamic range (the difference between the slightest audible tone and the loudest painless tone) of 140 dB. This is a range of 14 powers of 10. Davis and Silverman have said it well.

Hearing impairments are classified by severity as follows. The average hearing threshold at 500, 1000 and 2000 Hz is measured and compared with the average normal thresholds shown in Figs. 11.2 and 11.3. Deviations from the average thresholds are quantified in dB HL (hearing level). Average thresholds of 0–26 dB HL are termed normal, those between 27 and 92 dB HL are termed hard of hearing and those above 92 dB HL are termed deaf. These classifications are summarised in Table 11.1. The cause of the elevated thresholds can be either conductive or sensorineural hearing loss. A simple hole in the drum may cause only a 5–10 dB loss. Simple interruption of the train of ossicles reduces the sensitivity by about 60 dB. Conductive hearing loss is limited to about 60 dB (if no sensorineural loss is present) when bone conduction by-passes the inoperative middle ear.

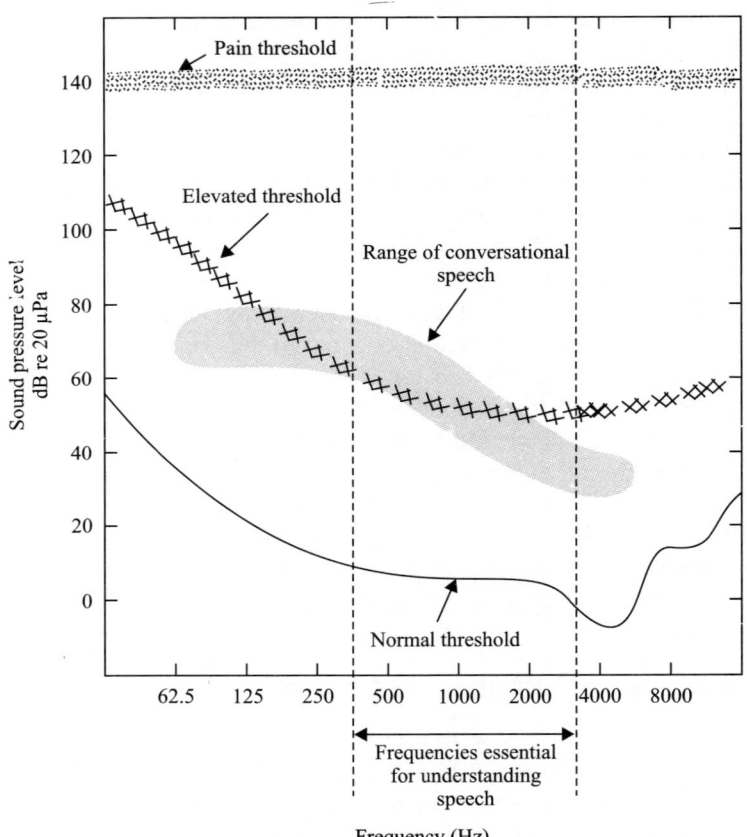

Fig. 11.2. Hearing curve with normal and elevated threshold due to conductive loss.

Table 11.1. Classification of hearing levels.

Average threshold	Classification
0–26 dB	Normal
27–92 dB	Hard of hearing
Above 92 dB	Deaf

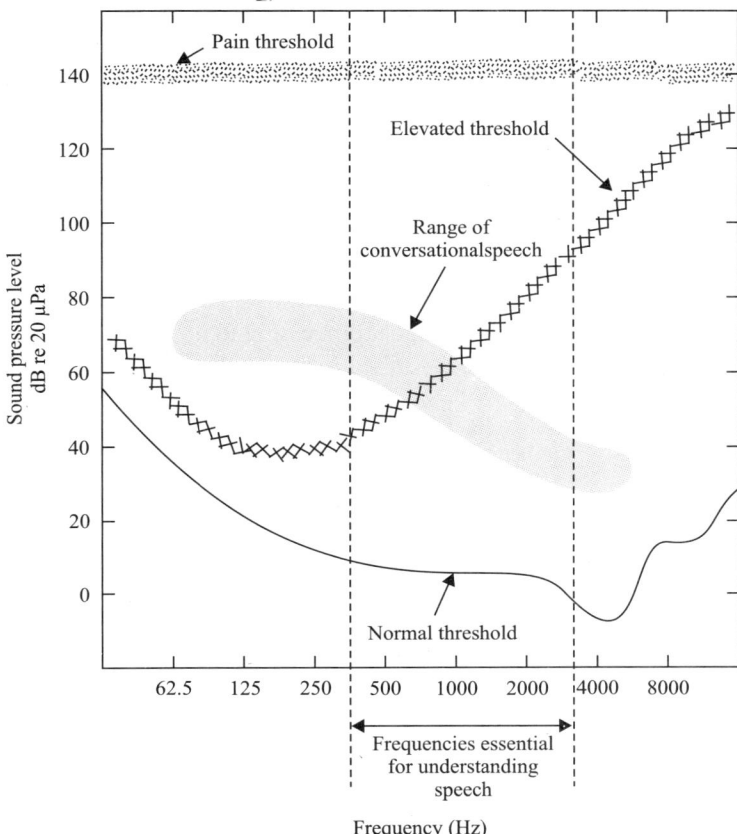

Fig. 11.3. Hearing curve with normal and elevated threshold due to sensorineural loss.

A traditional test to differentiate between conductive and sensorineural impairments is administered by presenting an oscillating tuning fork, first placing the vibrating fork next to the ear to test the air conduction and then applying the base of the vibrating fork to the skull to test the bone conduction. If bone conduction is normal and air conduction is reduced, it is likely that the patient has a conductive impairment. This is generally caused by either obstructing the outer ear canal (e.g., with wax) or restricting the motion of the drum and/or the ossicles. On the other hand, poor bone conduction does not always indicate a sensorineural loss because rigidity of the ossicles can hamper the transfer of bone-borne vibrations to fluid waves at the oval window.

Patients exhibiting elevated thresholds due to either conductive of sensorineural hearing impairments can usually benefit from hearing aids that amplify the sound presented to the outer ear. For example, Fig. 11.2 depicts the threshold curve for a patient with an elevated threshold due to conductive hearing loss. Note that the loss is fairly constant over the entire frequency range. A wideband amplifying hearing aid would benefit this patient. Figure 11.3 shows the threshold curve for a patient with an elevated high-frequency threshold due to a sensorineural hearing loss. A hearing aid that provides gain only in the high frequencies would be of great utility to this patient.

HEARING AID IMPLEMENTATION

Two types of hearing aids are presently in use. Conventional electronic amplification aids have been in use for decades and have evolved from vacuum tube body-worn designs to microelectronic behind-the-ear (BTE) and in-the-ear (ITE) designs. The evolution of these aids is summarised in Fig. 11.4, which indicates the shrinking size of electronic aids over the past six decades. More recently, the FDA has approved the use of a cochlear implant for profoundly deaf patients. The cochlear implant is a device that by-passes the outer, middle and inner ear by converting sound waves directly into auditory nerve pulses. Implantable aids that by-pass the outer ear by directly driving the ossicles of the middle ear with an electromechanical transducer have been developed. Less controversial and closer to public use are digital hearing aids that employ state-of-the-art digital signal processing to obtain superior frequency response and ease of fitting. These implementation are described in the sections that follow.

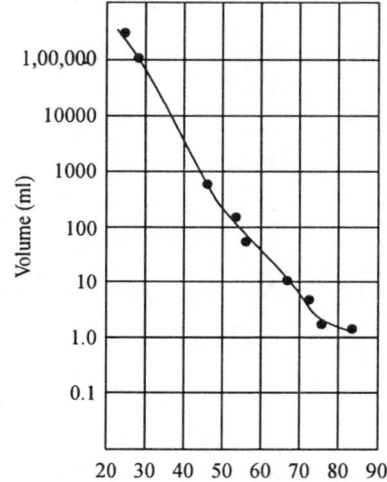

Fig. 11.4. Hearing aid sizes by year.

Regardless of the type of implementation, one measure of a hearing aid's performance is the difference in decibels between the sound pressure levels at the ear drum with and without the aid. This difference is called the insertion gain of the aid when measured acoustically; when measured behaviourally, it is called the functional gain. Due to the anatomical differences of the head, hair, external ear and impedance of the tympanic membrane among individuals, this is not simply the gain of the hearing aid in a test cavity.

Conventional Aids

As shown in the block diagram of Fig. 11.5, conventional electroacoustic hearing aids are composed of a microphone and associated pre-amplifier, an active filter, a power amplifier, an output transducer or receiver and a power supply or battery. These components are packaged in one of several housings: a body-worn aid, which places all of the components except the output transducer in a shirt-pocket-sized enclosure and features a wire connecting this module to the output transducer module worn in the ear; a BTE aid (sometimes referred to as a 'shrimp' aid because of its physical appearance) which houses all of the components in a curved module designed to fit comfortably behind the ear and an ITE design which is the least objectionable aid from a cosmetic viewpoint since it fits completely inside of the outer ear and in the case of a canal aid, completely inside the canal.

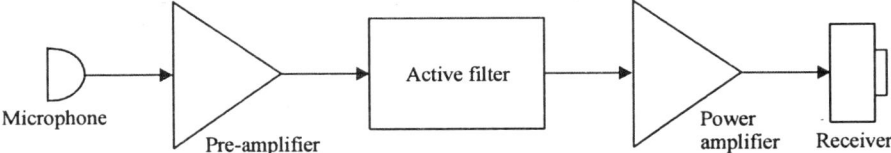

Fig. 11.5. Block diagram of generic electronic hearing aid.

The most common input transducer in use today is the electret microphone, which contains an integral field effect transistor (FET) pre-amplifier (Fig. 11.6). The FET pre-amplifier is housed in the metallic microphone case to shield its input from extraneous electromagnetic fields and thus reduce noise pick-up.

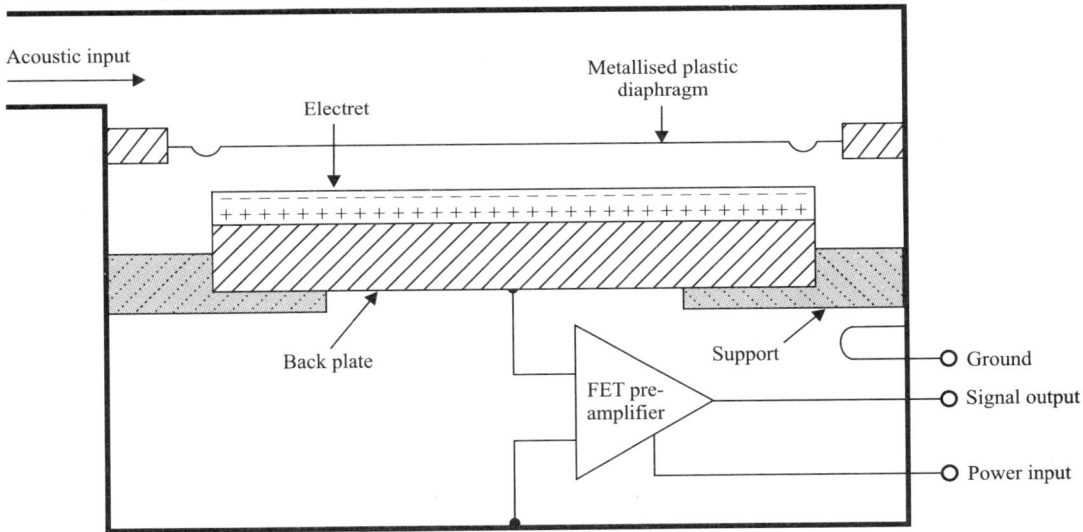

Fig. 11.6. Electret microphone.

The active filter accounts for the tunable nature of the aid. It may incorporate some type of compression technique to limit the power output and avoid uncomfortable loudness levels. Figure 11.7a presents the input/output function for a system that incorporates simple peak clipping to limit maximum power output. Any output signal that has a value greater than the peak clipping level (or compression threshold) is reduced to the clipping level. This accounts for the horizontal portion of the graph above the compression threshold. Other compression techniques introduce a gradual upward slope in the input/output curve for values greater than the compression threshold. A typical input/output curve for such a system is shown in Fig. 11.7b. These systems allow both the compression threshold value and the slope above it to be adjusted. All compression techniques introduce unavoidable distortion since they process the signal with non-linear operation. The extent to which an aid's frequency response can be altered is limited to the capabilities of the active filter section. The active filter is adjusted with tone controls that generally provide for low-frequency attenuation (since most hearing aid wearers require high frequency gain) of up to 30–40 dB relative to the high frequency response.

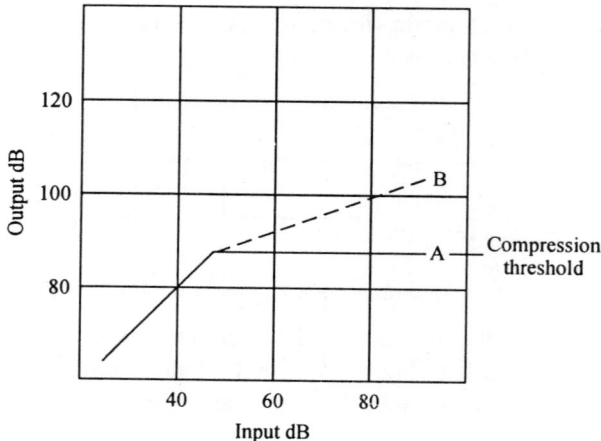

Fig. 11.7. Compression curves: A, peak clipping; and B, moderate compression.

The output transducer or receiver, is shown in Fig. 11.8. It is an electromagnetic device that features a miniature diaphragm connected by a drive pin to a movable armature. The acoustic output is routed to a custom-fitted ear mould through a short length of flexible tubing. The frequency response of the tubing can be altered to boost the high frequency by tapering its inside diameter from the ear mould back to the receiver port end. Tapered tubing is referred to as an acoustic horn.

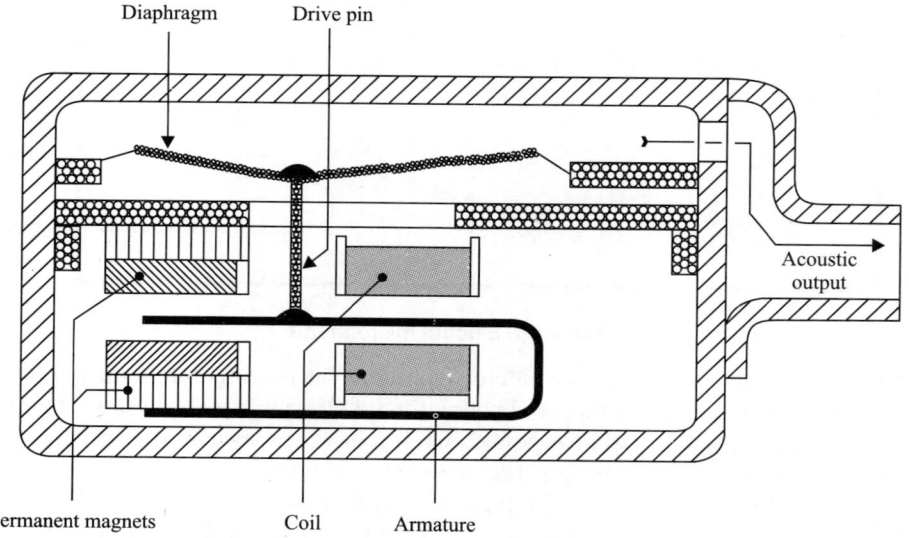

Fig. 11.8. Receiver cutaway.

The mechanical considerations involved in hearing aid designs are considerable. Most notable is the desire to provide large electroacoustic gain while avoiding the very annoying squeal caused by acoustic feedback. To accomplish this goal the output and input transducers must be isolated mechanically.

Although several types of cochlear implants have been proposed, they all share four components (Fig. 11.9): an input microphone, a microelectronic signal processor that converts the sampled sound into electrical signals, a system to transmit these signals from the external module to the implanted module and electrode(s) to convey the electrical signals to the auditory nerve. The signal processing unit splits the input signal into one or more channels or frequency bands for delivery to the auditory nerve. Being a single-channel device it enables the patient to sense sounds but not to understand speech. Multichannel devices may be able to restore speech intelligibility as well but are still in the research phase of their development.

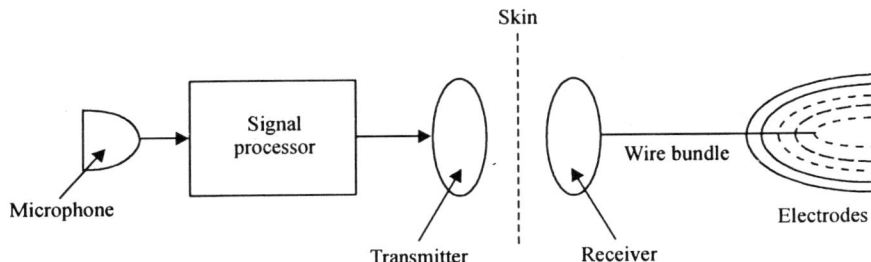

Fig. 11.9. Block diagram of cochlear implant.

Implantable Hearing Aids

An implantable hearing aid differs from the cochlear implant in that it provides a means for driving the ossicles directly and thus substitutes an implanted piezoelectric crystal or magnet attached to one of the ossicles for the receiver, tubing and ear mould of a conventional aid. The implanted output stage, be it magnetic or piezoelectric, is driven inductively by an external module that houses the input microphone, active filter, power amplifier and battery. The goal of such a system is to improve the sound fidelity compared with conventional aids. Because the outer ear canal is not obstructed by such an aid, improved speech discrimination is obtained. Furthermore, since the output transducer is electromechanical as opposed to acoustic, no acoustic feedback is produced. Implantable aids have been proposed to foster cosmetic acceptance, but the proponents of these devices have not yet been able to demonstrate sufficient improvements over conventional aids to warrant the cost and risk of the necessary surgery.

Digital Hearing Aids

Figure 11.10 shows the block diagram of a generic digital hearing aid. Sound waves picked up by the microphone and transformed into electrical signals are converted to a digital representation for processing by an analog-to-digital converter and the processed signals are converted back to analog by the digital-to-analog converter whose output drives the power amplifier. The promise of digital technology is to provide superior signal processing capabilities, ease of fit and unchanging long-term performance. The potential signal processing improvements include shaping the frequency response to invert the patient's hearing loss, effectively enhancing the signal-to-noise ratio with adaptive filtering, reducing or eliminating acoustic feedback and expanding and/or compressing signals while minimising distortion. The challenge is to incorporate effective digital signal processing capabilities while not exceeding a power budget that allows reasonable battery life. The advances in low-power, very large scale integrated (VLSI) circuit technology are expected to continue over the next few years to the point that micropower digital hearing aids will become practical.

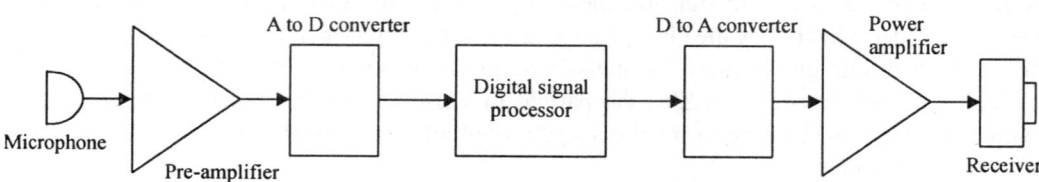

Fig. 11.10. Block diagram of digital hearing aid.

HEARING AID FITTING PROCEDURES

Several popular methods exist for fitting hearing aids to patients. These can be classified into the two major categories of selective and non-selective procedures. Non-selective procedures, which use a fixed frequency-gain characteristic, were once thought to serve most hearing-impaired individuals equally well with a single hearing aid response. More recently, the selective procedures, which can be sub-divided into comparative and descriptive types, have been overtaking the non-selective procedures.

The more popular selective procedure is the comparative method, in which an aid is chosen after several have been compared through the scores obtained by the patient in word-discrimination tests, the use of preference scales or combinations of these so-called objective and subjective ratings. Comparisons can be made between various aids or settings of a given aid. The patient's discomfort level for speech is used to set the maximum power output and the average gain is chosen to be about one-half of the hearing loss. The frequency response of the aid and the ear mould and tubing are selected with the intention of matching the inverted slope of the patient's threshold curve. However, since measurement is extremely difficult, until very recently the chosen aid has rarely been placed in the real ear to estimate the sound that is actually delivered.

The descriptive method of hearing aid fitting specifies an optimal aid response according to assumptions based on one or more of the following: the patient's threshold curve, his comfort levels and a desired relation between the average speech spectrum and the patient's residual dynamic range. The first uses the threshold curve alone to set the gains of the aid across the spectrum. This is known as mirroring the audiogram. The threshold levels can be biased by the average speech spectrum in an effort to enhance the patient's ability to understand speech. The second assumption is based on mirroring the equiloudness contour of the patient at his most comfortable listening level. The third assumption attempts to place the average speech spectrum within the patient's residual dynamic range at a comfortable level.

All fitting procedures are vexed by the inherent problems associated with: (i) making accurate measurements of the patient's threshold, most comfortable and uncomfortable levels; and (ii) predicting the frequency response of the selected hearing aid on the patient, given its response in a test cavity, which in general differs greatly.

The use of a probe microphone to measure the sound-pressure level in the ear canal has recently emerged as a solution to the problem of measuring accurately the patient's residual hearing curves. Although its use is generally limited to research clinics and has not yet achieved widespread acceptance with hearing aid dealers, rapid deployment of such systems is now underway. The problem of re-calibrating the aid on the patient, given its calibration parameters in a test cavity, can be avoided by making all measurements through the hearing aid, using the patient's own ear mould.

Recently a digital hearing aid, incorporating an integral probe microphone and a companion fitting procedure have been developed for rapid and accurate fitting of a wide variety of hearing disorders using a descriptive fitting method.

SECTION II
Medical Imaging Systems

Chapter 12

Medical X-Ray Equipment

INTRODUCTION

X-rays are well known even in ordinary experience. Almost everyone has been X-rayed at one time or another by a medical doctor, dentist or radiologist. In fact, it was the medical applications that caused the X-ray industry to grow. Besides medical uses, however, they are also used in industry for quality control purposes and by researchers in the scientific fields of chemistry, physics and biology. X-rays are a means for photographing the interior structures of objects normally opaque to visible light.

It was not until November 8, 1895, however, that X-rays were even known. Even then, their discoverer, W.K. Roentgen, only called them X-rays because their nature was not known. The name has persisted even until today, despite the fact that considerably more is known about them. In honour of their discoverer, since 1925 the internationally accepted unit for X-ray quantity has been called the Roentgen.

PROPERTIES OF X-RAYS

Before discussing the types of diagnostic X-ray apparatus commonly found in hospitals, let's first review briefly the physics of X-rays. These 'rays' are actually electromagnetic waves, much like radio signals and light. Figure 12.1 shows a spectrum chart giving the relationship of the respective frequencies in the electromagnetic spectrum. Electromagnetic waves are different from other types because they can travel in a vacuum and are thereby propagated even through outer space. Electromagnetic waves are said to have the following properties, some of them in common with other types of waves:

1. They obey the relationship $V = F\lambda$.
2. The relative intensity of electromagnetic waves will obey the inverse square law: their intensity is proportional to $1/D^2$.
3. They propagate rectilinearly.
4. They are not deflected by magnetic fields.
5. They produce interference and diffraction phenomena.

Thus, the velocity of wave propagation is equal to the product of frequency and wavelength. In the case of electromagnetic waves, this velocity is the speed of light, denoted by the letter c and equal to approximately 3×10^8 meters per second.

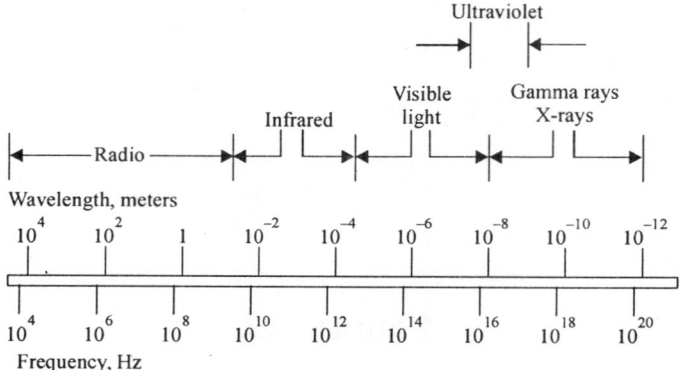

Fig. 12.1. Electromagnetic spectrum chart showing the relative wavelengths of radio, light and X-ray waves.

The inverse square law states that the field intensity falls off as the reciprocal of the square of the distance, $I = 1/D^2$. This simply means that doubling the distance from a point-source radiator will cause the relative intensity to diminish to a quarter of the previous intensity. This effect can be demonstrated with an ordinary flashlight. Turn the switch on and shine the light onto a nearby wall. Note the intensity when the light source is a small distance, say one foot and then back off to four feet. You will note that the reduction in the intensity is quite a bit—to about one sixteenth. The amount of energy has not changed, but at a longer distance, it must illuminate a much larger area of the wall. This particular phenomenon must be taken into account when working with X-ray equipment. It was in the study of electromagnetic phenomena, namely black body thermal radiation, that modern physics broke with the classical physics then prevalent. In the later part of the nineteenth century, it became apparent that Newtonian physics could not account for observed facts concerning electromagnetic phenomena. Whenever scientists find that observations in nature or in the experimental laboratory contradict a theory, then that theory must be either modified or scrapped to make room for a new all-encompassing theory.

Modern physics began in the year 1900 when a classical physicist named Max Planck proposed, in a paper presented before the German Physical Society, the notion that electromagnetic energy must be quantised. That is to say, it can only exist in certain discrete packages now called photons. According to this view, photon energy follows the relationship:

$$E = hF = hc/\lambda$$

where,

    E = energy
    F = frequency
    h = Planck's constant (6.62×10^{-34} joule-second)
    c = speed of light (3×10^8 m/sec)
    λ = wavelength in meters.

In the next section we shall discuss certain quantum phenomena, but only as they relate to the understanding of medical X-ray equipment.

PHOTOELECTRIC EFFECT

The photoelectric effect was first noted by Heinrich Hertz in 1887 during an experiment to confirm one of Maxwell's predictions. Photoelectric effect is the emission of electrons from a clean metallic surface when electromagnetic radiation falls onto that surface. There are at least four different phenomena which can cause electrons to be released from a metallic surface. Besides photoelectric effect there is also thermionic emission, field emission and secondary emission.

Thermionic emission is the process that creates the electron current in vacuum tubes. The metal object is heated to incandescence and this imparts thermal energy to the free electrons. Some of the more energetic surface electrons actually 'boil off' from the surface into space.

Field emission is the attraction of electrons from the surface by a strong electric field.

Secondary emission is a problem in ordinary vacuum tubes and the mode of operation of X-ray generator vacuum tubes. This occurs when a rapidly moving electron strikes the metallic plate, imparting some of its kinetic energy to electrons in the plate. If enough energy is transferred to these electrons, they may jump off the surface, creating a secondary emission of electrons.

Figure 12.2 shows an experiment used to study the photoelectric effect. When light strikes the positive anode, electrons will be emitted. These electrons will be moving with a kinetic energy of:

$$E = \tfrac{1}{2} m_e v^2$$

where, m_e = mass of an electron (9.11×10^{-31} kg)
$\quad\quad v$ = velocity of the electrons in meters per second.

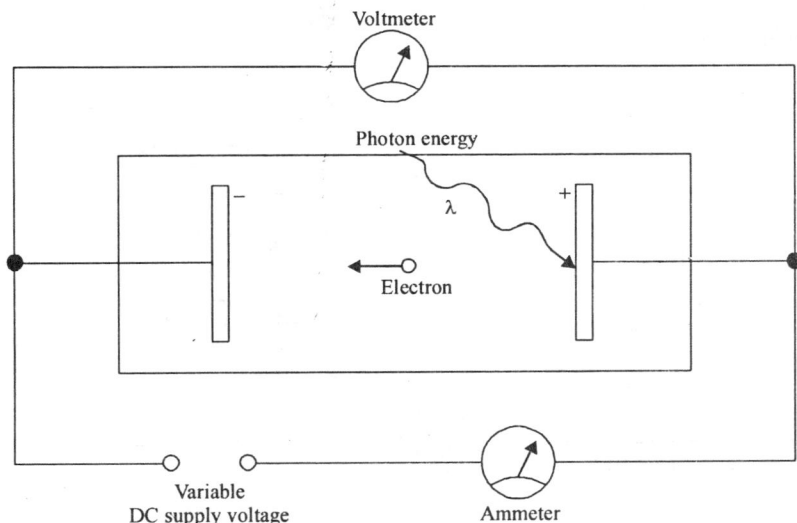

Fig. 12.2. Apparatus used to demonstrate the photoelectric effect.

The external power supply creates an electric field that opposes the electrons and creates a retarding influence on their motion. At some potential V_0 even the most energetic electrons will be retarded so that no current flows in the external circuit. The energy situation under these circumstances is:

$$eV_0 = \tfrac{1}{2} m_e v_M^2$$

where, e = electron charge
$\quad\quad V_0$ = external voltage
$\quad\quad v_M$ = velocity of the most energetic electrons

One interesting aspect of the photoelectric effect is that V_0 is independent of light intensity but is dependent upon the frequency (colour) of the impinging light wave. Light photons striking the metallic surface have an energy $E = hF$ presented earlier. Each photon can only give up all of its energy to a single electron (fractions are not permitted), so we can write:

$$hF = \tfrac{1}{2}\, m_e\, v_M^2 + hF_0$$

The extra term, hF_0, is called the work function and is a property of the particular material comprising the metallic cathode surface. Frequency F_0 is the critical frequency that must be exceeded for the photoemission of electrons to occur. Photoemission can only occur if hF is greater than hF_0.

COMPTON EFFECT

The Compton effect is a phenomenon by which a photon can impart only a part of its energy to a charged particle such as an electron. This situation is illustrated in Fig. 12.3. In part (a) of the figure, an electron is at rest and lying in the path of an incident photon with energy level hF. This photon 'collides' with the electron and some of its energy is imparted to the electron. This, incidentally, implies that photons carry momentum. In fact, the momentum of the photon is equal to:

$$P = E/c = hF/c = h/\lambda$$

where,

$$
\begin{aligned}
E &= \text{energy} \\
F &= \text{frequency of the photon} \\
c &= \text{speed of light} \\
h &= \text{Planck's constant} \\
\lambda &= \text{wavelength}
\end{aligned}
$$

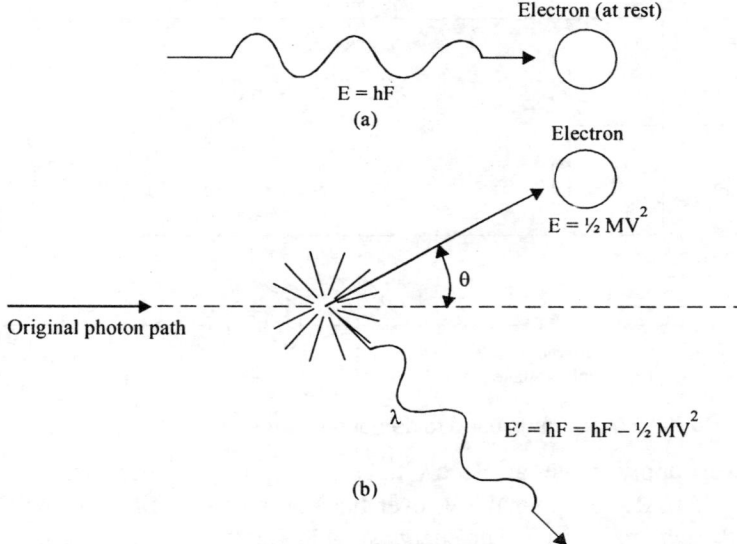

Fig. 12.3. The Compton effect is a means by which an incident photon can give up only part of its energy to a nearby electron.

The photon will still exist after the collision because it only imparts a portion of its energy to the electron. It will, however, exist at a lower frequency (longer wavelength) because of the lost energy. The energy lost to the electron will become kinetic energy, setting the electron in motion.

A particle at rest has a potential energy of $U = mc^2$, so by conservation of energy:

$$hF + U = hF' + U'$$

where U' is the potential energy of the re-coiling electron and the other terms have been previously defined.

The loss of energy means that photon hF' has a longer wavelength, λ'. The difference in wavelength, $\Delta\lambda$, is given by:

$$\Delta\lambda = 1/F - 1/F' = (h/Mc) (1 - \cos(\theta))$$

where θ is the angle of deflection shown in Fig. 12.3.

The kinetic energy of the moving electron is:

$$E = hF\left(\frac{\Delta\lambda}{\lambda + \Delta\lambda}\right)$$

BREMSSTRAHLUNG

The word Bremsstrahlung is German for braking radiation. An example of Bremsstrahlung is shown in Fig. 12.4. An electron with kinetic energy E_1 approaches and is deflected by the heavy nucleus of a nearby atom. After the deflection, the electron has a new level of energy, E_2. By considerations of energy conservation:

$$E_1 - E_2 = hF$$

X-rays are generated by Bremsstrahlung and they are merely photons (electromagnetic waves) with a wavelength of approximately one angstrom (10^{-10} meters).

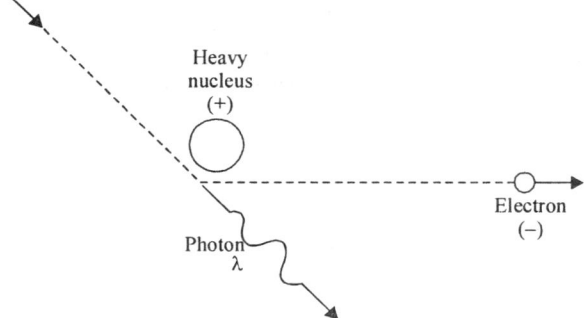

Fig. 12.4. Diagram of a Bremsstrahlung collision by which X-rays are produced.

X-RAY TUBE

The X-ray tube is simply a glass-enclosed vacuum tube diode consisting of a cathode that thermally emits electrons and an anode that attracts these electrons. A functional diagram of an X-ray tube is given in Fig. 12.5, which shows a filament-heated cathode, an anode and a glass vacuum enclosure. The filament source voltage V_F causes a current I_F to flow through the filament coil, heating the cathode metal. Electrons in the cathode are boiled off the metal into the vacuum. In an X-ray the anode voltage V_A is high enough that these electrons are swept across to the anode and form the beam current, I_B. V_A on the tube is very high, on the order of 100 kV. This high voltage impels the electron to a very high velocity. Approximately

1 per cent of the electrons upon entering the anode collide with atoms and produce X-rays. The X-rays then pass through the tube into space.

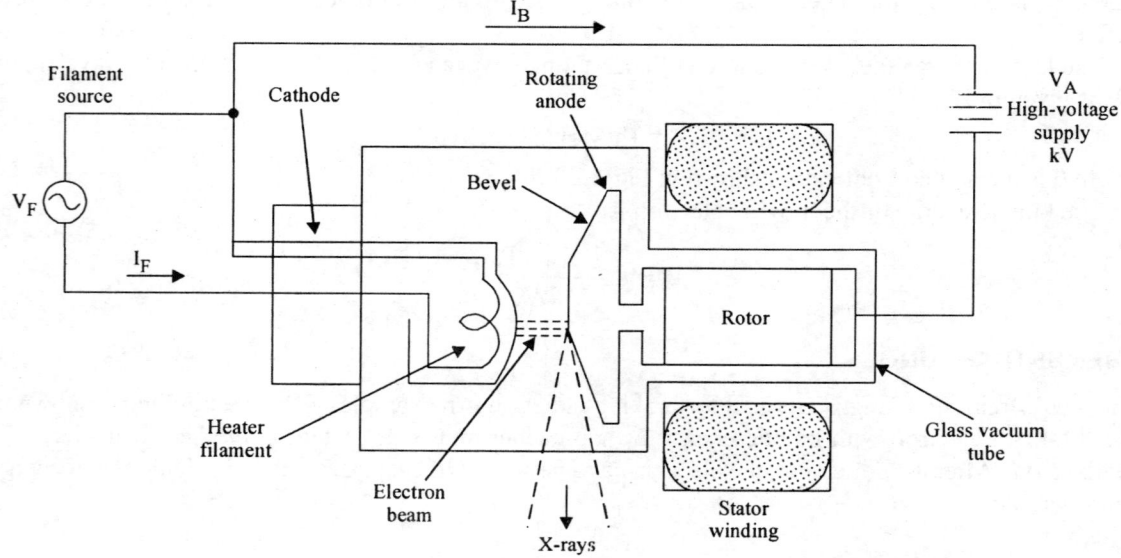

Fig. 12.5. An X-ray tube with a rotating anode.

To understand how X-rays are produced it is necessary to first consider the beam current. Electrons are boiled off the heated cathode because thermal agitation gives them enough energy to escape from the bonding forces into tube vacuum. The value of that energy, called the work function, E_W, differs among metals (Table 12.1). The value of the current in amperes due to thermal agitation, I_B, is derived from quantum mechanical considerations as

$$I_B = C_0 A_C T^2 e^{-11600 E_W /T} \qquad\qquad ...(12.1)$$

where A_C is the cathode area in meters squared and C_0 is the cathode material coefficient. Values of C_0 for several materials used in cathodes are listed in Table 12.1.

Table 12.1. X-ray tube cathode material coefficients and work functions.

Cathode	$C_0 \left(\dfrac{A}{m^2 K^2} \right)$	E_W (eV)
Tungsten	60×10^4	4.52
Thoriated tungsten	3×10^4	2.63
Oxide coated	0.01×10^4	1

Equation (12.1) calculates the beam current only under the assumption that the anode voltage V_A is large enough to sweep all electrons boiled off the cathode across the vacuum. This is usually the case in X-ray tubes. The current computed by Equation (12.1) is limited by the temperature, T and is called the thermally limited current. If V_A is not high enough, however, a space charge of electrons will form around the cathode and they will simply fall back into it. In that case Equation (12.1) does not compute the correct value of beam current. Rather, the current would be determined by the anode voltage and is called the electronic current, I_{BE}. Of course, when the X-ray tube voltage V_A is turned off, such a space charge is formed around the cathode.

Example 12.1. An X-ray tube has no space charge around the cathode. The cathode is tungsten and it has a surface area of 1 cm². Plot the beam current versus temperature.

Solution. Using the valves for tungsten from Table 12.1 in Equation (12.1) gives

$$I_B = (60 \times 10^4) A_C T^2 e^{-11600(4.52)/T}$$

The area is then $A_C = (1 \text{ cm}^2)(1 \text{ m}/100 \text{ cm})^2 = 10^{-4} \text{ m}^2$.

Therefore, $$I_B = 60 T^2 e^{-52432/T} \qquad \text{(in A)}$$

A plot of I_B is given in Fig. 12.6.

Figure 12.6 shows that the beam current can be controlled with the temperature of the cathode. In X-ray tubes, this method is used. This is done by keeping the anode voltage high enough to prevent a space charge build-up around the cathode. To control the cathode temperature, the operator normally varies the filament voltage. This allows the operator to change the beam current while holding the anode voltage constant.

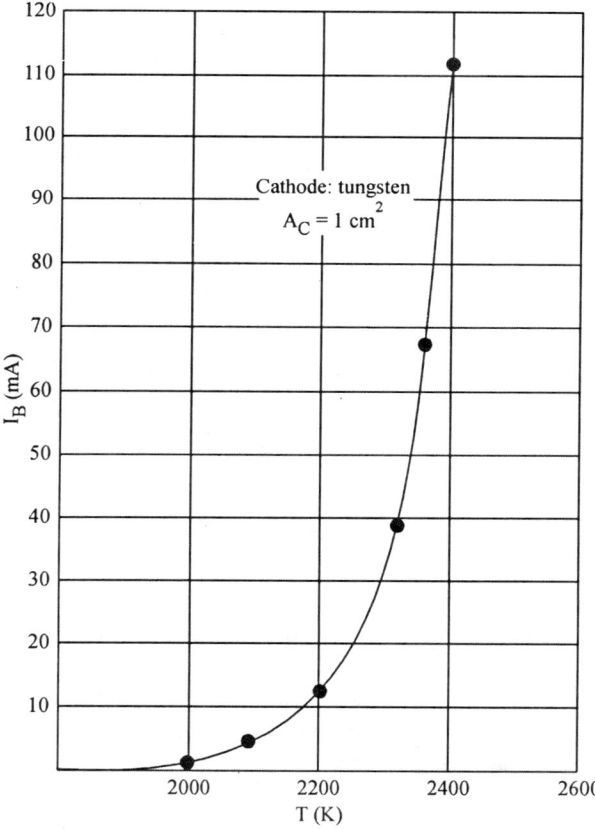

Fig. 12.6. The thermally limited beam current versus cathode temperature of a tungsten cathode.

Nature of X-Rays

An X-ray is produced by an electron beam when one of the electrons collides with an atom in the anode. The collision causes one of the orbiting electrons of the atom to shift to a higher energy orbit. It then falls back to its rest state and emits a photon of X-ray. This is known as characteristic radiation. The energy shifts, K_α and K_β, illustrated in Fig. 12.7, represent different orbital shifts in the atom. Characteristic radiation is used to study the atomic structure of materials and is not typically used in medical X-ray applications. A second type of collision, scattering of the incident electron, produces a spectrum of X-ray radiation, called Bremsstrahlung radiation. This radiation is caused by changes in the velocity of the beam electron that reduce its kinetic energy by a factor equal to the energy in the X-ray.

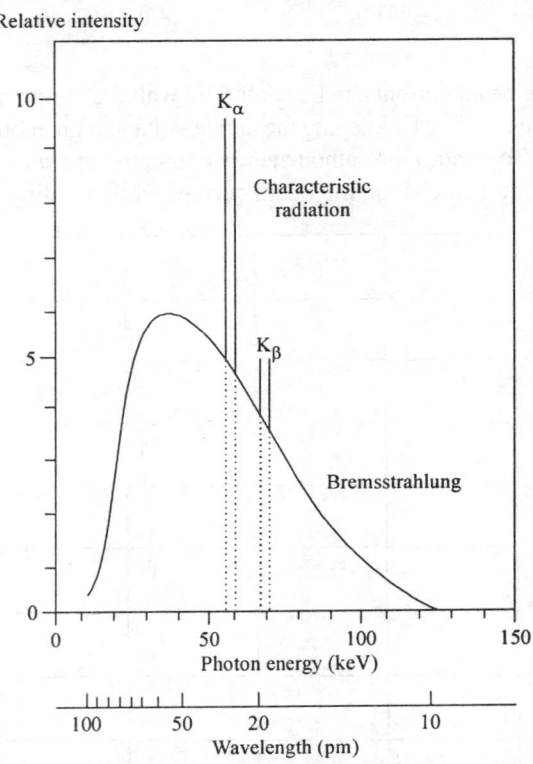

Fig. 12.7. X-ray spectrum emitted by a tungsten anode at 130 kV.

Bremsstrahlung radiation contains most of the X-ray energy. For this reason it is most important in medical applications, which are based on energy absorption rather than on the measurement of particular wavelengths, as in crystallographic studies using X-rays.

The effect of the anode voltage on the radiated photon energy is shown in Fig. 12.8. Increased anode voltage at a constant beam current produces high-energy electrons in the beam. In fact, the energy of the electron, E_E, when it strikes the anode is given by

$$E_E = eV_A \qquad \qquad ...(12.2)$$

where e is the electronic charge on an electron [e = 1.602×10^{-19} coulomb (C)]. E_E is measured in units of electron-volts (eV). An electron-volt is defined as the energy acquired by an electron as it is accelerated through one volt. When the electron collides with an atom in the anode, it produces a photon of X-ray having an energy, in accordance with quantum mechanics, given by

$$E_P = hf \qquad \qquad ...(12.3)$$

where h is Planck's constant (h = 6.625×10^{-34} J.s) and f is the photon frequency. No radiated photon can have more energy than the electron that produces it in collision. Therefore, in Fig. 12.8, the photon Bremsstrahlung energies do not exceed eV_A and are limited by the anode voltage.

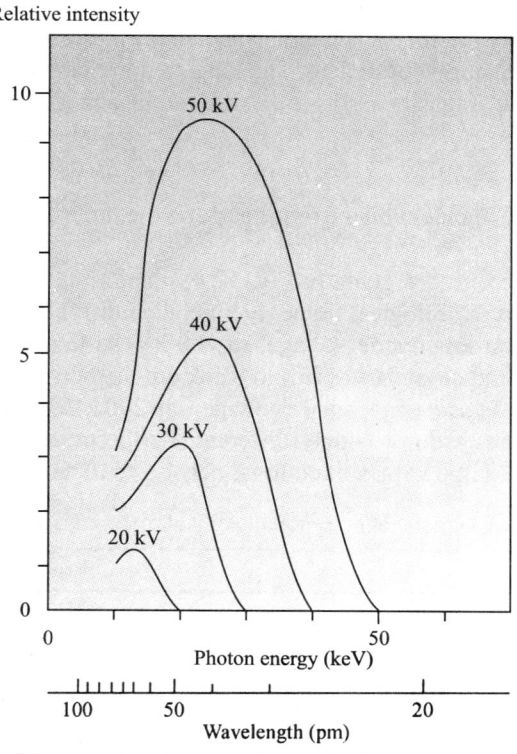

Fig. 12.8. The effect of the anode voltage on the emission spectrum from an X-ray tube.

Example 12.2. For a 40kV anode voltage, find the maximum photon energy of the radiated X-ray.

Solution. The maximum energy in the electron of the beam is eV. So the maximum electron energy = 1.602×10^{-19} (40×10^3).

$$E_{Pmax} = 6.408 \times 10^{-15} \quad \text{(in J)}$$

X-ray photons have a frequency given by

$$f = c/\lambda \qquad \qquad ...(12.4)$$

where c is the speed of light (3×10^8 m/s) and λ is the wavelength of the radiation in meters.

X-Ray Absorption

Medical X-ray imaging is done by applying X-rays to the surface of the body and measuring how much passes through. That is, the amount of X-rays absorbed by the body is measured by taking the difference of the input and output radiation energies. X-ray absorption is the basic mechanism for discrimination between organs in a body under X-ray observation. Bone tissue, for example, absorbs more X-ray than muscle and therefore can be easily distinguished from it. Exactly how much X-ray is absorbed by different tissues are determined by Lambert's law. Lambert observed that with X-rays, equal thicknesses of material absorb equal proportions of radiation $\Im$. In other words, the fraction of X-ray energy absorbed is proportional to the thickness of the material absorbing it. Lambert's law is stated mathematically as

$$\frac{d\Im}{\Im} = -\mu\rho \; ds \qquad\qquad ... (12.5)$$

where ρ is the medium density (g/cm^3), s is the distance through the material and μ is a proportionality constant called the mass attenuation coefficient. The units of μ are cm^2/g. The symbol $d\Im$ represents the differential change in the X-ray intensity and ds is the differential change in distance. Solution of equation (12.5) yields the formula

$$\Im = \Im_0 e^{-\mu\rho s} \qquad\text{(in W/m}^2\text{)} \qquad\qquad ... (12.6)$$

where $\Im_0$ is the X-ray intensity incident on the tissue and $\Im$ is the intensity of X-rays that emerge from the tissue of thickness s.

Values for μ in units of cm^2/g are given in Fig. 12.9, illustrating the relative values for bone and muscle. Also, typical densities of biological tissues are included in Table 12.2. It is apparent that to study bone a physician should use a low anode voltage, say 60 kV, so that it is easy to distinguish it from muscle. On the other hand, if the physician wishes to blank out the bone to distinguish underlying muscle tissue from fat, he or she should use a high anode voltage, say 200 kV. It is apparent from Table 12.2 that the densities of the soft tissues are not widely different. Furthermore, the μ values are nearly equal. Therefore, it is difficult to get large values of contrast between soft tissues using X-ray.

Table 12.2. Density of common biological materials.

Material	Density (g/cm^3)
Air	0.0013
Water	1.0
Muscle	1.06
Fat	0.91
Bone	1.85

Example 12.3. Suppose the incident X-ray intensity on water is 1 W/cm^2. Compute the intensity that emerges from a container of water 2 cm thick. The photon energy is 20 keV and the corresponding mass attenuation is 0.523 cm^2/g.

Solution.

$$\Im_{H_2O} = 1 \; W/cm^2 e^{-(0.523 \; cm^2/g)(1 \; g/cm^3)(2 \; cm)}$$

$$= e^{-2(0.523)} = 0.3513 \; W/cm^2$$

Example 12.4. Suppose the incident X-ray on bone is 1 W/cm^2. Compare the energy emerging from bone with a density of 1.2 g/cm^3 having the dimensions of Example 12.3, with the result 0.3513 W/cm^2 for $\Im_{H_2O}$. At 20 kV, the mass attenuation constant for bone is 2.51 cm^2/g.

Solution.

$$\Im_B = 1 \; e^{-(2.51)(1.2)(2)} = 0.0024 \; W/cm^2$$

Notice that the ratio of

$$\frac{\Im_B}{\Im_{H_2O}} = \frac{0.0024}{0.3513} = 0.0068 \ (-21.7 \ dB)$$

and that this is a power ratio.

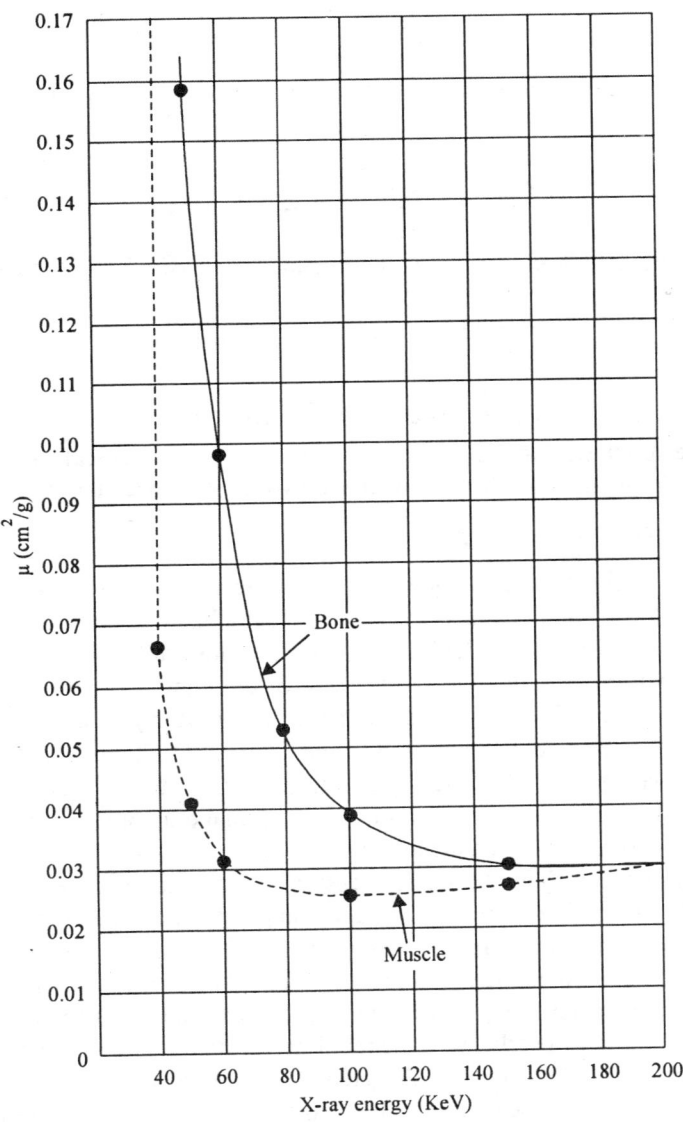

Fig. 12.9. The mass attenuation coefficient versus the X-ray photon energy.

Obviously the X-ray intensity emitted from water is far greater than that emitted from bone. This means that the bone absorbs more X-ray energy than water. Furthermore, this difference in X-ray intensities on film will produce an image having good contrast properties.

Tissue Contrast

The contrast in the image on film made by two tissues is defined in terms of the relative intensities of the X-rays that reach the film. $\mathfrak{I}_1$ is the intensity of X-rays emitted from tissue 1 and $\mathfrak{I}_2$ is the intensity of X-rays emitted from tissue 2. The contrast between the two tissues is then defined by the equation

$$C_{12} = 10 \log \frac{\mathfrak{I}_1}{\mathfrak{I}_2} \qquad \text{(in dB)} \qquad \qquad \dots (12.7)$$

Here the multiplier 10 is used because the ratio $\mathfrak{I}_1$ to $\mathfrak{I}_2$ is a power ratio. Applying Equation (12.6) then yields

$$C_{12} = 10 \log \frac{\mathfrak{I}_0 e^{-\mu_1 \rho_1 s_1}}{\mathfrak{I}_0 e^{-\mu_2 \rho_2 s_2}}$$

where s_1 is the thickness of tissue 1 and s_2 is the thickness of tissue 2. Manipulation of this equation yields

$$C_{12} = 10 (\log e) (\mu_2 \rho_2 s_2 - \mu_1 \rho_1 s_1)$$

or

$$C_{12} = 4.3429 (\mu_2 \rho_2 s_2 - \mu_1 \rho_1 s_1) \text{ dB} \qquad \qquad \dots (12.8)$$

From this equation we conclude that the contrast between two tissues depends on their mass attenuation coefficient, density and thickness. In fact, C_{12} increases with differences between these parameters.

X-RAY EQUIPMENT BLOCK DIAGRAM

The basic components that must be part of any medical diagnostic X-ray unit are shown in Fig. 12.10. In general, the purpose of these components is to create an X-ray image of high density, high contrast and high sharpness on film or other imaging device. This must be done while minimising the dose of ionising radiation given to the patient. The density or darkness, of the image is proportional to the amount of X-rays that penetrate the film and would increase in proportion to X-ray tube beam current, for example. Contrast is a measure of the darkness of a desired image compared to its surroundings and it is basically determined by the relative attenuation of the object. This factor is often directly affected by X-ray beam voltage. Sharpness or clarity of the edges, is reduced in an image by blurring due to distortions in the X-ray beam as it passes from the X-ray tube to the patient.

A high-voltage source from 20 to 200 kV is necessary in order to produce X-rays at the X-ray tube anode. However, the duration of time the high voltage is applied to the tube must be carefully limited, in order that the patient does not receive an excessive dose, the film does not become overexposed and the X-ray tube does not overheat. Since the X-ray tube is operated in its thermally limited mode, the X-ray intensity in watts per square meter is adjusted by the X-ray tube filament current. As a protection against overheating, the temperature of the tube anode is monitored with a temperature detector. If it exceeds a specified value, a thermal overload will be detected and the high-voltage supply will be turned off automatically. This will eliminate the source of heat and cause the X-ray tube to turn off. Most X-ray tube anodes are rotated by induction-motor action in order to limit the beam power on any one spot and to help cool the anode. The voltage level from the high-voltage source in Fig. 12.10 is amplified passively by a high-voltage transformer to the 20–200 kV level. It is then rectified and passed through the X-ray tube, which will pass conventional current in only one direction, from anode to cathode. X-rays produced by the tube anode are either absorbed in lead or collimated through the X-ray tube opening. Since most of the power in the medical X-ray is Bremsstrahlung radiation, it contains a broad range of frequencies. The X-rays at unwanted frequencies only increase the patient dose and decrease image contrast. Aluminium filters cut to an appropriate thickness absorb lower X-ray frequencies and reduce these negative effects. The intensity of low-frequency or soft, X-rays incident on the patient is reduced by use of an aluminium filter. Soft X-rays do not contribute significantly to diagnostic data in many procedures, but they do increase the overall dose.

Thus, the aluminium serves an important function. Another means of reducing patient dose is to confine the X-rays to the region of interest on the body. An external collimator between the patient and the filters serves this function by limiting the mass of the body exposed to X-rays.

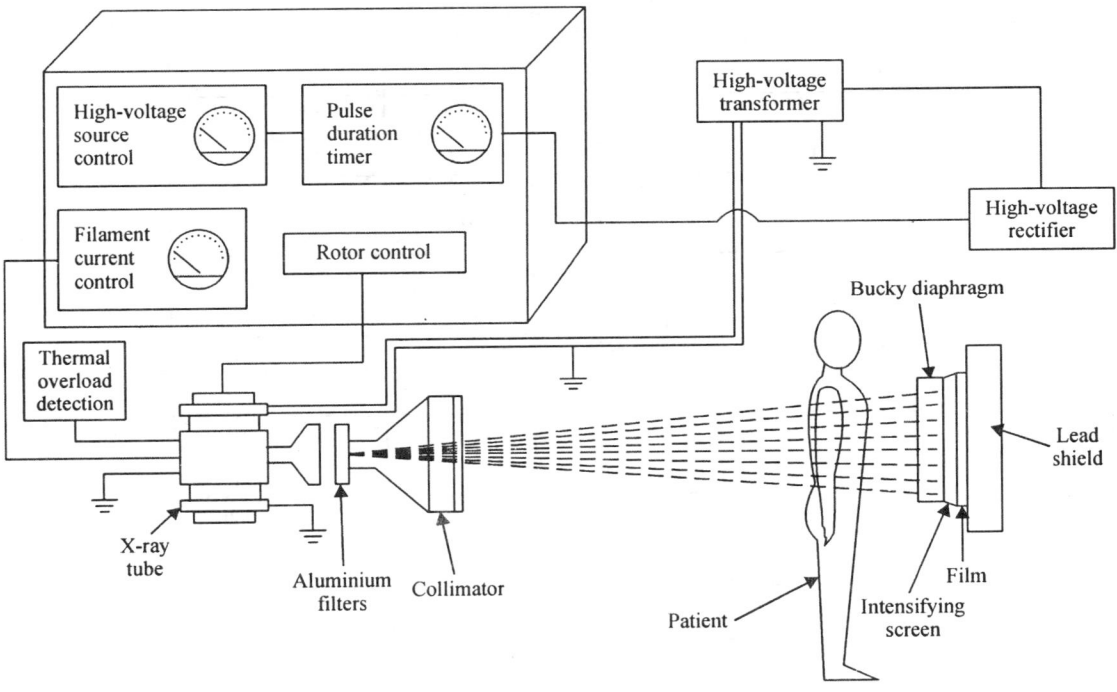

Fig. 12.10. A block diagram of an X-ray machine.

X-rays inside the patient create X-ray scattering, which tends to blur the images. To absorb the scattered X-rays and eliminate the subsequent blurring, the radiologist uses a lead grid called a Bucky diaphragm, which is tapered to pass the X-rays incident on the patient. Radiation following these X-ray paths strikes the film and leaves an image as desired, while the scattered X-rays are absorbed by the Bucky.

As already mentioned in the beginning of chapter an X-ray tube is an expensive wearing element in medical radiological equipment, costing thousands of dollars and requiring replacement as often as twice a year in many X-ray machines. The wearing mechanism is the tungsten of the cathode, which boils off to produce the electron beam. The approximately 1 per cent efficiency of the tube means that 99 per cent of the electron beam energy must be dissipated as heat. This heat flow through the anode, caused by the electron beam striking it, raises its temperature to destructive levels if it is not limited. Rotating the anode at speeds ranging from 3600 to 10000 rpm, with an electric motor armature, spreads the heat over a larger mass and allows it to be dissipated by radiation.

For any tube, the amount of heat that can be dissipated is fixed. This means that the joules of heat energy that can be absorbed by the anode of a given tube over a given time period are also fixed. Since the energy absorbed by the anode is proportional to the product of the anode voltage V_A, the beam current I_B and the exposure time T_D, a set of curves called the X-ray tube rating chart must be consulted to find the maximum exposure time for a given tube V_A or I_B. An example curve is given in Fig. 12.11 for a hypothetical tube.

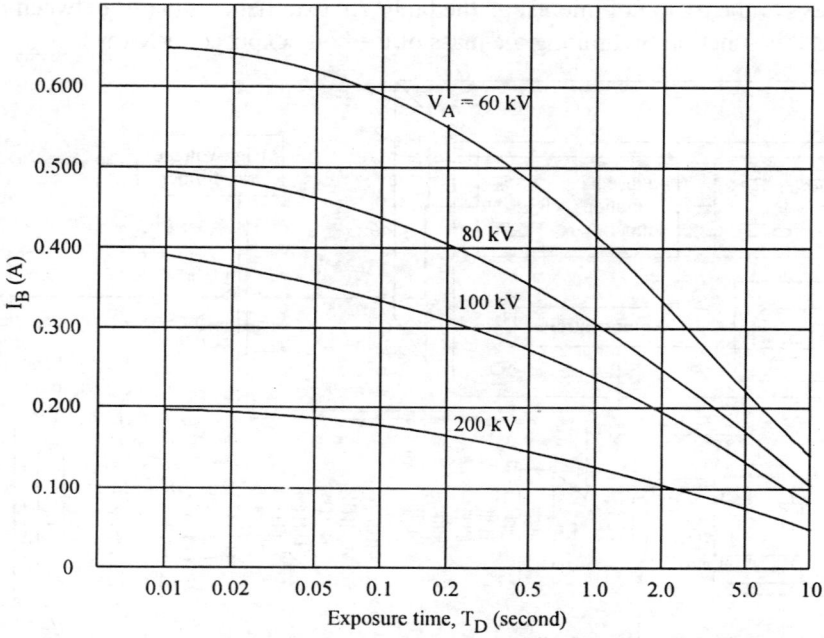

Fig. 12.11. The tube exposure time limit at given current and anode voltage levels.

The efficiency, η, of the X-ray tube is equal to the ratio of the power emitted in the X-ray beam to the power in the electron beam producing X-rays. That is, the power of the X-ray beam, P_X, is proportional to V_A^2. Also, large values of both I_B and the atomic number of the material, Z, increase the probability of a collision of the beam electron with an atom of the anode material. Therefore, the power, P_X, in the X-ray beam is proportional to all of these factors, as

$$P_X = kI_B Z V_A^2$$

where k is a proportionality constant. The power in the electron beam is just $V_A I_B$. The tube efficiency, η, is defined as the ratio of P_X to the power in the electron beam. Therefore

$$\eta = \frac{kI_B Z V_A^2}{I_B V_A} \qquad \qquad \text{... (12.9)}$$

$$= kZV_A$$

Empirically the constant k is determined to be k = 1.4×10^{-9}, in units of V^{-1}.

The anode is bevelled, as shown in Fig. 12.5. The bevel directs the X-rays out the side of the tube. The desired X-rays pass through a slot into a collimator arranged as shown in Fig. 12.10. Some of the X-rays from the anode scatter about in the tube and are absorbed by lead shielding.

Collimator

In order to reduce the dose of X-rays to the patient, the beam should not strike any more of the body than necessary. The necessary shaping of the X-ray beam is done with a collimator, as illustrated in Fig. 12.12. The shutters consist of a heavy metal to absorb unwanted X-rays. A lamp and reflective mirror that make a visible pattern on the patient, so that the attendant can tell where the X-rays will strike, can be used to align the beam.

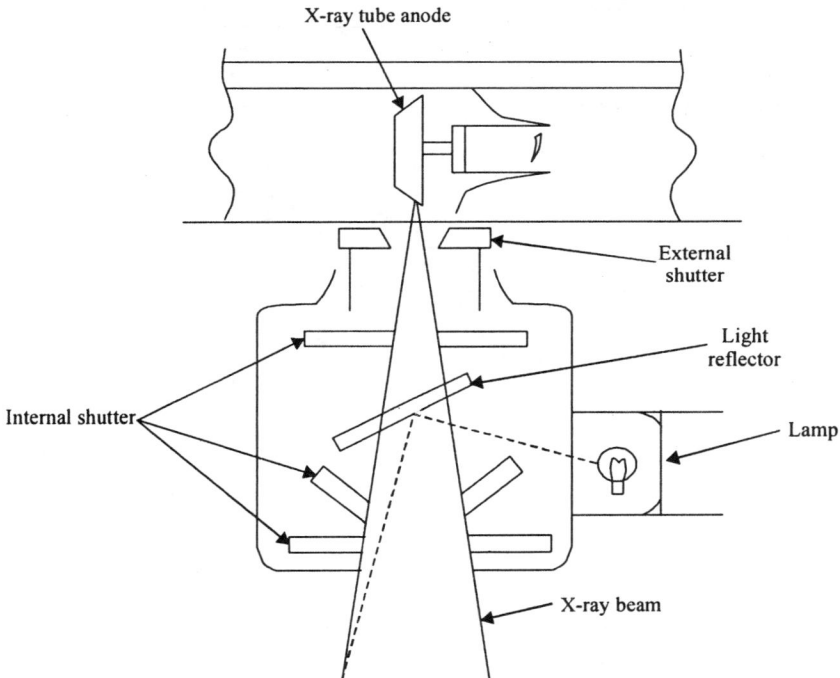

Fig. 12.12. A collimator for directing X-rays at the patient.

Bucky Grid

After X-rays enter a patient, some rays are deflected off their straight-line course by close encounters with atoms. This is called scattering and it causes a smearing of the image at the edges and deteriorates image sharpness. The sharpness of the image is recovered by use of a Bucky grid, illustrated in Fig. 12.13. Here slots are arranged in lead so that rays travelling in straight lines from the X-ray tube through the patient will strike the film whereas scattered radiation will strike the lead lining the slots and be absorbed. Since some X-rays are lost by this process, the density of the image will be diminished and slots themselves will block some of the film and reduce the image resolution. The Bucky grid is part of the vertical Bucky stand illustrated in Fig. 12.14.

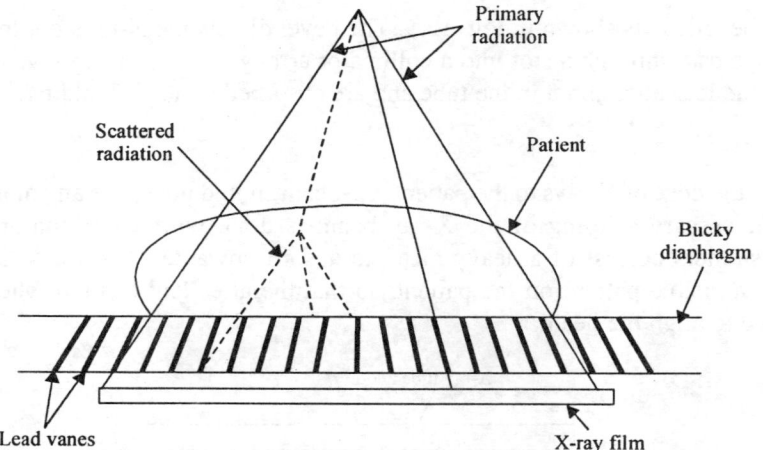

Fig. 12.13. A Bucky grid for reducing the effects of X-ray scattering in the patient.

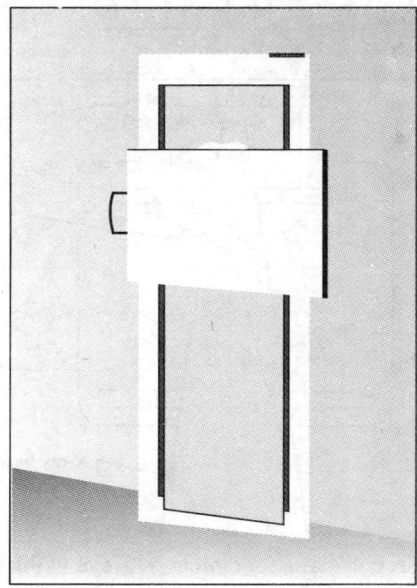

Fig. 12.14. A vertical Bucky stand for patient-erect radiographic studies of the chest.

X-Ray Detector

The X-rays now pass into a film sensitive to both X-rays and light, such as silver bromide. Since the film is relatively insensitive to X-ray, a phosphor coating, such as shown in Fig. 12.15, is used to produce light when hit by X-rays. The amount of X-rays captured is increased by placing a material with a high atomic number, called a Hi-Z screen above the phosphor. This introduces secondary radiation by the scattering process. Although this scattering would tend to decrease the image sharpness, the effect is minimal because the high-Z screen is immediately adjacent to the phosphor and the deflected X-rays travel only a small distance.

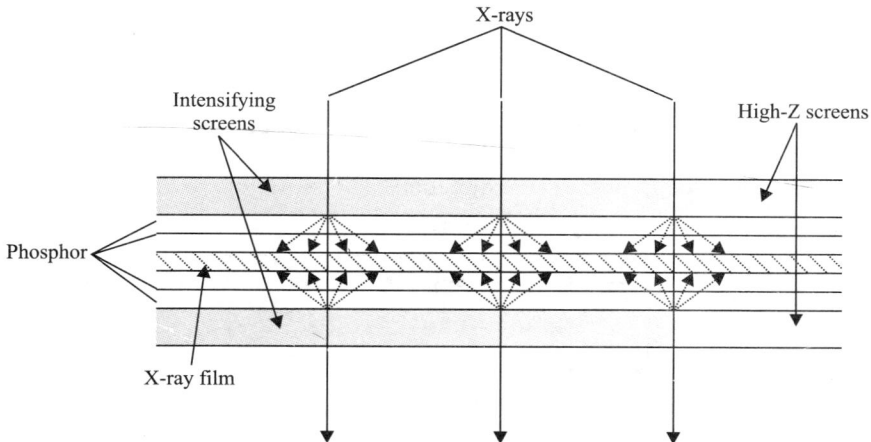

Fig. 12.15. An image-intensifying film.

A special-purpose X-ray machine for radiographic studies of the female breast, called a mammograph. The patient stands to the left of the shield and the attendant stands behind it to operate the controls.

Power Supply

The power supply for an X-ray machine plays a crucial and active role in X-ray production. The radiation is turned on and off in the power supply. It is used to control the X-ray energy and consequently the image contrast, as well as the beam current and consequently the image density. Thermal overload from the X-ray tube anode creates signals that turn the power supply off as appropriate. The power supply must be large to handle several kilowatts of power and several hundred kilovolt levels. At such high voltages, safety precautions are necessary. The voltage breakdown of air at sea level is 75 kV/inch. Therefore, at X-ray voltages, a conductor, such as a technician's hand, within several inches of a high-voltage terminal can draw a deadly arc of voltage. As a safety precaution when working on X-ray power supplies, a technician should turn off all power supplies, if possible and the capacitors should be discharged before components are touched.

A simplified X-ray block diagram for a single-phase power supply is shown in Fig. 12.16. The kV to the X-ray tube are controlled by adjusting N_2 on the low-voltage autotransformer varactor T_A. The low voltage prevents arcing of the transformer wiper arm. High voltage of about 100 kV is then produced by a fixed high-voltage transformer, T_H. The filament heater is controlled by a step-down transformer T_F. Adjusting the turns ratio N_6 sets the mA, beam current, of the X-ray tube by increasing the heat to the filament and boiling off more electrons for the thermally limited current.

Considering the transformers T_A, T_F and T_H to be ideal, the following voltage relationships hold:

$$V_2 = \frac{N_2}{N_1} V_1$$

$$V_3 = \frac{N_3}{N_1} V_1$$

$$V_5 = \frac{N_7}{N_6} V_3$$

$$V_4 = \frac{N_5}{N_4} V_2$$

The full-wave rectifier in Fig. 12.16 has diodes 2 and 4 conducting when the voltage drop V_4 is positive, producing a positive tube current I_B. When V_4 is negative, diodes 1 and 3 conduct and the others are off, again producing I_B in the same direction.

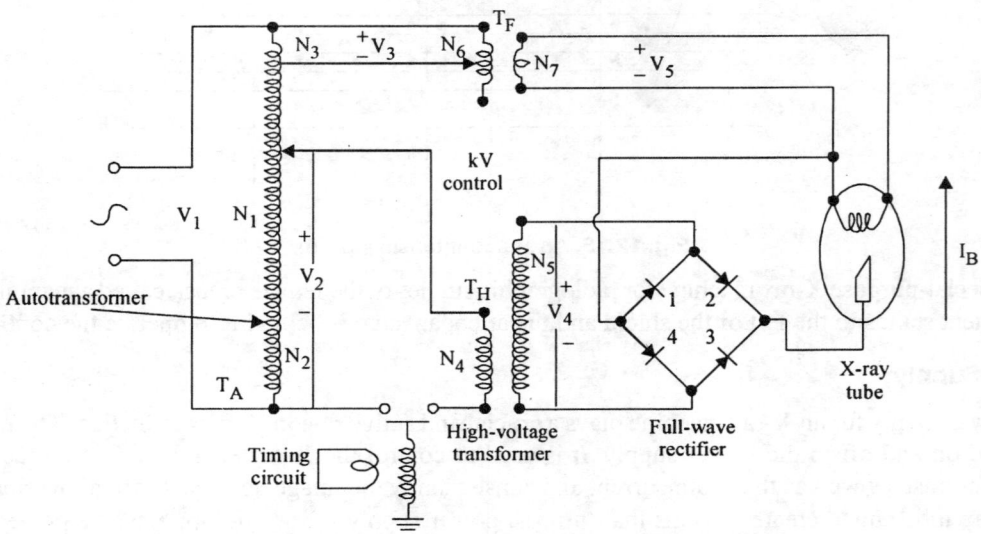

Fig. 12.16. A single-phase high-voltage power supply.

The single-phase power supply described above is limited in its efficient power-handling capability. High-power equipment often uses a three-phase power source. The crucial change in the power supply for three phases is in the high-voltage transformer, illustrated in Fig. 12.17. In a three-phase voltage system, V_{AB}, V_{BC} an V_{CA} are the same magnitude and are displaced in phase by 120° from each other, as illustrated in the Fig. 12.17. The current I_B is always in the same positive direction and is determined at any instant in time by the voltage V_{AB}, V_{BC} or V_{CA}, whichever has the highest absolute value. To verify that I_B is always positive, you may trace the current through the circuit and verify the following table:

Voltage polarity		Diodes on
V_{AB}	Positive	2, 3
	Negative	1, 4
V_{BC}	Positive	4, 5
	Negative	3, 6
V_{CA}	Positive	1, 6
	Negative	2, 5

For example, when V_{AB} is positive, diodes 2 and 3 conduct, provided also that V_{AB} is greater than both V_{BC} and V_{CA} at the instant considered.

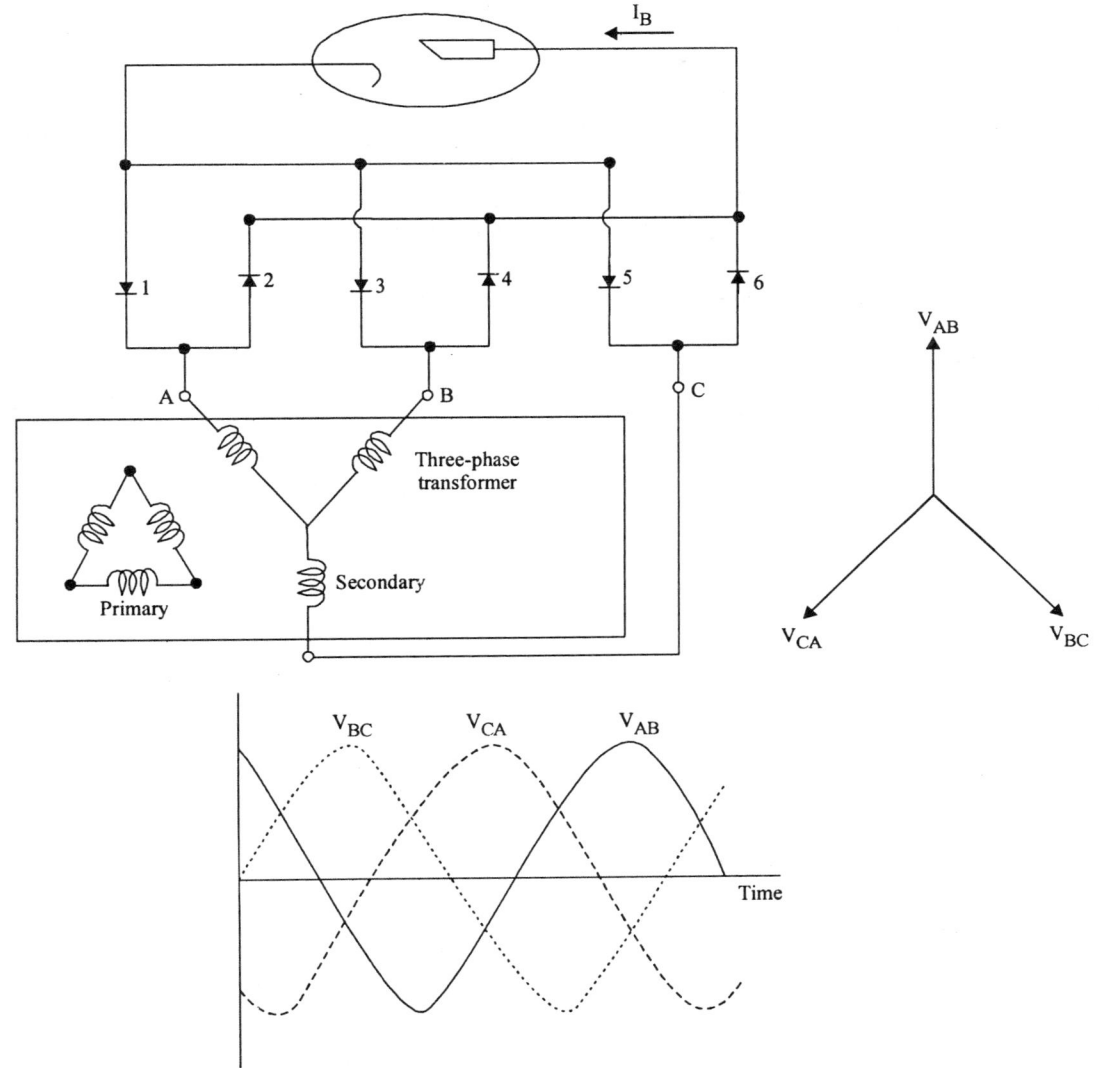

Fig. 12.17. A three-phase X-ray tube power supply.

FLUOROSCOPIC SYSTEM

In various medical procedures, physicians view an X-ray image instantly so they can monitor movements of organs and other objects put into the body. In a cardiac catheterisation procedure, the physician may wish to watch the catheter as it is moved through the veins into the heart ventricle. Or when a kidney stone is being pulverised with ultrasonic waves, it may be monitored using X-rays. Such instantaneous fluoroscopic pictures are called realtime images, such as we see on live television broadcasts.

The basic components of the fluoroscopic unit are the X-ray tube, fed by a high-voltage supply and control unit under the table. The patient is placed on the table top. A lead shield protects the operator from radiation. An image intensifier amplifies the image and converts the X-ray into light. A television camera then picks up the image and transfers it to the television monitor for viewing by the radiologist or operator. A block diagram of a typical digital fluoroscopic system appears in Fig. 12.18. In this system, information about the image density is fed to an automatic exposure control so that if the image begins to fade, the beam current on the X-ray tube will automatically increase.

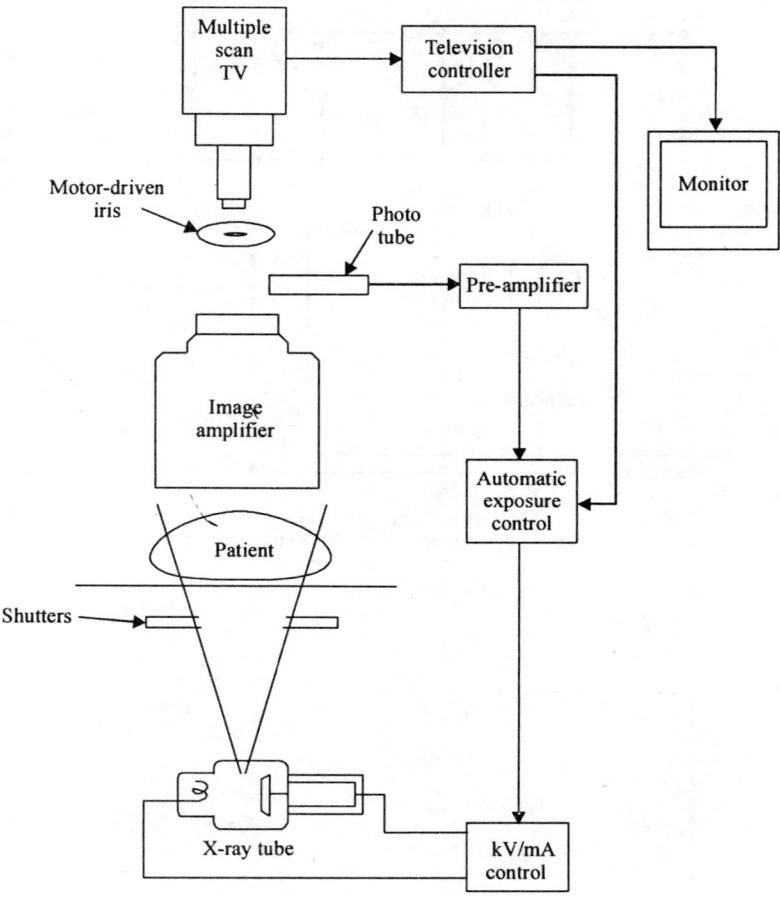

Fig. 12.18. A typical digital fluoroscopic system.

The unique component of a fluoroscopic system is the image intensifier, shown in Fig. 12.19. The X-rays strike a fluorescent screen, producing light. The light then strikes the photocathode, which produces electrons. The electrons are accelerated by a 25 kV potential and are focused on the fluorescent screen, which produces increased light and a denser image. This light image can then be photographed or picked up with a television camera. The fluorescent screens consist of many 2–3 μm phosphor crystals that emit light when bombarded by high-energy particles.

For example, a medium-short persistence of blue colour is produced by ZnS:Ag(Ni) crystals. If light photons with sufficient energy strike a photocathode, electrons are emitted, known as photoelectrons. Common photocathode materials consist of alloys of cesium and tin.

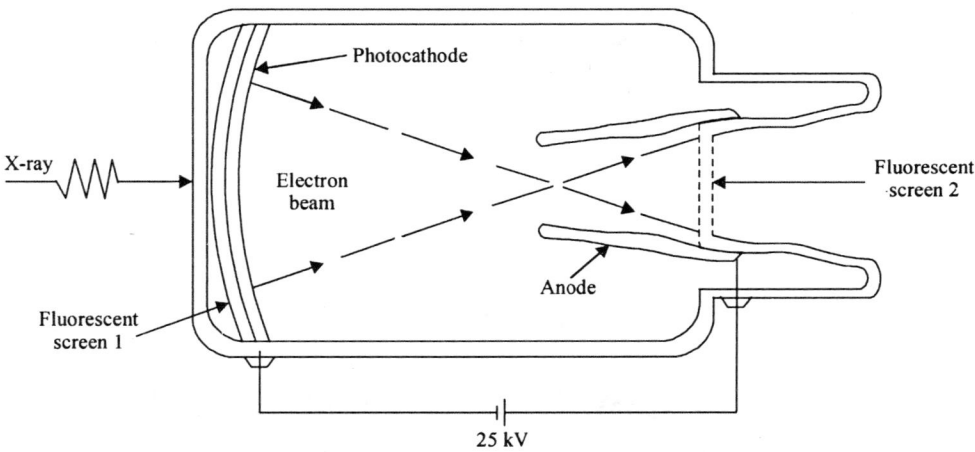

Fig. 12.19. An image intensifier.

Chapter 13

X-ray Computed Tomography

INTRODUCTION

The invention of the computer tomography (CT) scanner was made possible by a previously established mathematical insight and by the development of the dedicated minicomputer. The mathematical basis for producing an image of the cross-section of the body is that if one measures the total attenuation along rows and columns of a matrix, one can compute the attenuation of the matrix elements at the intersections of the rows and columns. The number of mathematical operations necessary to yield clinically applicable and accurate images is so large that a computer is essential to do them. This is the main reason why the CT scanner is a primary example of a medical instrument for which the computer is an indispensable component.

Figure 13.1 illustrates the block diagram of a typical CT scanner. The timing, anode voltage kV and beam current mA are controlled by a dedicated microcomputer through a control bus. The high-voltage DC power supply drives an X-ray tube that can be mechanically rotated along the circumference of a gantry. The X-rays pass through the patient, who is lying in a tube through the center of the gantry and impinge upon several of as many as 1000 detectors fixed in place around the circumference of the gantry. The microcomputer senses the position of the tube and samples the output of the detector along a diameter line opposite the tube. A calculation based on data from a complete scan of the tube is made by the computer. The output unit then produces a visual image of a transverse plane cross-section of the patient. The output may then be displayed on a cathode-ray tube and/or photographed with a camera to produce a hard-copy record.

CT SCANNERS AND DETECTORS

The detectors may consist of ionisation chambers, filled with a gas such as xenon, sealed at both ends and having two conductors forming a capacitor on the sides. A high DC voltage is applied to the capacitor. An X-ray entering the chamber ionises a xenon atom, causing it to migrate to the capacitor plate and causing a current in the high-voltage lead. This current is proportional to the radiation and is fed to the computer as data for computing the image.

A simplified example calculation called back projection reconstruction will now be presented in order to illustrate how the attenuation values along the surface of a transverse slice can be computed from knowledge of externally measured attenuation factors. A detailed rationale for the steps is not presented, but the specific illustration demonstrates the manner of analysis involved in the calculations.

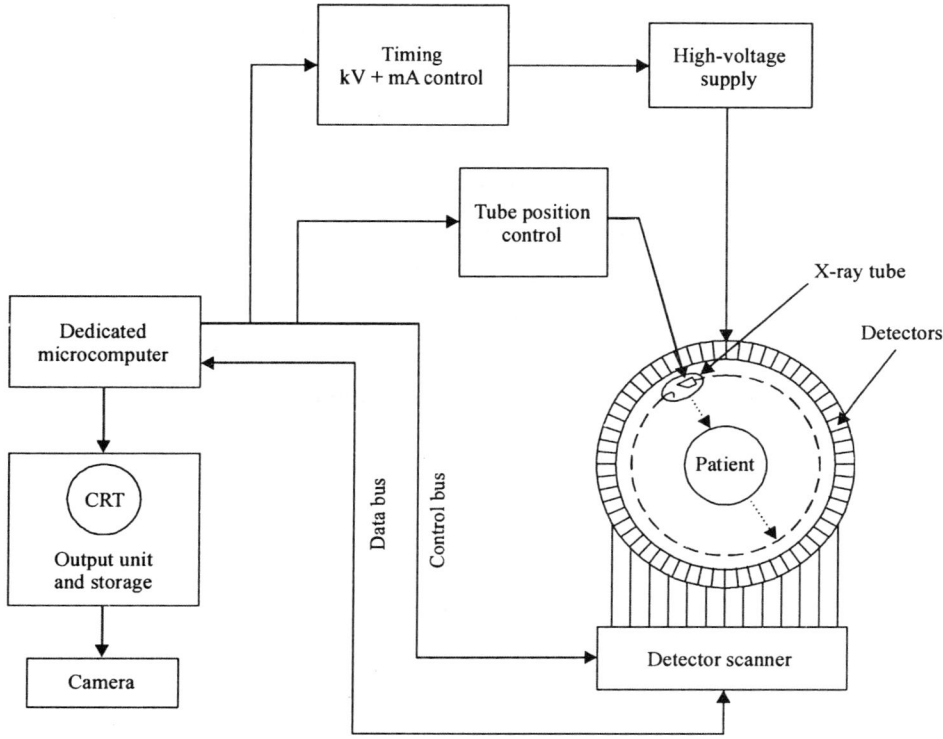

F!g. 13.1. A block diagram for a CT scanner.

Suppose the actual attenuation values, normalised to zero, are

$$\begin{bmatrix} 0 & 2 \\ 3 & 4 \end{bmatrix}$$

Each number in the matrix represents the attenuation of the space where it is located. For example, here the '2' is a measure of the attenuation in the upper right-hand corner of the matrix. The attenuation values are measured from the outside as those seen along the rows, 2 and 7. Using these as the first estimate, we have attenuation numbers

$$\begin{bmatrix} 2 & 2 \\ 7 & 7 \end{bmatrix}$$

1st estimate

The second estimate is obtained from the values measured along the columns, giving the sums, 3 and 6:

$$\begin{bmatrix} 3 & 6 \\ 3 & 6 \end{bmatrix}$$

Adding this to the first estimate yields a second estimate:

$$\begin{bmatrix} 5 & 8 \\ 10 & 13 \end{bmatrix}$$

2nd estimate

A third estimate results from values measured along the northeast diagonal:

$$\begin{bmatrix} 0 & 5 \\ 5 & 4 \end{bmatrix}$$

Adding this to the second estimate yields a third estimate:

$$\begin{bmatrix} 5 & 13 \\ 15 & 17 \end{bmatrix}$$

3rd estimate

The fourth estimate results from measurements of total attenuation along the north-west diagonal:

$$\begin{bmatrix} 4 & 2 \\ 3 & 4 \end{bmatrix}$$

Adding this to the third estimate gives

$$\begin{bmatrix} 9 & 15 \\ 18 & 21 \end{bmatrix}$$

4th estimate

Now we normalise this to zero by subtracting 9 from each element:

$$\begin{bmatrix} 0 & 6 \\ 9 & 12 \end{bmatrix}$$

Then we divide by 3 to yield

$$\begin{bmatrix} 0 & 2 \\ 3 & 4 \end{bmatrix}$$

Final image

The final matrix is the same as the first one. The numbers in the matrix correspond to the attenuations of locations on a tissue slice, having the same spatial relationship as the matrix numbers.

Thus the final image has the same attenuation values as the actual transverse slice, but the values were obtained from external measurements of attenuation alone. The CT scan X-ray is used to measure these values externally; the computer finds the matrix values. The illustration is for a 2 × 2 matrix that could be done by hand. The computer is needed to calculate larger, more accurate matrices.

Advanced models of the CT scanner create images at an angle other than 90° to the body axis. These reconstructed image is displayed as a two-dimensional matrix, with each pixel corresponding to the CT number of the tissue at that spatial location.

Scanner Instrumentation

Several components of the CT system such as the X-ray source, collimator and antiscatter grid are very similar to the instrumentation described previously for planar X-ray radiography. Over the past 30 years single-slice CT scanners have developed from systems with a single source and single detector, which took many minutes to acquire an image, to single-source, multiple-detector instruments, which can acquire an image in 1 second or less. Multislice systems have also been developed. The principles of data acquisition and processing for CT can be appreciated by considering the development from the earliest, so-called 'first-generation scanners' to the third and fourth-generation systems found in most hospitals today. A schematic of the basic operation of a first-generation scanner is shown in Fig. 13.2.

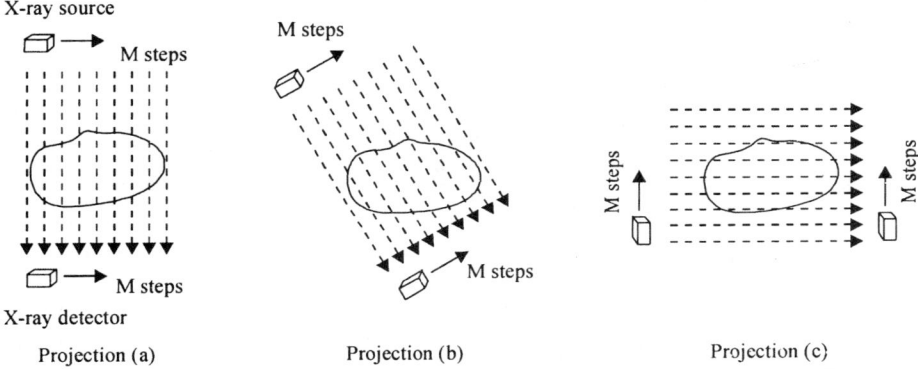

Fig. 13.2. The mode of operation of a first-generation CT scanner. The source and the detector move in a series of linear steps and then both are rotated and the process repeated. Typically, the number of projections and the number M of steps in each projection are equal in value.

Motion of the X-ray source and the detector occurred in two ways, linear and rotational. In Fig. 13.2, M linear steps were taken with the intensity of the transmitted X-rays being detected at each step. This produced a single projection with M data points. Then both the source and detector were rotated by (180/N) degrees, where N is the number of rotations in the complete scan and a further M translational lines were acquired at this angle. The total data matrix acquired was therefore M × N points. The spatial resolution could be increased by using finer translational steps and angular increments, up to a limiting value dictated by the effective X-ray focal spot size, but this resulted in a longer imaging time. Collimation of the X-ray beam gave a certain beam width in the axis perpendicular to the axis of rotation and this determined the thickness of the slice. Typical data matrix sizes were 180 × 180 and scanning times were 4–5 minutes. Image reconstruction algorithms were based upon back-projection. In second-generation scanners, instead of the single beam used in the first-generation scanners, a thin 'fan beam' of X-rays was produced from the source and multiple X-ray detectors were used rather than a single one. The major advantage of the second-generation scanner, shown in Fig. 13.3, was the reduction in total scanning time, which, for example, made abdominal imaging feasible within a single breath-hold. Image reconstruction required the development of 'fan-beam' back-projection reconstruction algorithms.

Third-generation scanners, also shown in Fig. 13.3, use a much wider X-ray fan beam and a sharply increased number of detectors, typically between 512 and 768, compared to the second-generation systems. Two separate collimators are used in front of the source. The first collimator restricts the beam to an angular width of roughly 45°. The second collimator, placed perpendicular to the first, restricts the beam to the desired slice thickness, which is typically 1–5 mm. An intense pulse of X-rays is produced for a time period of 2 to 4 ms for each projection and the X-ray tube/detector unit rotates through 360°. The scanner usually operates at a kV_p of 140 kV, with filtration giving an effective X-ray energy of 70–80 keV and a tube current between 70 and 320 mA. The focal spot size is between 0.6 and 1.6 mm. Typical operating conditions are a rotation speed of once per second, a data matrix of either 512 × 512 or 1024 × 1024 and a spatial resolution of ~0.35 mm.

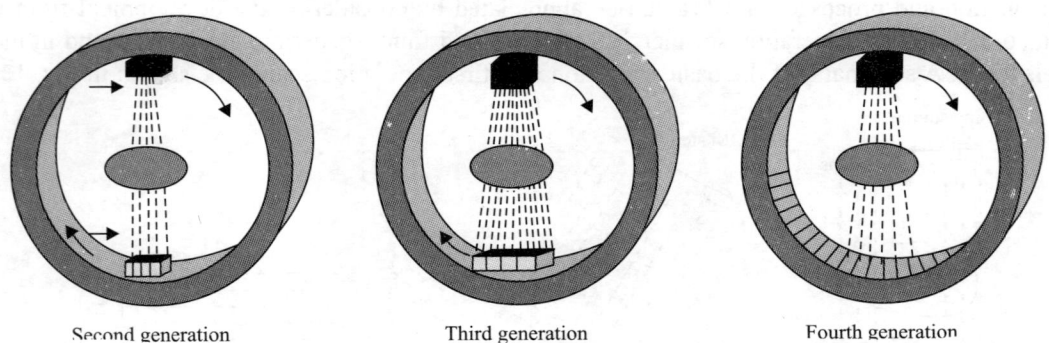

Second generation   Third generation   Fourth generation

Fig. 13.3. A schematic showing the development of second, third and fourth-generation CT scanners.

In the fourth-generation scanner a complete ring of detectors surrounds the patient. The X-ray tube rotates through 360° with a wide fan beam. There is no intrinsic decrease in scan time for fourth-generation with respect to third-generation scanners. In fact, the vast majority of scanners in hospitals are third generation.

Detectors for Computed Tomography

The most common detectors for CT scanners are xenon-filled ionisation chambers, shown in Fig. 13.4. Because xenon has a high atomic number of 66, there is a high probability of photoelectric interactions between the gas and the incoming X-rays. The xenon is kept under pressure at ~20 atmosphere to increase further the number of interactions between the X-rays and the gas molecules. An array of interlinked ionisation chambers, typically 768 in number (although some commercial scanners have up to 1000), is filled with gas, with metal electrodes separating the individual chambers. X-rays transmitted through the body ionise the gas in the detector producing electron-ion pairs. These are attracted to the electrodes by an applied voltage difference between the electrodes and produce a current which is proportional to the number of incident X-rays. Each detector electrode is connected to a separate amplifier and the outputs of the amplifiers are multiplexed through a switch to a single A/D converter. The digitised signals are logarithmically amplified and stored for subsequent image reconstruction. In this design of the ionisation chamber, the metal electrode plates also perform the role of an antiscatter grid, with the plates being angled to align with the focal spot of the X-ray tube. The plates are typically 10 cm in length, with a gap of 1 mm between adjacent plates.

IMAGE PROCESSING FOR COMPUTED TOMOGRAPHY

Image reconstruction takes place in parallel with data acquisition in order to minimise the delay between the end of data acquisition and the display of the images on the operator's console. As the signals corresponding to one projection are being acquired, those from the previous projection are being amplified and digitised and those from the projection previous to that are being filtered and processed.

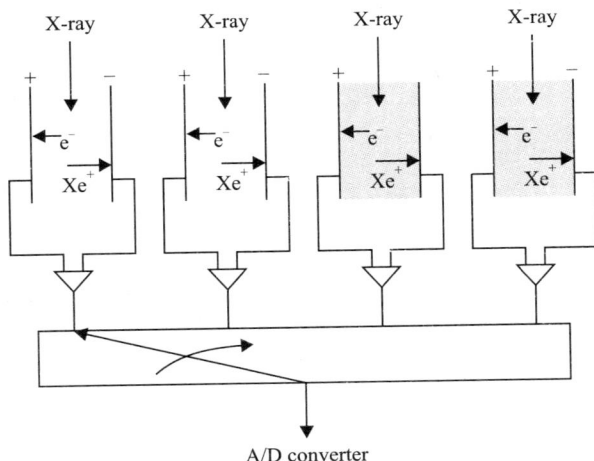

Fig. 13.4. A schematic of the Xe-filled detectors used in computed tomography and the switched connections between multiple detectors and a single analog-to-digital converter.

In order to illustrate the issues involved in image reconstruction, consider the raw projection data that would be acquired from a simple object such as an ellipse with a uniform attenuation coefficient, as shown in Fig. 13.5. The reconstruction goal is illustrated on the right of Fig. 13.5 for a simple 2×2 matrix of tissue attenuation coefficients: given a series of intensities I_1, I_2, I_3, I_4, what are the values of the attenuation coefficients $\mu_1, \mu_2, \mu_3, \mu_4$?

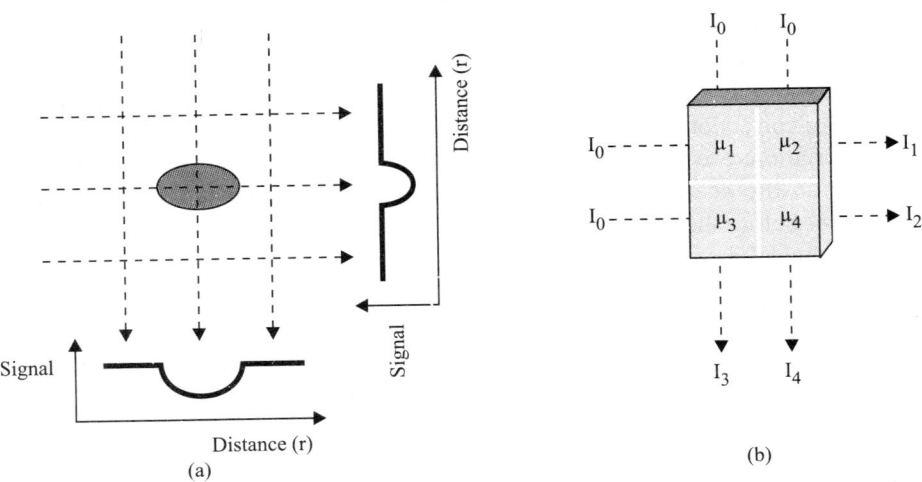

Fig. 13.5. (a) Two projections acquired from an elliptical test object. (b) Two projections acquired from an object consisting of a simple 2×2 matrix of tissue attenuation coefficients.

For each projection, the signal intensity recorded by each detector depends upon the attenuation coefficient and the thickness of each tissue that lies between the X-ray source and that particular detector. For the simple case shown on the right of Fig. 13.5, two projections are acquired, each consisting of two data points: projection 1 (I_1 and I_2) and projection 2 (I_3 and I_4). If the image to be reconstructed is also a two-by-two matrix, then the intensities of the projections can be expressed in terms of the linear attenuation coefficients by:

$$I_1 = I_0 e^{-(\mu_1 + \mu_2)x}$$

$$I_2 = I_0 e^{-(\mu_3 + \mu_4)x}$$

$$I_3 = I_0 e^{-(\mu_1 + \mu_3)x}$$

$$I_4 = I_0 e^{-(\mu_2 + \mu_4)x} \qquad \qquad \text{... (13.1)}$$

where x is the dimension of each pixel. It might seem that this problem could be solved by matrix inversion or similar techniques. These approaches are not feasible, however, first due to the presence of noise in the projections (high noise levels can cause direct inversion techniques to become unstable) and second because of the large amount of data collected. If the data matrix size is, for example, 1024 × 1024, then matrix inversion techniques become very slow. Image reconstruction, in practice, is carried out using either back-projection algorithms or iterative techniques, both of which are covered in the following sections.

Pre-processing Data Corrections

Image reconstruction is preceded by a series of corrections to the acquired projections. The first corrections are made for the effects of beam hardening, in which the effective energy of the X-ray beam increases as it passes through the patient due to greater attenuation of lower X-ray energies. This means that the effective linear attenuation coefficient of tissue decreases with distance from the X-ray source. If not corrected, beam hardening results in significant artifacts in the reconstructed images. Correction algorithms typically assume a uniform tissue attenuation coefficient and estimate the thickness of the tissue through which the X-rays have travelled for each projection. These algorithms work well for images containing mainly soft tissue, but can give problems in the presence of bone.

The second type of correction is for imbalances in the sensitivities of individual detectors and detector channels. If these variations are not corrected, then a ring or halo artifact can appear in the reconstructed images. Imbalances in the detectors are usually measured using an object with a spatially uniform attenuation coefficient before the actual patient study. The results from this calibration scan can then be used to correct the clinical data.

Radon Transform and Backprojection Techniques

The mathematical basis for reconstruction of an image from a series of projections is the Radon transform. For an arbitrary function f(x, y), its Radon transform R is defined as the integral of ρ(x, y) along a line L, as shown in Fig. 13.6:

$$R\{f(x, y)\} = \int_L f(x, y)\, dl \qquad \qquad \text{... (13.2)}$$

Each X-ray projection p(r, φ) can therefore be expressed in terms of the Radon transform of the object being studied:

$$p(r, \phi) = R\{f(x, y)\} \qquad \qquad \text{... (13.3)}$$

where p(r, φ) refers to the projection data acquired as a function of r, the distance along the projection and φ, the rotation angle of the X-ray source and detector.

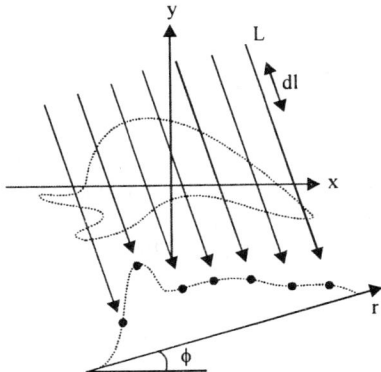

Fig. 13.6. A representation of the X-ray line integrals defining the Radon transform of an object.

Reconstruction of the image therefore requires computation of the inverse Radon transform of the acquired projection data. The most common methods of implementating the inverse Radon transform use backprojection or filtered backprojection algorithms.

After reconstruction, the image is displayed as a map of the tissue CT number, which is defined by

$$CT_0 = 1000 \frac{\mu_0 - \mu_{H_2O}}{\mu_{H_2O}} \qquad \qquad ...\ (13.4)$$

where CT_0 is the CT number and μ_0 is the linear attenuation coefficient of the tissue. The reconstructed image consists of CT numbers varying in value from +3000 to –1000. The image display screen typically has only 256 gray levels and thus some form of non-linear image windowing is used to display the image. Standard sets of contrast and window parameters exist for different types of scan.

Fan-Beam Reconstruction

The backprojection reconstruction methods outlined in Appendix B assume that each line integral corresponds to a parallel X-ray path from the source to detector. In third and fourth-generation scanners, the geometry of the X-rays is a fan beam, as shown previously in Fig. 13.3. Since the X-ray beams are no longer parallel to one another, image reconstruction requires modification of the backprojection algorithms to avoid introducing image artifacts. The simplest modification is to 'rebin' the acquired data to produce a series of parallel projections, which can then be processed as described previously. For example, in Fig. 13.7, the X-ray beam from source position S_1 to detector D_3 is clearly not parallel to the beam from S_1 to detector D_1. However, when the source is rotated to position S_2, for example, the X-ray beam from S_2 to D_3 is parallel to that from S_1 to D_1. By re-sorting the data into a series of composite datasets consisting of parallel X-ray paths, for example, S_1D_1, S_2D_3, etc., one can reconstruct the image using standard backprojection algorithms. Alternatively, filtered backprojection can be used directly on the fan-beam data, but each projection must be multiplied by the cosine of the fan beam angle and this angle is also incorporated into the convolution kernel for the filter.

Iterative Algorithms

An alternative approach to image reconstruction involves the use of iterative reconstruction algorithms. These algorithms start with an initial estimate of the two dimensional matrix of attenuation coefficients.

By comparing the projections predicted from this initial estimate with those that are actually acquired, changes are made to the estimated matrix. This process is repeated for each projection and then a number of times for the whole datasets until the residual error between the measured data and those from the estimated matrix falls below a pre-designated value. Iterative schemes are used relatively sparingly in standard CT scanning, where the SNR is sufficiently high for filtered backprojection algorithms to give good results. They are, however, used extensively in nuclear medicine tomographic techniques. There is a large number of methods for iterative reconstruction, most of which are based on highly complicated mathematical algorithms. One very simple illustrative method, called a ray-by-ray iteration method, is shown here.

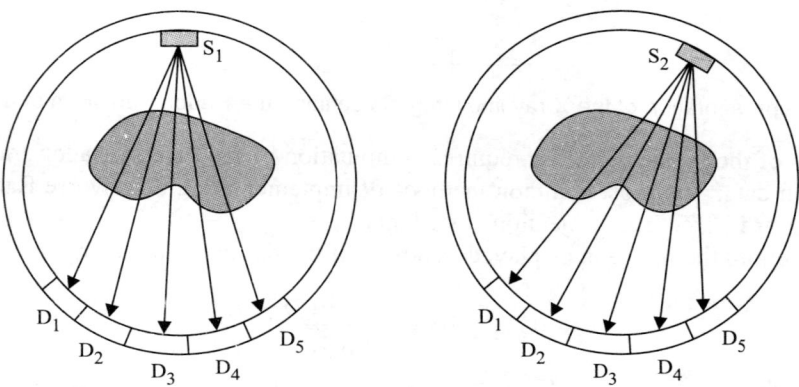

Fig. 13.7. Fan-beam projection data corresponding to two positions S_1 and S_2 of the X-ray source. By re-sorting the data from different positions of the source to produce composite data sets consisting of parallel X-ray beams, standard backprojection algorithms can be applied for image reconstruction.

Figure 13.8 shows two four-point projections from a two-dimensional matrix of tissue attenuation coefficients, μ_1–μ_{16}. In generating an initial estimate, the components of the horizontal projection, $0.2I_0$, $0.4I_0$, $0.3I_0$ and $0.1I_0$, are considered first (this choice is arbitrary). In the absence of prior knowledge, an initial estimate is formed by assuming that each pixel has the same X-ray attenuation coefficient. If the pixel dimensions are assumed to be square with height = length = 1 for simplicity, then the following equations can be written:

$$0.2I_0 = I_0 e^{-4\mu_A}, \quad \mu_A = \mu_1 = \mu_2 = \mu_3 = \mu_4$$

$$0.4I_0 = I_0 e^{-4\mu_B}, \quad \mu_B = \mu_5 = \mu_6 = \mu_7 = \mu_8$$

$$0.3I_0 = I_0 e^{-4\mu_C}, \quad \mu_C = \mu_9 = \mu_{10} = \mu_{11} = \mu_{12}$$

$$0.1I_0 = I_0 e^{-4\mu_D}, \quad \mu_D = \mu_{13} = \mu_{14} = \mu_{15} = \mu_{16} \qquad \text{... (13.5)}$$

This gives the first iteration of the estimated matrix, shown in Fig. 13.9. Clearly the individual data points of the vertical projection calculated from this iteration do not agree with the measured data, $0.4I_0$, $0.5I_0$, $0.1I_0$ and $0.3I_0$. The mean squared error (MSE) per pixel is calculated as:

$$\text{MSE / pixel} = \frac{1}{4} I_0[(0.4 - 0.22)^2 + (0.5 - 0.22)^2 + (0.1 - 0.22)^2 + (0.3 - 0.22)^2] \qquad \text{... (13.6)}$$

The value of the MSE per pixel after the first iteration is approximately $0.0325I_0$. The next iteration forces the estimated data to agree with the measured vertical projection. Consider the component that passes through pixels μ_1, μ_5, μ_9 and μ_{13}. The measured data is $0.4I_0$, but the calculated data using the first iteration is $0.22I_0$. The values of the attenuation coefficients have been overestimated and must be reduced. The exact amount by which the attenuation coefficients μ_1, μ_5, μ_9 and μ_{13} should be reduced is unknown and again the simple assumption is made that each value should be reduced by an equal amount. Applying this procedure to all four components of the horizontal projection gives the estimated matrix shown on the right of Fig. 13.9. Now, of course, the estimated projection data do not agree with the measured data of the horizontal projection but the MSE per pixel has been reduced to $0.005I_0$.

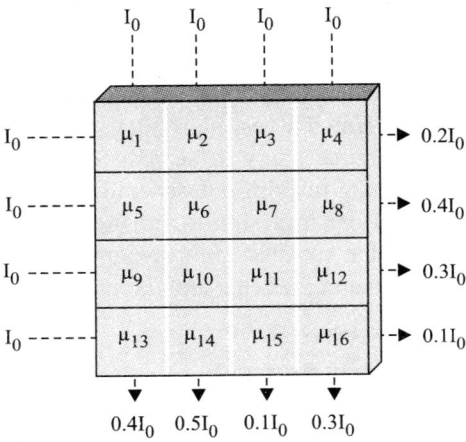

Fig. 13.8. The starting point for a ray-by-ray iterative reconstruction method. Two measured projections, each containing four data points, are shown. The aim is to use these data to estimate the values of $\mu_1 - \mu_{16}$.

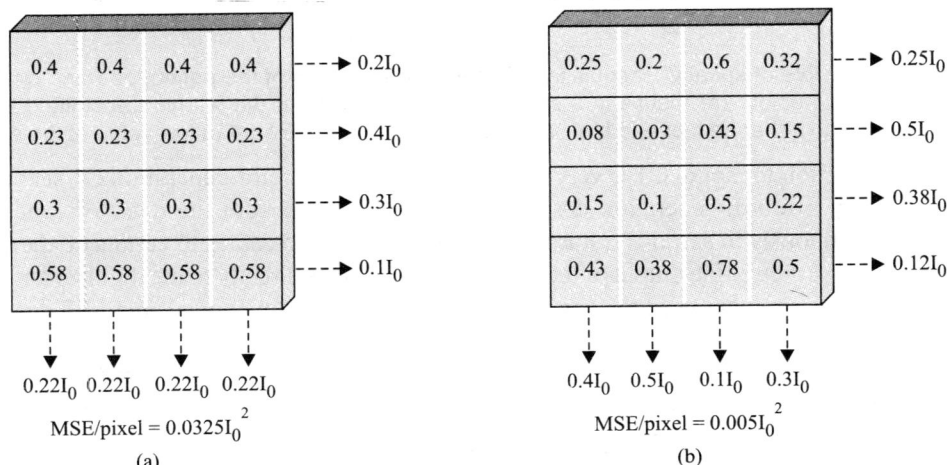

Fig. 13.9. (a) The results from the first-pass iterative reconstruction based on the horizontal projection; and (b) The second-pass iteration incorporating the measured data from the vertical projection.

In a practical realisation of a full ray-by-ray iterative reconstruction, many more projections would be acquired and processed. After a full iteration of all of the projections, the process can be repeated a number of times until the desired accuracy is reached or further iterations produce no significant improvements in the value of the MSE.

SPIRAL/HELICAL COMPUTED TOMOGRAPHY

In the conventional CT systems described thus far, only a single slice can be acquired at one time. If multiple slices are required to cover a larger volume of the body, the entire thorax, for example, then the patient table is moved in discrete steps through the plane of the X-ray source and detector. A single slice is acquired at each discrete table position, with an inevitable time delay between obtaining each image. This process is both time-inefficient and can result in spatial misregistrations between slices if the patient moves. In the early 1990s a technique called spiral or helical, CT was developed to overcome these problems by acquiring data as the table position is moved continuously through the scanner, as shown in Fig. 13.10. The trajectory of the X-ray beam through the patient traces out a spiral or helix: hence the name. This technique represented a very significant advance in CT because it allowed scan times for a complete chest and abdominal study to be reduced from ~10 minutes to ~1 minute. In addition, a full three-dimensional vascular imaging dataset could be acquired very shortly after injection of an iodinated contrast agent, resulting in a significant increase in the SNR of the angiograms. Incorporation of this new technology has resulted in three-dimensional CT angiography becoming the method of choice for diagnosing disease in the renal and the pulmonary arteries as well as the aorta.

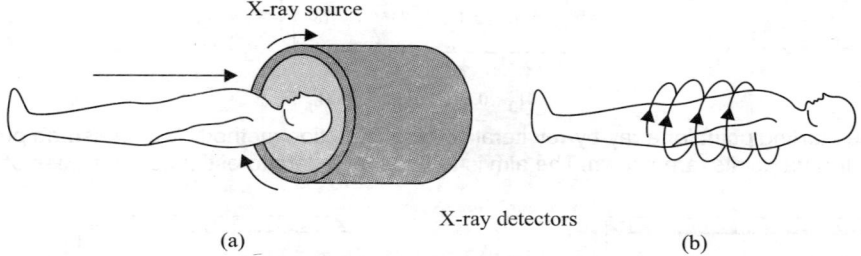

Fig. 13.10. The principle of spiral CT acquisition. Simultaneous motion of the patient bed and rotation of the X-ray source and detectors (a) results in a spiral trajectory; and (b) of the X-rays transmitted through the patient. The spiral can either be loose (a high value of the spiral pitch) or tight (a low value of the spiral pitch).

The instrumentation for spiral CT is very similar to conventional third-generation CT scanners (some companies employ a fourth-generation design). However, because both the detectors and the X-ray source rotate continuously in spiral CT, it is not possible to use fixed cables to connect either the power supply to the X-ray source or the output of the photomultiplier tubes directly to the digitiser and computer. Instead, multiple slip-rings are used for power and signal transmission. Typical spiral CT scanners have dual-focal spot X-ray tubes with three kV_p settings possible.

The main instrumental challenge in spiral CT scanning is that the X-rays must be produced continuously, without the cooling period that exists between acquisition of successive slices in conventional CT. This requirement leads to very high temperatures being formed at the focus of the electron beam at the surface of the anode. Anode heating is particularly problematic in abdominal scanning, which requires higher values of tube currents and exposures than for imaging other regions of the body. Therefore, the X-ray source must be designed to have a high heat capacity and very efficient cooling. If anode heating is too high, then the tube current must be reduced, resulting in a lower number of X-rays and a degraded image SNR. X-ray detector design is also critical in spiral CT because highly efficient detectors reduce the tube currents needed and help to alleviate issues of anode heating. The detectors used in spiral CT are either solid-state, ceramic scintillation crystals or pressurised xenon-filled ionisation chambers, described previously. Scintillation crystals, usually made from bismuth germanate (BGO), have a high efficiency (75–85 per cent) in converting X-rays to light and subsequently to electrical signals via coupled photomultiplier tubes. Gas-filled ionisation chambers have a lower efficiency (40–60 per cent), but are much easier and cheaper to construct. The total number of detectors is typically between 1000 (third-generation scanners) and 5000 (fourth-generation systems).

A number of data acquisition parameters are under operator control, the most important of which is the spiral pitch p. The spiral pitch is defined as the ratio of the table feed d per rotation of the X-ray source to the collimated slice thickness S:

$$p = \frac{d}{S} \qquad \dots (13.7)$$

The value of p lies between 0 and 2 for single-slice spiral CT system. For p values less than 1, the X-ray beams of adjacent spirals overlap, resulting in a high tissue radiation dose. For p values greater than 2, gaps appear in the data sampled along the long axis of the patient. For large values of p, image blurring due to the continuous motion of the patient table during data acquisition is greater. A large value of p also increases the effective slice thickness to a value above the width of the collimated X-ray beam: for example, at a spiral pitch value of 2, the increase is of the order of 25 per cent. The value of p typically used in clinical scans lies between 1 and 2, which results in a reduction in tissue radiation dose compared to a single-slice scan by a factor equal to the value of p.

Due to the spiral trajectory of the X-rays through the patient, modifications of the backprojection reconstruction algorithm is necessary in order to form images that correspond to those acquired using a single-slice CT scanner. Reconstruction algorithms use linear interpolation of data points 180° apart on the spiral trajectory to estimate the data that would have been obtained at a particular position of a stationary patient table. Images with thicknesses greater than the collimation width can be produced by adding together adjacent reconstructed slices. Images are usually processed in a way which results in considerable overlap between adjacent slices. This has been shown to increase the accuracy of lesion detection, for example, because with overlapping slices there is less chance that a significant portion of the lesion lies between slices.

MULTISLICE SPIRAL COMPUTED TOMOGRAPHY

The efficiency of spiral CT can be increased further by incorporating an array of detectors in the z direction that is, the direction of table motion. Such an array is shown in Fig. 13.11. The increase in efficiency arises from the higher values of the table feed per rotation that can be used. Multislice spiral CT can be used to image larger volumes in a given time or to image a given volume in a shorter scan time, compared to single-slice spiral CT. The collimated X-ray beam can also be made thinner, giving higher quality three-dimensional scans. The spiral pitch p_{ms} for a multislice CT is defined slightly differently from that for a single-slice CT system:

$$p_{ms} = \frac{d}{S_{single}} \qquad \dots (13.8)$$

where S_{single} is the single-slice collimated beam width. For a four-slice spiral CT scanner, the upper limit of the effective spiral pitch is increased to a value of eight. In multislice spiral CT scanning the effective slice thickness is dictated by the dimensions of the individual detectors, rather than the collimated X-ray beam width.

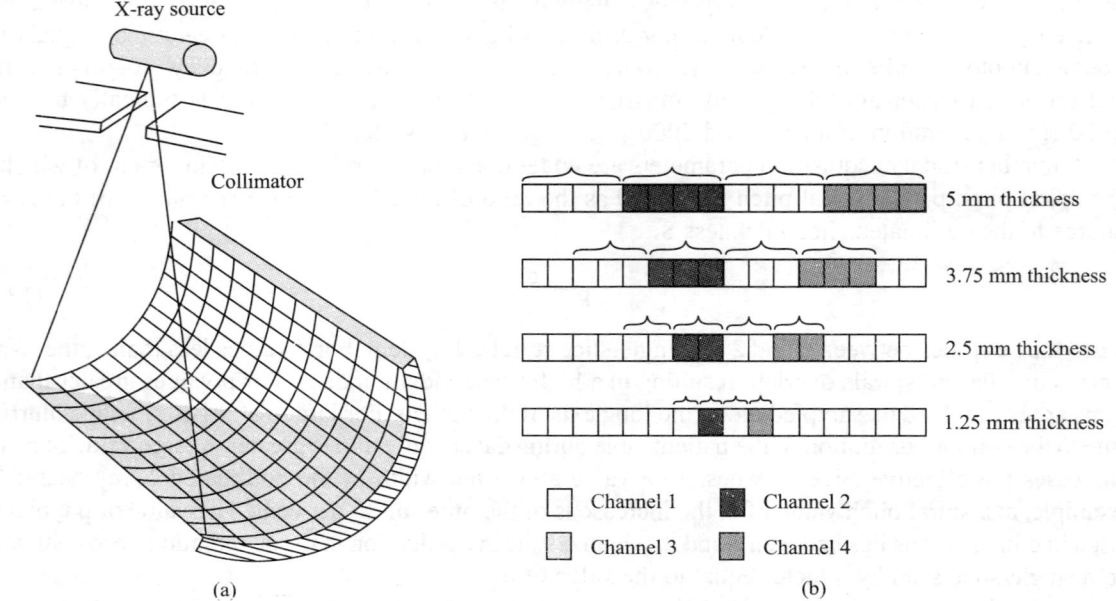

(a)   (b)

Fig. 13.11. (a) A schematic of a fixed-array detector geometry for a multislice spiral scanner; (b) Four configurations connecting the data acquisition channels to single or multiple elements of the arrayed detectors produce four different slice thicknesses. For 5 mm slices, the collimated beam shown in (a) covers all 16 detectors. The degree of collimation can be increased progressively to cover only the central 12 (four 3.75 mm slices), the central 8 (four 2.5 mm slices) or the central 4 (four 1.25 mm slices) detectors.

In a multislice system the focal-spot-to-isocentre and the focal-spot-to-detector distances are shortened compared to those in a single-slice scanner and the number of detectors in the longitudinal direction is increased from one long element to a number of shorter elements. There are two basic types of detector arrangements, called fixed and adaptive. The former consists of 16 elements, each of length 1.25 mm, giving a total length of 2 cm. The signals from sets of four individual elements are typically combined. With the set-up shown in Fig. 13.11, four slices can be acquired with thicknesses of 1.25, 2.5, 3.75 or 5 mm. These types of systems are typically run in either high-quality (HQ) mode with a spiral pitch of 3 or high-speed (HS) mode with a spiral pitch of 6. The second type of detector system is the adaptive array, which consists of eight detectors with lengths 5, 2.5, 1.5, 1, 1, 1.5, 2.5 and 5 mm, also giving a total length of 2 cm. As for the fixed detector system, four slices are usually acquired with 1, 2.5 or 5 mm thickness. Unlike the fixed detector system, in which only specific pitch values are possible, the pitch value in an adaptive array can be chosen to have any value between 1 and 8.

Fan-beam reconstruction techniques, in combination with linear interpolation methods, are used in multislice spiral CT. One important difference between single-slice and multislice spiral CT is that the slice thickness in multislice spiral CT can be chosen retrospectively after data acquisition, using an adaptive axial algorithm. The detector collimation is set to a value of 1, 2.5 or 5 mm before the scan is run. After the data have been acquired, the slices can be reconstructed with a thickness between 1 and 10 mm. Thin slices can be reconstructed to form a high-quality three-dimensional image, but the same dataset can also be used to produce a set of 5 mm thick images with a high SNR. In Fig. 13.12, the projections p_{ZR} acquired at every position z_R are averaged using a sliding filter $w(z)$ to give an interpolated set of projections p_{ZR}^{int} given by:

$$p_{ZR}^{int} = \frac{\sum_i w\,(Z_i - Z_R)\,p\,(z_i)}{\sum_i w\,(Z_i - Z_R)} \qquad \text{... (13.9)}$$

The width of the filter, which is usually trapezoidal in shape, determines the thickness of the reconstructed slice.

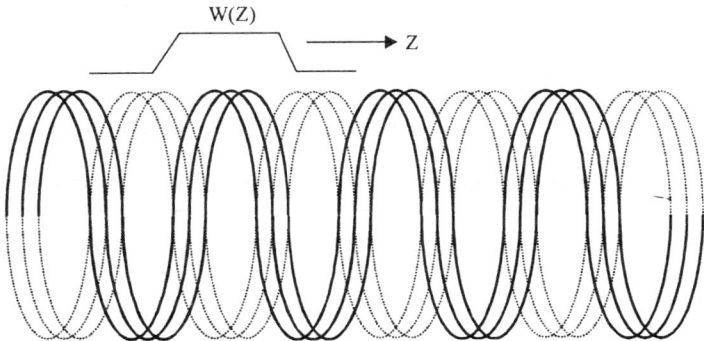

Fig. 13.12. The basic principle of data reconstruction using z-interpolation in multislice spiral CT. The solid lines show the acquired data and the dotted lines represent the rebinned data from opposite rays. The projections are averaged at each z position by weighting the projections by the filter w(z).

RADIATION DOSE

Ionising radiation can cause damage to tissue in a number of ways. The largest risk is that of cancer arising from genetic mutations caused by chromosomal aberrations. The effects of radiation are both deterministic and stochastic. Deterministic effects are produced by high doses and are associated with cell death. These effects are characterised by a dose threshold below which cell death does not occur. In contrast, stochastic effects occur at lower radiation doses, but the actual radiation dose affects only the probability of damage occurring, that is, there is no absolute dose threshold.

The absorbed dose D is equal to the radiation energy E absorbed per unit mass. The value of D is given in units of grays (Gy), where 1 Gy equals 1 J/kg. Many publications still refer to absorbed dose in units of rads: 1 Gy is equal to 100 rads. The patient dose is often specified in terms of the entrance skin dose, with typical values of 0.1 mGy for a chest radiography and 1.5 mGy for an abdominal radiograph. Such measurements, however, give little overall indication of the risk to the patient. The most useful measure of radiation dose is the effective dose equivalent H_E, which sums the dose delivered to each organ weighted by the radiation sensitivity w of that organ with respect to cancer and genetic risks:

$$H_E = \sum_i w_i H_i \qquad \text{... (13.10)}$$

where i is the number of organs considered and H_i is the dose equivalent for each of the i organs. The value of H is given by the absorbed dose D multiplied by the quality factor (QF) of the radiation. The QF has a value of 1 for X-rays (and also for γ-rays), 10 for neutrons and 20 for α-particles. The unit of H and H_E is the sievert (Sv). Older radiation literature quotes the units of dose equivalent and effective dose equivalent in units of rems: 1 Sv equals 100 rems. Typical values of w for the calculation of H_E are: gonads, 0.2; lung, 0.12; breast, 0.1; stomach, 0.12; skin, 0.01; and thyroid, 0.05.

In CT, the radiation dose to the patient is calculated in a slightly different way because the X-ray beam profile across each slice is not uniform and adjacent slices receive some dose from one another. For example, in the United States, the Food and Drug Administration (FDA) defines the computed tomography dose index (CTDI) for a 14 slice examinations to be:

$$\text{CTDI} = \frac{1}{T} \int_{-7T}^{+7T} D_z \ dz \qquad \qquad ... \ (13.11)$$

where D_z is the absorbed dose at position z and T is the thickness of the slice. In terms of assessing patient risk, again the value of H_E is a better measure. Table 13.1 lists typical values of H_E for standard clinical examinations. The limit in annual radiation dose under federal law in the United States is 0.05 Sv (5000 mrem). This limit corresponds to over 1000 planar chest X-rays, 15 head CTs or 5 full-body CTs.

Table 13.1. Effective dose equivalent H_E for clinical X-ray CT examinations.

Clinical examinations	H_E (mSv)
Breast	0.05
Chest X-ray	0.03
Skull X-ray	0.15
Abdominal X-ray	1.0
Barium fluoroscopy	5
Head CT	3
Body CT	10

CLINICAL APPLICATIONS OF COMPUTED TOMOGRAPHY

CT is used for a wide range of clinical conditions. The following list and series of images is by no means exhaustive. There are a large number of books devoted solely to the clinical applications of CT.

Cerebral Scans

One of the most important applications of CT is in head trauma, where it is used to investigate possible skull fractures, underlying brain damage or haemorrhage. Haemorrhage shows up on CT scans as areas of increased signal intensity due to higher attenuation from the high levels of protein in haemoglobin. Edema, often associated with stroke, shows up as an area of reduced signal intensity on the image. For brain tumors, CT is excellent at showing calcification in lesions such as meningiomas or gliomas and can be used to investigate changes in bone structure and volume in diseases of the sinus. Figure 13.13 shows an example of the sensitivity of CT, in this case able to detect a sub-acute infarct. In well-vascularised tumours such as meningiomas, iodinated contrast agents are often injected and increase the signal intensity of the tumor. In healthy brain tissue, the blood brain barrier (BBB) selectively filters the blood supply to the brain, allowing only a limited number of naturally occurring substrates to enter brain tissue. If the brain is damaged, by a tumor, for example, the BBB is disrupted such that the injected contrast agent can now enter the brain tissue. As tumors grow, they develop their own blood supply and blood flow is often higher in tumors, particularly in the periphery of the tumor, than in normal tissue. Abscesses, for example, often show a distinctive pattern in which the centre of the pathology appears with a lower signal than surrounding tissue, but is encircled by an area of higher signal, a so-called 'rim enhancement'.

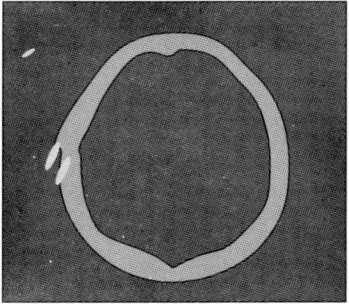

Fig. 13.13. CT image of a sub-acute infarct, which appears as a large area of low signal intensity on the left of the brain.

Pulmonary Disease

CT is particularly useful in the detection of pulmonary disease because lung imaging is extremely difficult using ultrasound and magnetic resonance imaging. CT can detect pulmonary malignancies as well as emboli and is often used to diagnose diffuse diseases of the lung such as silicosis, fibrosis and emphysema. Cystic fibrosis can also be diagnosed, as shown in Fig. 13.14.

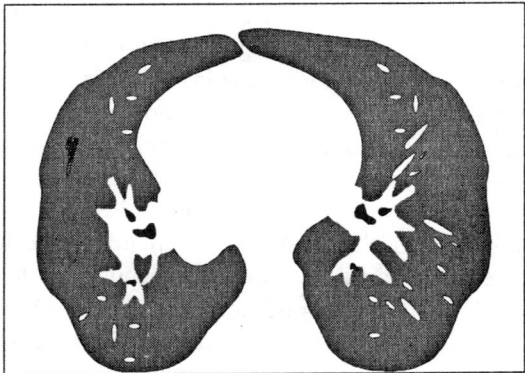

Fig. 13.14. CT image of a patient with cystic fibrosis. The disease can be diagnosed by the thickening of the airways and the presence of small, opaque areas filled with mucus.

Abdominal Imaging

Compound fractures in organs such as the pelvis, which occur commonly in elderly patients, can be visualised in three dimensions using CT. CT is also very useful in the detection of abdominal tumors and ulcerations in the liver. Most of these latter studies use an iodinated contrast agent. Pathologies such as hepatic hemangiomas can be detected by acquiring a series of images after injection of the agent: the outside of the hemangioma increases in signal intensity very soon after injection, but within 30 minutes there is uniform enhancement of the whole tumour.

Chapter 14

Nuclear Medical Imaging Systems

INTRODUCTION

In contrast to X-ray, ultrasound and magnetic resonance, nuclear medicine imaging techniques do not produce an anatomical map of the body, but instead image the spatial distribution of radiopharmaceuticals introduced into the body. The complementary role of nuclear medicine diagnoses arises from the fact that most pathological conditions are initiated by a change in the basic chemistry and biochemistry of tissue. In time, these chemical changes lead to deficiencies in organ function and changes in the physical properties of the tissue. Examples include cell swelling and the formation of edema, tumour enlargement and metastasis and changes in tissue morphology. Imaging techniques that are sensitive to these early biochemical changes form an important part of clinical diagnosis. Nuclear medicine detects these early indicators of disease by imaging the uptake and biodistribution of radioactive compounds introduced into the body in very small amounts (typically nanograms) via inhalation into the lungs, direct injection into the bloodstream, sub-cutaneous administration or oral administration. These 'radiopharmaceuticals', also termed radiotracers, are compounds consisting of a chemical substrate linked to a radioactive element. The chemical structure of the particular radiopharmaceutical determines the biodistribution of the complex within the body and a large number of radiopharmaceuticals are used clinically in order to target specific organs. Abnormal tissue distribution or an increase or decrease in the rate at which the radiopharmaceutical accumulates in a particular tissue is a strong indicator of disease. Radiation, usually in the form of γ-rays, from the radioactive decay of the radiopharmaceutical is detected using an imaging device called a gamma camera.

Figure 14.1 shows the basic principles and instrumentation involved in image formation. The radiopharmaceutical is shown in Fig. 14.1 to be localised in a specific organ in the body. Decay of the radioactive element produces γ-rays, which emanate in all directions. Attenuation of γ-rays in tissue occurs via exactly the same mechanisms as for X-rays, namely coherent scattering, Compton scattering and photoelectric interactions. In order to determine the position of the source of the γ-rays, a collimator is placed between the patient and the detector so that only those components of radiation that have a trajectory at an angle close to 90° to the detector plane are recorded. Rather than using film, as in planar X-ray imaging, to record the image, a scintillation crystal is used to convert the energy of the γ-rays that pass through the collimator into light. These light photons are in turn converted into an electrical signal

276

by photomultiplier tubes (PMTs). The image is formed by analysing the spatial distribution and the magnitude of the electrical signals from each PMT. Planar nuclear medicine images are characterised, in general, as having a poor SNR and low spatial resolution (~5 mm), but extremely high sensitivity, being able to detect very small amounts of radioactive material and very high specificity because there is no background radiation in the body.

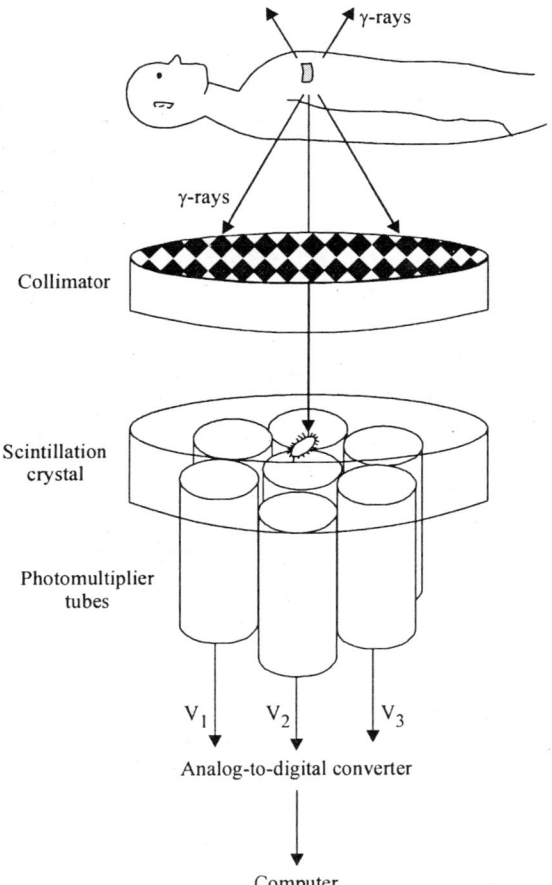

Fig. 14.1. A general schematic of the instrumentation required for the formation of nuclear medicine images using a gamma camera.

Three-dimensional nuclear medicine images can be produced using the principle of tomography. A rotating gamma camera is used in a technique called single photon emission computed tomography (SPECT). As in X-ray CT, the increase in image dimensionality increases the diagnostic power of the technique significantly. This is particularly true in cases where the radiopharmaceutical is distributed in more than one overlying organ. The most recently developed technique in nuclear medicine is positron emission tomography (PET), which is based on positron-emitting radiopharmaceuticals. Due to the nature of the processes involved in positron-emitting radiopharmaceuticals. Due to the nature of the processes involved in positron annihilation and subsequent emission of two γ-rays, PET has a sensitivity advantage over SPECT of between two and three orders of magnitude.

^{99m}Tc-based radiopharmaceuticals are listed in Table 14.1.

Table 14.1. ^{99m}Tc radiopharmaceuticals and corresponding clinical applications.

Radiopharmaceutical	Clinical application
^{99m}Tc-macroaggregated albumin	Pulmonary perfusion
^{99m}Tc-diphosphonate	Skeletal
^{99m}Tc-glucoheptonate	Brain tumours
^{99m}Tc-sulphur colloid	Liver and spleen, sentinel node location
^{99m}Tc-DTPA	Renal, pulmonary ventilation
^{99m}Tc-HMPAO	Brain perfusion
^{99m}Tc-Sestamibi	Myocardial perfusion
^{99m}Tc-MAG$_3$	Renal

INSTRUMENTATION: THE GAMMA CAMERA

The gamma camera, shown in Fig. 14.2, is the instrumental basis for all nuclear medicine imaging studies. The roles of each of the separate components are covered in the following sections.

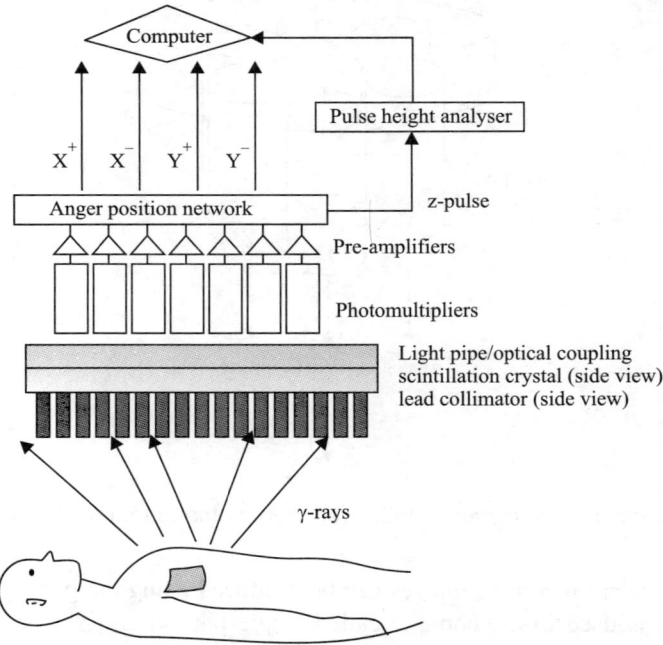

Fig. 14.2. Schematic diagram of a gamma camera positioned above the patient. The distribution of the radiopharmaceutical is indicated by the shaded region within the body.

Collimators

Many types of collimator are used in nuclear medicine, but the most common geometry is a parallel-hole collimator, which is designed such that only γ-rays travelling at angles close to 90° to the collimator surface are detected. The collimator thus reduces the contribution from γ-rays that have been Compton-scattered in tissue; these contain no useful spatial information and reduce the image CNR. The collimator is usually constructed from thin strips of lead, through which transmission of γ-rays is negligible. The normal pattern of the lead strips is a hexagonally based 'honeycomb' geometry, as shown in Fig. 14.3.

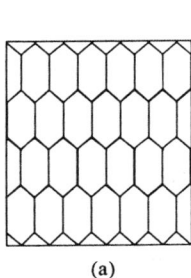

(a)

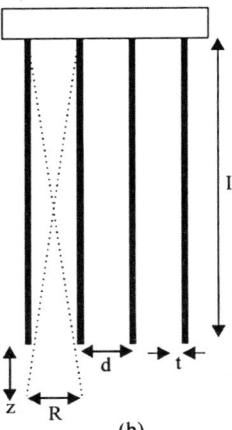

(b)

Fig. 14.3. (a) A top view of a hexagonal geometry lead collimator placed directly on the surface of the scintillation crystal. (b) A side view of the collimator and crystal: the values of L, t, d and z determine the closest separation R at which two sources of radioactivity can be resolved.

Scintillation Crystal and Coupled Photomultiplier Tubes

The most common γ-ray detector is based on a single crystal of thallium-activated sodium iodide, NaI(Tl). The thallium creates imperfections in the crystal structure of the NaI such that atoms within the crystal can be excited to elevated energy levels. When a γ-ray strikes the crystal, it loses energy through photoelectric and Compton interactions with the crystal. The electrons ejected by these interactions lose energy in a short distance by ionising and exciting the scintillation molecules. Deexcitation of these excited states within the scintillation crystal occurs via emission of photons with a wavelength of 415 nm (visible blue light), corresponding to a photon energy of ~4 eV. The intensity of the light is proportional to the energy of the incident γ-ray. The light emission decay constant, which is the time for the excited states to return to equilibrium, is 230 ns for NaI(Tl). This means that count rates of $10^4 - 10^5$ γ-rays per second can be recorded accurately. The linear attenuation coefficient of NaI(Tl) at 140 keV has a high value, 2.22 cm^{-1} and so 90 per cent of the γ-rays that strike the scintillation crystal are absorbed in a 1 cm thickness. Overall, approximately 13 per cent of the energy deposited in the crystal via γ-ray absorption is emitted as visible light. One disadvantage of the NaI(Tl) crystal is that it is hygroscopic and so must be hermetically sealed.

The choice of crystal thickness in nuclear medicine involves the same trade-off between spatial resolution and sensitivity for intensifying screens in X-ray imaging. When a γ-ray strikes the NaI(Tl) crystal, light is produced from a very small volume determined by the range, typically 1 mm, of the photoelectrons or Compton-scattered electrons. The thicker the crystal, the broader is the light spread function and the poorer is the spatial resolution. For obtaining ^{99m}Tc or ^{201}Tl nuclear medicine images, the optimal crystal thickness is approximately 0.6 cm. However, this value is too small for detecting, with high sensitivity, the higher energy γ-rays associated with radiopharmaceuticals containing gallium, iodine and indium and so a compromise crystal thickness of 1 cm is generally used in these cases.

The second step in forming the nuclear medicine image involves detection of the light photons emitted by the crystal by hexagonal PMTs, which are closely coupled to the scintillation crystal. This geometry gives efficient packing and also has the property that the distance from the centre of one PMT to that of each neighbouring PMT is the same: this property is important for determination of the spatial location of the scintillation event using an Anger position network. Arrays of 61, 75 or 91 PMTs, each with a diameter of between 25 and 30 mm, are typically used. The basic design of a PMT is shown in Fig. 14.4. Light photons pass through the transparent window of the PMT and strike the photocathode, which is made of a bialkali material with a spectral sensitivity matched to the light-emission characteristics of the scintillation crystal. Provided that the photon energy is greater than the photoelectric work function of the photocathode, free electrons are generated in the photocathode via photoelectric interactions. These electrons have energies between 0.1 and 1 eV. A bias voltage of between 300 and 5000 V applied between the first anode (also called a dynode) and the photocathode attracts these electrons toward the anode. If the kinetic energy of this incident electron is above a certain value, typically 100–200 eV, when it strikes the anode a large number of electrons are emitted from the anode for every incident electron: the result is effectively noise-free amplification. A series of 10 successive accelerating dynodes produces between 10^5 and 10^6 electrons for each photoelectron, creating an amplified current at the output of the PMTs. This current then passes through a series of low-noise pre-amplifiers and is digitised using an A/D converter.

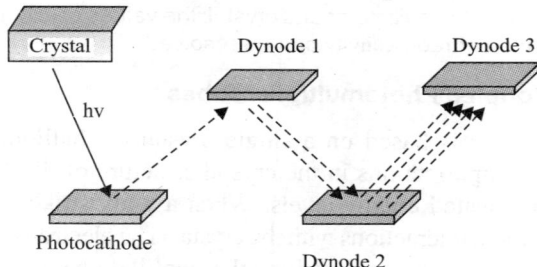

Fig. 14.4. A schematic of a photomultiplier tube. Light emitted by the scintillation crystal is converted into a current at the output of the photomultiplier tube. Only 3 dynodes are shown; typically up to 10 are present. For every electron striking a dynode, a significantly greater number of electrons is emitted.

Each PMT should ideally have an identical energy response, that is, the output current as a function of the energy of the γ-ray. If this is not the case, then artifacts are produced in the image. For planar nuclear medicine scans, a variation in uniformity of up to 10 per cent can be tolerated; however, for SPECT imaging, covered later in this chapter, this value should be less than 1 per cent. In practice, calibration of the PMTs is performed using samples of uniform and known radioactivity and automatic data correction algorithms are applied to the data. More recently, continuous monitoring of individual PMTs during the nuclear medicine scan has become possible using a light-emitting diode (LED) calibration source for each PMT.

New types of gamma cameras, based on multiple-crystal detectors, are currently being developed and may become standard in the near future. In one such design, a two-dimensional array of long, thin crystals is situated in front of a single position-sensitive PMT (PSPMT). The signal from the PSPMT is digitised using a high-speed A/D converter, with this signal carrying information on the energy of the detected γ-ray, as well as the x and y co-ordinates of the scintillation event. In this set-up, each crystal in the two-dimensional array represents one pixel in the re-constructed nuclear medicine scan. In a further development of the crystal-array concept, the NaI(T1) crystals can be replaced by a semi-conductor, cadmium zinc telluride (CZT), which has a much greater energy resolution and can measure much higher count rates.

IMAGE CHARACTERISTICS

As outlined in the introduction to this chapter, the characteristics of nuclear medicine scans are a low SNR and poor spatial resolution, but an extremely high CNR, compared to other imaging modalities. Various forms of data post-processing are used to increase the image SNR, although this degrades further the spatial resolution.

Signal-to-Noise Ratio

Radioactive decay is a statistical process in that there is no way to predict exactly which atom will decay at a particular time. The number of disintegrations per unit time fluctuates around an average value described by a Poisson statistical distribution. The SNR is proportional to the square root of the total number of counts and therefore the greater the number of γ-rays detected, the higher is the SNR. Factors which affect the SNR include the following:

1. The radioactive dose administered: The number of γ-rays detected is proportional to the dose of radiopharmaceutical, but there are clearly patient safety limits to the dose that can be used.
2. The effectiveness of the radiopharmaceutical at targeting a specific organ: The higher the organ specificity of the radiopharmaceutical, the higher is the accumulated dose in that particular organ and the greater is the SNR.
3. The total time over which the image is acquired: The greater the time, the larger is the number of γ-rays detected. The time is limited by patient comfort and the radioactive and biological half-lives of the radiopharmaceutical.
4. Tissue attenuation: The closer the organ being imaged is to the surface of the patient, the less is the degree of γ-ray attenuation. For different radionuclides, the higher the energy of the γ-ray emitted, the lower is the attenuation in tissue and the higher is the image SNR.
5. The intrinsic sensitivity of the gamma camera: For a given system, increasing the scintillation crystal thickness increases the SNR because more γ-rays are detected (however, this decreases the spatial resolution). Similarly, decreasing the length or thickness of the lead septa increases the SNR. The geometry of the collimator, that is, pinhole, converging, diverging etc., also affects the image SNR.
6. Post-acquisition image filtering: Due to the relatively low SNR of nuclear medicine images, processing of the final image to aid diagnosis is standard clinical practice. Normally this processing consists of applying a low-pass filter to the image. This filter reduces the contribution of high spatial frequencies, that is, reduces the noise level, but also blurs the image. The degree to which the image is low-pass-filtered depends on the SNR of the acquired image. Because the intrinsic image spatial resolution is relatively poor, quite strong filtering can be applied without introducing significant blurring.

Spatial Resolution

There are four major contributions to the spatial resolution of a nuclear medicine scan:

1. The intrinsic spatial resolution of the gamma camera (excluding the collimator) R_{gamma}: This reflects the uncertainly in the exact location at which light is produced in the scintillation crystal.

2. The geometry of the collimator: The spatial resolution resulting from the use of a parallel-hole collimator is determined by the length and the spacing between, the lead septa.
3. The degree of Compton scattering of γ-rays within the patient: The deeper the targeted organ lies within the body, the greater is the number of γ-rays that will be Compton-scattered, the lower is the CNR and the poorer is the spatial resolution.
4. Post-acquisition image filtering.

Contrast-to-Noise Ratio

The intrinsic image contrast is extremely high in nuclear medicine because there is no background signal from tissues in which the radiopharmaceutical has not distributed. In this case, the image CNR is essentially equal to the image SNR. However, the presence of Compton-scattered γ-rays does contribute to some degradation of the image SNR. If the spatial resolution is poor, then the CNR is reduced because image blurring cause signal 'bleed' from areas of high signal intensity to those where no signal should be present. This phenomenon is referred to as the partial volume effect and is particularly pronounced for small structures.

CLINICAL APPLICATIONS OF NUCLEAR MEDICINE

The major clinical applications of nuclear medicine are the measurement of blood perfusion in the brain, the diagnosis of tumours in various organs and the assessment of cardiac function. The following descriptions are not exhaustive, but outline the development of a wide variety of different radiopharmaceuticals for the detection of many different types of disease.

Brain Imaging

Planar scintigraphy is used in the brain scanning to detect tumours using either injected ^{99m}Tc-diethylenetriaminetetraacetic acid (DTPA) or ^{99m}Tc-glucoheptonate. As described earlier, in healthy brain tissue the blood brain barrier (BBB) selectively filters the blood supply to the brain, allowing only a limited number of naturally occurring substrates, such as glucose, to enter brain tissue. If the brain is damaged, the BBB is disrupted such that injected radiopharmaceuticals can now enter the brain tissue. Because blood flow is often higher in tumours than in healthy tissue, injected radiopharmaceuticals tend to show higher uptake in tumours than surrounding tissue. Planar scintigraphy is also used to confirm brain death. If the brain is functionally dead, then the carotid arteries are visualised on nuclear medicine scans, but are cut off at the base of the skull. The sagittal and venous sinuses are not visualised.

Ceretec is used to diagnose a large range of diseases that cause altered perfusion in the brain. The normal brain has symmetric blood perfusion patterns in the two hemispheres, with higher blood flow in cortical gray matter than white matter. Diseases that cause altered perfusion patterns include epilepsy, cerebral infarction, schizophrenia and dementia. Brain tumours can also be identified using SPECT imaging of labelled amino acids such as ^{123}I-α-methyl-L-tyrosine (IMT), which is taken up in tumours by a specific amino acid transport system. This agent accumulates in tumours to a much higher degree than in surrounding cortical gray matter due to this active transport mechanism.

Bone Scanning and Tumour Detection

Whole-body scanning using ^{99m}Tc phosphonates such as methylenediphosphonate (MDP) or hydroxymethylenediphosphonate (HMDP, Osteoscan) can be used to detect bone tumours and also soft-tissue tumours that cause deformation and re-modelling of bone structure. The mode of concentration of these agents in bone is thought to involve the affinity of diphosphonate for the metabolically active bone mineral hydroxyapatite, which exhibits increased metabolic turnover during bone growth. The usual response of bone to a tumour is to form new bone at the site or in the periphery of the tumour. For example, spinal tumours, which consist of metastatic lesions growing in the spinal marrow space, cause the bone structure of the spine to re-model. This results in local uptake of the radiopharmaceutical. Scanning starts 2–3 hours after injection of the radiopharmaceutical, to allow accumulation within the skeletal structure and 10 or more scans are used to cover the whole body. If any suspected tumour sites show up, then more-localised scans can be acquired. Bone infarctions or aggressive bone metastases often show up as signal voids in the nuclear medicine scan because bone necrosis has occurred and there is no blood flow to deliver the radiopharmaceutical to the region.

Radiopharmaceuticals can also be designed to target specific sites present during the cell cycle of the cancerous tissue. For example, it is a well established that somatostatin receptors are overexpressed in a number of human tumours. Monoclonal antibodies and fragments have also been used to target tumours.

Cardiac Imaging

Cardiac SPECT scans are performed to measure blood flow patterns in the heart and to detect coronary artery disease and myocardial infarcts. Unlike most other applications, the cardiac SPECT system usually contains only two rotating gamma cameras, with the detectors situated at 90° to one another. Typically, only a 180° rotation is used to form the image because the heart is positioned close to the front of the thorax and well to the left of the body and therefore views in which the detector is far away from the heart would essentially contribute only scattered γ-rays.

The most common type of scan measures myocardial perfusion and is referred to as a cardiac stress test.

A further class of agents used to assess cardiac disease comprises radiopharmaceuticals that are formed from fatty acids. Fatty acids are a major source of energy in normal myocardium, but fatty acids oxidation is suppressed in ischemic and post-ischemic myocardium. Therefore, the biodistribution of a radiolabelled fatty acid is indicative of the metabolic state of the myocardium. Radioactive iodinated analogs of fatty acids such as 15-(p-iodophenyl)-3-(R,S)-methylpentadecanoic acid (BMIPP) are used most commonly.

Respiratory System

The roles of the lungs are to add oxygen to and remove carbon dioxide from, the blood supply to the rest of the body. These processes occur at the blood-air interface in the alveoli of the lungs. Blood flows to the lungs through the pulmonary arteries and veins and via the bronchial arteries. Air enters the lungs via the pharynx into the trachea. Different respiratory diseases can either cause disruptions to blood flow (perfusion), air flow (ventilation) or both.

Perfusion (Q) and ventilation (V) scans are often carried out in the same examination. A so-called 'V/Q mismatch', in which ventilation is normal, but perfusion is abnormal, is indicative of the presence of an obstruction such as a pulmonary embolism.

If both perfusion and ventilation are abnormal, referred to as a V/Q-matched abnormality, this is indicative of diseases such as bronchitis, asthma or pulmonary edema.

Liver and Reticuloendothelial System

The functions of the liver include detoxification of the blood supply, formation of bile and the metabolism and synthesis of a variety of proteins. The most common diseases of the reticuloendothelial system (RES) are cirrhosis and fatty infiltrations of the liver, the presence of tumours (hepatomas) and abscesses, obstructions to hepatobiliary clearance and hemangiomas.

When a disease such as cirrhosis of the liver is present, then the liver is unable to phagocytise the particles fully and an increased level of radioactivity is seen in the spleen and the bone marrow. The colloids are preferentially localised in normal tissue, with almost no radioactivity found in abnormal lesions (focal nodular hyperplasia is an exception) and so diseases such as metastatic tumours, cysts, abscesses and hematomas can be visualised by the lack of the radioactivity in these areas, so-called 'cold spots' in the image.

Renal Imaging

Radiopharmaceuticals used in brain scanning can also be used to image renal function because these agents are excreted through the kidneys. Whichever agent is used, the normal diagnostic procedure is to acquire a time series of images in order to build up a profile of the increase and subsequent decay of the radiopharmaceutical concentration. Abnormal kinetics during one or both of the stages is indicative of specific physiological defects in the kidneys. For example, a prolonged retention of the agent in one or both of the kidneys is associated with renal artery stenosis. Renal infarction, on the other hand, is associated with a very slow build-up of the agent.

POSITRON EMISSION TOMOGRAPHY

Positron emission tomography (PET) is one of the fastest growing imaging modalities in modern clinical diagnosis. Similar to SPECT, PET is a tomographic technique that is used to measure physiology and function, rather than gross anatomy, the fundamental difference between the two imaging techniques is that the injected or inhaled radiopharmaceuticals used in PET emit positrons, which, after annihilation with an electron in tissue, result in the formation of two γ-rays. The fact that two γ-rays are detected, rather than one as in SPECT, allows the instrumentation used in PET to be designed to produce images with much higher SNR and spatial resolution than in SPECT.

PET is used clinically mainly in oncology, cardiology and neurology. The spatial distribution, extent of uptake, rate of uptake and rate of washout of a particular radiopharmaceutical are all quantities which can be used to distinguish diseased from healthy tissue. The major disadvantages of PET revolve around its high cost and the need to have a cyclotron on-site to produce positron-emitting nuclides, because the half-lives of these nuclides are so short.

General Principles

As outlined above, PET is a diagnostic imaging technique used to map the biodistribution of positron-emitting radiopharmaceuticals within the body. These radiopharmaceuticals must be synthesised using a cyclotron and are structural analogs of a biologically active molecule, such as glucose, in which one or more of the atoms has been replaced by a radioactive atom.

The spatial resolution in PET depends upon a number of factors including the number and size of the individual crystal detectors: typical values of the overall system spatial resolution are ~3–5 mm.

Radionuclides Used for PET

All the radionuclides used in PET are produced by a cyclotron. The most commonly used radionuclides are ^{18}F, ^{11}C, ^{15}O and ^{13}N, which are incorporated into biologically active molecules before being injected into or inhaled by the patient. These radionuclides can all be produced from relatively small cyclotrons using protons with an energy of ~10 MeV or deuterons with an energy ~5 MeV. The radioactive properties of these four radionuclides are summarised in Table 14.2.

Table 14.2. Properties of the most common radionuclides used for PET.

Radionuclide	Half-life (min.)
^{11}C	20.4
^{15}O	2.07
^{13}N	9.96
^{18}F	109.7

After production of the particular radionuclide it must be incorporated, via rapid chemical synthesis, into the corresponding radiopharmaceutical. For speed and safety considerations the synthesis should ideally be carried out robotically.

Instrumentation for PET

The major differences in PET instrumentation compared to that in SPECT are the scintillation crystals needed to detect 511-keV γ-rays efficiently and the additional circuitry needed for coincidence detection.

RADIOISOTOPES AND RADIOPHARMACEUTICALS

Early nuclear scientists at the turn of the century discovered three types of radiation emitted spontaneously from matter. These were arbitrarily called alpha, α, beta, β and gamma, γ, rays. Alpha rays are positively charged helium nuclei that do not penetrate tissue very well and so are not very useful in nuclear medicine.

Beta rays consist of negatively charged electrons and like alpha rays, are particle radiation. Gamma rays are electromagnetic radiation, with energy levels above those of medical X-rays. Example of radionuclides that produce clinically significant amounts of beta and gamma rays are listed in Table 14.3.

Table 14.3. Example radionuclides.

Isotope	Half-life	Typical radiation	Typical target organs
Phosphorus 32 (^{32}P)	14.3 days	Beta	Liver
Chromium 51 (^{51}Cr)	27.8 days	Gamma	Red blood cells; urinary
Barium 131 (^{131}Ba)	11.6 days	Gamma	Intestinal
Iodine 131 (^{131}I)	8.1 days	Gamma	Thyroid; blood
Technetium 99m (^{99m}Tc)	6.0 hours	Gamma	Brain; lung

Because of the low tissue-penetrating capability of beta radiation, most procedures using it are done *in vitro*, that is, in a glass tube. *In vivo* procedures, on the other hand, are done on the tissue directly. These radiation procedures are frequently done using the high tissue-penetrating characteristic of gamma radiation. The central element of nuclear medicine imaging equipment is the detector, which can localise radiation and measure the dose.

Radiation Detectors

The most simple and basic radiation detector for X-rays and gamma rays, as well as for alpha and beta rays, consists of a parallel plate capacitor in air, connected through an ammeter to a battery, as shown in

Fig. 14.5. The radiation will produce either positive or negative ions in the air, helium or argon gas between the capacitor plates. The ions will be attracted by the voltage on the capacitor plates and will cause a current in the ammeter. The current has units of coulombs per second (C/s) and roentgens have units of coulombs per kilogram (C/kg). Therefore, the ammeter can be calibrated to read roentgens per second (R/s) of radiation. Depending upon the voltage level applied to the capacitor plates, the unit serves different functions, as indicated in Fig. 14.5b.

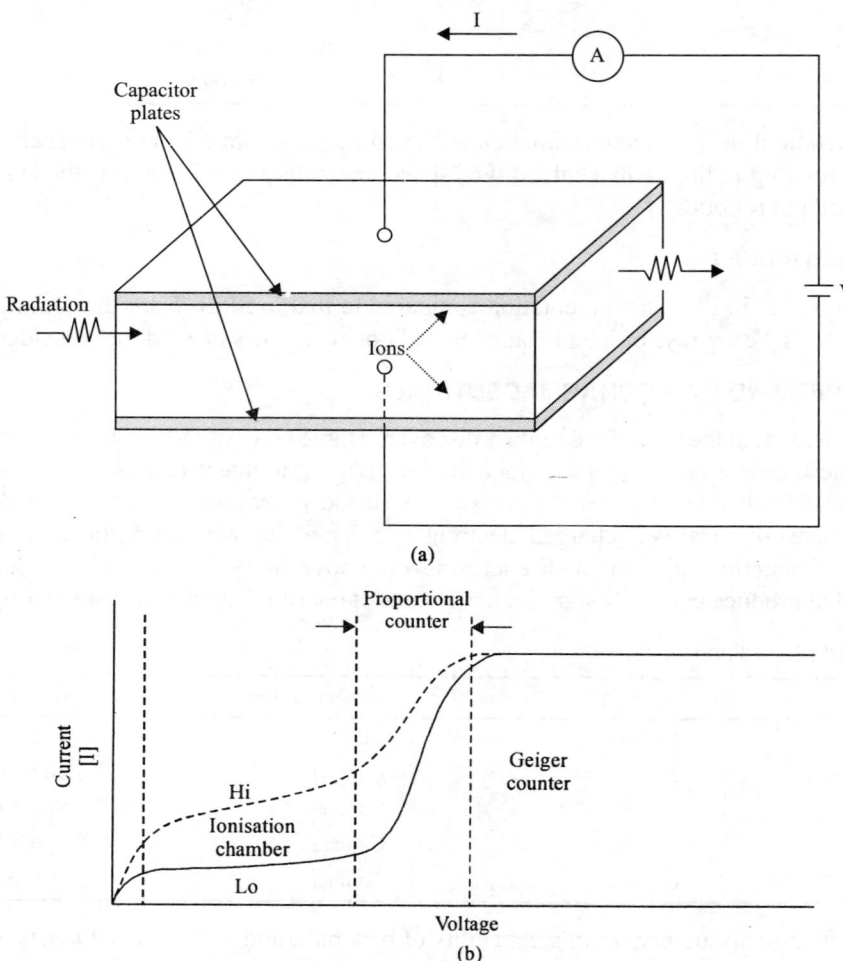

(a)

(b)

Fig. 14.5. A basic ionisation chamber.

For low voltages of about 100 V/cm, every ion produced between the plates will be conducted to the plate and produce the same current regardless of changes in the applied voltage V. This is the ionisation chamber mode of operation, in which the current I is proportional to the radiation intensity. Large radiation follows the Hi curve and small radiation follows the Lo curve. As voltage V is increased, the ions have secondary collisions and produce more ions, amplifying the current due to the radiation in proportion to the radiation intensity. This is called the proportional counter mode. If the voltage is increased so high that any radiation pulse causes all atoms in the chamber to ionise by a general avalanche effect, the chamber is operating as a Geiger counter. In the Geiger counter mode each ionising event causes the same-value pulse output. The radiation intensity is measured by counting the number of pulses per second. Personnel exposed to radiation need to know their accumulated dose so they can keep their level below the Occupational Safety and Health Administration (OSHA) restriction of 5 rads per year. A measurement of one rad of radiation means the body has absorbed 0.01 joules per kilogram (J/kg) of X-ray radiation. Convenient pocket-size radiation detectors are available to make this measurement. In Fig. 14.6, a charged-capacitor-type radiation monitor is shown.

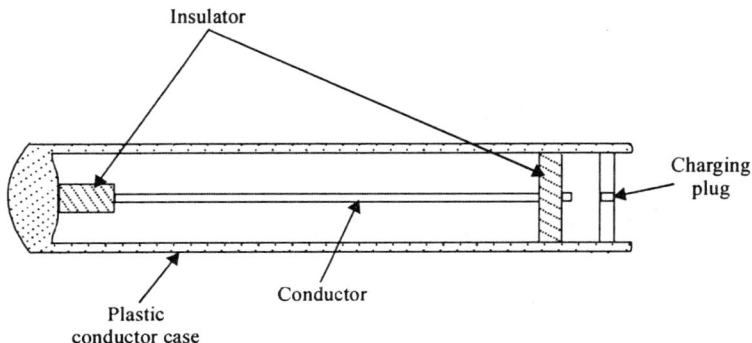

Fig. 14.6. A capacitor radiation monitor.

To operate the capacitor radiation monitor, the charging plug is moved against the centre conductor and a high voltage is applied. Then the charging plug is moved away. The centre conductor will hold its charge, being insulated by high-quality insulators. The outside conductor is a conductive plastic that passes radiation, which ionises the space between the two conductors. These ions cause a current that lowers the charge on the centre conductor. After exposure to radiation, the charging plug is put in contact with the centre conductor and the voltage is read. The change in voltage is then a measure of the radiation exposure since it was charged.

Another common personal radiation detector is a film badge. Ionisation radiation causes a darkening of the silver halide in the photographic emulsion. A photoelectric densitometer may then be used to measure the radiation exposure of the film.

The detectors we have discussed tend to be insensitive because, being gas or film, they do not capture all of the radiation incident upon them. Crystal scintillation tends to be more sensitive and because it takes place in a solid which absorbs more radiation, is widely used in electronic imagers.

Crystals of sodium iodide (NaI), laced with traces of thallium, produce light when irradiated by X-ray or gamma-ray photons. A photodetector may then be used to measure the light intensity. NaI crystal detectors are used in nuclear medicine systems and in particular, in conjunction with a photo-multiplier tube.

Photomultiplier Tube

A photomultiplier tube consists of a photocathode that produces electrons when light impinges on it. Then a set of plates amplify the electron beam by a process of secondary emission, as illustrated in Fig. 14.7.

A photocathode consists of an opaque substrate coated with a cesium lead compound. Typical sensitivities run from 3 to 150 microamps per lumen (μA/lm). The supply voltage, V_B, causes equal voltage drops across successive dynodes or plates, numbered 1, 2, 3, 4, 5 and so on. These voltages accelerate the electrons from the photocathode, causing secondary emission from each dynode, such that the beam current increases successively from dynode 1 to dynode 5. The output current through R_L is thus amplified and may be detected with a differential amplifier.

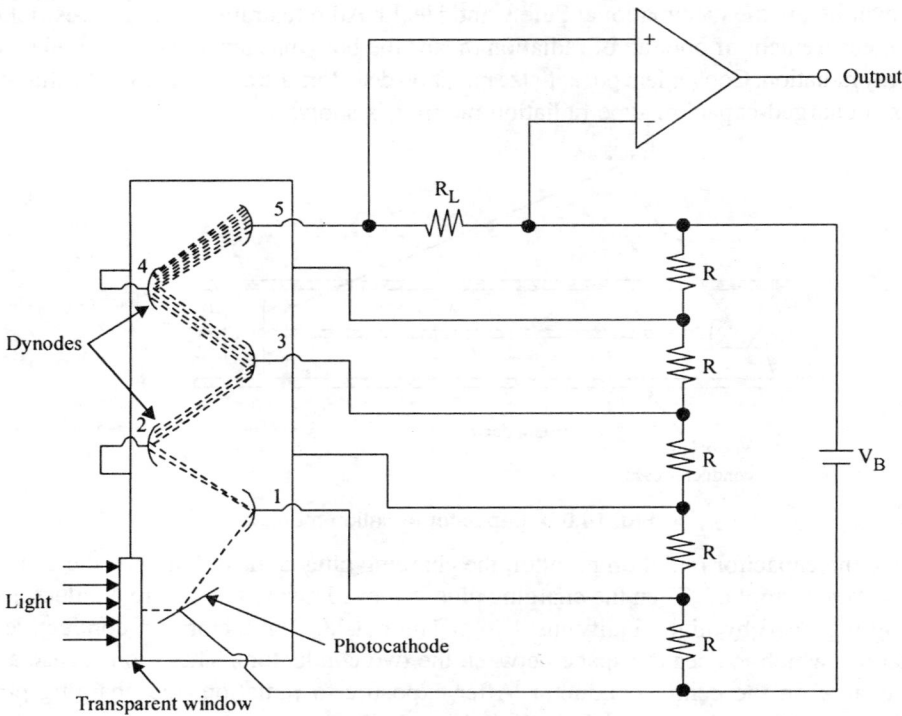

Fig. 14.7. A photomultiplier tube circuit.

Gamma-Ray Camera

A gamma-ray camera, sometimes called an Anger scintillation camera after its inventor Hal O. Anger, is used to localise and measure the gamma rays from a patient who has been injected with a radionuclide. The block diagram in Fig. 14.8 illustrates a patient under a gamma-ray scanner.

If, for example, a radiopharmaceutical such as barium 131 (^{131}Ba) is taken into the intestine, the camera head would be placed over the patient's abdomen. Radiation from the ^{131}Ba isotope is passed through a pinhole collimator to eliminate scattering effects and directed into a large (15 inch diameter) sodium iodide (NaI) scintillation crystal optically coupled to an array of 14 photomultiplier tubes. The light flashes from the crystal create a current in the photomultipliers. Each photomultiplier is successively scanned. The photomultiplier puts out a corresponding pulse of current. The pulse height is measured by the A/D converter shown in Fig. 14.8. Larger pulses will turn on more of the AND gate outputs, producing a binary number output that can be processed by a microprocessor that correlates it with the position of the photomultiplier in the camera head. A digital output unit may produce a dot-matrix printout showing the large concentrations of radiopharmaceutical as an increased density of dots on an x-y plot. The data may also be displayed on a cathode-ray tube on which the x-y position is fixed, as on an oscilloscope and the intensity of the image would correspond to the radiation intensity on the appropriate position.

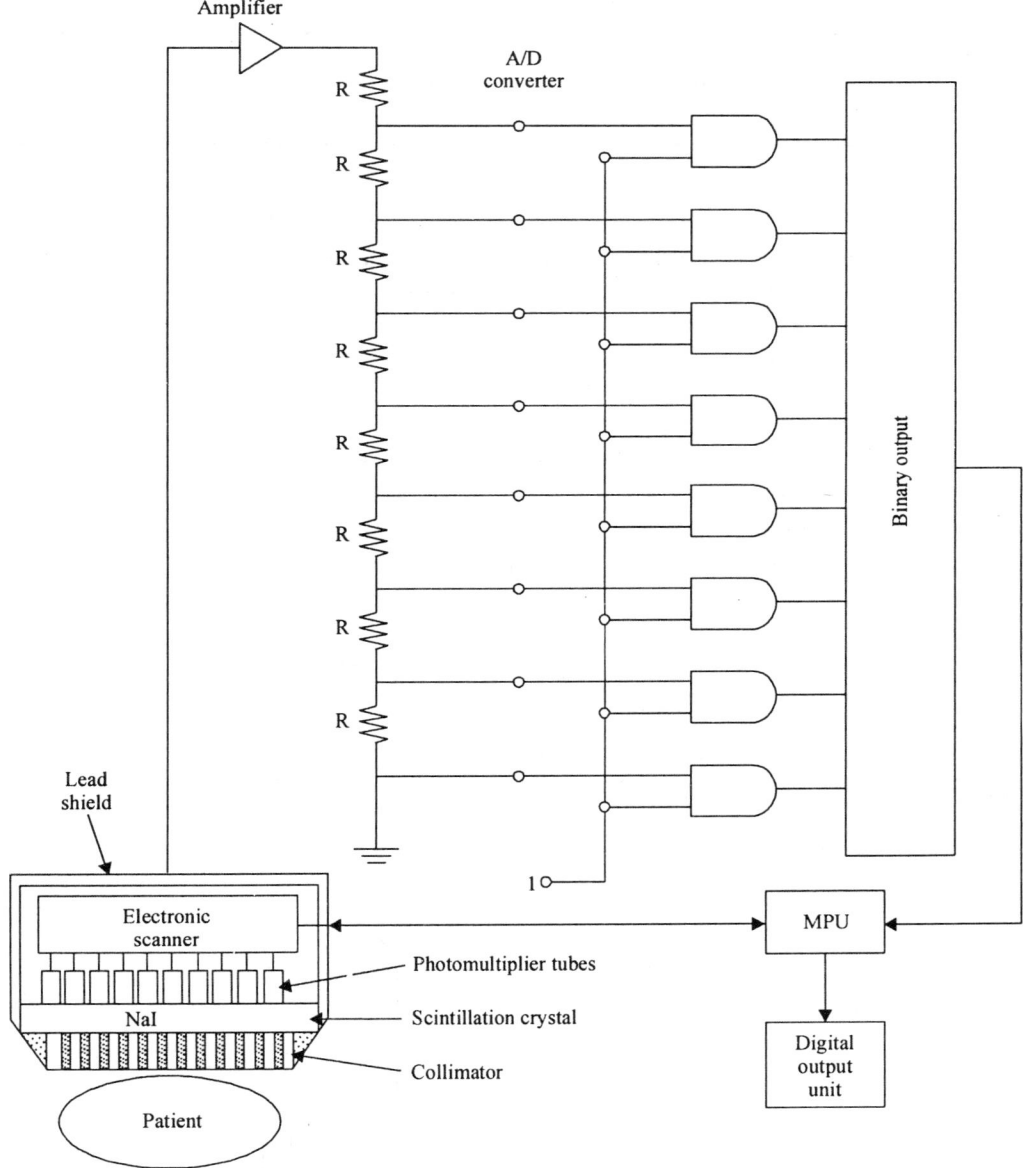

Fig. 14.8. A gamma-ray camera circuit.

RADIATION DOSE

One of the side effects of x-radiation or nuclear medicine is the dose absorbed by the patient and those using the X-ray machinery. The dose can be computed from a knowledge of the X-ray beam current, anode voltage and radiation pattern. It is most important to carefully define the units of ionising radiation as follows:

Quantity	Name	Units	Conversion
Activity	Becquerel (Bq)	s^{-1}	1 curie (Ci) = 3.7 (10^{10}) Bq
Exposure	roentgen (R)	C/kg	1 R = 2.58 × 10^{-4} C/kg
Dose	rad	J/kg	1 rad = 0.01 J/kg

To correlate the various types of ionising radiation, we define roentgen equivalent man (rem): the dosage of ionising radiation that will have the same biological effect as one roentgen of x or gamma radiation.

Example 14.1. The x-radiation incident on a 50 kg man is 0.5 W/m² and the radiation intensity that emerges from him is 0.05 W/m². How many rads does he receive during a 50 ms exposure over a body surface of 0.5 m²?

Solution. The joules of energy absorbed are

$$(0.5 - 0.05) \ (\text{W/m}^2) \ (0.5 \ \text{m}^2) \ (0.05 \ \text{s}) = 0.0113 \ \text{J}$$

The dose, D, is

$$D = (0.0113 \ \text{J/}50.00 \ \text{kg}) = 2.26 \times 10^{-4} \ \text{J/kg}$$
$$= (2.26 \times 10^{-4} \ \text{J/kg}) \ [1 \ \text{rad/}(0.01 \ \text{J/kg})] = 2.26 \times 10^{-2} \ \text{rad}$$

The dose is therefore 22.6 mrad.

To compute the dose of radiation left in a volume of tissue, refer to Fig. 14.9, which depicts a tissue with density ρ. The dose equals the joules per kilogram of X-ray left in the tissue. To derive a formula for dose we first find the power loss in the tissue, then we compute the energy loss in joules and divide by the tissue mass in kilograms:

$$\text{Power in tissue} = \mathfrak{J}_0 A - \mathfrak{J}_0 A e^{-\mu \rho s}$$

For an X-ray pulse of duration T_D seconds,

$$\text{Energy in the tissue} = \mathfrak{J}_0 A T_D \ (1 - e^{-\mu \rho s})$$

Since the tissue mass = $A s \rho$, we have

$$\text{Dose} = \frac{\mathfrak{J}_0 T_D (1 - e^{-\mu \rho s})}{\rho s}$$

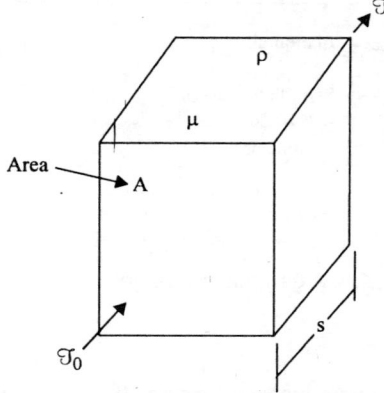

Fig. 14.9. A geometric model for dose calculations.

The dosage from ionising radiation is cumulative because the probability of cell damage increases as more X-rays pass through the body. Government regulations require that occupationally induced X-rays, which are absorbed by the whole-body, should not exceed a cumulative dose (CD) of

$$CD = 5 \ (n - 18) \ rad \qquad\qquad \text{... (14.1)}$$

where n is the worker's age in years. A one-year exposure should not exceed 5 rad. In medical application to patients, physicians may decide to exceed these limits when they feel the risk to the patient from disease exceeds the risk of X-ray exposure. The number of rads of dose absorbed from a given exposure to radiation depends upon the material as well as the photon energy level. Figure 14.10 gives data on the ratio of rads/roentgen (rad/R) for bone and muscle. Rads nearly equal roentgens in the soft tissue of the body. Since soft tissue makes up most of the body, we can say that in human the dose in rads is approximately equal to the exposure in roentgens.

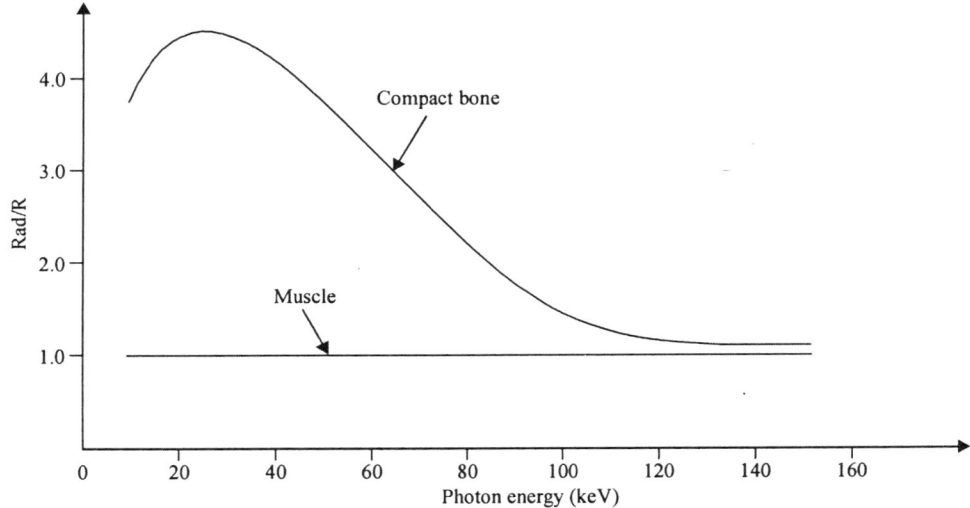

Fig. 14.10. The relationship of an absorbed dose to exposure in body tissues over the diagnostic energy range.

Government regulations on the allowed X-ray dose have become more stringent as long-term effects have become apparent. In 1900, the permissible whole-body dose was 10 rem per day. This is now reduced by nearly one thousand times, to 5 rem per year. The reason for these regulations is summarised by the description of the effects of ionising radiation on human.

Since X-ray is a carcinogen, it is essential to reduce dose levels due to stray X-rays to less than 5 rads per year. This is usually done with shielding by a massive material such as lead, iron or concrete. Since the dose in rads is proportional to the X-ray intensity in watts per meter squared (W/m^2), it follows that the dose out of a shield D_{OUT} is related to the dose into the shield, D_{IN}, in rads, by

$$D_{OUT} = D_{IN}e^{-\mu\rho s} \qquad\qquad \text{... (14.2)}$$

where s is the thickness of the shield.

Anyone who has worn a lead shield during X-ray procedures has probably wondered if a lighter material is available to shield X-rays. Unfortunately, material less dense than lead must be thicker, keeping the weight about the same.

The thickness of lead required for radiation protection may be deduced from Table 14.4.

Table 14.4. Thickness of lead required to reduce useful beam to 5 per cent.

Potential (kV)	Required lead thickness (mm)
60	0.1
100	0.16
140	0.70
200	1.0
250	1.7
400	2.3

Chapter 15

Magnetic Resonance Imaging

INTRODUCTION

Magnetic resonance imaging (MRI) is a non-ionising technique with full three-dimensional capabilities, excellent soft-tissue contrast and high spatial resolution (~1 mm). In general, the temporal resolution is much slower than for ultrasound or computed tomography, with scans typically lasting between 3 and 10 minutes and MRI is therefore much more susceptible to patient motion. The cost of MRI scanners is relatively high. The major uses of MRI are in the areas of assessing brain disease, spinal disorders, angiography, cardiac function and musculoskeletal damage.

The MRI signal arises from protons in the body, primarily water, but also lipid. The patient is placed inside a strong magnet, which produces a static magnetic field typically more than 10000 times stronger than the earth's magnetic field. Each proton, being a charged particle with angular momentum, can be considered as acting as a small magnet. The protons align in two configurations, with their internal magnetic fields aligned either parallel or antiparallel to the direction of the large static magnetic field, with slightly more found in the parallel state. The protons precess around the direction of the static magnetic field, in an analogous way to a spinning gyroscope under the influence of gravity. The frequency of precession is proportional to the strength of the static magnetic field. Application of a weak radiofrequency (RF) field causes the protons to precess coherently and the sum of all of the protons precessing is detected as an induced voltage in a tuned detector coil.

Spatial information is encoded into the image using magnetic field gradients. These impose a linear variation in all three dimensions in the magnetic field present within the patient. As a result of these variations, the precessional frequencies of the protons are also linearly dependent upon their spatial location. The frequency and the phase of the precessing magnetisation is measured by the RF coil and the analog signal is digitised. An inverse two-dimensional Fourier transform is performed to convert the signal into the spatial domain to produce the image. By varying the data acquisition parameters, differential contrast between soft tissues can be introduced, as shown in Fig. 15.1.

NUCLEAR MAGNETISM

In MRI the patient is placed inside a very strong magnet for scanning. A typical value of the magnetic field, denoted B_0, is 1.5 T (15000 G), which can be compared to the earth's magnetic field of approximately

50 µT (0.5 G). The MRI signal arises from the interaction between the magnetic field and hydrogen nuclei or protons, which are found primarily as water in tissue and also lipid. This interaction can be described in terms of the nuclear magnetism, either from a quantum mechanical or a classical approach, both of which are described in the following sections.

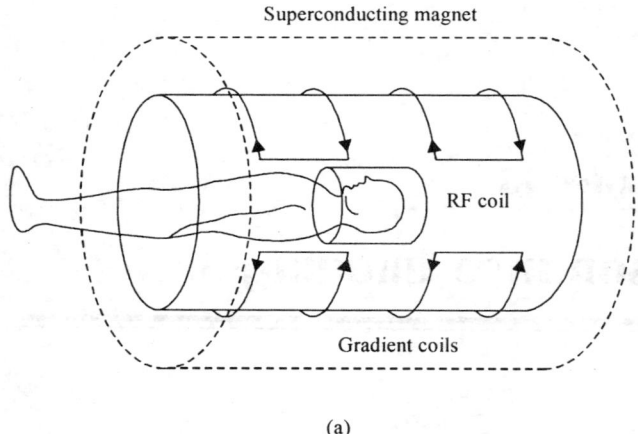

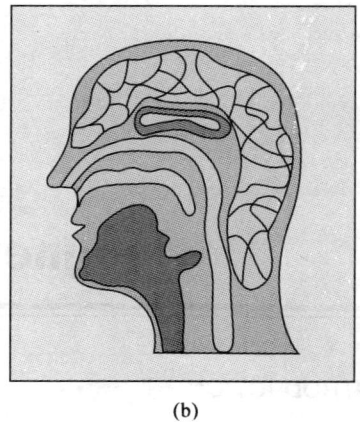

(a)   (b)

Fig. 15.1. (a) The instrumentation involved in MRI consists of a superconducting magnet, three sets of magnetic field gradients (only one is shown) and a radiofrequency coil. (b) A single-slice MRI of the brain showing excellent soft-tissue contrast between gray and white matter and high spatial resolution.

Quantum Mechanical Description

All nuclei with an odd atomic weight and/or an odd atomic number possess a fundamental quantum mechanical property termed 'spin'. For MRI the most important nucleus is the hydrogen nucleus or proton.

Shown in Table 15.1 are the values of γ and I for naturally occurring nuclei within the body. Neither of the major isotopes of carbon (^{12}C) nor oxygen (^{16}O), both abundant in the body, gives an MRI signal. It is possible to detect these elements, but only the isotopes ^{13}C and ^{17}O, which exist in very low natural abundance, 1.1 per cent and 0.048 per cent, respectively.

Table 15.1. Properties of nuclei found at high abundance in the body.

Nucleus	Atomic number	Atomic Mass	I	$\gamma/2\pi$ (MHz/T)	MRI signal
Proton	1	1	½	42.58	Yes
Phosphorus	15	31	½	17.24	Yes
Carbon	6	12	0	–	No
Oxygen	8	16	0	–	No
Sodium	11	23	3/2	11.26	Yes

Classical Description

The quantum mechanical model describes the basics of nuclear magnetism, but becomes cumbersome when analysing complicated MRI pulse sequences. A more intuitive approach is to consider the interactions of protons with magnetic fields purely in terms of classical mechanics.

Radiofrequency Pulses and the Rotating Reference Frame

In order to obtain an MRI signal, transitions must be induced between the protons in the parallel and the antiparallel energy levels. The energy required to do this is supplied by an oscillating electromagnetic field.

VECTOR DESCRIPTION OF MAGNETIC RESONANCE

So far a simple quantum mechanical approach has been used to describe NMR. But to use quantum mechanics to explain the phenomenon in more detail, it is necessary to use complex mathematics. An alternative approach, that is easier to visualise but less rigorous, is the so-called vector model. This description, which represents the average properties of all the nuclei in a sample as simple vectors, will be used from now on. As discussed, when a sample is placed in a magnetic field, the nuclei populate two states, with a net excess in the lower state; in the vector model this net magnetisation is represented as a magnetisation vector (Fig. 15.2). The individual nuclear spin vectors interact with the magnetic field and precess, much in the way that a gyroscope precesses in the earth's gravitational field. It can be shown that the precession frequency is the same Larmor frequency predicted by quantum mechanics.

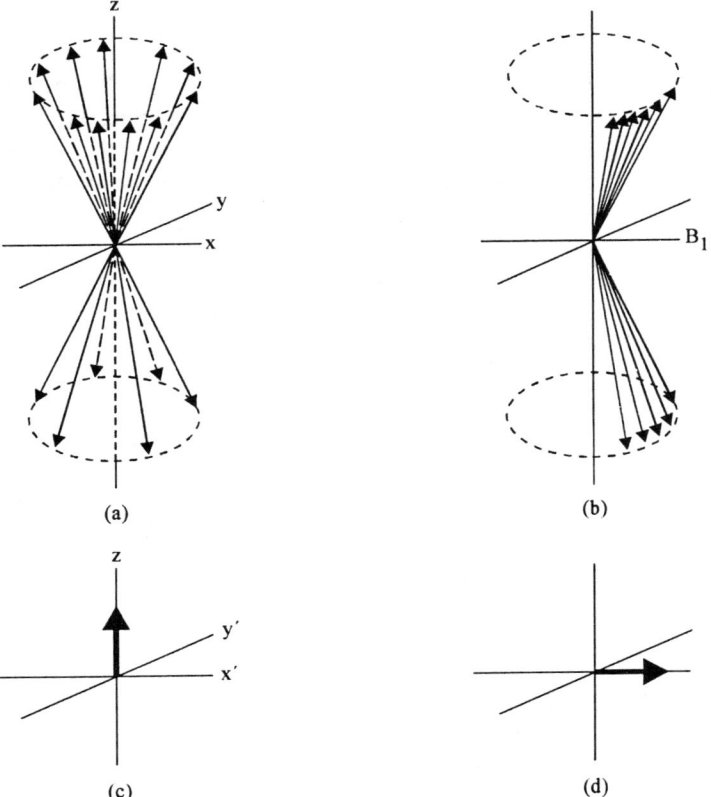

Fig. 15.2. (a) Vector model of magnetic resonance represents the nuclear spins as vectors processing about the magnetic field. (b) Following a pulse the population are changed (equalised for a 90° pulse) and a phase coherence generated. (c,d). In the rotating-frame modification for the conditions (a) and (b), the spin states are represented as simple net vectors.

The vector description can be further simplified by using a set of axes that rotate about the magnetic field axis (z axis) at the Larmor frequency. The net magnetisation is now a simple static vector along the z axis (M_z). The length of this vector corresponds to the population difference between the levels. In the presence of a second magnetic field B_1, that is, at the Larmor frequency, quantum mechanics tells us that energy is absorbed and that nuclei are promoted to the excited state (i.e., M_z is reduced). To perturb M_z, B_1 must be orthogonal to the z axis. In the rotating frame, since B_1 is at the Larmor frequency, it is a static field along the x' axis (prime indicates it is a rotating axis). In the presence of B_1, M_z rotates about the x' axis by an angle and hence M_z reduces as cos α. Simultaneously, a y' component of the magnetisation is produced proportional to sin α. The angle of rotation produced depends on the value of B_1 and the duration τ of the applied field:

$$\alpha = \gamma B_1 \qquad \qquad \dots (15.1)$$

τ is usually a short period, hence the concept of a 90° pulse, which is one that produces maximum M'_y and zero M_z. A 180° pulse is one that produces—M_z (i.e., a population inversion) but no M'_y.

The rotating frame can be defined only for one Larmor frequency. If there are nuclei present with a different resonant frequency, then they appear to precess at this frequency difference, that is, any transverse magnetisation is represented as M'_y vectors precessing about the z-axis.

After excitation, the spin system returns to equilibrium. In the vector description this corresponds to an exponential decline in M'_y and an exponential return of M_z to its equilibrium values. As is explained later in the chapter these processes do not always happen at the same rate. M_z cannot grow faster than M'_y decays since this would imply a net gain of magnetisation during relaxation; but M'_y can and frequently does decay faster than M_z grows. The phenomenon can be visualised (Fig. 15.3) as a loss of coherence in M'_y due to the effects of local inter- and intramolecular magnetic fields. The M'_y vector fans out in the x'y' plane; whereas the sum of M_z and the 'total' transverse magnetisation stay constant, the phase coherent or net transverse magnetisation can decay faster than M_z recovers. Since, as will be discussed, the signal detected by an NMR system is proportional to the phase coherent component of the transverse magnetisation (i.e., M'_y), the signal following an excitation pulse dies away exponentially.

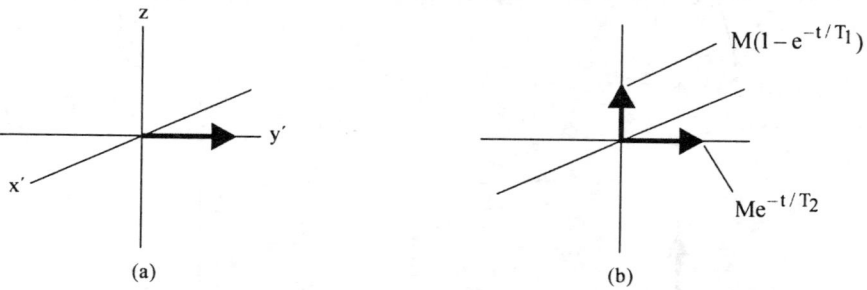

(a)   (b)

Fig. 15.3. (a) Following a 90° pulse, all the nuclear magnetisation is along the y' axis; and (b) at time t second later, M_y has decreased and M_z increased.

TWO DOMAINS

The NMR signal detected following a pulse is a function of time. In the simple case of having one type of nucleus in a uniform magnetic field, it is a single exponentially decaying signal whose frequency depends on its resonance frequency. This signal is termed the free induction decay (FID). If there are several groups of nuclei in the sample, in different local magnetic fields, as is the case when field gradients are used to produce an image, then the signal is more complex. In this case the signal is the sum of the signals from the nuclei in these differing fields that are precessing at their own frequencies and decaying at their own relaxation rates. Such a complex signal is difficult if not impossible to interpret. What is necessary is to analyse this signal into its individual frequency components, which can be achieved by a Fourier transform. The transform of a simple exponential decay is a Lorentzian line. The result in a more general case is a spectrum that is a display of nuclear magnetisation as a function of frequency, which, if a gradient field has been added, is a projection. This procedure is illustrated in Fig. 15.4 for the simple case of two types of nucleus, each of which has its own Larmor frequency.

The relationships between functions of time and frequency (i.e., in the time and frequency domains) are very important in magnetic resonance (MR). These two domains are related by a Fourier transform that has the analytical form x,

$$M(y) = \int_{-x}^{x} m(x) \exp(-2\pi i x y) \, dx \qquad \qquad \dots (15.2)$$

which is normally carried out digitally in a computer using the fast Fourier transform or Cooley-Tukey algorithm. One example of a Fourier pair is shown in Fig. 15.4, the simple exponential and a Lorentzian line; a second is given in Fig. 15.5, that of the pulse and the sinc function. The sinc function/pulse Fourier pair is important in understanding two important concepts in MRI. First, it has been assumed that we have applied a single frequency to excite the system, even when it is known that the sample contains nuclei that have a range of Larmor frequencies, typically spread over many kilohertz. This effect is achieved by applying the excitation in the form of a pulsed, high-frequency wave, a procedure previously assumed with no rationale. As can be seen from Fig. 15.5, if x is time and y is frequency, then, if the excitation is a short function of time, say 10–100 µsec it acts as a spread of frequency that is 100 Hz to 10 kHz wide centered on the basic frequency. Thus a short enough pulse excites all the nuclei equally.

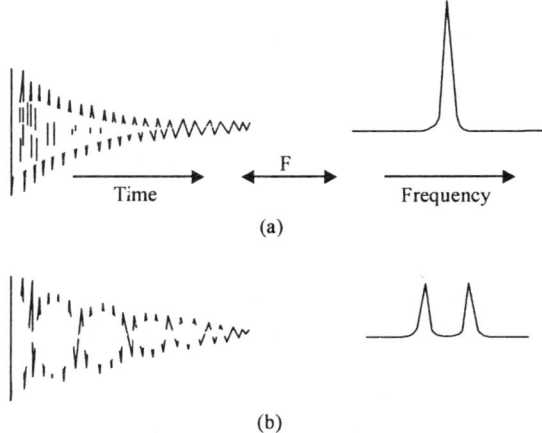

Fig. 15.4. The detected signal following excitation is a decaying cosine wave. (a) In Fourier transformation this yields a single horizontal line. (b) If two frequencies are present in the decay, then the signal is a more complex beat pattern and in transformation shows two lines.

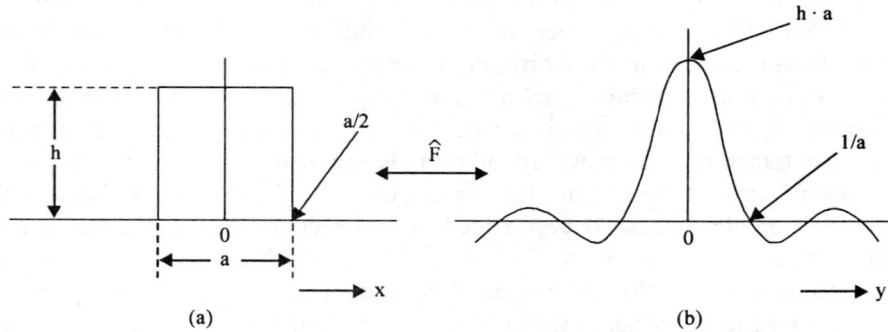

Fig. 15.5. Two functions frequently encountered are (a) the pulse and (b) the sin x/x (or sinc x). These functions are related by a Fourier transform.

The second area in which the Fourier pair concept is important is that of selective excitation. For example, for slice selection in MRI it is necessary to produce an excitation that contains only a discrete range of frequencies, as opposed to the wide spread of frequencies produced by a short rectangular pulse. If the excitation pulse is shaped like a sinc function (i.e., y now time), then it contains only a specific range of frequencies.

SIGNAL EXCITATION AND DETECTION

Nothing has been said about how, in practice, the energy is applied to the sample (patient) or how the signal is detected. The energy is applied by means of a coil wire wrapped around the patient and the signal is detected by the voltage induced in that coil by the transverse nuclear magnetism generated.

To stimulate resonance, the excitation field B_1 must be orthogonal to the main magnetic field and rotate in the correct sense. This can be achieved by applying either a sinusoidal or a true rotating field, the former being the simplest experimental approach. The sinusoidal field can be considered to be resolved into two components; one is of the correct sense and frequency and corresponds to a static vector in the rotating frame. The other component precesses at frequency v in the opposite sense and has no effect on the nuclear spins; it does, however, use power.

In MRI the patient usually lies parallel to the magnetic field; hence a simple solenoid coil cannot be used for excitation and detection since it produces a field parallel to its axis. A coil structure based on a Helmholtz pair (i.e., two mechanically parallel coils separated by a radius wired in electrical series) is usually used since this produces a reasonably uniform field in the correct direction. A schematic diagram is shown in Fig. 15.6.

It is possible to produce a true rotating magnetic field by driving two pairs of Helmholtz type coils orthogonal to each other, with voltages 90° out of phase (i.e., in quadrature). This approach, although more complex, has two advantages. First, it uses half the power of a simple system, since it does not produce the unwanted counter-rotating component; and second, the two coils can be arranged so that each produces a signal. These signals can be summed to produce twice the signal, since they are coherent, while producing only a $\sqrt{2}$ increase in noise. At frequencies above about 20–30 MHz, especially when imaging the body, simple coils of the type outlined above are difficult if not impossible to tune because they tend to self-resonante. Above these frequencies, resonator-type devices are used. Their principle of operation is, however, the same as outlined above.

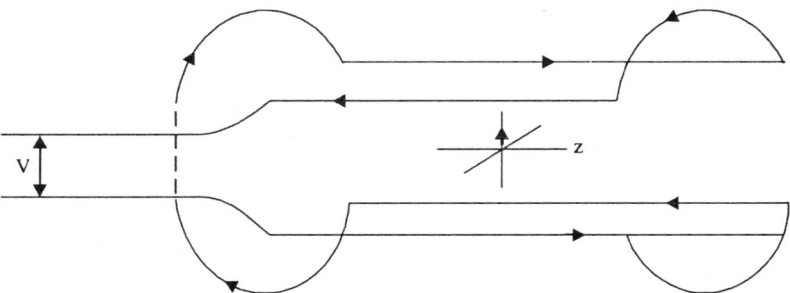

Fig. 15.6. If the basic magnetic field used is parallel to the patient axis, the rf coil has to be based on the Helmholtz pattern (i.e., two coils with opposing senses) to generate a field orthogonal to the main field. The exact dimensions and layout are critical in obtaining a uniform B_1 field.

Coherent transverse magnetisation M_y is generated by the excitation pulse. As M_y precesses it induces a voltage in the rf coil, oscillating at Larmor frequency. This voltage is phase detected with respect to the excitation and amplified to produce a signal that is proportional to M' (i.e., magnetisation in the rotating frame). The signal is then digitised to permit a Fourier transformation and to allow signal averaging.

As discussed previously, NMR signals are weak and contain a considerable quantity of noise. The signal-to-noise ratio (SNR) of the signal can be improved, at the expense of data collection time, by repeating the experiment and averaging the results. Signals from consecutive experiments, being coherent, add, whereas noise (by definition is incoherent) increases only as the square root of the number of data sets added together.

RELAXATION

The energy absorbtion by the sample is almost instantaneous; however, relaxation (loss of energy) is not spontaneous. It occurs only when it is stimulated by local magnetic fields having components at the Larmor frequency. These fields, produced by local magnetic fields the molecules themselves are modulated by molecular motion and structure. Two distinct types of nuclear relaxation must be considered. Both are thought of as first-order or simple exponential processes; that is, the effects of decay can be described as

$$M \propto \exp\left(-\frac{t}{TC}\right) \qquad \qquad ... (15.3)$$

where, TC is a time constant.

The first relaxation process is the loss of the excess energy resulting from the pulse to the surroundings (lattice) as thermal energy. This process is called spin-lattice relaxation and the time constant is T_1. Thus T_1 describes the rate of return to equilibrium of the M_z magnetisation from the value it has following excitation (e.g., from 0 if a 90° pulse has been used) and is typically hundreds of milliseconds for protons in human tissue. If a second excitation pulse is applied on a time scale less than or even equal to T_1, then the detectable signal produced by the second 90° pulse ($\propto M_z$) is less than that produced by the first, since M_z has not relaxed to its full value and if a series of pulses is applied, a steady state is set up. The effect is called saturation and can be used as a source of contrast in MR imaging.

The second relaxation time that can be used as a source of contrast is the spin-spin relaxation time or T_2 and is more difficult to visualise. Following the pulse, all the nuclei are in phase, that is, their vectors are all parallel with the y' axis. As time proceeds, they interact with each other in such a way that they gradually get out of phase. As the nuclei get out of phase, their net M'_y magnetisation decays as $\exp(-t/T_2)$. This process is different from the T_1 process, which is the return to equilibrium of the population difference M_z and is an energy effect; T_2, on the other hand, describes the loss of phase coherence (i.e., M'_y) induced by the excitation pulse, which is an entropy effect. Since it is only the phase coherent part of the transverse magnetisation that can produce a signal, it is T_2 that describes the decay of the detectable signal following a pulse. The two relaxation processes are shown in Fig. 15.3 following a 90° pulse. In general, in biological samples $T_2 < T_1$. For pure liquids $T_1 = T_2$.

Relaxation times in the solid and gaseous phases differ greatly from those in liquids due to the greatly differing degrees of nuclear motion. In the solid state, T_2 relaxation is very short (less than 1 msec), whereas T_1 can be very long (more than 1 minute). In the liquid state, relaxation is in the hundredths of a millisecond region with T_1/T_2 in the range 1–10. With the instrumentation used for MRI, signals are detected only from molecules in the liquid phase and even here only from small molecules, such as water, with rapid nuclear motion. The signals from macromolecules and bone decay too quickly to produce a detectable signal.

SPIN ECHO

As stated previously, the detected NMR signal depends on M_y, which decays by T_2 effects. However, M_y also decays because of magnet inhomogeneities. To explain the latter in more detail, the sample is considered to consist of an assembly of extremely small regions called isochromats. Within each isochromat, field inhomegeneities are neglible. Following a pulse, each isochromat precesses at its own Larmor frequency; thus some rotate faster and some slower than the mean (Fig. 15.7). This results in a fanning out of the isochromats and decrease in net M_y; that is, the signal decays. Magnet inhomogeneity does not affect the total transverse magnetisation M_y, which decays only by T_2 processes.

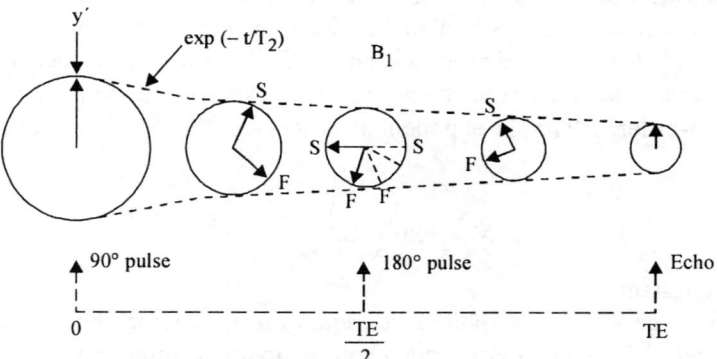

Fig. 15.7. In the presence of a non-uniform magnetic field, each isochromat moves at its own rate, some faster than the mean, some slower. A 180° pulse (at time TE/2) reverses the order of the isochromats; the fastest is now behind the mean and vice versa. At time TE, field inhomogeneities are re-focused and a spin echo is produced.

If at some time TE/2 second after excitation an 180° pulse is applied, then, as shown in Fig. 15.8, the relative positions of these vectors are reversed; the fast are behind the mean and vice versa. At a time TE second after the 90° pulse, therefore, the effects of magnet inhomogeneity are re-focused and the so-called spin echo is produced. The magnitude of the echo has, of course, been reduced by T_2 relaxation to $\exp(-TE/T_2)$, but the unwanted effects of magnet inhomogeneities have been removed.

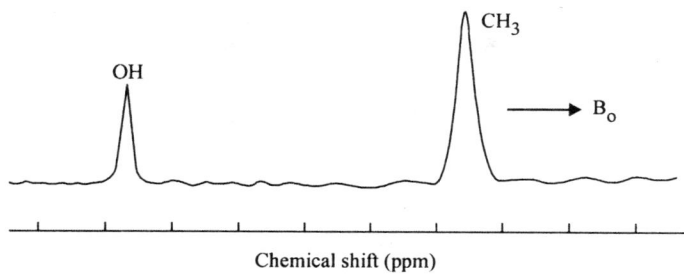

Fig. 15.8. Proton NMR spectrum of methanol (CH_3OH).

NMR SPECTRUM

Five years or so after the first demonstrations of NMR, as the uniformity of the magnets were improved, it was discovered that not all nuclei of an isotope resonated at exactly the same frequency. This effect was shown to depend on the chemical environment of the nuclei involved and was termed the chemical shift.

Figure 15.8 illustrates the chemical shift for the case of methanol, which has two types of protons, those bonded to the carbon atom and those bonded to oxygen. The magnetic field seen by these two groups of protons is the basic field screened to a very small extent by the electrons in the molecules. Thus the resonance frequencies are given by

$$v(CH_3) = B_0(1 - \sigma_{CH_3}) \qquad \qquad ... (15.4a)$$

$$v(OH) = B_0(1 - \sigma_{OH}) \qquad \qquad ... (15.4b)$$

where σ is the screening constant. The difference between these frequencies is the chemical shift δ between the nuclei. The chemical shift is very small (parts per million) and if expressed as a simple frequency, would depend on the magnetic field used. Although it is easy to measure frequencies accurately, magnetic fields can be measured with sufficient accuracy only by NMR; so a circular problem occurs. Chemical shifts are therefore always expressed with respect to a reference line, either already present in or added to the sample:

$$\delta_i = \frac{v_i - v_{ref}}{v_{ref}} \times 10^6 \qquad \qquad ... (15.5)$$

Dividing by the frequency of the reference makes the chemical shift independent of the basic field of the NMR system.

Under conditions of very high resolution (i.e., when using a very homogeneous magnet) where there are very narrow lines, a smaller field-independent effect called spin-spin coupling can be observed.

Spin-spin coupling takes place when nuclei 'sense' the spin state of neighbouring nuclei via the bonding electrons; the result is that resonances are split into multiplets. Under these conditions NMR spectra contain many lines, which may be assigned to specific nuclear types, yielding extensive information of detailed molecular structure.

When the 'sample' is a human, the lines observed are much broader than those from simple solutions and small effects such as coupling constants are usually lost in the increased line width. The line broadening is a result of many factors, including intrinsic relaxation effects and the problems of obtaining a sufficiently homogeneous field over the required volume in the presence of such heterogeneous body.

The proton spectrum of a human consists of two main features, the largest being the resonance of water and the minor feature being the multiple resonances of the CH_2 protons in the alkyl chains of the mobile triglycerides. The ratio of these features depend on the region from which the signal arises. More chemically informative data can be obtained using ^{31}P spectroscopy. The typical ^{31}P NMR spectrum of a human shows resolved resonances from the phosphorus nuclei in ATP, phosphocreatine and inorganic phosphate; study of their relative concentrations can yield detailed information concerning tissue metabolism.

PRINCIPLES OF NMR IMAGING

So far the origin of the signal has been considered without attention to how spatial localisation can be achieved. Spatial information is coded onto the detected signal by the use of field gradients. These gradients, whose properties are summarised in Fig. 15.9, cause the local magnetic field and thus the resonant frequency to be functions of position. Consider the simple case (Fig. 15.10) of a phantom consisting of two tubes of water in a magnetic field. In a uniform field the 'spectrum' following excitation, detection and transformation is a single line. If, however, a linear x-gradient is applied to the field, then, since each tube is now in a different local field, the 'spectrum' consists of two lines whose difference in frequency is related to the difference in their x co-ordinates. The spectrum is the projection of the phantom onto the x axis. To construct an image of two tubes it is necessary to have more information than the single projection onto the x axis indicated above. A simple y gradient would produce a second projection, which would be adequate for the simple case of two tubes; but in general more information would be necessary.

Make magnetic field depend on position

$$B_{(x,y,z,)} = \begin{vmatrix} xG_x \\ yG_y \\ zG_z \end{vmatrix} B_0 \quad G_x = \frac{\partial B_z}{\partial X}$$

Must exceed magnet inhomogeneities
Must have high linearity
Need a short rise time (~ 1 ms)

Fig. 15.9. Required properties of magnetic field gradients.

One approach, the original one used by Lauterbur, is to use a mixture of x and y gradients to produce a series of projections and to re-construct an image by the filtered backprojection methods of X-ray CT. For may reasons, some of which will be discussed later, this method is now little used in MRI.

The imaging methods currently used are based on the ideas of Ernst and on the properties of Fourier transforms. Collecting a series of n data points in the presence of an x gradient produces following transformation: a series of n spatially encoded data points. To define a planar image, spatial information about the y axis must also be encoded onto the signal. In Ernst's original proposal this was achieved by varying the duration of the time t_2 during which a y gradient was applied (Fig. 15.11a). The duration of t_2 defines the phase of signal at the start of the period t_1: 0° phase shift in t_2 being a cosine function, 90° being a sine function and so on. Repeating the procedure and collecting n data points during t_1 for m values of t_2 produces an m × n data array. Performing a double or two-dimensional (2-D) Fourier transform produces an m × n data set that now represents equally spaced points in the xy plane; that is, if the intensity of each data point is converted into a gray-scale value, the result is an image of the plane. To use the fast FT algorithm, m and n must be whole powers of 2 (e.g., 256 or 512).

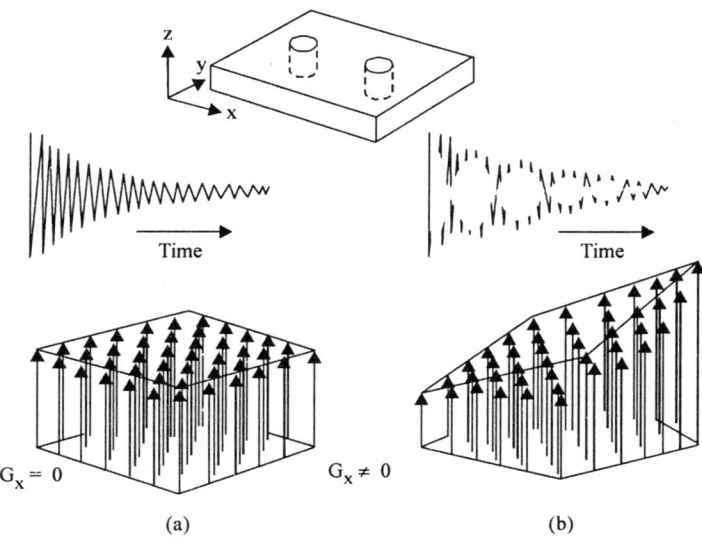

Fig. 15.10. Two-tube water phantom. (a) In the absence of a field gradient both tubes resonate at the same frequency. (b) In the presence of a gradient each resonates at its own frequency and the detected signal contains two frequencies whose difference is directly related to their separation along the x axis.

The drawback to the simple 2-D FT method is that the signal present at the start of t_1 depends on the duration of t_2, which by definition is changing during the procedure. This drawback can be minimised by using the so-called spin-wrap or phase-encoding method. The phase that is coded onto the start of the data depends on the product of the field gradient used and the duration of t_2. In the spin-wrap method, t_2 is held constant and the value of the y gradient is incremented by m equal steps over the full range (Fig. 15.11b).

The basic procedure for generating a magnetic resonance image is the following.

1. Excite the spin system.
2. Apply a phase-encoding gradient g_y for a fixed time t_2.
3. Apply a read gradient g_x and collect n data points.
4. Increment the value of g_y and repeat steps 1, 2 and 3 m times.
5. Perform a 2-D Fourier transform on the data, which produces an m by n image.

The larger the number of points collected, the smaller the separation between them and the more precise the image will be. Since axes are defined by gradient coils, all axes should be equal and sagittal and coronal images can be produced just as simply as the more familiar axial image found in CT.

It is relevant at this stage to comment on the time required to obtain an MR image. As is discussed later, steps 1, 2 and 3 take only a few tens of milliseconds; however, the spin physics demands that, to avoid complete saturation, excitation can be repeated only on a time scale of seconds. The time between successive excitations, termed TR, must therefore be of that order. Since steps 1, 2 and 3 are repeated m times, where m is the number of phase-encoding steps (i.e., rows in the final image), the total time required for an imaging procedure is m × TR. If averaging is used, then this time is increased by the number of averages taken. The number n of data points collected during the read period has effectively no influence on the total imaging time. This distinction between the effect of the number of data points collected in a read period on total imaging and the effect of the number of data points produced by phase encoding is very significant.

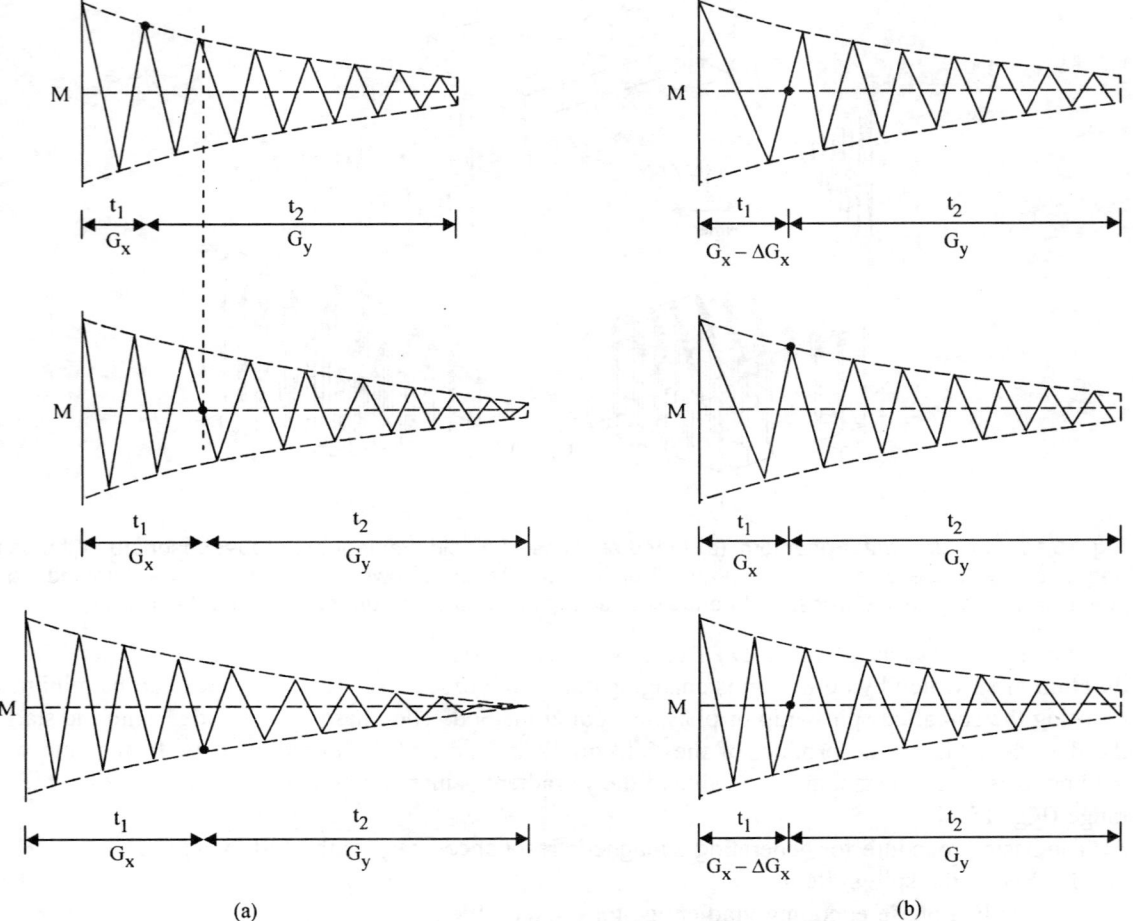

Fig. 15.11. (a) The basic 2-D FT imaging technique; and (b) the spin-wrap variation. Data are collected during the period t_2, which contains y spatial information. The x information is phase encoded during the time t_1.

MULTIPLE SLICE VERSUS VOLUME IMAGING

In the above discussion the third (z) axis was ignored; that is, the sample was assumed to be uniform in that direction. It is possible to generalise the basic procedure so far described to three dimensions by using two phase-encoding gradients prior to the read period. If l points are required on the z axis, then, the imaging procedure takes l times longer than for a planar image (i.e., $l \times m \times TR$). If $l = m = n$, then this time penalty is great, but a true isotropic image can be obtained which permits enormous flexibility with respect to image display, for example, generation of oblique slices.

Frequently there is one axis that does not require as many points; for example, a study may be satisfactorily performed with a series of, say, 20 contiguous slices (axial, coronal or sagittal). If the straightforward 3-D approach is applied, by reducing l to 20, then considerable problems due to undersampling or line spread are encountered and poor image quality results. A better and more time efficient compromise is to use a multislice approach.

In MRI, slice selection can be achieved by exciting in the presence of a pulse that contains only a discrete band of frequencies. Thus a sinc-shaped pulse applied in the presence of a z gradient excites spins only in an xy plane. The thickness of this slice depends on the strength of the gradient and the shape of the pulse (see Fig. 15.5). If the slices were studied truly sequentially, then this would increase the imaging time significantly, simply l times the time for one slice. The technique of multislice imaging minimises this effect (Fig. 15.12). In this mode, one line of slice 1 is excited and the n read points collected; but then, rather than wait (until TR) for relaxation to occur, since to a first approximation it was unaffected by the first pulse, line 1 of slice 2 is excited and so on, until time TR is reached when line 2 of slice 1 is interrogated and so on. The number of multiple slices that can be obtained depends on the time required for excitation, data collections and some data handling divided into TR. Typically, 10–20 slices are possible for a TR in the order of one second; 10–20 images can thus be obtained in the time required for a single-slice image to be obtained in the more straightforward way.

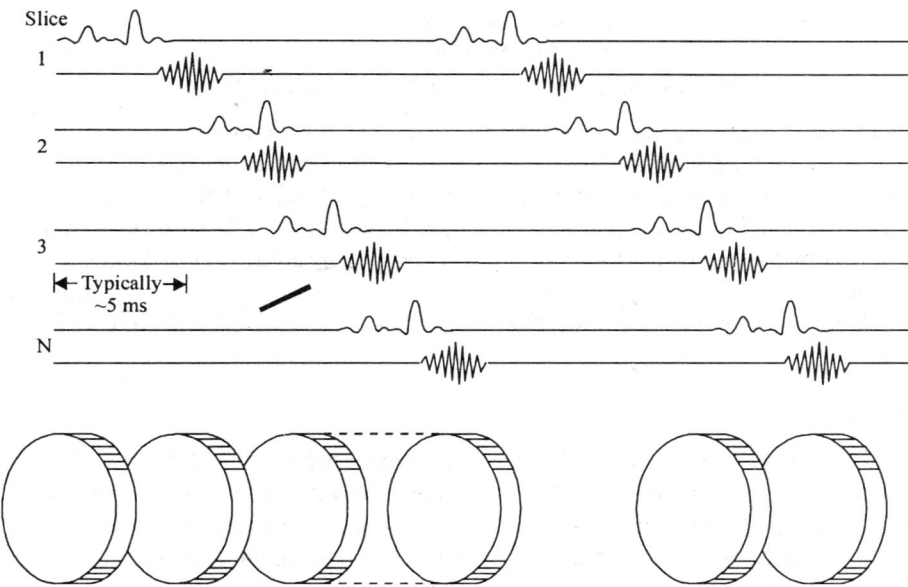

Fig. 15.12. The principle of multislice imaging. Slices are excited in sequence until time TR expires; then the first slice is excited for the second time and so forth.

IMAGING PULSE SEQUENCE

It is now appropriate to look in some detail at a practical imaging experiment. A typical imaging pulse sequence is built up from a series of building blocks, combined so as to produce a signal at the desired time and weighted by the appropriate spin properties (i.e., T_1, T_2, etc.). These blocks are non-selective rf pulse, selective rf pulse, field gradient and data collection period.

rf Pulses

The properties of the two classes of rf pulse used in MRI are summarised in Fig. 15.13. A non-selective pulse, as its name suggests, is designed to excite all nuclei equally. Such a pulse is a simple, short rectangular pulsed rf; that is, the rf comes on quickly, stays on with a constant amplitude and phase and then goes off quickly. A rectangular pulse is non-selective over a frequency range centered at its basic frequency, which approximately equals the reciprocal of its duration. If the imaging system uses a 0.5 g/cm gradient, this means that a 20 cm diameter sample in the middle of the field of view extends over ± 5 G or ± 20 kHz. A truly non-selective pulse (i.e., to within a few per cent) must therefore be less than about 50 µsec. Depending on its amplitude (or duration) a non-selective pulse can be a 90 or 180° pulse. However, if it has to last longer than the time indicated above, it is no longer truly non-selective in so much as if affects the parts of the sample at the edges less than those in the middle.

Non-selective pulse
Short (µsec)
Rectangular
Large bandwidth (~ duration^{-1})

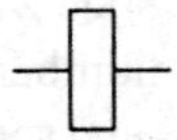

Selective pulse
Relatively long (msec)
Shaped (usually sin t/t)
Narrow in bandwidth

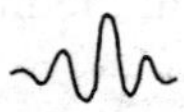

Fig. 15.13. Characteristics of rf pulses used in MRI.

A selective pulse is more complex. Here the rf is not simply switched on and off; the amplitude is shaped in such a way that it does not produce a continuous band of frequencies but only a limited band of frequencies; thus, in the presence of a gradient, only limited parts of the sample are affected. The major use of selective pulses is in the presence of a z gradient to select a slice: if, for example, the pulses sample in the xy plane from z_1 to z_2. The pulse is usually shaped by a function of the form (sin x)/x $\equiv$ sinc x and the narrower the required frequency range of the pulse, the longer and more complex the shaping required. Typical selective pulses are millisecond in duration compared with microseconds for non-selective pulses.

Field Gradients

The purpose of field gradients is to encode spatial information onto the NMR signal; this they do by making the frequency response characteristic of position. Field gradients have two effects on an NMR signal: the wanted one given above and the unwanted one of dephasing the signal. The two are intimately related. Following a 90° pulse, the vector representing all the nuclear spins is pointing along the y' axis. If the field is non-uniform (e.g., has a gradient), this vector will fan out in the x'y' plane as some components move faster than the average and some slower. This is called dephasing and it is the degree of this dephasing that gives us the spatial information we want. Dephasing does, however, also reduce the detectable signal. A balance has to be struck between sufficient dephasing to allow an analysis of the individual components (which ultimately become pixels in the final image) and not so much dephasing that the signal decays too far to be useful. The properties of field gradient are summarised in Fig. 15.9.

Fortunately, if, as is sometimes the case (e.g., in slice selection), we have 'finished' with a field gradient early in the sequence, we can reverse the unwanted dephasing by a 'time-reversal' gradient, that is, a gradient of equal magnitude but opposite sign to the one we would apply to achieve the desired effect. Under the influence of a time-reversal gradient, the dephasing caused by the first gradient is reversed and signal grows again. This effect is similar to, but distinct from, the spin echo, in which the vectors are interchanged by a 180° pulse, it is called time reversal because reversing the sign of the gradient can be thought of as reversing the direction of dephasing with respect to time. In other words, real-time dephasing becomes re-phasing.

Data Collection Period

The final component of an imaging sequence is the period during which the signal is detected in the presence of a read gradient g_x. The NMR signal then contains a mixture of frequencies whose range depends on the size of the object and the gradients used. If the object is central and 20 cm in diameter, then with 0.5 g/cm gradients the NMR signal contains frequencies of $\pm$ 20 kHz about the basic frequency of the pulse. A fundamental theorem of data processing (Nyquist theorem) tells us that to record a signal unambiguously we must sample at twice the maximum frequency present in the signal, that is, 40 kHz in the above example.

This can be converted into two rules of thumb.

1. The rate of data acquisition $\propto$ (field gradient used) $\times$ (field of view) $\times \gamma / 2\pi$.
2. The duration of NMR signal acquisition $\propto$ to

$$\frac{\text{number of pixel columns in final image}}{(\text{field of view}) \times (\text{field gradient})} \approx 5 \text{ msec}$$

In practice the data-acquisition time is usually kept constant and the gradients adjusted to match the field view.

The imaging sequence currently most commonly used is to hold the duration of the phase-encoding gradient constant and vary its amplitude. The sequence can be divided into five stages as shown in Fig. 15.14. For the case of a planar sequence the stages are described in the following paragraphs.

Stage 1: The first stage in obtaining a 2-D or planar image is to select a slice. This selection is achieved by applying a field gradient on the z axis and a selective 90° pulse. This result in all the nuclei in the appropriate xy plane being excited. If a narrow slice is required, then a high gradient and a long selection pulse are required; during this selection period a large amount of unwanted phasing occurs and only a small signal results. The gradient is present only to permit slice selection; once that is over, its presence and consequences are no longer required. Thus dephasing is an unwanted consequence of slice selection.

Stage 2: Since the dephasing in Stage 1 is unwanted after slice selection has been achieved, it is now removed (as discussed previously) with a time-reversal gradient. At the end of this time-reversal period, a much larger signal is obtained than without the reversal gradient. The signal has decayed only by spin-spin relaxation during the time elapsed.

Stage 3: After a slice is selected, the next stage is to encode spatial information onto it. This is achieved for one axis by applying a read gradient during the collection of the FID. The detected signal now decays much faster than previously since it is collected in the presence of a gradient, but it contains the x information we require. After transform and so on, this signal corresponds to the projection of the signal from the selected xy plane onto the x axis. If a second gradient G_y is simultaneously applied such that $G_x = \sin \theta$ and $G_y = \cos \theta$ and θ is incremented, then a series of projections of the object can be obtained. This is the simple projection-reconstruction imaging experiment. The projections obtained for various values of θ are backprojected and so on, as in the case of X-ray CT.

In the case of 2-D FT, the two gradients are applied in sequence and hence the data set produced is a projection on the x axis by row and the y axis by column; re-construction now is simpler and less sensitive to instrumental problems such as magnet inhomogeneity. The procedure is repeated for as many values of G_y as required to define the y axis of the final image.

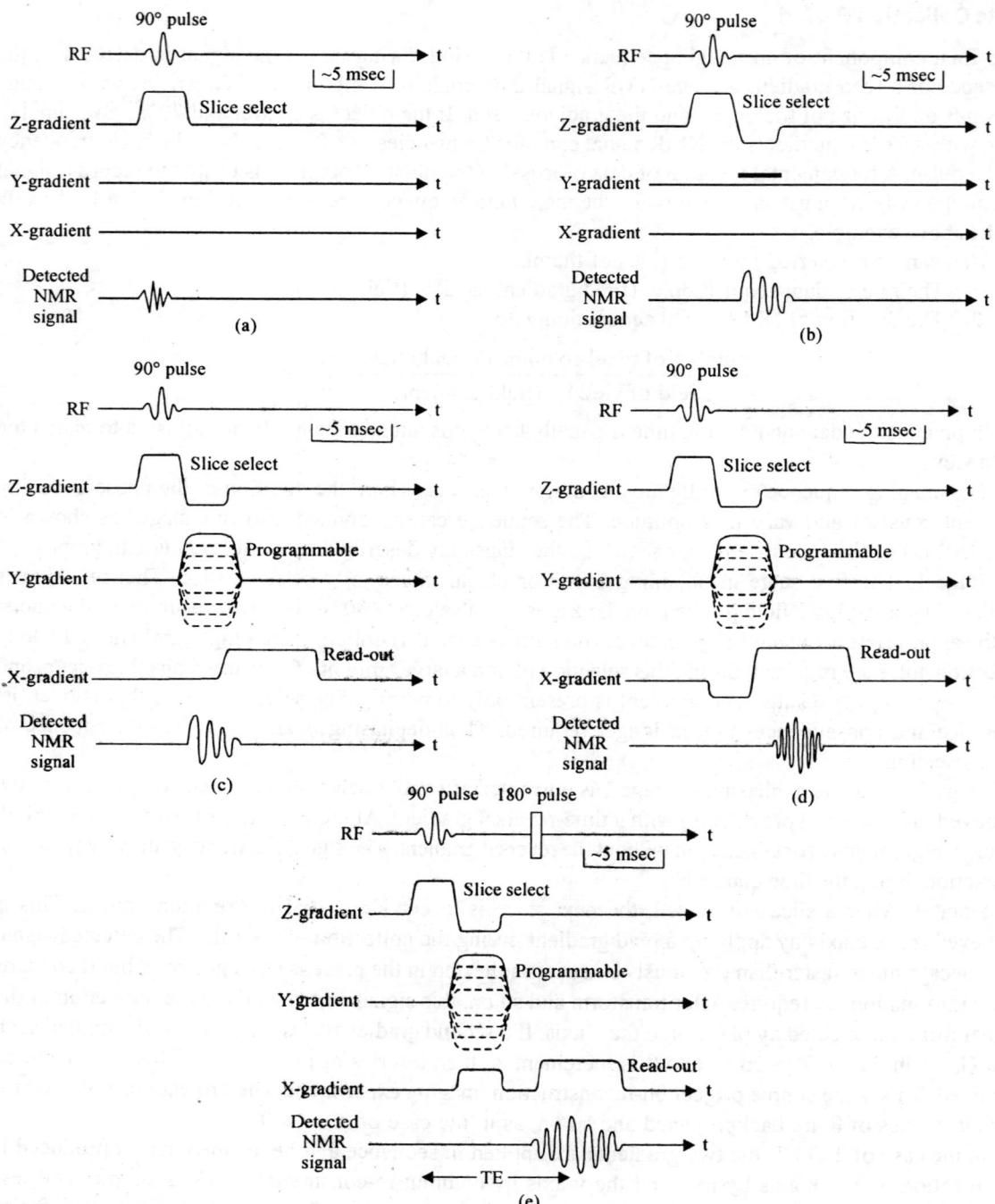

Fig. 15.14. The five basic stages of spin a imaging sequence. (a) Select slice. (b) Re-phase spins. (c) Apply phase-encoding and read-out gradients. (d) Dephase prior to read-out gradient. (e) Generate spin echo to overcome magnet inhomogeneities.

Stage 4: The problem with the simple sequence shown in Stage 3 is an instrumental one. Gradients do not switch as quickly as is implied in the drawing. It is a short time, but since the signal is decaying rapidly, a significant time, before they stabilise and accurate data can be collected. This can be overcome by applying a time-reversal gradient before the read gradient, at the time that the unwanted consequences of G_z are being corrected. The signal recovery from the initial dephasing occurs during the read period and an echo like signal, called a field echo, appears, as shown. This echo can be considered as two back-to-back FIDs and is transformed to produce a projection in the same way as discussed above. The reversal gradient, like the y encoding gradient, is frequently given a gaussian shape to optimise the shape of lines in the frequency spectrum used to construct the image.

Stage 5: The final level of sophistication is to use a 180° pulse, as shown in Fig. 15.14e, to produce a spin echo. The use of a spin echo re-focuses the unwanted defocusing due to magnet inhomogeneity up to the time of data collection, which is defined by the field echo produced by the time reversal-gradient period discussed in Stage 4. If the spin and field echoes do not coincide, then chemical shift effects are introduced (see later). Note that the sign of the time-reversal gradient is inverted to allow for the effect of the 180° pulse.

All pulses applied in an imaging sequence are imperfect; that is, they do not produce the exact degree of magnetisation change required over all the sample. These imperfections are due to both timing and shaping errors and to the fact that pulses are not infinitely powerful. The consequences of these imperfections are not too serious for 90° pulses, because the effect of a 180° pulse is not too different from that of a 90° pulse. Imperfections are, however, very important for a 180° pulse, which is required to produce zero transverse magnetisation. Deviation from this condition produces some magnetisation which cause subsequent problems. Residual transverse magnetisation can be minimised by applying short, intense field gradients (so-called homospoil pulses) immediately after a 180° pulse to destroy any unwanted residual xy magnetisation.

FACTORS AFFECTING IMAGE APPEARANCE

Many factors affect the appearance of an image. The purpose of this section is to outline briefly the effects of some of the extrinsic variables on the final image. Straightforward effects such as non-linear gradients producing geometrically distorted images or changing display parameters (e.g., window and level) will not be considered, neither will the changing of image contrast due to differential proton density (defined as [H]) T_1 and T_2 weighting.

Signal-to-Noise Ratio

To produce an acceptable image, a signal-to-noise ratio (SNR) in the order of 20:1 is necessary; above this level the eye perceives little improvement. The major factors affecting both signal and noise are listed in Fig. 15.15. The significance of those parameters affected by field are discussed in next section.

Voxel size and read gradient strength affect the noise by their affect on the receiver bandwidth necessary, whereas reducing the size of the voxel reduces the size of the signal resulting from it. The net result is that for a given set of conditions, the SNR in an image scales linearly with voxel size.

Voxel Size

Apart from its effect on SNR the size of the voxel also affects image appearance through partial-volume effects. If the pixel is larger than the structural homogeneity of the tissue being imaged, then the signal that makes up any voxel is an average; so small structures are lost.

Parameters affecting signal to noise[1]

	Signal	Noise
Magnet field	B_0[2]	
Operating frequency	ω_0[3]	ω_0[4]
Voxel size	Volume	(No. of cols)$^{-1/2}$
Number of averages	N	$N^{1/2}$
Read-out gradient		$G_x^{-1/2}$

1. Assuming constant imaging time	2. Induced frequency
3. Boltzman effect	4. Patient noise

Fig. 15.15. Summary of the factors affecting SNR, assuming constant imaging time.

Motion Artifacts

As with any imaging modality, patient motion during the procedure produces artifacts. Motion during the actual period of data collection (which is only a few milliseconds long) is negligible; however, motions on the time scale of the whole imaging sequence (i.e., m × TR) are significant. Such motions result in phase modulation of the data and are thus seen as ghosts in the phase-encoding direction only. Their displacement is proportional to the frequency of the motion and their intensity to the amplitude of the displacement.

Regular or semi-regular involuntary motion artifacts can be minimised by synchronisation, for example, to the ECG signal in the case of cardiac motion. Since the periodicity of the cardiac cycle is comparable to TR, the time penalty is slight; however, this is not the case for respiratory motion in which simple gating to collect data during the period of minimum thoracic motion slows the imaging procedure significantly. To compensate for breathing motion, chest position has to be sensed and software procedures used. With sophisticated algorithms, only a time overhead of about 5–10 per cent is necessary to compensate for respiratory motion.

Effect of Field Strength in MRI

The strength of the magnetic field used to polarise the nuclear spins affects MR images in three ways: by increasing the SNR, by changing the absolute and relative values of T_1 and by increasing chemical shift effects. Increasing the magnetic field applied to the nuclear spin system increases, proportionally, the energy difference ΔE between the ground and the excited state, which consequently increases their population difference; this in turn increases the magnitude of the detected signal. Parallel with increasing field is increasing Larmor frequency. This in turn proportionally increases the detected signal because of more efficient coupling of the nuclear magnetisation to the detection coil; thus the signal increases as B^2 or v^2. Unfortunately, noise also increases with operating frequency; thus,

$$\text{noise} \propto (a \cdot v^{1/2} + b \cdot v^2)^{1/2} \qquad \text{... (15.6)}$$

where 'a' is the noise generated by circuit resistance and b the noise generated by the patient, who is a large conducting body. Except at frequencies below about 10 MHz the patient noise is dominant and hence noise scales with frequency. The SNR thus scales linearly with operating field.

The above discussion is superficial and many assumptions have been made, such as constant receiver bandwidth; however, the linear increase in SNR with field is empirically supported.

Spin-spin relaxation is effectively constant for biological tissues in the frequency used for imaging; spin-lattice relaxation, however; has a dependence on field of the form

$$T_1 \propto Av^B \qquad \qquad \text{... (15.7)}$$

where A and B are tissue specific constants, B being in the range 0.2–0.4.

In a T_1 weighted image, therefore, contrast changes with operating field. The exact change depends on the tissue interface considered and the pulse sequence used. Since the SNR increases with field, the ability to differentiate tissue interfaces (i.e., contrast to noise) increases with field. However, the magnitude of the gain in contrast to noise depends on the pulse timing used and the specific interface considered.

The effects of the chemical shift on imaging are dealt with in later section of this chapter. All that is necessary here is to point out that chemical shift differences increase proportionally to the applied magnetic field.

PULSE SEQUENCES AND IMAGE CONTRAST

The origin of contrast in an MR image is a complex topic that depends on many intrinsic parameters such as proton density [H], T_1, T_2, flow and chemical shift (in chemical shift imaging).

If the image is formed from data collected with an interval between the 90° pulses (TR) that is long compared with T_1 and a short TE, then only proton density affects the image. The differences in proton density among the various soft tissues is, however, relatively small compared with the differences in T_1 and T_2. Image contrast can therefore be enhanced if relaxation effects are brought into play.

The signal contributing an image can be expressed in terms of the times between successive 90° pulses (TR) and the time at which signal is detected (TE); thus,

$$M_y \propto [H]\left(1 - 2\exp\left[-\frac{(TR - TE/2)}{T_1}\right]\right) + \exp\left(-\frac{TR}{T_1}\right)\exp\left(-\frac{TE}{T_2}\right) \qquad \text{... (15.8)}$$

Two limiting cases are normally considered. The first is the so-called partial saturation sequence when $TE \ll T_2 \ll TR$ and Eq. (15.9) reduces to:

$$M_y \propto [H](1 - \exp(-TR/T_1)) \qquad \qquad \text{... (15.9)}$$

that is, an image weighted by proton density and T_1 is produced. The second is the spin echo sequence where TE becomes comparable to T_2 but still much less than TR. If TR is long compared with T_1, then an image weighted by proton density and T_2 results:

$$M_y \propto [H]\exp(-TE/T_2) \qquad \qquad \text{... (15.10)}$$

The simplest way to use relaxation effects for image contrast is to use the partial saturation sequence and apply the second 90° pulse before the spin system has fully relaxed, while keeping TE very short. As is shown in Fig. 15.16, the tissues with a long T_1, such as cerebrospinal fluid, have their signal saturated more than those with a short T_1, such as white matter and contrast is enhanced.

An alternative approach for adding relaxation contrast is to make TR long (i.e., remove T_1 effects) but lengthen TE (Fig. 15.17), which introduces T_2 contrast into the image. When using a spin echo sequence, one can generate multiple echoes by applying more than one 180° pulse, producing further echoes and thus obtaining a series of images with progressively greater T_2 induced contrast (but with progressively lower signal due to signal decay). Obviously, if TR is shortened, then contrast can be introduced by T, in addition to T_2.

A third sequence used in MRI is the inversion recovery sequence, in which the equilibrium magnetisation is inverted by a 180° pulse and then the image is produced by a 90° pulse TI seconds later (Fig. 15.18). During the period between the inversion and reading pulses the signal relaxes from $-M_z$ toward M_z as $[1 - 2 \exp(-TI/T_1)]$. This sequence produces images with high T_1 contrast but takes longer than the other two sequences.

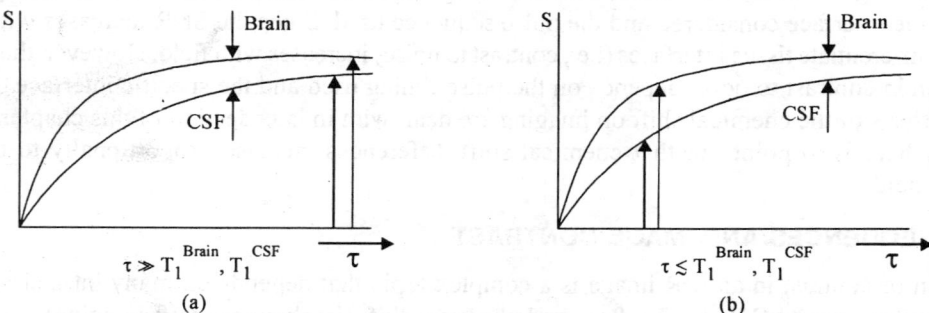

(a)   (b)

Fig. 15.16. Growth showing the source of contrast in a partial separation sequence.

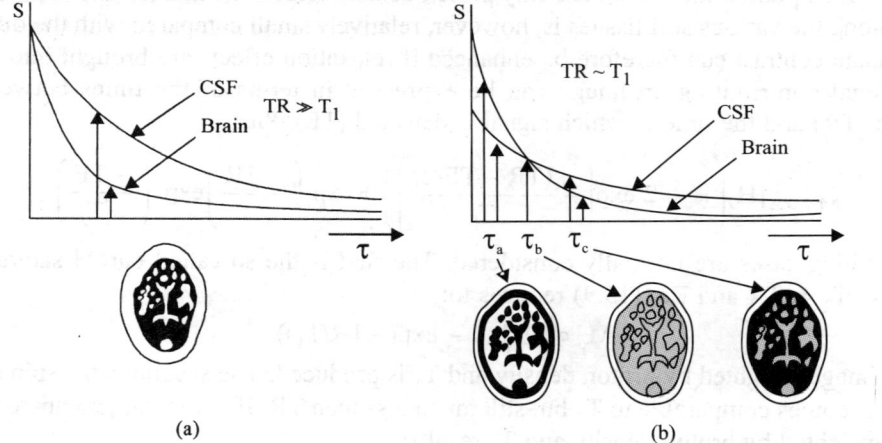

(a)   (b)

Fig. 15.17. Graphs showing the source of contrast in a spin echo sequence (a) with no T, weighting; (b) with T, weighting.

Choosing the most efficient sequence and optimising the parameters to produce the best image is a complex procedure. Various pathologies are best seen utilising various processes; for example, the long I_2 of edema makes it show well in images with a long TE. A very simplistic approach is to define TR to optimise T_1 effects (or TI if T_1 is very important)—typically TR is 1–2 seconds—and then use this time to collect as many image planes or echoes as the system allows. The choice of the number of TE/slice and thus the value, depends on the significance of T_2 in showing the pathology of interest.

EFFECT OF FLOW ON MAGNETIC RESONANCE IMAGES

MR images are affected by flow in a complex way. In a simple planar imaging protocol using PS techniques, a flowing liquid appears bright since unsaturated blood is flowing into the imaging plane.

Axial flow can be made a source of contrast in two basic ways. First, a plane downstream of the imaging plane can be subjected to a 180° pulse and an image collected some T seconds later. If this image is subtracted from an image taken without perturbing the downstream plane, then only areas in which nuclei from the downstream plane have flowed into the imaging plane appear in the subtraction image. By varying the position of the plane and the time T, one can obtain detailed flow information.

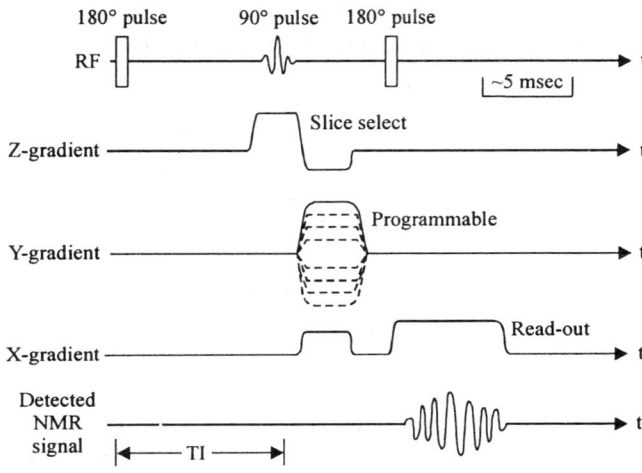

Fig. 15.18. Inversion recovery sequence.

A second method is to apply an extra gradient period, followed by an equal time period with the opposite gradient, before the data collection echo occurs. To first order for non-flowing liquids, this has no effect on the image; the second period re-phases the dephasing of the first period. Flowing liquids, by definition, are not a constant position and since there is a gradient present, spins in a flowing liquid are not in the same field during the second or re-phasing, period as they were during the first period. They are therefore subject to net dephasing, that is, loss of signal. Appropriate data processing produces an image in which a scale indicates flow velocity.

When multiple-echo images are obtained, they are sensitive to flow within the plane. Basically, even echoes re-focus any transverse flow effects; therefore, images obtained by subtracting images obtained from odd and even echoes in a multiple-echo sequence illustrate transverse or in-plane flow.

CHEMICAL SHIFT IMAGING (CSI)

In the imaging methods discussed so far the data were collected in the presence of a read gradient. This read gradient tends to swamp the small differences that arise from chemical shift effects. As already discussed the proton signal from a patient consists, to a first approximation, of two signals: that from water and that from triglycerides in fatty tissue. When one is using high-field systems, this chemical shift effect, if uncorrected (see later), can lead to a shift or ambiguity of about 1 or 2 pixels at the boundary of tissue that has a large different fat content, typically in the abdomen. Chemical shift effects appear only in the read direction.

The full chemical shift information (i.e., the NMR spectrum) can be recovered if data are collected in the absence of a field gradient. The most general approach is to phase-encode spatial information and collect the final data set without a gradient (Fig. 15.19).

A 3-D Fourier transform yields a planar image in which each pixel (i.e., xy value) has an n-point NMR spectrum; n is typically 512 or 1024 points. Such an image is termed as chemical shift image. Since each additional phase-encoding value takes a further TR, high spatial resolution images take a long time; for example; a 32×32 image with TR = 1 second takes about 17 minutes per average. Furthermore, to achieve a satisfactory SNR in the frequency (chemical shift) domain, several averages are often required. The data set, even for a planar image, is now three dimensional (i.e., x, y, δ). The information can be presented either as a spectrum from each pixel [M $(\delta)_{xy}$] or as an image for each chemical shift $(M_{(xy)}\delta)$.

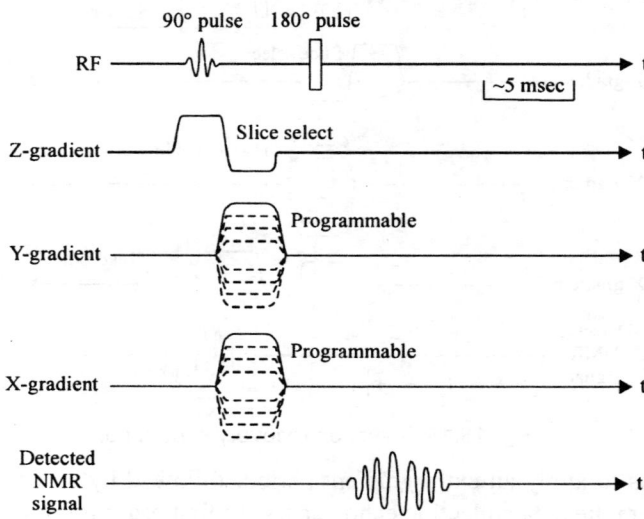

Fig. 15.19. Pulse sequence used to obtain chemical-shift images.

The reason for using the above sequence is that full definition of all the lines in an NMR spectrum requires many points; for example, for high-resolution spectra of a solution, up to 16 or 32 thousand, may be required. Increasing the number of read data points does not cost time. On the other hand, from a simple, clinical proton-imaging view point, separation of images from the two major components (i.e., water and fat) may well be sufficient. To do so requires only two data points. Under these circumstances it is more time efficient to phase encode the chemical shift information.

Chemical shift information can be phase encoded onto the image data set by making the field echo and the spin echo occur at different times. At the time of the spin echo, all the vectors, such as those from water and fat, are in phase. Thus, if the field echo and the spin echo coincide, then the signal is water and fat. Following this echo, the vectors get out of phase with each other at a rate that depends on their chemical shift difference Δ. As already discussed, the data collection period is defined by the timing of the field echo. Thus, if the field echo occurs when the two vectors are 180° out of phase, ½Δ second after the spin echo, the image corresponds to water minus fat. Having sum and difference images makes it trivial to obtain the two images separately, as shown in Fig. 15.19. This method can be extended to more than two components if their relative chemical shifts are known beforehand. By shifting the water and lipid images by the appropriate number of pixels and adding an image corrected for chemical shift problems induced of tissues boundaries can be generated. The latter technique can be called chemically selective imaging and is more time effective than full chemical shift imaging if there are only a few components of comparable concentrations to be separated. Since the technique uses subtraction, there can be problems looking for minor components. If multiple or unknown components are to be studied, then true shift imaging is the preferred method.

INSTRUMENTATION

Three basic components make up the MRI scanner: the magnet, three magnetic field gradient coils and an RF coil. The magnet polarises the protons in the patient, the magnetic field gradient coils impose a linear variation on the proton Larmor frequency as a function of position and the RF coil produces the oscillating magnetic field necessary for creating phase coherence between protons and also receives the MRI signal via Faraday induction. Each MRI system has a number of different-sized RF coils, used according to the particular part of the body being imaged, which are placed on or around the patient. The gradient coils are fixed permanently inside the bore of the superconducting magnet.

In addition to these three elements there is a series of electronic components used to turn the gradients on and off, to pulse the B_1 field and to amplify and digitise the signal. A simplified block diagram of a system is shown in Fig. 15.20. Various components are discussed further in the following sections.

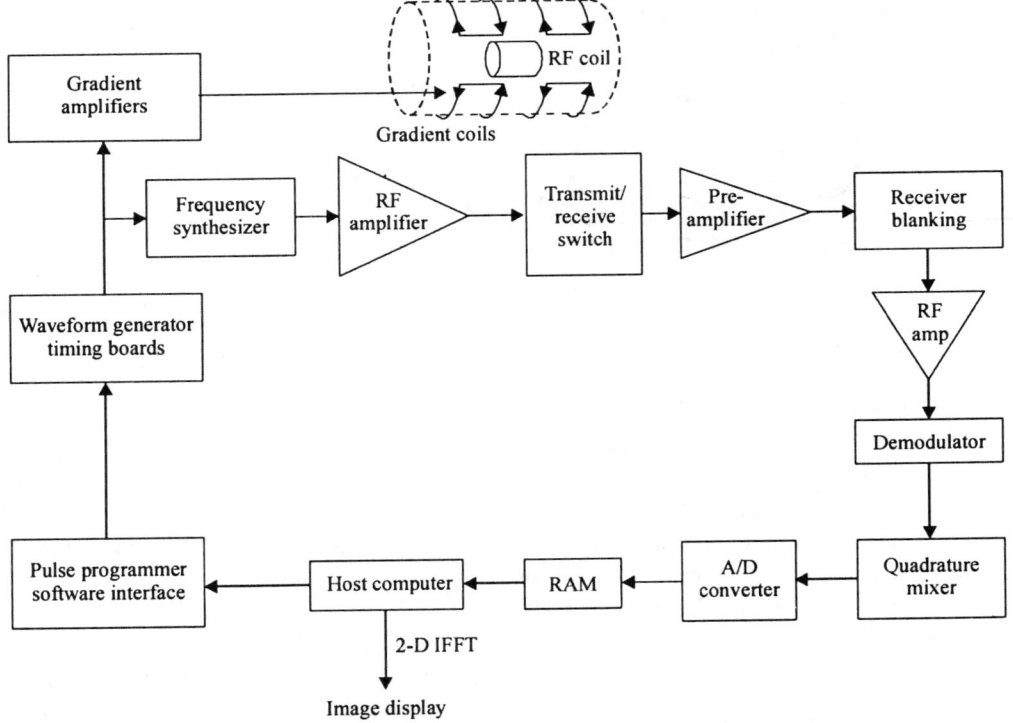

Fig. 15.20. A block diagram of the electronic and computer components making up an MRI systems.

Magnet Design

The purpose of the magnet is to produce a strong, temporally stable and homogeneous magnetic field within the patient. A strong magnetic field increases the amplitude of the MRI signal, a homogeneous magnetic field is required so that the tissue T_2 value is not too short and images are not distorted by B_0

inhomogeneities and high stability is necessary to avoid introducing unwanted artifacts into the image. There are three basic types of magnet: permanent, resistive and superconducting.

For magnetic fields of approximately 0.35 T or less, either resistive or permanent magnets can be used. Permanent magnet systems are usually constructed of rare earth alloys such as cobalt-samarium. Their advantages include relatively low cost, ease of siting due to very limited stray magnetic fields present outside the magnet, the lack of a requirement for cooling the magnet and a reduced susceptibility to patient claustrophobia due to their open nature, as can be seen in Fig. 15.21. Permanent magnet systems are used widely for interventional MRI, in which surgical procedures are carried out in the magnet simultaneously with imaging. The disadvantages of permanent magnets are the very large weight of such magnets and the fact that the field homogeneity and temporal stability are highly temperature-dependent, meaning that sophisticated thermal regulation must be used.

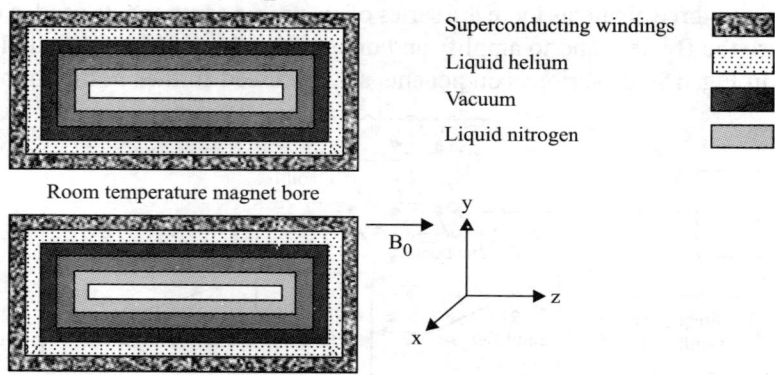

Fig. 15.21. A schematic of the construction of a superconducting magnet.

In resistive magnets, the magnetic field is created by the passage of a constant current through a conductor as copper. The strength of the magnetic field is directly proportional to the magnitude of the current and thus high currents are necessary to create high magnetic fields. However, the amount of power dissipated in the wire is proportional to the resistance of the conductor and the square of the current. Because the power is dissipated in the form of heat, cooling the conductors is a major problem and ultimately limits the maximum current and therefore magnetic field strength, that can be achieved with a resistive magnet. As with permanent magnets, the field homogeneity and the temporal stability of resistive magnets are highly temperature-dependent.

The solution to the problem of conductor heating is to minimise the resistance of the conductor by using the phenomenon of superconductivity, in which the resistance of many conductors becomes zero at very low temperature. In order to create high static magnetic fields, it is still necessary for the conductor to carry a large current when it is superconducting and this capability is only possessed by certain alloys, particularly those made from niobium-titanium. Below a critical temperature (9 K) and critical magnetic field (10 T), once current has been fed into such an alloy, this current will run through the wire with constant magnitude essentially indefinitely. Superconducting magnets are used for most systems above 0.35 T. The most common field for clinical scanning is 1.5 T, although 3 T systems are becoming increasingly common, particularly for brain scanning and experimental systems operating at 7 and 8 T now exist for human study. Figure 15.20 shows a typical clinical 1.5 T scanner, with a moveable bed used to position the patient at the centre of the magnet.

The superconducting alloy is usually fashioned into multistranded filaments within a conducting matrix because this arrangement can support a higher critical current than a single, larger-diameter superconducting wire. This superconducting matrix is housed in a stainless steel can containing liquid helium at a temperature of 4.2 K. This can is surrounded by a series of radiation shields and vacuum vessels to minimise the boil-off of the liquid helium. Finally, an outer container of liquid nitrogen is used to cool the outside of the vacuum chamber and the radiation shields. Because heat losses cannot be completely contained, liquid nitrogen and liquid helium must be replenished on a regular basis.

The exact placement of the superconducting filaments within the magnet is designed to give the maximum B_0 homogeneity over the patient region. The basic design consists of a number of solenoids of different diameters and separations, each wound along the major axis of the magnet. Slight errors in positioning the wires can lead to large variations in the field uniformity and so additional coils of wire are added in series with the main coil as 'correction coils.' After the magnet has been energised by passing current into the major filament windings, the current can be changed in these correction coils to improve the homogeneity. Final fine tuning is performed by using a series of independently wired coils, termed shim coils. The operator can adjust the current in these coils of each clinical examination and so the magnet homogeneity can be optimised for individual patients.

Magnetic Field Gradient Coils

The basic principle of MRI requires the generation of magnetic field gradients, in addition to the static magnetic field, so that the proton resonant frequencies within the patient are spatially dependent. Such gradients are achieved using 'magnetic field gradient coils,' a term usually shortened to simply 'gradient coils.' Three separate gradient coils are required to encode the x, y and z dimensions of the image. The requirements for gradient coil design are that the gradients are linear over the region being imaged, that they are efficient in terms of producing high gradient strengths per unit current and that they have fast switching times for use in rapid imaging techniques.

As in the case of magnet design, a magnetic field gradient is produced by the passage of current through conducting wires. Unlike the design of the magnet, however, the geometry of the conductors for the three gradient coils must be optimised to produce a linear gradient, rather than a uniform field. The value of the gradient is relatively small compared to the strength of the main magnetic field, with typical values of 4 G/cm for clinical scanners. Copper at room temperature can therefore be used as the conductor, with chilled-water cooling being sufficient to remove the heat generated by the current. Because the gradient coils fit directly inside the bore of the cylindrical magnet, the geometrical design is usually cylindrical. The simplest configuration for the coil producing a gradient in the z direction is a 'Maxwell pair,' shown in Fig. 15.22, which consists of two separate loops consisting of multiple turns of wire. The two loops are wound in opposite directions around a cylindrical former and the loops are spaced by a separation of $\sqrt{3}$ times the radius of the loop. The magnetic field produced by this gradient coil is zero at the centre of the coil and is linearly dependent upon position in the z direction over about one-third of the separation of the two loops. The gradient strength is proportional to the square of the number of turns. The x and y-gradient coils are completely independent from the z-gradient coils and each gradient coil is connected to a separate gradient amplifier. From symmetry considerations the same basic design can be used for coils producing gradients in the x and y directions with the geometries simply rotated by 90°. The most common configuration is the 'saddle coil' arrangement, with four arcs, as shown in Fig. 15.22. Each arc subtends an angle of 120°, the separation between the arcs along the z axis is 0.8 times the radius of the gradient coil and the length of each arc is 2.57 times the radius.

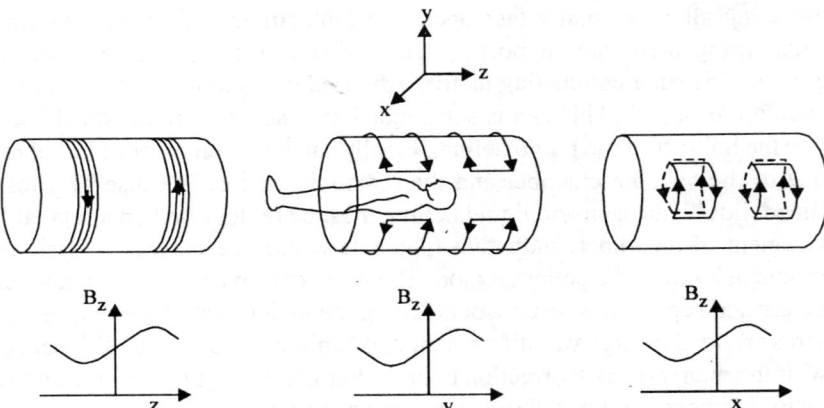

Fig. 15.22. The basic design of magnetic field gradient coils used for MRI. The arrows indicate the direction of current flow. (Left) A z-gradient coil, (centre) a y-gradient coil and (right) an x-gradient coil. Each coil consists of multiple turns of wire, which for clarity are only shown for the z-gradient coil. The useable region of the magnet effectively corresponds to the volume over which the gradients are linear.

A second design criterion is that the current in the gradient coils should be switched on and off in the shortest possible time. This reduces the time which must be allowed for gradient stabilisation in imaging sequences. This criterion is achieved by minimising the inductance of the gradient coils. A related issue is achieving high minimising the inductance of the gradient coils. A related issue is achieving high efficiency, that is, a high gradient per unit current, which corresponds to minimising the resistance of the gradient coils. When the gradients are switched rapidly, they induce eddy currents in nearby conducting surfaces such as the radiation shield in the magnet. These currents, in turn, produce additional unwanted gradients, which may decay only very slowly, even after the original gradients have been switched off. All gradient coils in commercial MRI systems are now 'actively shielded' to reduce the effects of eddy currents. Active shielding uses a second set of coils placed outside the main gradient coils, the effect of which is to minimise the stray gradient fields.

Radiofrequency Coils

As described previously, in order to produce an MRI signal, magnetic energy must be supplied to the protons at the Larmor frequency in order to stimulate transitions between the parallel and the antiparallel nuclear energy levels, thus creating precessing transverse magnetisation. The particular piece of hardware that delivers this energy is called an RF coil, which is usually placed directly around or next to, the tissue to be imaged. The same RF coil is also usually used to detect the NMR signal via Faraday induction. The power needed to generate the RF pulses for clinical systems can be many kilowatts and the receiver is designed to detect signals only on the order of 1–10 V. Therefore, it is important that during signal transmission there is no possibility of signal 'leaking' through to the receiver and damaging the electronics. A transmit/receive switch and active receiver blanking, both shown in Fig. 15.20, are used to ensure that the leakage is minimised.

Superficially, the RF coil could be thought of as performing in a similar way to a conventional radio antenna, but there are several important differences in its function and design. An antenna is designed to radiate a large fraction of its input power into the far field. An RF coil, on the other hand, should be designed to store as much of its magnetic energy as possible in the near-field region, that is, within the patient. The most efficient coil design is based on resonant electric circuits, in which where there is a resonant frequency ω_r at which the magnetic energy stored in the coil is a maximum.

In terms of the electrical properties of the coil, this frequency is given by

$$\omega_r = \frac{1}{\sqrt{LC}} \qquad \qquad ...\,(15.11)$$

where L is the inductance of the RF coil. The value of C represents both the intrinsic capacitance of the coil and also the capacitance that is added, in the form of discrete capacitors, to the circuit for tuning the resonance to ω_r and also matching the input impedance to 50 Ω for maximum operational efficiency. A well-designed coil efficiently converts power from a frequency source and RF amplifier into an oscillating magnetic field, thereby minimising the power deposited in the patient. It also detects the precessing nuclear magnetisation efficiently, resulting in a high image SNR. Examples of RF coil geometries for imaging different body parts are—'birdcage' coil, 'volume coil' designed to give a spatially uniform magnetic field over the entire volume of the coil. It is typically used for brain, abdominal and knee studies. The circular loop coil, is a 'surface' coil, used to image objects at the surface of the body with high sensitivity. The third type of coil, is a 'phased array,' which consists of a series of surface coils. These coils are typically used to image large structures such as the spine. A phased array maintains the high sensitivity of a small coil, but, by using a large number of coils, the FOV can be made much larger than for a single coil. A phased array needs a system with multiple receiver channels, one for each coil.

The design of volume coils aims to produce a spatially uniform B_1 field across, for example, the entire volume of the head. From electromagnetic theory, a perfectly homogeneous B_1 field transverse to the cylindrical axis can be generated in an infinitely long cylinder by surface currents running parallel to the axis of the cylinder. The required current density is proportional to the sine of the azimuthal angle ϕ, as shown in Fig. 15.23. A practical realisation of this theoretical result is the 'birdcage coil,' shown schematically in Fig. 15.23, which uses a large number of parallel conductors, typically between 16 and 32.

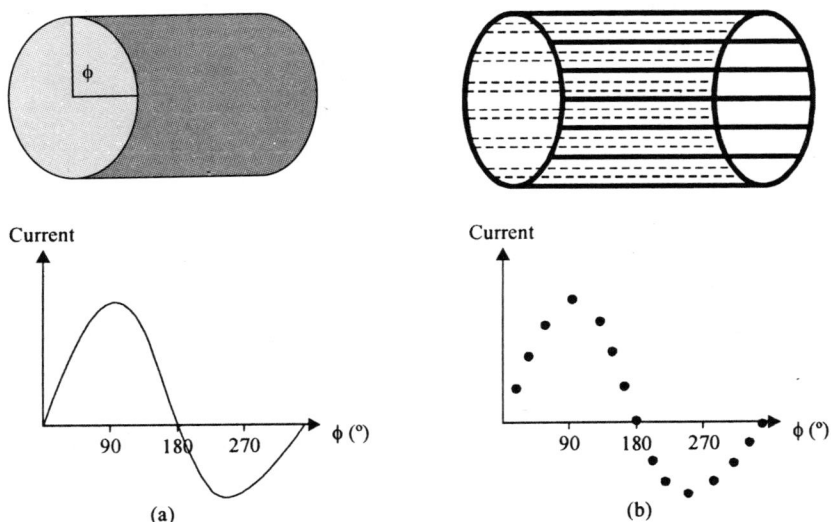

Fig. 15.23. (a) The ideal current density needed to produce a spatially uniform B_1 field across a sample placed in the cylindrical coil. A practical realisation of the theoretical model is the birdcage design with multiple parallel conductors.

Many clinical studies only need to look at tissues close to the surface of the body. In this case, the best RF coil design is a surface coil. The simplest design is basically a loop of wire, with additional capacitance added to resonate the coil at the required frequency. This coil has very high efficiency close to the coil, but suffers from extremely poor B_1 homogeneity due to its geometry, as shown in Fig. 15.24. The normal mode of operation is that the RF pulses are applied by a large volume coil surrounding the patient and the signal is received from the surface coil. Crossed diodes are included in the coil networks to decouple the two coils during signal transmission and reception.

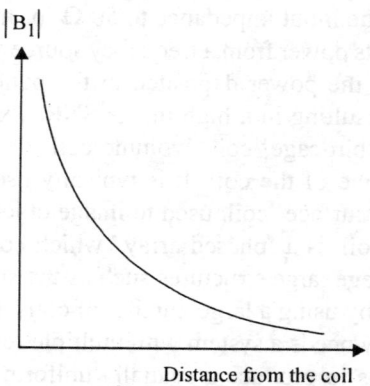

Fig. 15.24. A plot of the magnitude of the B_1 field versus distance from the coil for a surface coil. Very high signal can be obtained close to the coil, but the signal from tissues deep in the patient is very low.

Chapter 16

Ultrasonic Imaging Systems

INTRODUCTION

Medical ultrasonics is a field that, by all accounts, is expected to expand by a large margin over the next few years. It encompasses a large number of different instruments or devices that are diagnostic or therapeutic. In most electronic specialities, the words ultrasonic and ultrasound usually denote a signal that has a frequency above the range of human hearing but below something loosely termed radio frequency. For most applications, this will mean 20000 to 1,50,000 Hz, the exact limits being dependent upon who is setting them and for what purpose they are needed. Medical ultrasound, however, usually involves frequencies ranging from approximately 20 kHz to well over 10 MHz.

Some physical therapy 'ultrasound' is actually radio-frequency waves well into the UHF region. This latter, though, is more properly relegated to the field of diathermy. The use of frequencies to 10 MHz under the heading 'ultrasound' is not really a contradiction because it assumes another factor and that is the nature of the physical wave generated. To be sure, a 2500 kHz or 10 MHz electrical signal would generate an electromagnetic radio wave that would propagate into space if the signal source was coupled to a radio antenna of appropriate dimensions. This is not, however, the case in medical ultrasonics. In this class of instruments, the generated wave is purely sonic and any sonic wave, ultra or otherwise, is a mechanical disturbance in some medium such as air, water or human tissue.

A significant number of medical diagnostic and testing instruments use ultrasonic waves to provide information required about the patient's condition. The ultrasonic images are often superior to X-rays.

THERAPEUTIC AND DIAGNOSTIC EQUIPMENT

Ultrasonic equipment serves a variety of functions in medicine. It is used for imaging internal organs non-invasively. It is used to apply massage and deep-heat therapy to muscle tissue. And it is used to measure blood flow and blood pressure non-invasively.

The principle of imaging or making pictures of internal organs, is that of ultrasonic wave reflection. Ultrasonic waves reflect from the boundaries of two tissues, just as waves reflect from an object in water. Because the amount of reflection differs in different tissues, it is possible to distinguish between materials and make images of them using ultrasonics.

The quality that makes ultrasonic waves therapeutic is that they cause tissue matter to vibrate and heat up. It is the heat that has therapeutic effects. For use as therapy, it is necessary to couple relatively high power (up to approximately 5 W/cm^2) into the tissue.

Blood pressure and blood flow are measured by application of the Doppler effect. This effect is the increase in frequency of a sound reflected by a body approaching the source of the sound. To observe this effect, sing a steady tone, then move your hand rapidly toward your mouth. You will hear the increase in the pitch due to the motion of your hand.

Therapeutic Ultrasonic Equipment

Therapeutic ultrasonic equipment consists of a sinusoidal voltage generator driving a piezoelectric crystal pressed against the body tissue, as illustrated in Fig. 16.1. The sinusoidal voltage generator in the figure produces a voltage to be applied to the crystal transducer. The requirement of the generator is that it generate a voltage high enough to produce between 1 and 10 W on the transducer in the frequency range from 1 to 10 MHz. The piezoelectric effect causes the crystal to change its size and shape slightly when the electric field intensity changes, as driven by the voltage generator. The electric forces on the crystal atoms cause the atoms to move. Since the applied voltage is sinusoidal, it sets up sinusoidal vibrations in the crystal that are called ultrasound.

To get these sound waves into the tissue efficiently, it is necessary to match the impedance of the transducer to the impedance of the tissue, because of the maximum power transfer theorem. The acoustic impedance or the impedance to sound waves, is higher in the transducer than in body tissue, such as muscle. That is, the transducer, being ceramic, is hard, while the muscle is relatively soft. The acoustic impedance of materials often increases as a function of increased hardness.

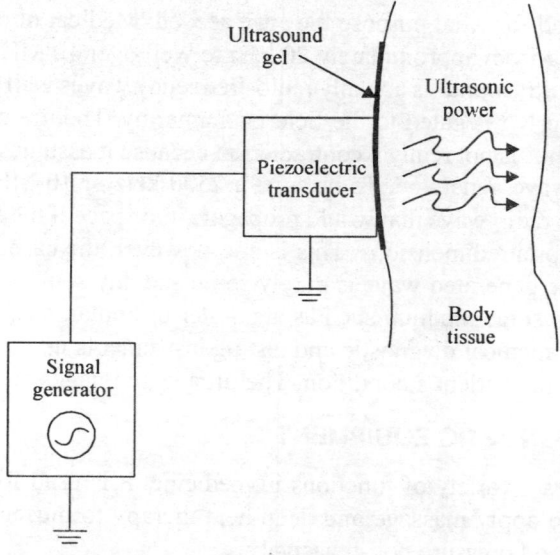

Fig. 16.1. Therapeutic ultrasonic equipment.

The impedance is matched by filling all of the voids between the tissue surface and filling the transducer with a gel. If this gel is not properly applied, the transducer can be damaged and skin burns can occur because too much energy will stay in the transducer and overheat it.

Besides resulting from overheating, failures can also arise from breakage. The crystals are relatively brittle and the metal adhesives may dry out or come loose. If epoxy is used in the construction, it also may deteriorate or break.

Piezoelectric Transducers

The piezoelectric crystal used for ultrasound occurs naturally as quartz. Practical transducers are constructed of ammonium dihydrogen phosphate (ADP) or lead zirconate titanate (PZT). ADP dissolves in water, but it can be used in high power applications. PZT is a commonly used transducer made from ceramic. The crystal is cut to one half wavelength, $\lambda/2$, at the frequency of the ultrasonic signal. This causes it to resonate at that frequency and give its maximum power output. In order to get the electric field throughout the crystal, the two ends perpendicular to the half wavelength axis are metalised. This forms a parallel plate capacitor, as illustrated in Fig. 16.2. These are wired to the voltage generator and the structure is covered with electrical insulation. In order to direct the energy out of one surface of the crystal, a backing material is applied to the surface opposite the tissue. This reflects ultrasonics; therefore, waves travel out of only one surface of the transducer. The impedance matching of the crystal may be adjusted by fixing a container of oil between the crystal and the tissue contact surface. The acoustic impedance of oil can be adjusted by changing its viscosity, that is, by diluting it. In other words, just as you can match the impedance of an amplifier to that of an antenna by adjusting the turns in a transformer connecting them, so you can impedance-match an ultrasonic transducer to skin by adjusting the viscosity of oil at the interface.

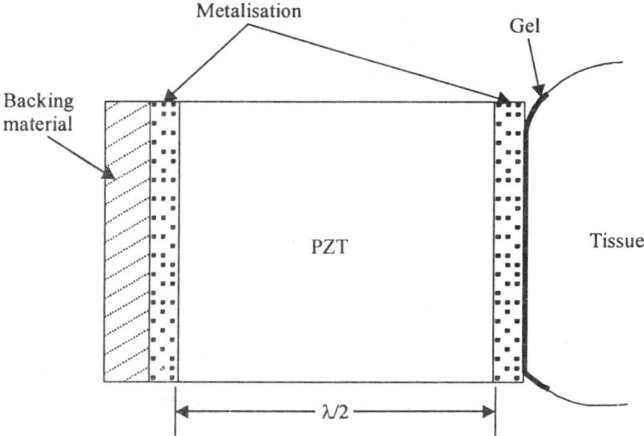

Fig. 16.2. A PZT ultrasonic transducer.

Ultrasonic Imaging Equipment

The voltage generator in ultrasonic imaging devices hits the piezoelectric transducer with a short pulse and causes it to oscillate at its resonant frequency. It is also possible to use a pulse-modulated generator to drive the piezoelectric crystal. The pulse generated would be long compared to the period of the 1 to 10 MHz ultrasonic oscillation. It would be short, however, compared to the acoustic transmission time in the tissue. Sound velocity in the body averages about 1540 m/s. Therefore, 1 mm in distance requires 0.65 μs on the average.

The pulse of ultrasonic energy travels into the tissue. It is reflected from tissue boundaries, causing echoes. By the time the echoes reach the transducer, the pulse generator has turned off and the echo creates an oscillation in the transducer again. The echo is like that of a drum beat reverberating off a wall, except the drum operates at a lower, audible frequency. The electronic signal from the transducer induced by the ultrasonic echo would go into the limiter in Fig. 16.3. The function of the limiter is to protect the receiver from the transmitted pulse. The small echo, from 40 to 100 dB below the transmitted pulse, is passed by the limiter. However, the transmitter pulse is severely clipped off to provide the protection.

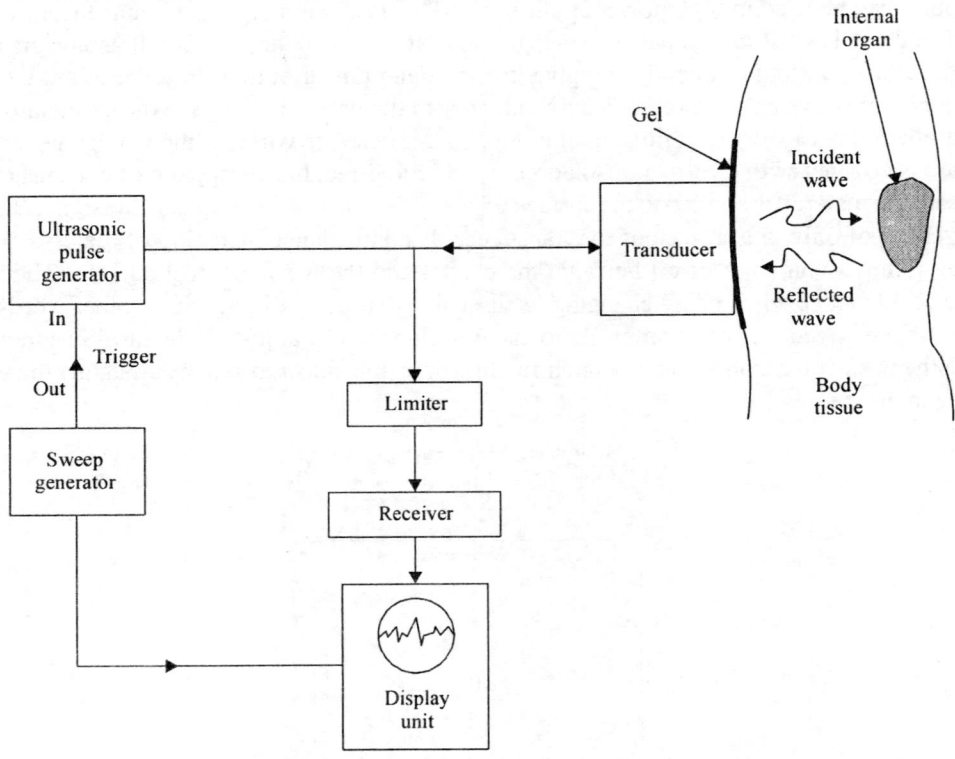

Fig. 16.3. A block diagram of ultrasonic imaging equipment.

The receiver is a conventional radio frequency (RF) unit operating in the 1 to 10 MHz range. It contains a detector circuit that filters out the ultrasonic frequencies and delivers the pulse to the output. The reflected pulse then appears on the display unit.

Display Unit

A simple image display can be made from a conventional oscilloscope. This is called an A-mode display. A trigger from the pulse generator initiates the horizontal sweep when the pulse is transmitted. The beam then travels along the horizontal axis as shown in Fig. 16.4. The horizontal scale is calibrated approximately according to the speed of sound in most body tissue. Based on the 1540 m/s average speed, it takes 1 μs for ultrasound to pass through 1.54 mm of tissue one way. On the A-scope it makes a round trip. Therefore 1 μs on the A-scope horizontal display is equivalent to 0.77 mm of tissue thickness. Controls at the receiver may be set so that the receiver gain increases in proportion to the distance along the sweep. This tends to make the echoes equal in size and compensates for tissue attenuation of the ultrasound echo.

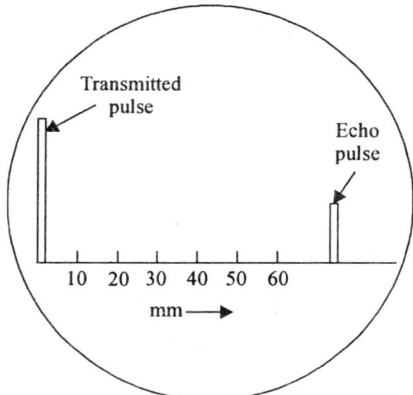

1 μs = 0.77 mm tissue thickness, round trip

Fig. 16.4. An A-mode display.

Scanning-Type Displays

The A-mode display gives information about the distance between tissue boundaries. For example, it may be used to measure organ thickness. In order to add a dimension and give breadth information, scanning-type displays are used.

A B-mode display may be generated by pivoting the transducer on an axis, causing it to rotate through an arc. The rotational speed, being mechanical, is slow compared with the time required for each sweep. The transmitted pulse appears at the origin in Fig. 16.5. The depth is proportional to the distance along each radial line. Ultrasonic echoes appear as an intensity-modulated dot, as indicated in the figure. The result is an outline of the body tissue in two dimensions.

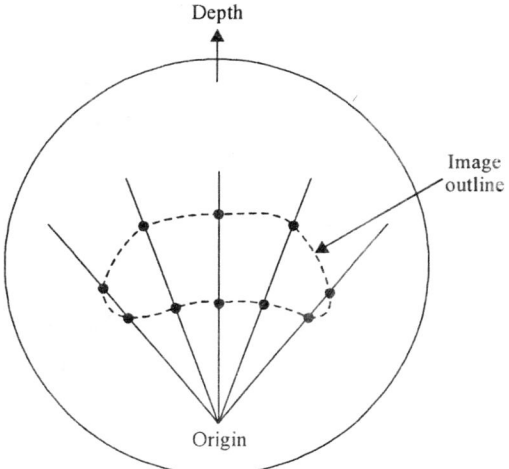

Fig. 16.5. A B-mode display.

A B-mode display may also be generated with a phased array transducer, illustrated with an ultrasonic imager in Fig. 16.6. A phased array transducer consists of a set of piezoelectric transducers placed along a line. Each transducer is pulsed successively in time. Depending upon the time between the firing of each transducer, constructive interference of the transmitted wave will occur along a particular radial line. The direction of the radial line is varied by changing the firing time between successive transducers in the display.

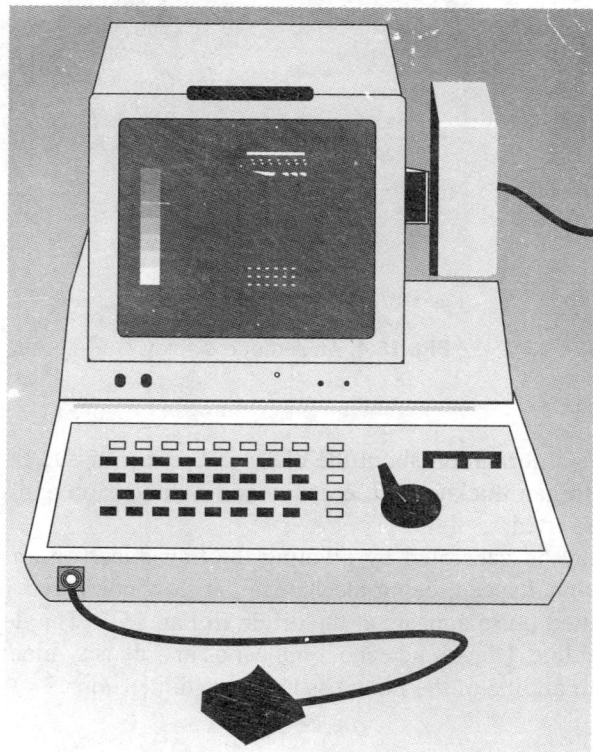

Fig. 16.6. An ultrasound imager with a phased array transducer.

The phased array transducer can be scanned faster than the rotating transducer, because the control pulses are electronic and travel at the speed of light. In a practical application, a linear phased array may be useful for getting images of the heart from a site between the ribs, for example.

A single transducer is used to generate an M-mode display (Fig. 16.7), where the M stands for motion, because it measures the motion of the tissue. As with the B-mode display, the intensity of the reflections from the tissue is recorded as an intensity of the spot on the CRT. The horizontal axis of the CRT is slowly scanned so that if the tissue is moving, as in the case of a heart valve, the new position will be recorded on successive scans. From the scan rate, usually on the order of seconds per scan, it is possible to calculate the rate of motion of the tissue. Several transducers of different shapes are illustrated in Fig. 16.8. The flat single transducer matches the impedance of the skull in brain midline studies. A rounded transducer can be placed near the apex of the heart for heart valve studies. In Fig. 16.8, a trans-anal transducer suitable for insertion into the colon is shown.

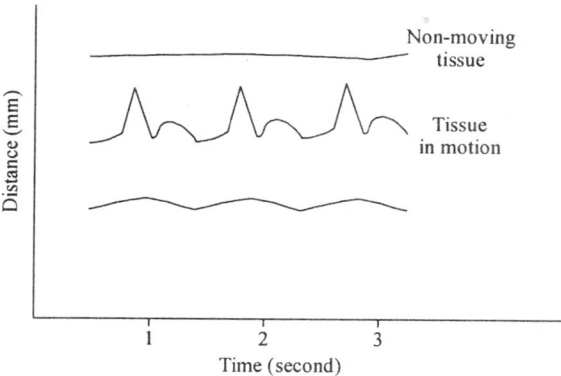

Fig. 16.7. An M-mode display.

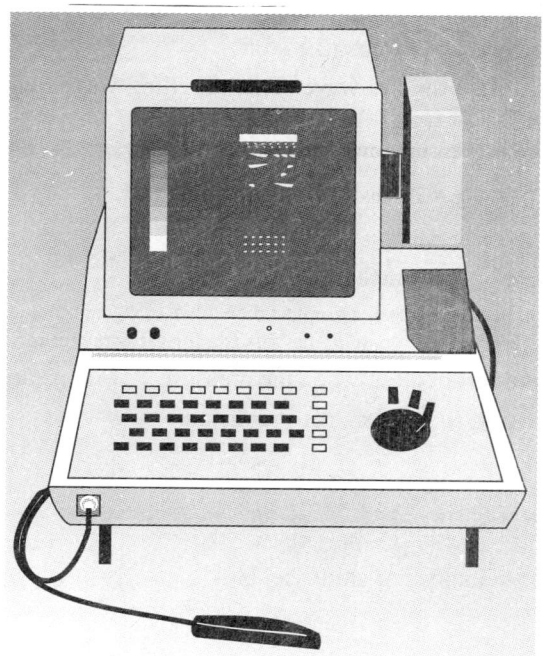

Fig. 16.8. An ultrasonic imager showing a trans-anal transducer attached to a patient cable.

ULTRASONIC WAVES

Ultrasonic equipment is used to generate and measure ultrasonic waves. To understand the equipment and its operation, it is necessary to understand ultrasonic wave mechanics. Ultrasonic waves are similar to the pressure and flow waves. A pressure difference, p, across two points in matter, whether air, tissue or metal, causes a displacement of the atoms, giving them a velocity, v. The atoms do not move very far because they are bound by elastic forces. However, the energy of one atom is transferred to other atoms and it propagates through the matter at its own velocity, c.

There exists an analogy of ultrasonic waves to voltage waves: ultrasonic pressure, p, is analogous to voltage and the particle velocity, v, of ultrasonic waves is analogous to current. Furthermore, the acoustic impedance is analogous to the impedance of an electrical circuit. Therefore, knowledge of electrical circuits will help to understand ultrasonics.

An ultrasonic wave is a travelling pressure wave. If you were to drop a rock into a smooth lake, waves would propagate out from the point of impact. We have all observed how these waves travel. The force that causes the undulation of the water that we observe is a pressure wave. A mathematical expression that describes it is

$$p = P_0 e^{-\alpha x} \cos (\beta x - \omega t) \qquad \qquad \text{... (16.1)}$$

This is the mathematical expression for a travelling sinusoidal wave. In this equation, p is pressure, β is the phase constant, x is position, $\omega = 2\pi f$ is the radian frequency, t is time and α is an attenuation constant. For clarity of presentation and because it is not of primary importance in ultrasonic imaging, we will restrict ourselves to the case that $\alpha = 0$, the lossless case. The description of the travelling wave is then taken as

$$p = P_0 \cos (\beta x - \omega t) \qquad \qquad \text{... (16.2)}$$

where P_0 is the magnitude of the pressure wave. The travelling-wave behaviour of Equation (16.2) is illustrated in Example 16.1.

Example 16.1. (a) Plot the following pressure wave equation for the case

$$p = P_0 \cos (\beta x - \omega t)$$

where $\beta = 1$ rad/m, f = 1 Hz and $P_0 = 10$ N/m^2.

(b) Is this a forward-travelling wave or a backward-travelling wave?

Solution. See Fig. 16.9. Note that in the successive graphs taken at t = 0, $\frac{1}{8}$ and $\frac{1}{4}$ seconds, the crest of the wave has moved in position to the right. Therefore we conclude that this is a forward-travelling wave.

The crest velocity is derived from dx/dt when the pressure, p, is constant in Equation (16.2). That is,

$$\beta x - \omega t = \text{constant}$$

Differentiating both sides gives

$$\beta \frac{dx}{dt} - \omega = 0$$

Therefore, defining the crest velocity c = dx/dt yields

$$c = \frac{\omega}{\beta} \qquad \qquad \text{... (16.3)}$$

The wavelength, λ, is the distance between wave crests at any time t. For example, at t = 0, Equation (16.2) shows that

$$\lambda = \frac{2\pi}{\beta} \qquad \qquad \text{... (16.4)}$$

Then, combining Equations (16.3) and (16.4) gives

$$c = \lambda f \qquad \qquad \text{... (16.5)}$$

The wave in Fig. 16.9 travels in the positive x-direction. Changing the sign in the argument reverses the direction of the wave. That is,

$$p = P_0 \cos (\beta x + \omega t)$$

travels in the negative x-direction and is called a backward-travelling wave.

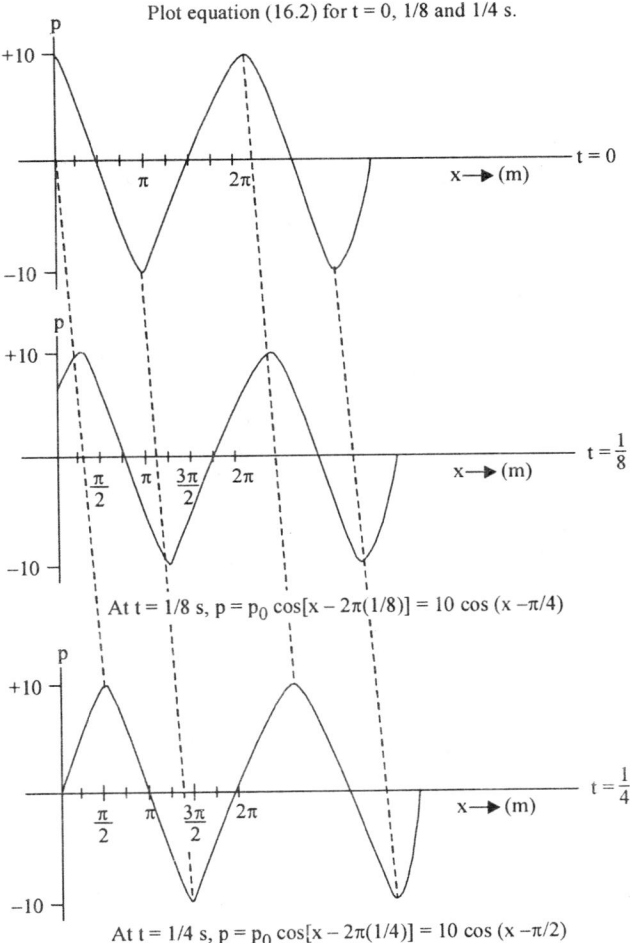

Plot equation (16.2) for t = 0, 1/8 and 1/4 s.

At t = 1/8 s, $p = p_0 \cos[x - 2\pi(1/8)] = 10 \cos (x - \pi/4)$

At t = 1/4 s, $p = p_0 \cos[x - 2\pi(1/4)] = 10 \cos (x - \pi/2)$

Fig. 16.9. A plot of a forward-travelling wave.

Because the wave crest travels through the medium, we call it a propagating wave. The propagating pressure wave causes a displacement of the particles of matter through which it travels. A mathematical expression describing the velocity, v, is

$$v = V_0 \cos (\beta x - \omega t) \qquad \dots (16.6)$$

Since Equation (16.6) has the same form as Equation (16.2), plotting it will show that it too is a propagating wave. It is analogous to the current in an electric wave, which is the velocity of charges. In a water wave caused by a splash, it represents the velocity of the water making the wave.

Completing the analogy, we can define the impedance of the forward travelling wave as the characteristic impedance, Z_0. That is,

$$Z_0 = \frac{p}{v} = \frac{P_0 \cos(\beta x - \omega t)}{V_0 \cos(\beta x - \omega t)}$$

and cancelling the cosine functions,

$$Z_0 = \frac{P_0}{V_0} \qquad \qquad \qquad ...(16.7)$$

In general, the characteristic impedance is defined as the wave impedance of a single wave travelling in one direction. It can also be shown that the characteristic impedance is a physical property of the medium supporting the travelling wave and is given by

$$Z_0 = \rho c \qquad \qquad \qquad ...(16.8)$$

where ρ is the material density in kg/m^3 and c is the velocity of sound in the medium in m/s. The units of Z_0 are then

$$\left(\frac{kg}{m^3}\right)\frac{m}{s} = \left(\frac{kg}{m^2 s}\right)$$

Wave Reflections

The key principle of operation for ultrasonic imaging equipment, as well as for most other ultrasonic equipment other than therapeutic massagers, is the principle of travelling wave reflection, commonly known in the audio spectrum as echo. Tissues are distinguished from one another by their relative reflected wave intensities. It is important to understand what property of the tissue influences reflection so that the proper uses and limitations of the equipment can be appreciated. We shall see that tissue density is the most distinctive feature in the ultrasonic spectrum. Although an exact analysis of reflections in biological tissue is very complex, to understand the principle and limitations of ultrasonic imaging, it is sufficient to consider only two tissues.

When a wave impinges on the boundary of two tissues, some of the wave is reflected back. For example, if the wave is travelling in tissue 1 with a characteristic impedance $Z_{01} = \rho_1 c_1$ and strikes a medium having a characteristic impedance $Z_{02} = \rho_2 c_2$, the pressure wave is reflected back. The situation is illustrated in Fig. 16.10, in which the dimension x is taken as positive going toward the left and x = 0 is the boundary between the two tissues. The wave incident on the boundary travels in the negative x-direction and has the formula

$$p_1 = P_{01} \cos (\beta_1 x + \omega t)$$

and the reflected wave is some fraction R of that as

$$p_2 = RP_{01} \cos (\beta_1 x + \omega t)$$

The minus sign on the ωt indicates the wave travels in the positive x-direction. R is called the reflection coefficient and is defined as

$$R = \frac{\text{Pressure magnitude reflected at the boundary x = 0}}{\text{Pressure magnitude incident on the boundary at x = 0}} \qquad ...(16.9)$$

The pressure in tissue 1 is the sum $p_1 + p_2$, or

$$p = P_{01} [\cos (\beta_1 x + \omega t) + R \cos (\beta_1 x - \omega t)] \qquad ...(16.10)$$

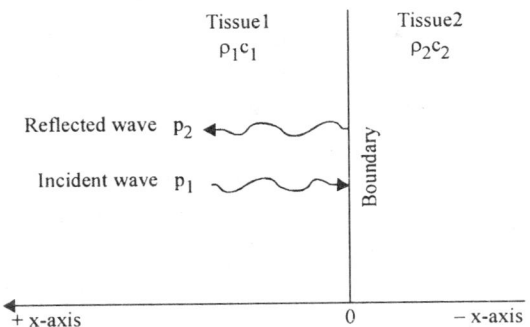

Fig. 16.10. Waves reflected from the boundary.

Each of these pressures causes a velocity and the velocity of the reflected wave is in a direction opposite to that of the incident wave, accounting for the minus sign preceding the R in the following equation for particle velocity:

$$v = V_{01} [\cos(\beta_1 x + \omega t) - R \cos(\beta_1 x - \omega t)] \qquad \ldots (16.11)$$

Because of the analogy already mentioned that pressure plays the role of voltage and particle velocity plays the role of current, the wave impedance Z is defined as

$$Z = \frac{p}{v} \qquad \ldots (16.12)$$

That is, wave impedance equals the pressure divided by the velocity of the wave composed of the sum of all incident and reflected waves. Notice that Z is equal to the characteristic impedance of Equation (16.7) only when there are no reflected waves and R = 0 in Equations (16.10) and (16.11).

A means of measuring the reflection coefficient is derived by considering the wave impedance at the boundary. First set x = 0 in Equations (16.10) and (16.11). Insert these into Equation (16.12) to yield

$$Z(0) = \frac{P_{01}[\cos(\omega t) + R \cos(-\omega t)]}{V_{01}[\cos(\omega t) - R \cos(-\omega t)]}$$

Here the cosines cancel because cos (ωt) = cos (−ωt). Also, using Equation (16.7) we have

$$Z(0) = Z_{01} \frac{1+R}{1-R}$$

where Z_{01} is the characteristic impedance of tissue 1. In addition, because there are no reflected waves to the right of the boundary, we note that Z (0) = Z_{02}, the characteristic impedance of tissue 2. Therefore we have

$$\frac{Z_{02}}{Z_{01}} = \frac{1+R}{1-R} \qquad \ldots (16.13)$$

This is solved for the reflection coefficient as

$$R = \frac{Z_{02} - Z_{01}}{Z_{02} + Z_{01}} \qquad \ldots (16.14a)$$

Now, using Equation (16.8),

$$R = \frac{\rho_2 c_2 - \rho_1 c_1}{\rho_2 c_2 + \rho_1 c_1} \qquad \text{... (16.14b)}$$

This equation shows that the reflection coefficient can be calculated from thy physical properties of the tissue, namely its density ρ and speed of sound c.

The data necessary to compute the reflection coefficient, R, in common biological tissues is given in Table 16.1.

Table 16.1. Physical parameters of tissues.

Material	Density, ρ (g/cm^3)	Speed of sound, c (m/s)
Air	0.001	331
Bone	1.85	3360
Muscle	1.06	1570
Fat	0.93	1480
Blood	1.00	1560

Example 16.2. Use Table 16.1 to compute the characteristic impedance of muscle tissue, Z_{0M}.

Solution. From equation (16.8),

$$Z_{0M} = \left(1.06 \frac{g}{cm^3}\right)\left(\frac{kg}{1000\ g}\right)\left(\frac{100\ cm}{m}\right)^3\left(1570 \frac{m}{s}\right)$$

$$= 1.66 \times 10^6 \text{ kg/m}^2\text{s}$$

Analysis of a Typical Ultrasonic Reflection

The typical ultrasonic equipment used for diagnosis propagates a pulse of ultrasonics into a tissue turns off the transmitter and waits for the reflection. Because of this, the incident and reflected curve can be treated separately.

Ultrasonic Power

Consistent with the analog of pressure for voltage and velocity for current, the power density, $\wp$, of an ultrasonic wave is given by:

$$\wp = PV$$

where P is the root-mean-square (rms) value of pressure and V the rms value of velocity. The power density is also given by

$$\wp = \frac{P^2}{Z_0} \qquad \text{... (16.15)}$$

Using Equation (16.7) for the characteristic impedance Z_{01}, we have

$$\wp_1 = \frac{P_{01}^2}{Z_{01}}$$

This is the power in the incident wave in tissue 1.

Likewise, the reflected power in tissue 1 is

$$\wp_2 = \frac{(RP_{01})^2}{Z_{01}}$$

Thus we see that the ratio of the reflected power density to the incident power is equal to the square of the reflection coefficient. Or

$$\frac{\wp_2}{\wp_1} = R^2 \qquad \qquad ... (16.16)$$

That is, the power reflection coefficient equals the square of the pressure reflection coefficient, R^2.

For an engineer or service professional, it is important to understand ultrasonic power, since that is the quantity that causes harmful side effects. Although ultrasonic radiation does not have a lasting cumulative effect as X-ray does and it does not cause cancer as X-ray can, high-power ultrasonics in excess of 1 W/cm^2 can cause injury to patients from overheating and can cause mechanical tissue damage due to cavitation. Fortunately, diagnostic ultrasound uses power well below the danger level. However, therapeutic ultrasound for muscle massage and the like may cause high-power side effects.

Attenuation in Ultrasonic Waves

In order to know how deep into the tissue the power penetrates in therapeutic ultrasound equipment, attenuation factors have been measured as given in Table 16.2.

Table 16.2. Attenuation factors in biological tissues.

Tissue	Attenuation factor (dB/cm/MHz)
Fat	0.63
Muscle	1.3
Bone	20
Lung	41

Typical ultrasonic frequencies range from 1 to 5 MHz. From Table 16.2, we see that attenuation at 1 MHz for muscle is 1.3 dB/cm and at 5 MHz it is 6.5 dB/cm. The operating technician may use this fact to selectively heat surface muscle by choosing a frequency that would distribute the power relatively evenly over the muscle. Note that attenuation of 3 dB absorbs half the power available.

ULTRASONIC BLOOD FLOW EQUIPMENT

Ultrasonic equipment is often used to measure the velocity of objects such as a stream of blood, a moving heart valve or the motion of an artery in response to a pressure pulse. Blood flow is monitored either by observing frequency shift due to the Doppler effect or by observing shifts in the transit time of waves going first upstream, then downstream through the blood. An analysis of the Doppler effect is considered first.

An Analysis of the Doppler Effect

The Doppler effect is simply what someone moving away from a source of sound, such as a whistle, experiences. That person will hear a pitch lower than the pitch heard by the person standing still. And likewise, someone moving toward the whistle will hear a higher pitch. The situation is illustrated in

Fig. 16.11. The sound waves produce compressions in air separated by a wavelength λ. The stationary observer hears a frequency given by Equation (16.5),

$$f = c/\lambda$$

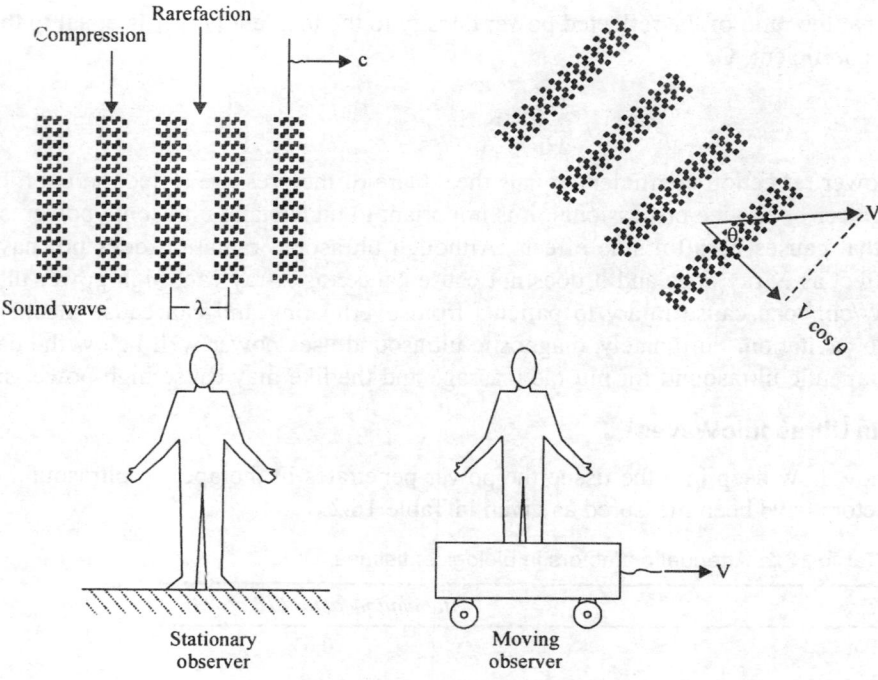

Fig. 16.11. The Doppler effect.

The crest velocity observed by the person on the platform travelling at a velocity V, however, will be c – V. Furthermore, the wavelength of the sound, unaffected by the platform, remains the same. Therefore, the person hears a frequency f_p of

$$f_p = \frac{c - V}{\lambda}$$

Taking the ratio of these two equations gives

$$\frac{f_p}{f} = 1 - \frac{V}{c}$$

or

$$f_p = \left(1 - \frac{V}{c}\right)f$$

If the platform moves at an angle θ with respect to the sound wave, the platform projected velocity is V cos θ, so that

$$f_p = \left(1 - \frac{V}{c}\cos\theta\right)f \qquad \qquad ...\,(16.17)$$

The echo frequency of the ultrasound reflected from the moving platform, f_s, heard by the stationary observer, will be affected by the velocity $2V \cos \theta$, because the change in the path length is that due to the incident wave plus the reflected wave, so that

$$f_s = \left(1 - \frac{2V}{c} \cos \theta\right) f \qquad \qquad \text{... (16.18)}$$

Much of the ultrasonic equipment used in medicine responds to the difference between the signal frequency f and the echo frequency, called

$$\Delta f = f - f_s$$

Then, from Equation (16.18),

$$\Delta f = f - f \left(1 - \frac{2V}{c} \cos \theta\right)$$

or

$$\Delta f = \frac{2V}{c} f \cos \theta \qquad \qquad \text{... (16.19)}$$

The difference frequency can be measured by the circuit in Fig. 16.12 and the flow velocity V is computed from

$$V = \frac{\Delta f c}{2f \cos \theta} \qquad \qquad \text{... (16.20)}$$

where Δf is the difference frequency, f is the generator frequency, θ is the angle of the transducer as specified, c is the velocity of sound in blood or the fluid and V is the fluid velocity in m/s.

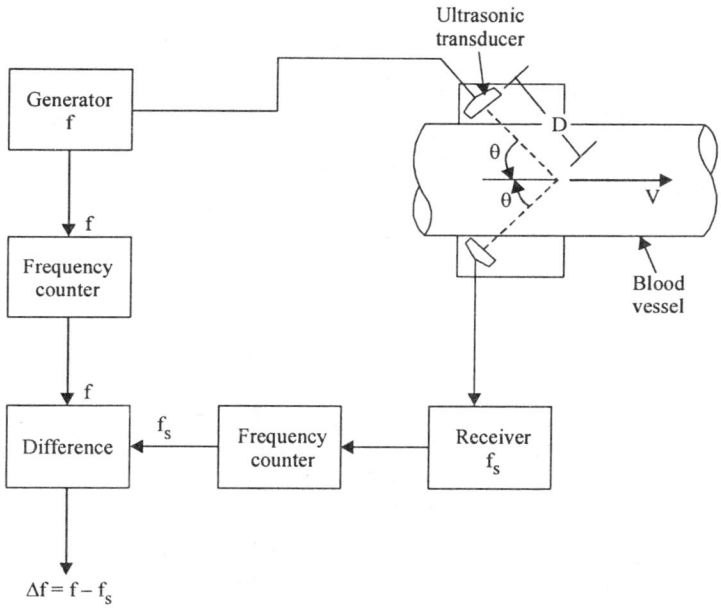

Fig. 16.12. An ultrasonic blood flow meter.

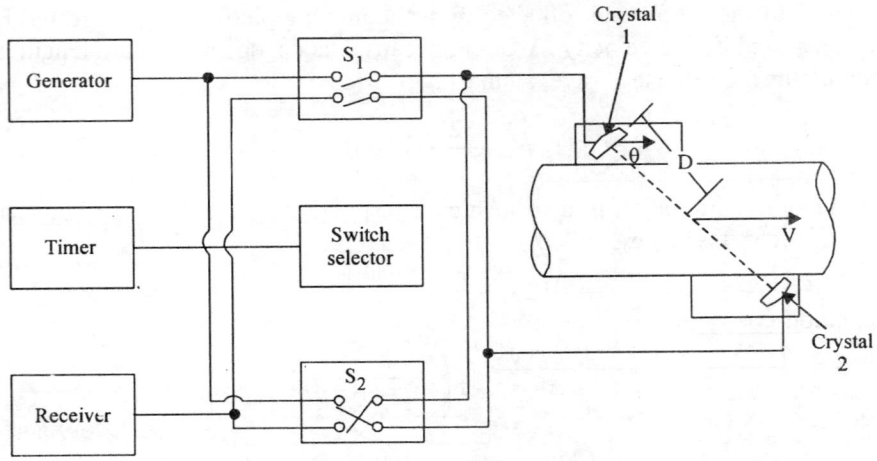

Fig. 16.13. Blood flow measurement by transit time difference.

An Analysis of Transit Time

Another measurement that can be made electronically to deduce the flow rate V is the transit time. In Fig. 16.13, the distance D the sound travels is related to the downstream transit time T_D as follows:

$$D = T_D (V \cos\theta + c)$$

In the downstream direction the velocity of the sound is increased by the velocity of the stream that carries it. This decreases the downstream transit time. The transit time upstream T_U, however, is increased so that

$$D = T_U (c - V \cos\theta)$$

The difference in transit time is then $\Delta T = T_U - T_D$ or

$$\Delta T = \frac{-D}{c + V \cos\theta} + \frac{D}{c - V \cos\theta}$$

$$= \frac{-(cD - VD \cos\theta) + Dc + VD \cos\theta}{c^2 - (V \cos\theta)^2}$$

For small values of V we have $V^2 \ll c^2$, so

$$\Delta T = \frac{2VD \cos\theta}{c^2}$$

The flow velocity V is then

$$V = \frac{\Delta T c^2}{2D \cos\theta} \qquad \qquad ...\ (16.21)$$

where ΔT is the difference between upstream and downstream transit time, θ is the angle of the transducer, c is the speed of sound in the fluid. A circuit for measuring the transit time difference ΔT is given in Fig. 16.13. The switch selector first closes S_1 and opens S_2. This connects the generator to crystal 1 and the receiver to crystal 2 and the upstream transit time is measured. Subsequently, the switch selector opens S_1 and closes S_2. This connects the generator to crystal 2 and the receiver to crystal 1 and measures the downstream transit time.

The difference ΔT between these two times is then measured and the blood velocity, V, is then read out according to Equation (16.21).

SAFETY AND BIOEFFECTS IN ULTRASONIC IMAGING

Under normal operating conditions, ultrasonic imaging is extremely safe, with no limit having been set by the FDA on the number of patient examinations over any given period of time. Increasingly sophisticated image acquisition processes such as compound scanning and power colour Doppler have, however, increased the amount of energy that is deposited in the body and there are a number of regulatory guidelines for recommended safety levels. Several measures are used to estimate the safety of an ultrasonic imaging protocol. However, as has been described, the majority of ultrasound experiments are carried out in pulsed mode. The 'duty cycle' in pulsed ultrasound is defined as the duration of the ultrasound pulse divided by the time between pulses. Temporal-averaged ultrasound intensity is calculated simply by multiplying the average intensity during the pulse by the duty cycle. The Gaussian beam profile can be accounted for by calculating the spatially averaged intensity I_{SA}. Common acronyms used for reporting ultrasound intensities for different procedures use a combination of these terms, for example, spatial average temporal average (SATA), spatial peak temporal average (SPTA), spatial peak pulse average (SPPA), spatial peak temporal peak (SPTP), spatial peak (SP) and spatial average (SA). The American Institute of Ultrasound in Medicine sets guidelines for these values, based on estimations on the tissue heating produced. For example, for fetal imaging, the current FDA regulatory limit for I_{SPTA} is 720 mW/cm^2.

It should be noted that ultrasound can be used therapeutically as a method for thermal destruction of tumours. Relatively low intensity ultrasound is used for hyperthermic tumour treatment, in which the tumour is heated to temperature between 42°C and 45°C in order to accelerate tumour cell destruction. Alternatively, very high intensities of ultrasound can be used for tumour thermoablation, in which the temperature in the tumour is raised rapidly to between 70°C and 90°C for a few seconds. The mechanism for this rapid heating involves cavitation effects, the formation and destruction of small air bubbles within the tumour.

CLINICAL APPLICATIONS OF ULTRASOUND

The non-invasive, non-ionising nature of ultrasonic imaging, its ability to measure blood velocity, together with real-time image acquisition and easy patient access mean that a very wide range of clinical protocols have ultrasonic imaging as an integral part. The most common use of ultrasound is in the abdomen and pelvis, imaging the gallbladder and renal system and transabdominal imaging of the uterus and ovaries in women and the testicles in men. As examples, applications to obstetrics, breast imaging, musculoskeletal damage and cardiac studies are outlined briefly below.

Obstetrics and Gynecology

Ultrasound is the only imaging technique routinely used for fetal studies. Parameters such as the size of the head and the brain ventricles (for diagnosis of hydrocephalus) and the condition of the spine are measured to assess the health of the fetus. If amniocentesis is necessary to detect disorders such as Down syndrome, then ultrasound is used for needle guidance. Doppler ultrasound is also used to measure fetal blood velocity.

Breast Imaging

In breast imaging, ultrasound is used in conjunction with the primary technique of X-ray mammography in the diagnosis of breast cancer. If mammography suggests that a 'lump' is present, then ultrasound can help to determine whether it is a fluid-filled cyst or a solid mass. Cysts typically have a round shape and anechoic interiors and acoustic enhancement is often seen behind the cyst. Since cysts are fluid-filled, the presence of acoustic streaming (fluid motion arising from the ultrasound pressure, detected using Doppler techniques) is also a useful diagnostic. Ultrasound is particularly valuable in women with dense breast tissue or young women because the tissue is relatively opaque to X-rays. If a needle biopsy is needed in order to determine whether a solid mass is cancerous or not, then real-time B-mode ultrasonic imaging can be used to guide the needle into the tumour. Ultrasound can also be used in the detection of microcalcifications, with spatial compound imaging being particularly useful due to the reduction in speckle.

Musculoskeletal Structure

Musculoskeletal damage can be quickly and effectively diagnosed using ultrasound, again most commonly with compound scanning for images with high spatial resolution and high SNR.

Cardiac Disease

Ultrasonic imaging of the heart can be used to diagnose disease such as mitral valve stenosis, regurgitation, congenital heart disease and the presence of cardiac tumours. It can also be used to assess left-ventricular function, often in combination with a stress test. Doppler techniques can be used to measure blood velocity in the arteries and veins in the heart. Contrast agents can be used to produce blood perfusion maps; myocardial infarcts often show reduced perfusion compared to areas of healthy tissue.

Therapeutic Equipment

Chapter 17

Cardiac Defibrillators

INTRODUCTION

No medical device so clearly represents emergency and in some aspects, intensive care medicine as much as the defibrillator. These are electric shock devices that are used to correct fatal cardiac arrhythmias such as ventricular fibrillation and ventricular tachycardia. Although usually characterised as a 'random' shallow beating of the heart, the process is known by more modern research to be actually 'chaotic' (which has very specific mathematical meaning in science).

Thousands of persons die of sudden cardiac arrest each year. If they could be treated with a defibrillator within one minute of the attack, 80 per cent would have an increased chance of survival. However, if this treatment is delayed by only ten minutes, the statistic falls from 80 per cent to 15 per cent, thus illustrating how important the defibrillator is and how important it is to have it available to the general population.

A defibrillator is an electronic device that creates a sustained myocardial depolarisation of a patient's heart in order to stop ventricular fibrillation or atrial fibrillation. These fibrillations occur because ectopic or out-of-place, stimulus sites take place in the heart and cause a disorganised cardiac muscle contraction. When this fibrillation happens to the ventricles, it causes a drastically reduced cardiac output of blood flow and results in death in a few minutes. An atrial fibrillation causes reduced cardiac output but is usually not fatal. The DC defibrillator is effective in treating both conditions.

Since 1 to 10 A of current can cause a sustained myocardial contraction. The early AC defibrillators proved unreliable and have since been replaced with more effective units, such as the DC defibrillator and biphasic units, which deliver DC pulses alternatively in opposite directions. A DC defibrillator is designed to deliver 50 to 400 joules (J) or watt-seconds (W-s), of energy through the thorax. The energy required depends upon the size of the patient and his or her skin resistance. The voltages required vary from 1000 to 6000 V, depending upon the duration of the DC pulse used. For example, if a 2000 V, 5 ms pulse is reduced in voltage, the duration must be extended to maintain the same energy delivery to the patient. The current level delivered by a defibrillator varies from 1 to 20 A. If the defibrillator pulse is applied directly to the heart during open-heart surgery or with an implanted defibrillator, the energy level is reduced to 15 to 50 J.

All defibrillators must have a mechanism for adjusting the energy level, by controlling either the amplitude or the duration of the defibrillator pulse. A schematic of the DC defibrillator like that introduced by Bernard Lown is given in Fig. 17.1. When the switch is in the charge position, current flows through the diode in one direction and charges the capacitor to its peak value, V_P. The voltage V_P can be varied by changing the setting on the varactor. The energy stored in the capacitor and available for defibrillation, W_A, is

$$W_A = \tfrac{1}{2}CV_P^2 \qquad\qquad ... (17.1)$$

Therefore the energy available from the defibrillator is varied by the varactor setting.

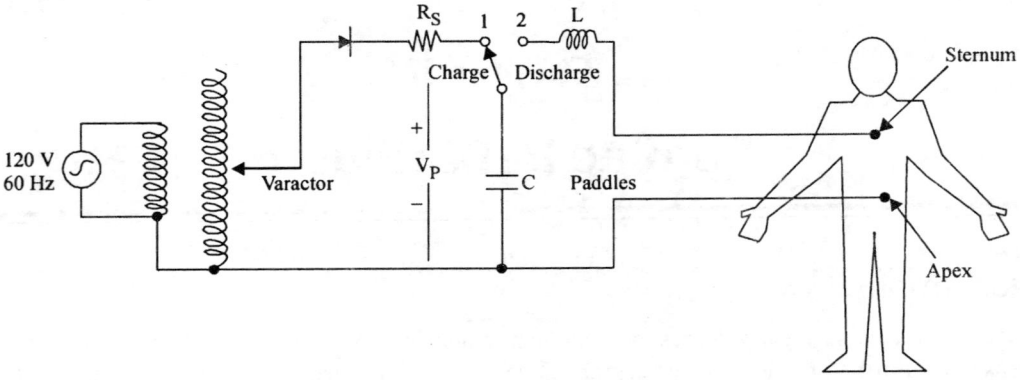

Fig. 17.1. Schematic of a DC defibrillator.

The defibrillator pulse is delivered by placing paddles covered with an electrode electrolyte gel against the skin of the patient and placing the switch in the discharge position. The paddles have a metal surface from 8 to 10 cm in diameter for adult patients. They may be placed either in the anterior-anterior position so that the current flows through the heart or in the anterior-posterior so that the current flows from the back to the chest through the heart. In the anterior-anterior position, one paddle is placed above the apex of the heart and the other is placed on the sternum. This causes the current to flow from the bottom to the top of the heart.

The discharge switch is usually mounted on the paddle. It is important that the attendants using the defibrillator avoid having the defibrillation pulse pass through their own bodies. For example, electrode gel on the paddle handle could provide a path for the defibrillation pulse through one arm of the attendant through the heart of the other arm. An attendant touching the patient is likewise in danger of a shock.

Because of the reduced surface resistance, the defibrillator pulse may be delivered to the open heart using paddles from 4 to 5 cm in diameter and the voltage levels may be reduced by one-third. For pediatric patients, the external paddles are approximately 5 cm in diameter and energy levels of about 50 J are delivered.

Defibrillation is indeed a hazardous procedure, since it involves stopping the heart; and if applied incorrectly, it could induce fibrillations in a normal heart. Therefore, it is essential that a diagnosis be made by trained specialists to ensure that the patient needs the treatment before it is initiated. In order to reduce this risk and to make the defibrillator available for more cardiac arrest victims more quickly, diagnostic circuitry is used to assess that a fibrillation is in fact occurring before the defibrillation pulse is applied to a patient. This then makes it safe for attendants with less training to use the defibrillator.

Figure 17.2 shows the generic block diagram of a defibrillator capable of diagnosing fibrillation. An ECG instrument is attached to the patient. If ventricular fibrillation is suspected, the switch is placed in the defibrillator position. A QRS detector consists of a threshold circuit that would pass an R-wave if such a wave is present. When the attendant energises the switch to deliver a defibrillation pulse, the signal passes through a logical AND gate, which is a digital circuit that provides an output signal only when an appropriate input appears on the two input nodes simultaneously. In this case the two inputs are the R-wave from the QRS detector and a signal from the attendant's switch. If both are present, the defibrillator is inhibited and will not deliver the pulse. A defibrillator pulse is delivered only if the fibrillation detector produces an output at the same time that the attendant energises the switch. The fibrillation detector searches the ECG signal for frequency components above 150 Hz. If they are present, fibrillation is probable. Under this condition, when the attendant energises the switch the defibrillation voltage would actually be delivered to the patient.

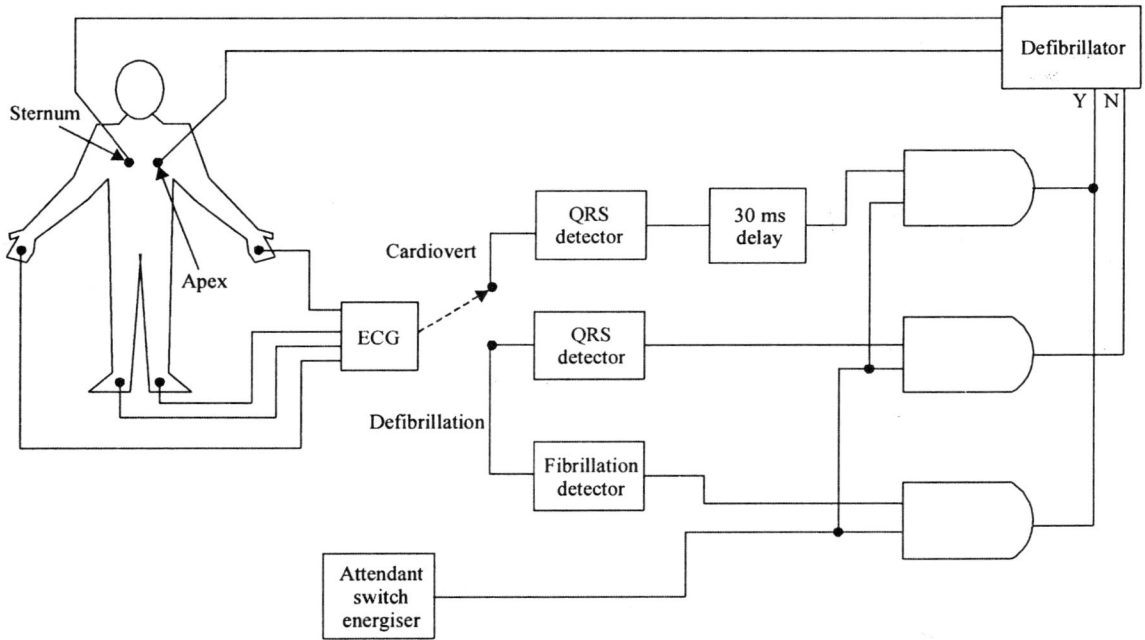

Fig. 17.2. Defibrillator/cardioverter block diagram.

A second mode of operation, cardioversion, is used, for example, when atrial fibrillation is diagnosed. After a diagnosis is made by specialists, treatment may be initiated. The ECG signal in the instrument is delivered to a QRS detector. The signal is used to time the delivery of the defibrillation pulse with a delay of 30 ms. At this time, the ventricles will be in a uniform state of depolarisation and the normal beat will not be disturbed. If the pulse were applied during the T-wave between 50 and 150 ms after the QRS complex, for example, while the heart is in the process of re-polarising, it would be possible to introduce a fibrillation into the heart. Therefore the 30 ms delay allows the attendant to defibrillate the atrium with a low risk of inducing a ventricular fibrillation. Coming within 30 ms of the low risk of inducing a ventricular fibrillation. Coming within 30 ms of the R-wave, the defibrillation pulse will occur before the period of ventricular vulnerability to fibrillation, namely during the T-wave.

Such diagnostic circuitry has been further developed to make it possible to permanently implant a defibrillator and attach it to a patient's diseased heart. If the heart fibrillates, a defibrillator pulse is automatically applied to the surface of the heart.

Example of Defibrillators

Commercially available defibrillators typically have specifications with the following ranges:

Weight	7 to 50 lbs (typically 30)
Maximum delivered energy	320 to 450 J
Charge time	1 to 22 seconds
Battery capability	20 to 80 discharges
Battery recharge time	1 to 16 hours

Because the defibrillator delivers therapeutic current to critically ill patients, reliability is crucial. The unit is tested as often as every day in many hospitals. Also, to facilitate testing it immediately before use, test circuits are built into the unit. The test procedure requires (i) turning on the line power; (ii) setting the energy selector to maximum; (iii) charging the unit; and (vi) discharging the paddles into their holders, as placed in the illustration. The defibrillator is automatically discharged into a 50 Ω load connected to the paddle holders in the defibrillator. An indicator light then verifies that the proper energy was discharged into the test load.

Defibrillation of a patient is performed by personnel trained and authorised to use the defibrillator. After a diagnosis is made using an ECG, an electrode gel is applied to the paddles. The defibrillator is then recharged to the proper energy level. The paddles may then be placed on the sternum and apex, respectively, of the patient's chest. Both discharge buttons on the paddles are engaged to defibrillate the patient. The paddles are usually isolated electrically from ground so that ground loops are eliminated that could injure the patient or attendants.

Cardioversion is done with the use of the ECG. The amplitude of the ECG is increased until a marker appears on the R-wave. This assures the user that the instrument will synchronise to the R-wave. To perform cardioversion, the user selects the cardioversion mode on the instrument by pushing the SYNC switch. The defibrillator is then charged to the proper energy level and the defibrillator pulse is delivered to the patient approximately 30 minutes after the R-wave peak, as explained earlier.

PADDLES

Energy is transferred from the defibrillator to the patient through a pair of electrodes called paddles. Several common types of defibrillator paddles are shown in Fig. 17.3. The form shown in Fig. 17.3a is the standard (if older design) anterior paddle. This type of paddle is designed to be applied directly to the chest. The posterior paddle is shown in Fig. 17.3b. This form of paddle is used on the patient's back. In typical applications, the posterior paddle is smeared with an electrolytic cream to make better electrical contact and is then inserted under the patient. The patient's weight makes electrical contact possible. Some defibrillators are equipped with an anterior/anterior pair, while others are equipped with anterior/posterior electrodes. None is equipped with a posterior/posterior pair.

The electrode shown in Fig. 17.3c is a D-ring anterior electrode. This form is probably the most common form used today, especially on portable models. The D-ring shape is superior for most applications because it is easier and more natural to hold in the strained position under which defibrillators are usually used. A final form of paddle is the interior paddle. The defibrillator used for direct application of electrical charge to the open heart (which is used during open heart surgery) will have a pair of these electrodes. Pediatric paddles are similar, except for a minor difference in shape and a size.

The push-button discharge switch is sometimes mounted on the front panel of the defibrillator, but in most cases, it is mounted on one or both paddles. On most modern machines there are two discharge switches wired together in an AND-gate manner as shown in Fig. 17.4. Both switches must be pressed before the defibrillator will fire and this is a significant safety device. A prematurely fired defibrillator is a hazard to both the patient being re-suscitated and the medical staff attending the patient.

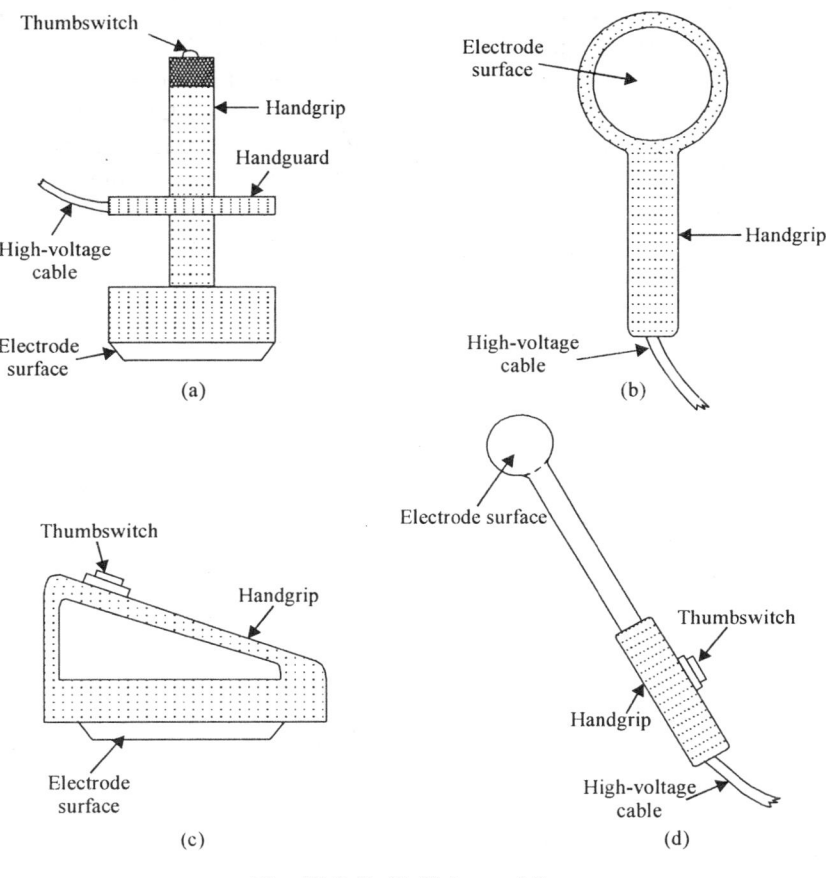

Fig. 17.3. Defibrillator paddles.

Fig. 17.4. Machine showing two discharge switches wired together.

DEFIBRILLATOR ENERGY DELIVERY

Proper distribution of energy is crucial in the use of a defibrillator, since energy that is directed to body tissue other than the heart can cause discomfort or injury to the patient. Most important, energy absorbed by the skin at the paddle can cause burns, since it is there that the current density is highest and the I^2R

heat losses are concentrated. This resistance can be reduced by proper application of electrode gel and proper pressure (approximately 30 lb), variables that depend on the operator. Hence, improper operator technique can cause injury to the patient.

To quantify the energy delivery, we may consider a defibrillator that produces a square pulse. Such a circuit has been constructed using digital circuits that shunt out the defibrillator capacitor as it discharges so as to square up the pulse. The square wave may also serve as a first-order approximation to a Lown-type defibrillator pulse. An equivalent circuit representing the square pulse defibrillator is shown in Fig. 17.5, where R_D is the internal resistance of the defibrillator, R_E is the electrode-skin resistance and R_T is the thorax resistance. The energy in the pulse, W_D, equals the instantaneous power times the pulse duration T_D. That is,

$$W_D = T_D V_D I_D \qquad \text{... (17.2)}$$

The total circuit resistance is

$$R_{TOT} = R_D + 2R_E + R_T \qquad \text{... (17.3)}$$

The resistance between the cables attached to the patient is

$$2R_E + R_T$$

Therefore,

$$W_D = \frac{V_D^2}{2R_E + R_T} T_D \qquad \text{... (17.4}$$

$$= I_D^2 T_D (2R_E + R_T)$$

where

$$I_D = \frac{V_D}{2R_E + R_T}$$

Since the current is equal through each of the resistances, the energy in each resistance is as follows:

Energy loss in the defibrillator:

$$W_L = I_D^2 R_D T_D \qquad \text{... (17.5)}$$

Energy loss in each electrode and skin:

$$W_E = I_D^2 R_E T_D \qquad \text{... (17.6)}$$

Energy delivered to the thorax:

$$W_T = I_D^2 R_T T_D \qquad \text{... (17.7)}$$

Energy available from the capacitor:

$$W_A = I_D^2 R_{TOT} T_D \qquad \text{... (17.8)}$$

The available energy is given by

$$W_A = W_T + 2W_E + W_L$$

Putting Equations (17.5), (17.6) and (17.7) into Eq. (17.8)

$$W_A = (R_T + 2R_E + R_D) I_D^2 T_D$$

Multiplying the right side by R_T/R_T and using Equation (17.8) yields

$$W_T = \frac{R_T}{R_T + 2R_E + R_D} W_A \qquad \text{... (17.9)}$$

Thus, the energy delivered to the thorax, W_T, is diminished from the available energy by the effects of both R_E and R_D.

Example 17.1. A defibrillator produces a square pulse of 3000 V with a duration of 5 ms. The instrument resistance $R_D = 10\ \Omega$, the skin-electrode resistance $R_E = 30\ \Omega$ and the thorax resistance $R_T = 30\ \Omega$. Compute the energy delivered to the patient's thorax when the defibrillator is connected as in Fig. 17.5(a).

Solution. The current from the defibrillator during the pulse is given by the voltage divided by the sum of the resistances as

$$I_D = \frac{3000}{10 + 2(30) + 30} = 30\ A$$

The energy absorbed by the thorax from Equation (17.7) is

$$W_T = (30^2)\,(30)\,(5 \times 10^{-3}) = 135\ J$$

Example 17.2. For the case in Example 17.1, calculate the energy absorbed by the two electrodes.

Solution. From Equation (17.6),

$$W_E = 2(30)^2\,(30)\,(5 \times 10^{-3}) = 270\ J$$

Notice that in these examples, more energy is absorbed by the skin at the electrodes than is delivered to the thorax. If the resistance is reduced by half, either by use of a larger electrode, by better contact with electrode gel or by increased pressure on the electrode, the energy absorbed by the skin would be reduced. This illustrates how proper electrode use and design can reduce the likelihood of tissue injury due to use of a defibrillator.

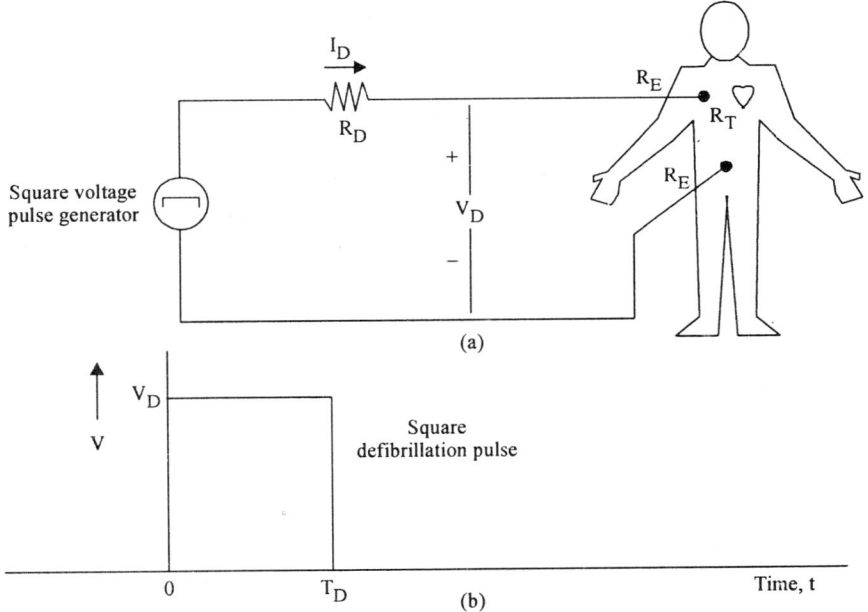

Fig. 17.5. An idealised square-wave defibrillator.

EXTERNAL DEFIBRILLATORS

As already discussed defibrillators are devices used to supply a strong electric shock (often referred to as a countershock) to a patient in an effort to convert excessively fast and ineffective heart rhythm disorders to slower rhythms that allow the heart to pump more blood. External defibrillators have been in common use for many decades for emergency treatment of life-threatening cardiac rhythms as well as for elective treatment of less threatening rapid rhythms. Figure 17.6 shows an external defibrillator.

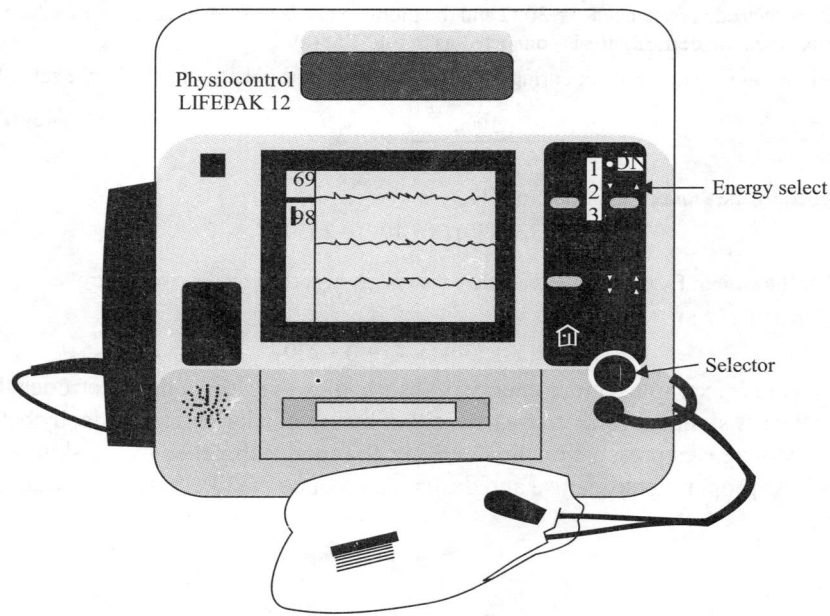

Fig. 17.6. Photograph of a trans-chest defibrillator.

Cardiac arrest occurs in more than 5,00,000 people annually in the United States and more than 70 per cent of the out-of-hospitals are due to cardiac arrhythmia treatable with defibrillators. The most serious arrhythmia treated by a defibrillator is ventricular fibrillation. Without rapid treatment using a defibrillator, ventricular fibrillation causes complete loss of cardiac function and death within minutes. Atrial fibrillation and the more organised rhythms of atrial flutter and ventricular tachycardia can be treated on less emergent basis. Although they do not cause immediate death, their shortening of the interval between contractions can impair filling the heart chambers and thus decrease cardiac output. Conventionally, treatment of ventricular fibrillation is called defibrillation, whereas treatment of the other tachycardias is called cardioversion.

Mechanism of Fibrillation

Fibrillation is chaotic electric excitation of the myocardium and results in loss of co-ordinated mechanical contraction characteristic of normal heart beats. These rhythm disorders are commonly held to be a result of re-entrant excitation pathways within the heart. The underlying abnormality that leads to the mechanism is the combination of conduction block of cardiac excitation plus rapidly recurring depolarisation of the membranes of the cardiac cells. This leads to rapid repetitive propagation of a single excitation wave or of multiple excitatory waves throughout the heart. If the waves are multiple, the rhythm may degrade into total loss of synchronisation of cardiac fibre contraction. Without synchronised contraction, the chamber affected will not contract and this is fatal in the case of ventricular fibrillation. The most common cause of these conditions and therefore of these rhythm disorders, is cardiac ischemia or infarction as a complication of atherosclerosis. Additional relatively common causes include other cardiac disorders, drug toxicity, electrolyte imbalances in the blood, hypothermia and electric shocks (especially from alternating current).

Mechanism of Defibrillation

The corrective measure is to extinguish the rapidly occurring waves of excitation by simultaneously depolarising most of the cardiac cells with a strong electric shock. The cells then can simultaneously re-polarise themselves and thus they will be back in phase with each other.

Despite years of intensive research, there is still no single theory for the mechanism of defibrillation that explains all the phenomena observed. However, it is generally held that the defibrillating shock must be adequately strong and have adequate duration to affect most of the heart cells. In general, longer duration shocks require less current than shorter duration shocks. This relationship is called the strength-duration relationship and is demonstrated by the curve shown in Fig. 17.7. Shocks of strength and duration above and to the right of the current curve (or above the energy curve) have adequate strength to defibrillate, whereas shocks below and to the left do not. From the exponentially decaying current curve an energy curve can also be determined (also shown in Fig. 17.7), which is high at very short durations due to high current requirements at short durations, but which is also high at longer durations due to additional energy being delivered as the pulse duration is lengthened at nearly constant current. Thus, for most electrical waveforms there is a minimum energy for defibrillation at approximate pulse durations of 3–8 minutes. A strength-duration charge curve can also be determined as shown in Fig. 17.7, which demonstrates that the minimum charge for defibrillation occurs at the shortest pulse duration tested. Very-short-duration pulses are not used, however, since the high current and voltage required is damaging to the myocardium. It is also important to note that excessively strong or long shocks may cause immediate re-fibrillation, thus failing to restore the heart function.

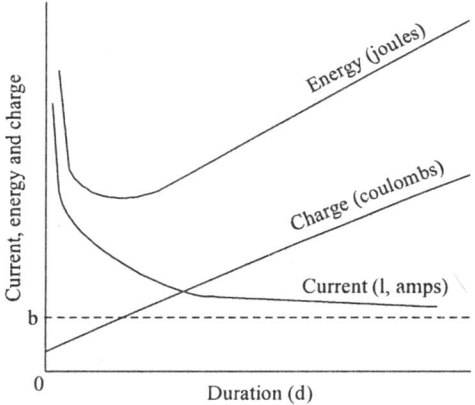

Fig. 17.7. Strength-duration curves for current, energy and charge. Adequate current shocks are above and to the right of the current curve.

In practice, for a shock applied to electrode on the skin surface of the patient's chest, durations are on the order of 3–10 milliseconds and have an intensity of a few thousand volts and tens of amperes. The energy delivered to the subject by these shocks is selectable by the operator and is on the order of 50–360 joules for most defibrillators. The exact shock intensity required at a given duration of electric pulse depends on several variables, including the intrinsic characteristics of the patient (such as the underlying disease problem or presence of certain drugs and the length of time the arrhythmia has been present), the techniques for electrode application and the particular rhythm disorder being treated (more organised rhythms require less energy than disorganised rhythms).

Clinical Defibrillators

Defibrillator design has resulted from medical and physiological research and advances in hardware technology. It is estimated that for each minute that elapses between onset of ventricular fibrillation and the first shock application, survival to leave hospital decreases by about 10 per cent. The importance of rapid response led to development of portable, battery-operated defibrillators and more recently to automatic external defibrillators (AEDs) that enable emergency responders to defibrillate with minimal training. All clinical defibrillators used today store energy in capacitors. Desirable capacitor specifications include small size, light weight and capability to sustain several thousands of volts and many charge-discharge cycles. Energy storage capacitors account for at least one pound and usually several pounds of defibrillator weight.

Figure 17.8 shows a block diagram for defibrillators. Most have a built-in monitor and synchroniser (dashed lines in Fig. 17.8). Built-in monitoring speeds up diagnosis of potentially fatal arrhythmias, especially when the ECG is monitored through the same electrodes that are used to apply the defibrillating shock. The great preponderance of defibrillators for trans-chest defibrillation deliver shocks with either a damped sinusoidal waveform produced by discharge of an RCL circuit or a truncated exponential decay waveform (sometimes called trapezoidal). Basic components of exemplary circuits for damped sine waveform and trapezoidal waveform defibrillators are shown in Figs. 17.9 and 17.10.

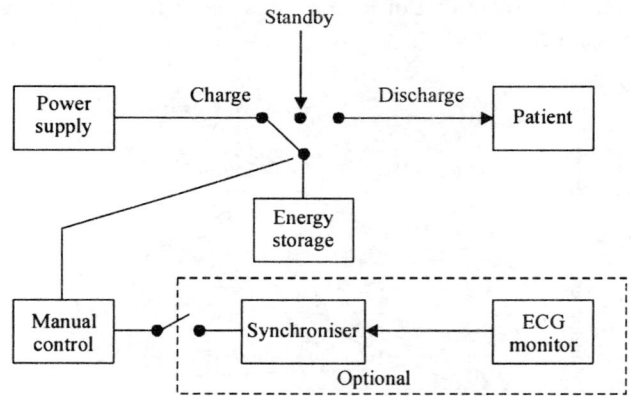

Fig. 17.8. Block diagram of a typical defibrillator.

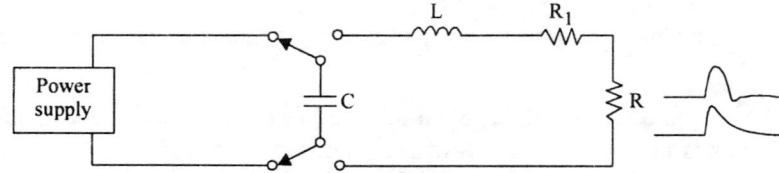

Fig. 17.9. Resister-capacitor-inductor defibrillator. The patient is represented by R.

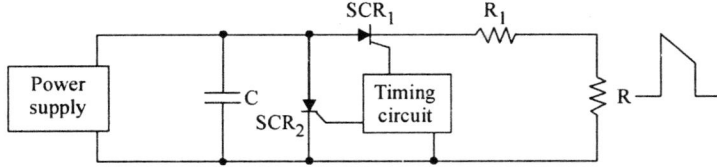

Fig. 17.10. Trapezoidal wave defibrillator. The patient is represented by R.

The shape of the waveforms generated by RCL defibrillators depend on the resistance of the patient as well as the energy storage capacitance and resistance and inductance of the inductor. When discharged into a 50 Ω load (to stimulate the patient's resistance), these defibrillators produce either a critically damped sine waveform or a slightly underdamped sine waveform (i.e., having a slight reversal of waveform polarity following the main waveform) into the 50 Ω load. Both RCL and trapezoidal waveforms defibrillate effectively. Implantable defibrillators now use alternative waveforms such as a biphasic exponential decay waveform, in which the polarity of the electrodes is reversed part way through the shock. Use of the biphasic waveform has reduced the shock intensity required for implantable defibrillators but has not yet been extended to trans-chest use except on an experimental basis. RCL defibrillators are the most widely available. They store up to about 440 joules and deliver up to about 360 joules into a patient with 50 ohm impedance. Several selectable energy intensities are available, typically from 5–360 J, so that pediatric patients, very small patients or patients with easily converted arrhythmias can be treated with low-intensity shocks. The pulse duration ranges from 3–6 ms. Because the resistance (R) varies between patients (25–150 ohms) and is part of the RCL discharge circuit, the duration and damping of the pulse also varies; increasing patient impedance lengthens and dampens the pulse. Figure 17.11 shows waveforms from RCL defibrillators with critically damped and with underdamped pulses.

Electrodes

Electrodes for external defibrillation are metal and from 70–100 cm^2 in surface area. They must be coupled to the skin with an electrically c	ductive material to achieve low impedance across the electrode-patient interface. There are two types of electrodes: hand-held (to which a conductive liquid or solid gel is applied) and adhesive, for which an adhesive conducting material holds the electrode in place. Hand-held electrodes are re-usable and are pressed against the patient's chest by the operator during shock delivery. Adhesive electrodes are disposable and are applied to the chest before the shock delivery and left in place for re-use if subsequent shocks are needed. Electrodes are usually applied with both electrodes on the anterior chest as shown in Fig. 17.12 or in anterior-to-posterior (front-to-back) position, as shown in Fig. 17.13.

Synchronisation

Most defibrillators for trans-chest use have the feature of synchronisation, which is an electronic sensing and triggering mechanism for application of the shock during the QRS complex of the ECG. This is required when treating arrhythmias other than ventricular fibrillation, because inadvertent application of a shock during the T-wave of the ECG often produces ventricular fibrillation. Selection by the operator of the synchronised mode of defibrillator operation will cause the defibrillator to automatically sense the QRS complex and apply the shock during the QRS complex. Furthermore, on the ECG display, the timing of the shock on the QRS is graphically displayed so the operator can be certain that the shock will not fall during the T-wave (see Fig. 17.14).

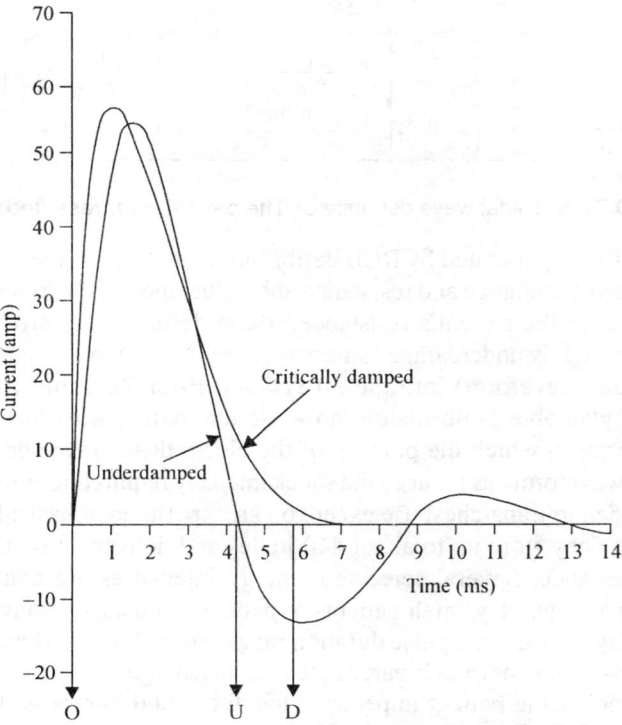

Fig. 17.11. The damped sine wave. The interval O–D represents a duration for the critically and overdamped sine waves. By time D, more than 99 per cent of the energy has been delivered. O–U is taken as the duration for an underdamped sine wave.

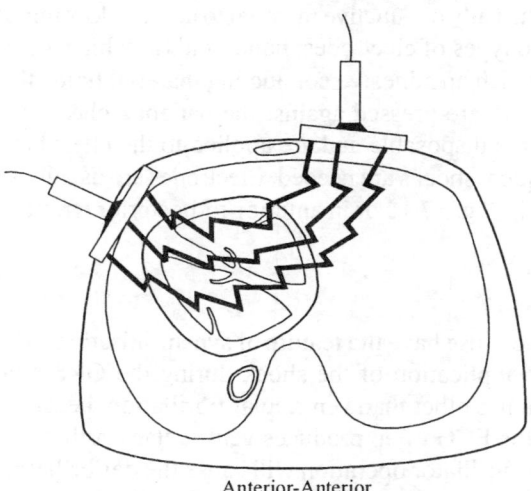

Anterior-Anterior

Fig. 17.12. Cross-sectional view of the chest showing position for standard anterior wall (pre-cordial) electrode placement. Lines of presumed current flow are shown between the electrodes on the skin surface.

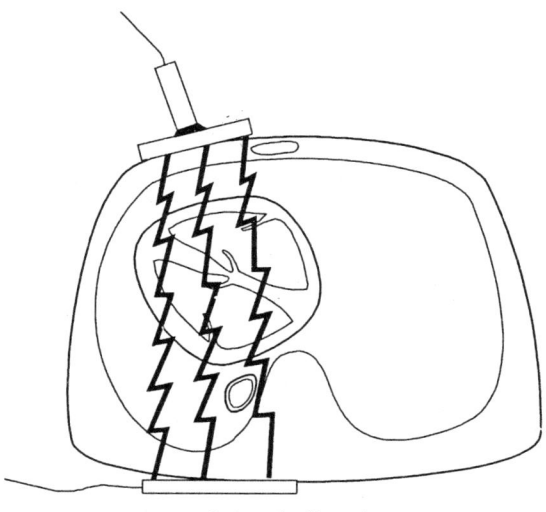

L-Anterior-Posterior

Fig. 17.13. Cross-sectional view of the chest showing position for front-to-back electrode placement. Lines of presumed current flow are shown between the electrodes on the skin surface.

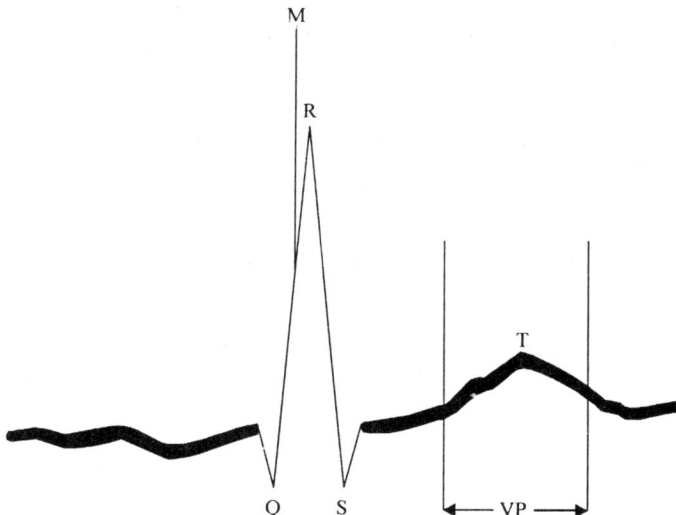

Fig. 17.14. Timing mark (M) as shown on a synchronised defibrillator monitor. The M designates when in the cardiac cycle a shock will be applied. The T-wave must be avoided, since a shock during the vulnerable period (VP) may fibrillate the ventricles. This tracing shows atrial fibrillation as identified by the irregular wavy baseline of the ECG.

Automatic External Defibrillators

Automatic external defibrillators (AEDs) are defibrillators that automatically or semi-automatically recognise and treat rapid arrhythmias, usually under emergency conditions. Their operation requires less training than operation of manual defibrillators because the operator need not know which ECG waveforms indicate rhythms requiring a shock. The operator applies adhesive electrodes from the AED to the patient and turns on the AED, which monitors the ECG and determines by built-in signal processing whether or not and when to shock the patient. In a completely automatic mode, the AED does not have a manual control as shown in Fig. 17.8 but instead has an automatic control. In semi-automatic mode, the operator must confirm the shock advisory from the AED to deliver the shock. AEDs have substantial potential for improving the chances of survival from cardiac arrest because they enable emergency personnel, who typically reach the patient before paramedics do, to deliver defibrillating shocks. Furthermore, the reduced training requirements make feasible the operation of AEDs in the home by a family member of a patient at high risk of ventricular fibrillation.

Defibrillator Safety

Defibrillator are potentially dangerous devices because of their high electrical output characteristics. The danger to the patient of unsynchronised shocks has already been presented, as has the synchronisation design to prevent inadvertent precipitation of fibrillation by a cardioversion shock applied during the T wave. There are other safety issues. Improper technique may result in accidental shocking of the operator or other personnel in the vicinity, if someone is in contact with the electric discharge pathway. This may occur if the operator is careless in holding the discharge electrode or if someone is in contact with the patient or with a metal bed occupied by the subject when the shock is applied. Proper training and technique is necessary to avoid this risk.

Another safety issue is that of producing damage to the patient by application of excessively strong or excessively numerous shocks. Although cardiac damage has been reported after high-intensity and repetitive shocks to experimental animals and human patients, it is generally held that significant cardiac damage is unlikely if proper clinical procedures and guidelines are followed.

Failure of a defibrillator to operate correctly may also be considered a safety issue, since inability of a defibrillator to deliver a shock in the absence of a replacement unit means loss of the opportunity to re-suscitate the patient. A recent review of defibrillator failures found that operator errors, inadequate defibrillator care and maintenance and to a lesser extent, component failure accounted for the majority of defibrillator failures.

IMPLANTABLE DEFIBRILLATORS

The implantable defibrillator is now an established and powerful therapeutic tool. The transition to pectoral implants with biphasic waveforms and efficient yet simple transvenous lead systems is simplifying the implant procedure and drastically reducing the number of unpleasant VF inductions required to demonstrate adequate system performance. These advances are making the implantable defibrillator easier to use, less costly and more acceptable to patients and their physicians.

The implantable cardioverter defibrillator (ICD) is a therapeutic device that can detect ventricular tachycardia or fibrillation and automatically deliver high-voltage (750 V) shocks that will restore normal sinus rhythm. Advanced versions also provide low-voltage (5–10 V) pacing stimuli for painless termination of ventricular tachycardia and for management of bradyarrhythmias. The proven efficacy of the automatic implantable defibrillator has placed it in the mainstream of therapies for the prevention of sudden arrhythmic cardiac death.

The newest devices can be implanted in the patient's pectoral region and use electrodes that can be inserted transvenously, eliminating the traumatic thoracotomy required for placement of the earlier epicardial electrode systems. Transvenous systems provide rapid, minimally invasive implants with high assurance of success and greater patient comfort. Advanced arrhythmia detection algorithms offer a high degree of sensitivity with reasonable specificity and extensive monitoring is provided to document performance and to facilitate appropriate programming of arrhythmia detection and therapy parameters. Generator longevity can now exceed 4 years and the cost of providing this therapy is declining.

Pulse Generators

The implantable defibrillator consists of a primary battery, high-voltage capacitor bank and sensing and control circuitry housed in a hermetically sealed titanium case. Commercially available devices weigh between 197 and 237 grams and range in volume from 113 to 145 cm^3. Clinical trials are in progress on devices with volumes ranging from 178 cm^3 to 60 cm^3 and weights between 275 and 104 grams. Further size reductions will be achieved with the introduction of improved capacitor and integrated circuit technologies and lead systems offering lower pacing and defibrillation thresholds. Progress should parallel that made with antibradycardia pacemakers that have evolved from 250 gram, non-programmable, VOO units with 600 μJ pacing outputs to 26 gram, multiprogrammable, DDDR units with dual 25 μJ outputs.

Implantable defibrillator circuitry must include an amplifier, to allow detection of the millivolt-range cardiac electrogram signals; non-invasively programmable processing and control functions, to evaluate the sensed cardiac activity and to direct generation and delivery of the therapeutic energy; high-voltage switching capability; DC-DC conversion functions to step up the low battery voltages; random access memories, to store appropriate patient and device data; and radiofrequency telemetry systems, to allow communication to and from the implanted device.

Monolithic integrated circuits on hybridised substrates have made it possible to accomplish these diverse functions in a commercially acceptable and highly reliable form.

Defibrillators must convert battery voltages of approximately 6.5 V to the 600–750 V needed to defibrillate the heart. Since the conversion process control cannot directly supply this high voltage at current strengths needed for defibrillation, charge is accumulated in relatively large ($\approx$85–120 μF effective capacitance) aluminium electrolytic capacitors that account for 20–30 per cent of the volume of a typical defibrillator. These capacitors must be charged periodically to prevent their dielectric from deteriorating. If this is not done, the capacitors become electrically leaky, yielding excessively long charge times and delay of therapy.

Early defibrillators required that the patient return to the clinic periodically to have the capacitors reformed, whereas newer devices do this automatically at pre-set or programmable times. Improved capacitor technology, perhaps ceramic or thin-film, will eventually offer higher storage densities, greater shape variability for denser component packaging and freedom from the need to waste battery capacity performing periodic reforming charges. Packaging density has already improved from 0.03 J/cm^3 for devices such as the early cardioverter to 0.43 J/cm^3 with some investigational ICDs. Capacitors that allow conformal shaping could readily increase this density to more than 0.6 J/cm^3.

Power sources used in defibrillators must have sufficient capacity to provide 50–400 full energy charges ($\approx$34 J) and 3 to 5 years of bradycardia pacing and background circuit operation. They must have a very low internal resistance in order to supply the relatively high currents needed to charge the defibrillation capacitors in 5–15 seconds. This generally requires that the batteries have large surface area electrodes and use chemistries that exhibit higher rates of internal discharge than those seen with the lithium iodide batteries used in pacemakers. The most commonly used defibrillator battery chemistry is lithium silver vanadium oxide.

Electrode Systems ('Leads')

Early implantable defibrillators utilised patch electrodes (typically a titanium mesh electrode) placed on the surface of the heart, requiring entry through the chest (Fig. 17.15). This procedure is associated with approximately 3–4 per cent peri-operative mortality, significant hospitalisation time and complications, patient discomfort and high costs. Although sub-costal, sub-xiphoid and thoracoscopic techniques can minimise the surgical procedure, the ultimate solution has been development of fully transvenous lead systems with acceptable defibrillation thresholds.

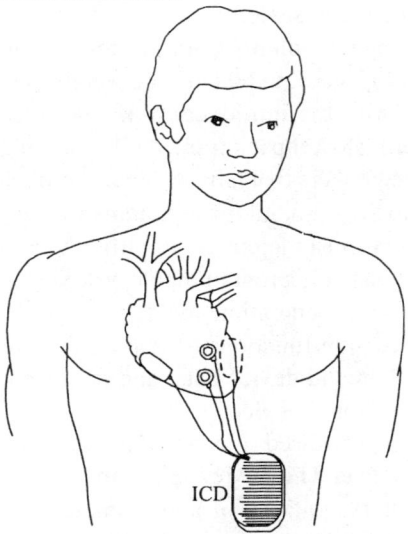

Fig. 17.15. Epicardial ICD systems typically use two or three large defibrillating patch electrodes placed on the epicardium of the left and right ventricles and a pair of myocardial electrodes for detection and pacing. The generator is usually placed in the abdomen.

Currently available transvenous leads are constructed much like pacemaker leads, using polyurethane or silicone insulation and platinum-iridium electrode materials. Acceptable thresholds are obtained in 67–95 per cent of patients, with mean defibrillation thresholds ranging from 10.9–18.1 J. These lead systems use a combination of two or more electrodes located in the right ventricular apex, the superior vena cava, the coronary sinus and sometimes, a sub-cutaneous patch electrode is placed in the chest region. These leads offer advantages beyond the avoidance of major surgery. They are easier to remove should there be infections or a need for lead system revision. The pacing thresholds of current transvenous defibrillation electrodes are typically 0.96 ± 0.39 V and the electrogram amplitudes are on the order of 16.4 ± 6.4 mV. The eventual application of steroid-eluting materials in the leads should provide increased pacing efficiency with transvenous lead systems, thereby reducing the current drain associated with pacing and extending pulse generator longevity.

Lead systems are being refined to simplify the implant procedures. One approach is the use of a single catheter having a single right ventricular low-voltage electrode for pacing and detection and a pair of high-voltage defibrillation electrodes spaced for replacement in the right ventricle and in the superior vena cava (Fig. 17.16a). A more recent approach parallels that used for unipolar pacemakers. A single-right ventricular catheter having bipolar pace/sense electrodes and one right ventricular high-voltage electrode is used in conjunction with a defibrillator housing that serves as the second high-voltage electrode (Fig. 17.16b). Mean biphasic pulse defibrillation thresholds with the generator-electrode placed in the patient's left pectoral region are reported to be 9.8 ± 6.6 J ($n = 102$). This approach appears to be practicable only with generators suitable for pectoral placement, but such devices will become increasingly available.

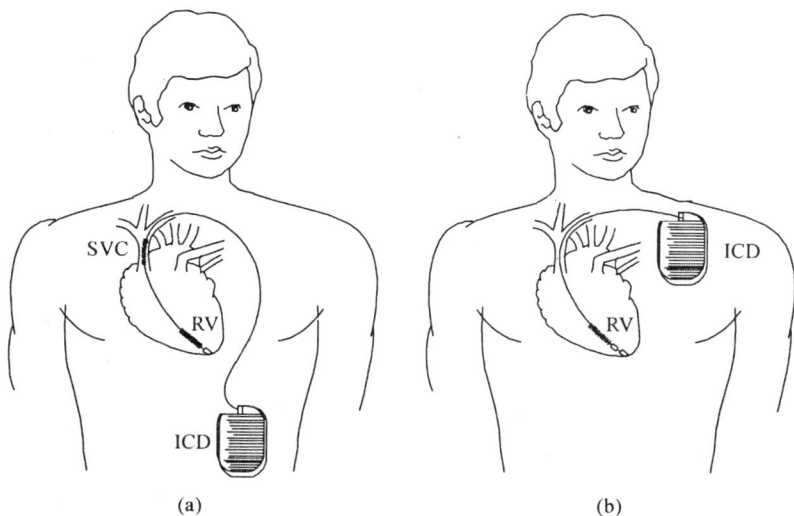

(a)   (b)

Fig. 17.16. The latest transvenous fibrillation systems employ a single catheter placed in the right ventricular apex. In panel (a), a single transvenous catheter provides defibrillation electrodes in the superior vena cava and in the right ventricle. This catheter provides a single pace/sense electrode which is used in conjunction with the right ventricular high-voltage defibrillation electrode for arrhythmia detection and antibradycardia/antitachycardia pacing (a configuration that is sometimes referred to as integrated bipolar). With pulse generators small enough to be placed in the pectoral region, defibrillation can be achieved by delivering energy between the generator housing and one high-voltage electrode in the right ventricle (analogous to unipolar pacing) as is shown in panel (b). This catheter provided bipolar pace/sense electrodes for arrhythmia detection and antibradycardia/antitachycardia pacing.

Arrhythmia Detection

Most defibrillator detection algorithms rely primarily on heart rate to indicate the presence of a treatable rhythm. Additional refinements sometimes include simple morphology assessments, as with the probability density function and analysis of rhythm stability and rate of change in rate.

The probability density function evaluates the percentage of time that the filtered ventricular electrogram spends in a window centered on the baseline. The rate-of-change-in-rate or onset evaluation discriminates sinus tachycardia from ventricular tachycardia on the basis of the typically gradual acceleration of sinus rhythms versus the relatively abrupt acceleration of many pathologic tachycardias. The rate stability function is designed to bar detection of tachyarrhythmias as long as the variation in ventricular rate exceeds a physician-programmed tolerance, thereby reducing the likelihood of inappropriate therapy delivery in response to atrial fibrillation. This concept appears to be one of the more successful detection algorithm enhancements.

Because these additions to the detection algorithm reduce sensitivity, some defibrillator designs offer a supplementary detection mode that will trigger therapy in response to any elevated ventricular rate of the prolonged duration. These extended-high-rate algorithms by-pass all or portions of the normal detection screening, resulting in low specificity for rhythms with prolonged elevated rates such as exercise-induced sinus tachycardia. Consequently, use of such algorithms generally increases the incidences of inappropriate therapies. Improvements in arrhythmia detection specificity are desirable, but they must not decrease the excellent sensitivity offered by current algorithms. The anticipated introduction of defibrillators incorporating dual-chamber pacemaker capability will certainly help in this quest, since it will then be possible to use atrial electrograms in the rhythm classification process. It would also be desirable to have a means of evaluating the patient's hemodynamic tolerance of the rhythm, so that the more comfortable pacing sequences could be used as long as the patient was not syncopal yet branch quickly to a definitive shock should the patient begin to lose consciousness.

Although various enhanced detection processes have been proposed, many have not been tested clinically, in some cases because sufficient processing power was not available in implantable systems and in some cases because sensor technology was not yet ready for chronic implantation. Advances in technology may eventually make some of these very elegant proposals practicable. Examples of proposed detection enhancements include extended analyses of cardiac event timing (PR and RR stability, AV interval variation, temporal distribution of atrial electrogram intervals and of ventricular electrogram intervals, timing differences and/or coherency of multiple ventricular electrograms, ventricular response to a provocative atrial extrastimuli), electrogram waveform analyses (paced depolarisation integral, morphology analyses of right ventricular or atrial electrograms), analyses of hemodynamic parameters (right-ventricular pulsatile pressure, mean right atrial and mean right ventricular pressures, wedge coronary sinus pressure, static right ventricular pressure, right atrial pressure, right ventricular stroke volume, mixed venous oxygen saturation and mixed venous blood temperature, left ventricular impedance, intramyocardial pressure gradient, aortic and pulmonary artery flow) and detection of physical motion.

Because defibrillator designs are intentionally biased to overtreat in preference to the life-threatening consequences associated with failure to treat, there is some incidence of inappropriate therapy delivery. Unwarranted therapies are usually triggered by supraventricular tachyarrhythmias, especially atrial fibrillation or sinus tachycardia associated with rates faster than the ventricular tachycardia detection rate threshold. Additional causes include non-sustained ventricular tachycardia, oversensing of T-waves, double counting of R-waves and pacing stimuli from brady pacemakers and technical faults such as loose lead-generator connections or lead fractures.

Despite the bias for high detection sensitivity, undersensing does occur. It has been shown to result from inappropriate detection algorithm programming, such as an excessively high tachycardia detection rate; inappropriate amplifier gain characteristics; and electrode designs that place the sensing terminals too close to the high-voltage electrodes with a consequent reduction in electrogram amplitude following shocks. Undersensing can also result in the induction of tachycardia should the amplifier gain control algorithm result in the undersensing of sinus rhythms.

Arrhythmia Therapy

Pioneering implantable defibrillators were capable only of defibrillation shocks. Subsequently, synchronised cardioversion capability was added. Antibradycardia pacing had to be provided by implantation of a standard pacemaker in addition to the defibrillator and if antitachycardia pacing was prescribed, it was necessary to use an antitachycardia pacemaker.

Several currently marketed implantable defibrillators offer integrated ventricular demand pacemaker function and tiered antiarrhythmia therapy (pacing/cardioversion/defibrillation). Various burst and ramp antitachycardia pacing algorithms are offered and they all seem to offer comparably high success rates. These expanded therapeutic capabilities improve patient comfort by reducing the incidence of shocks in conscious patients, eliminate the problems and discomfort associated with implantation of multiple devices and contribute to a greater degree of success, since the prescribed regimens can be carefully tailored to specific patient needs. Availability of devices with antitachy pacing capability significantly increases the acceptability of the implantable defibrillator for patients with ventricular tachycardia.

Human clinical trials have shown that biphasic defibrillation waveforms are more effective than monophasic waveforms and newer devices now incorporate this characteristic. Speculative examinations for biphasic superiority include the large voltage change at the transition from the first to the second phase or hyperpolarisation of tissue and re-activation of sodium channels during the initial phase, with resultant tissue conditioning that allows the second phase to more readily excite the myocardium.

Antitachycardia pacing and cardioversion are not uniformly successful. There is some incidence of ventricular arrhythmia acceleration with antitachycardia pacing and cardioversion and it is also not unusual for cardioversion to induce atrial fibrillation that in turn triggers unwarranted therapies. An ideal therapeutic solution would be one capable of preventing the occurrence of tachycardia altogether. Prevention techniques have been investigated, among them the use of precisely timed sub-threshold stimuli, simultaneous stimulation at multiple sites and pacing with elevated energies at the site of the tachycardia, but none has yet proven practical.

The rudimentary VVI antibradycardia pacing provided by current defibrillators lacks rate responsiveness and atrial pacing capability. Consequently, some defibrillator patients require implantation of a separate dual-chamber pacemaker for hemodynamic support. It is inevitable that future generations of defibrillators will offer dual-chamber pacing capabilities.

Atrial fibrillation, occurring either as a consequence of defibrillator operation or as a natural progression in many defibrillator patients, is a major therapeutic challenge. It is certainly possible to adapt implantable defibrillator technology to treat atrial fibrillation, but the challenge is to do so without causing the patient undue discomfort. Biphasic waveform defibrillation of acutely induced atrial fibrillation has been demonstrated in human with an 80 per cent success rate at 0.4 J using epicardial electrodes. Stand-alone atrial defibrillators are in development and if they are successful, it is likely that this capability would be integrated into the mainstream ventricular defibrillators as well. However, most conscious patients find shocks above 0.5 J to be very unpleasant and it remains to be demonstrated that a clinically acceptable energy level will be efficacious when applied with transvenous electrode systems to spontaneously occurring atrial fibrillation. Moreover, a stand-alone atrial defibrillator either must deliver an atrial shock with complete assurance of appropriate synchronisation to ventricular activity or must restrict the therapeutical energy delivery to atrial structures in order to prevent inadvertent induction of a malignant ventricular arrhythmia.

Implantable Monitoring

Until recently, defibrillator data recording capabilities were quite limited, making it difficult to verify the adequacy of arrhythmia detection and therapy settings. The latest devices record electrograms and diagnostic channel data showing device behaviour during multiple tachyarrhythmia episodes. These devices also include counters (number of events detected, success and failure of each programmed therapy and so on) that present a broad, though less specific. Monitoring capability in some of the newest devices appears to be the equivalent of 32 Kbytes of random access memory, allowing electrogram waveform records of approximately 2 minute duration, with some opportunity for later expansion by judicious selection of sampling rates and data compression techniques. Electrogram storage has proven useful for documenting false therapy delivery due to atrial fibrillation, lead fractures and sinus tachycardia, determining the triggers of arrhythmias; documenting rhythm accelerations in response to therapies and demonstrating appropriate device behaviour when treating asymptomatic rhythms.

Electrograms provide useful information by themselves, yet they cannot indicate how the device interpreted cardiac activity. Increasingly, electrogram records are being supplemented with event markers that indicate how the device is responding on a beat-by-beat basis. These records can include measurements of the sensed and paced intervals, indication as to the specific detection zone an event falls in, indication of charge initiation and other device performance data.

Follow-Up

Defibrillator patients and their devices require careful follow-up. In one study of 241 ICD patients with epicardial lead systems, 53 per cent of the patients experienced one or more complications during an average exposure of 24 months. These complications included infection requiring device removal in 5 per cent, post-operative respiratory complications in 11 per cent, post-operative bleeding and/or thrombosis in 4 per cent, lead system migration or disruption in 8 per cent and documented inappropriate therapy delivery, most commonly due to atrial fibrillation, in 22 per cent. A shorter study of eighty patients with transvenous defibrillator systems reported no post-operative pulmonary complications, transient nerve injury (1 per cent), asymptomatic sub-clavian vein occlusion (2.5 per cent), pericardial effusion (1 per cent), sub-cutaneous patch pocket hematoma (5 per cent), pulse generator pocket infection (1 per cent), lead fracture (1 per cent) and lead system dislodgement (10 per cent). During a mean follow-up period of 11 months, 7.5 per cent of the patients in this series experienced inappropriate therapy delivery, half for atrial fibrillation and the rest for sinus tachycardia.

Although routine follow-up can be accomplished in the clinic, detection and analysis of transient events depend on the recording capabilities available in the devices or on the use of various external monitoring equipment.

Economics

The annual cost of ICD therapy is dropping as a consequence of better longevity and simpler implantation techniques. Early generators that lacked programmability, antibradycardia pacing capability and event recording had 62 per cent survival at 18 months and 2 per cent at 30 months. Some recent programmable designs that include VVI pacing capability and considerable event storage exhibit 96.8 per cent survival at 48 months. It has been estimated that an increase in generator longevity from 2–5 years would lower the cost per life-year saved by 55 per cent in a hypothetical patient population with a 3 year sudden mortality of 28 per cent. More efficient energy conversion circuits and finer line-width integrated circuit technology with smaller, more highly integrated circuits and reduced current drains will yield longer-lasting defibrillators while continuing the evolution to smaller volumes.

Cost of the implantation procedure is clearly declining as transvenous lead systems become common-place. Total hospitalisation duration, complication rates and use of costly hospital operating rooms and intensive care facilities all are reduced, providing significant financial benefits. One study reported requiring half the intensive care unit time and a reduction in total hospitalisation from 26 to 15 days when comparing transvenous to epicardial approaches. Another centre reported a mean hospitalisation stay of 6 days for patients receiving transvenous defibrillation systems.

Increasing sophistication of the implantable defibrillators paradoxically contributes to cost efficacy. Incorporation of single-chamber brady pacing capability eliminates the cost of separate pacemaker and lead for those patients who need one. Eventually even dual-chamber pacing capability will be available. Programmable detection and therapy features obviate the need for device replacement that was required when fixed parameter devices proved to be inappropriately specified or too inflexible to adapt to a patient's physiologic changes.

Significant cost savings may be obtained by better patient selection criteria and processes, obviating the need for extensive hospitalisation and costly electrophysiologic studies prior to device implantation in some patient groups. One frequently discussed issue is the prophylactic role that implantable defibrillators will or should play. Unless a means is found to build far less expensive devices that can be placed with minimal time and facilities, the life-saving yield for prophylactic defibrillators will have to be high if they are to be cost-effective. This remains an open issue.

TROUBLESHOOTING DEFIBRILLATORS

Symptoms of defibrillator problems usually show up during routine testing procedures. Since it is an emergency-care device, capable of inflicting a fatal shock on patient or an attendant, procedures for its use must be fail-safe. Safety of the defibrillator is ensured by frequent testing and by proper training of the operators.

The defibrillator block diagram in Fig. 17.2 uses the signal from an ECG monitor. Test procedures that reveal problems in the blocks beyond the ECG are usually found with a defibrillator analyser. This device provides a 50 Ω resistance discharge path for the defibrillator paddles that simulates the torso resistance. The defibrillator electrodes are placed on the metal test pads. Energy levels of discharges into the test pads are measured up to 1000 J. The waveform of this discharge may be displayed on an oscilloscope. The defibrillator analyser generates an R-wave of an ECG pattern at approximately 60 bpm and it then displays the time between the leading edge of the R-wave and the cardioverter discharge. This measurement detects failures in the QRS detector and the 30 ms delay circuit in the block diagram.

In the defibrillator mode, the R-wave would be used along with the energise switch to ensure that the defibrillator properly inhibits unnecessary defibrillator pulses. The tester may also simulate a fibrillation waveform to ensure that a defibrillator discharge can be activated by the attendant switch as necessary. Any errors in the waveform or energy level would indicate problems in the defibrillator itself.

The wearing element that would yield low-energy output is the battery pack. The battery voltage should be tested under loaded conditions. In accordance with manufacturer specification, it should be periodically fully discharged (sometimes called 'deep discharged'). After re-charging, the battery will be capable of delivering its rated energy. Otherwise, polarisation on the battery terminals could limit its performance.

Chapter 18

Electrosurgical Devices

INTRODUCTION

An electrosurgical unit (ESU) passes high-frequency electric currents through biologic tissues to achieve specific surgical effects such as cutting, coagulation or desiccation. It has been used since the 1920s to cut tissue effectively while at the same time controlling the amount of bleeding. Cutting is achieved primarily with a continuous sinusoidal waveform, whereas coagulation is achieved primarily with a series of sinusoidal wave packets. The surgeon selects either one of these waveforms or a blend of them to suit the surgical needs. An electrosurgical unit can be operated in two modes, the monopolar mode and the bipolar mode. The most noticeable difference between these two modes is the method in which the electric current enters and leaves the tissue. In the monopolar mode, the current flows from a small active electrode into the surgical site, spreads through the body and returns to a large dispersive electrode on the skin. The high current density in the vicinity of the active electrode achieves tissue cutting or coagulation, whereas the low current density under the dispersive electrode causes no tissue damage. In the bipolar mode, the current flows only through the tissue held between two forceps electrodes. The monopolar mode is used for both cutting and coagulation. The bipolar mode is used primarily for coagulation.

BASIC ESU

The basic ESU, illustrated in Fig. 18.1, consists of a radio-frequency oscillator operating between 300 kHz and 3 MHz. The cutting electrode has a tapered edge that would be too dull to cut tissue without the RF current produced by the oscillator. When the electrode is held sufficiently far away from the body, no current flows and no cutting action occurs. Voltages on the electrode may range from 1000 to 10000 volts peak-to-peak (V_{pp}). As the electrode is brought closer to the skin at these voltages, a spark will jump across. The breakdown voltage of air is approximately 30 kV/cm, so if, for example, the electrode voltage is 10000 V, a spark 0.33 cm in length can be drawn. The existence of sparks in normal ESU application makes it a fire hazard in the presence of flammable anaesthetics or other flammable gases.

When the electrode touches the skin, no spark may be present. When the RF current is applied, it passes through individual cell membranes by capacitive coupling. At these high frequencies, large currents flow into the cell, causing it to vapourise and thereby cause a rupture of the tissue close to the cutting electrode. The current density a short distance from the cutting electrode on the way to the return electrode, as illustrated in Fig. 18.1, decreases quickly to harmless levels. These currents should not cause muscle contraction or heart fibrillation. The return electrode illustrated in Fig. 18.1 must have a large area to minimise the heating effect there and prevent surface burns. One of the hazards with ESU is burns at the return patient-plate electrode because of poor skin contact.

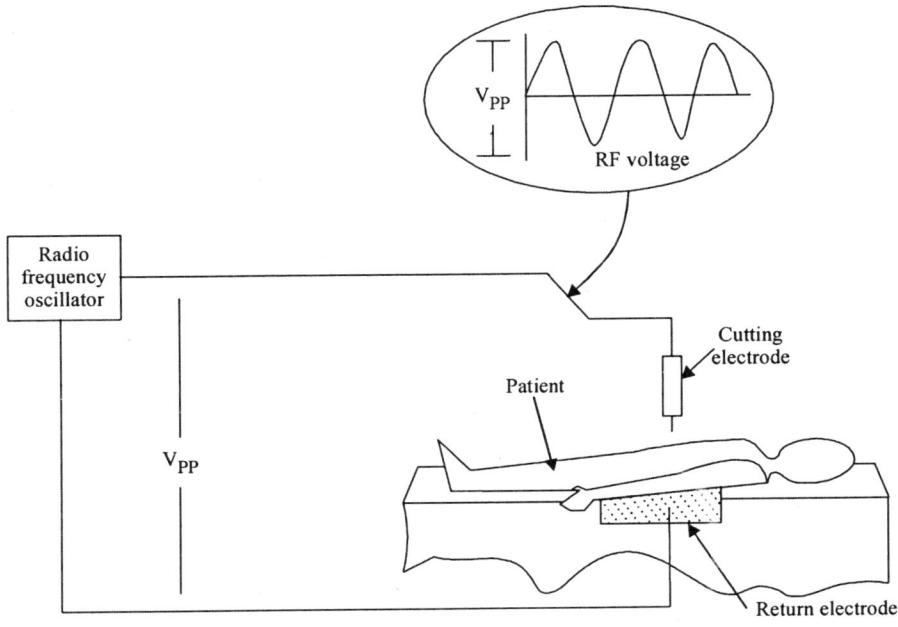

Fig. 18.1. The essential components of an ESU.

The ESU electrode has several advantages over the traditional stainless steel scalpel. It can often cut faster. Furthermore, the heating effect of the cutting currents and sparks has a cauterising effect on the tissue that inhibits bleeding. Therefore, the ESU can reduce blood loss and minimise the time the patient is in surgery.

This chapter discusses the theory of operation for electrosurgical units, outlines various modes of operation and gives basic design details for electronic circuits and electrodes. It then describes how improper application of electrosurgical units can lead to hazardous situations for both the operator and the patient and how such hazardous situations can be avoided or reduced through proper monitoring methods. Finally, the chapter gives an update on current and future developments and applications.

THEORY OF OPERATION

In principle, electrosurgery is based on the rapid heating of tissue. To better understand the thermodynamic events during electrosurgery, it helps to know the general effects of heat on biological tissue. Consider a tissue volume that experiences a temperature increase from normal body temperature to 45°C within a few seconds. Although the cells in this tissue volume show neither microscopic nor macroscopic changes, some cytochemical changes do in fact occur. However, these changes are reversible and the cells return to their normal function when the temperature returns to normal values. Above 45°C, irreversible changes take place that inhibit normal cell functions and lead to cell death. First, between 45°C and 60°C, the proteins in the cell lose their quaternary configuration and solidify into a glutinous substance that resembles the white of a hard-boiled egg. This process, termed coagulation, is accompanied by tissue blanching.

Further increasing the temperature up to 100°C leads to tissue drying; that is, the aqueous cell contents evaporate. This process is called desiccation. If the temperature is increased beyond 100°C, the solid contents of the tissue reduce to carbon, a process referred to as carbonisation. Tissue damage depends not only on temperature, however, but also on the length of exposure to heat. Thus, the overall temperature-induced tissue damage is an integrative effect between temperature and time that is expressed mathematically by the Arrhenius relationship, where an exponential function of temperature is integrated over time.

In the monopolar mode, the active electrode either touches the tissue directly or is held a few millimetres above the tissue. When the electrode is held above the tissue, the electric current bridges the air gap by creating an electric discharge arc. A visible arc forms when the electric field strength exceeds 1 kV/mm in the gap and disappears when the field strength drops below a certain threshold level. When the active electrode touches the tissue and the current flows directly from the electrode into the tissue without forming an arc, the rise in tissue temperature follows the bioheat equation:

$$T - T_0 = \frac{1}{\sigma \rho c} J^2 t \qquad \qquad ... (18.1)$$

where T and T_0 are the final and initial temperatures (K), σ is the electrical conductivity (S/m), ρ is the tissue density (kg/m^3), c is the specific heat of the tissue (Jkg^{-1}K^{-1}), J is the current density (A/m^2) and t is the duration of heat applications. The bioheat equation is valid for short application times where secondary effects such as heat transfer to surrounding tissues, blood perfusion and metabolic heat can be neglected. According to Eq. (18.1), the surgeon has primarily three means of controlling the cutting or coagulation effect during electrosurgery: the contact area between active electrode and tissue, the electrical current density and the activation time. In most commercially available electrosurgical generators, the output variable that can be adjusted in power. This power setting, in conjunction with the output power vs. tissue impedance characteristics of the generator, allow the surgeon some control over current. Table 18.1 lists typical output power and mode settings for various surgical procedures. Table 18.2 lists some typical impedance ranges seen during use of an ESU in surgery. The values are shown as ranges because the impedance increases as the tissue dries out and at the same time, the output power of the ESU decreases. The surgeon may control current density by selection of the active electrode type and size.

Table 18.1. Typical ESU power settings for various surgical procedures.

Power-level range	Procedures
Low power	
<30 W cutting	Neurosurgery
<30 W coagulation	Dermatology
	Plastic surgery
	Oral surgery
	Laparoscopic sterilisation
	Vasectomy
Medium power	
30–150 W cutting	General surgery
30–70 W coagulation	Laparotomies

Contd...

Power-level range	Procedures
	Head and neck surgery (ENT)
	Major vascular surgery
	Routine thoracic surgery
	Polypectomy
High power	
>150 W cutting	Transurethral resection procedures (TURPs)
>70 W coagulation	Thoracotomies
	Ablative cancer surgery
	Mastectomies

Note: Ranges assume the use of a standard blade electrode. Use of a needle electrode or other small current-concentrating electrode, allows lower settings to be used; users are urged to use the lowest setting that provides the desired clinical results.

Table 18.2. Typical impedance ranges seen during use of an ESU in surgery.

Cut mode application	Impedance range (Ω)
Prostate tissue	400–1700
Oral cavity	1000–2000
Liver tissue	
Muscle tissue	
Gall bladder	1500–2400
Skin tissue	1700–2500
Bowel tissue	2500–3000
Periosteum	
Mesentery	3000–4200
Omentum	
Adipose tissue	3500–4500
Scar tissue	
Adhesions	
Coagulation mode application	
Contact coagulation to stop bleeding	100–1000

MONOPOLAR MODE

A continuous sinusoidal waveform cuts tissue with very little hemostasis. This waveform is simply called cut or pure cut. During each positive and negative swing of the sinusoidal waveform, a new discharge arc forms and disappears at essentially the same tissue location. The electric current concentrates at this tissue location, causing a sudden increase in temperature due to resistive heating. The rapid rise in temperature then vapourises intracellular fluids, increases cell pressure and ruptures the cell membrane, thereby parting the tissue. This chain of events is confined to the vicinity of the arc, because from there the electric current spreads to a much larger tissue volume and the current density is no longer high enough to cause resistive heating damage. Typical output values for ESUs, in cut and other modes, are shown in Table 18.3.

Table 18.3. Typical output characteristics of ESUs.

	Output voltage range Open circuit, $V_{peak\text{-}peak}$ V	Output power range, W	Frequency, kHz	Crest factor $\left(\dfrac{V_{peak}}{V_{rms}}\right)$	Duty cycle
Monopolar modes					
Cut	200–5000	1–400	300–1750	1.4–2.1	100%
Blend	1500–5800	1–300	300–1750	2.1–6.0	25–80%
Desiccate	400–6500	1–200	240–800	3.5–6.0	50–100%
Fulgurate/spray	600–12000	1–200	300–800	6.0–20.0	10–70%
Bipolar mode					
Coagulate/desiccate	200–1000	1–70	300–1050	1.6–12.0	25–100%

Experimental observations have shown that more hemostasis is achieved when cutting with an interrupted sinusoidal waveform or amplitude modulated continuous waveform. These waveforms are typically called blend or blended cut. Some ESUs offer a choice of blend waveforms to allow the surgeon to select degree of hemostasis desired.

When a continuous or interrupted waveform is used in contact with the tissue and the output voltage current density is too low to sustain arcing, desiccation of the tissue will occur. Some ESUs have a distinct mode for this purpose called desiccation or contact coagulation.

In non-contact coagulation, the duty cycle of an interrupted waveform and the crest factor (ratio of peak voltage to rms voltage) influence the degree of hemostasis. While a continuous waveform re-establishes the arc at essentially the same tissue location concentrating the heat there, an interrupted waveform cause the arc to re-establish itself at different tissue locations. The arc seems to dance from one location to the other raising the temperature of the top tissue layer to coagulation levels. These waveforms are called fulguration or spray. Since the current inside the tissue spreads very quickly from the point where the arc strikes, the heat concentrates in the top layer, primarily desiccating tissue and causing some carbonisation. During surgery, a surgeon can easily choose between cutting, coagulation or a combination of the two by activating a switch on the grip of the active electrode or by use of a footswitch.

BIPOLAR MODE

The bipolar mode concentrates the current flow between the two electrodes, requiring considerably less power for achieving the same coagulation effect than the monopolar mode. For example, consider coagulating a small blood vessel with 3 mm external diameter and 2 mm internal diameter, a tissue resistivity of 360 Ωcm, a contract area of 2 × 4 mm and a distance between the forceps tips of 1 mm. The tissue resistance between the forceps is 450 Ω as calculated from R = ρL/A, where ρ is the resistivity, L is the distance between the forceps and A is the contact area. Assuming a typical current density of 200 mA/cm^2, then a small current of 16 mA, a voltage of 7.2 V and power level of 0.12 W suffice to coagulate this small blood vessel. In contrast, during monopolar coagulation, current levels of 200 mA and power levels of 100 W or more are not uncommon to achieve the same surgical effect. The temperature increase in the vessel tissue follows the bioheat equation, Eq. (18.1). If the specific heat of the vessel tissue is 4.2 Jg^{-1}K^{-1} and the tissue density is 1 g/cm^3, then the temperature of the tissue between the forceps increases from 37°C to 57°C in 5.83 seconds. When the active electrode touches the tissue, less tissue damage occurs during coagulation, because the charring and carbonisation that accompanies fulguration is avoided.

ESU DESIGN

Modern ESUs contain building blocks that are also found in other medical devices, such as microprocessors, power supplies, enclosures, cables, indicators, displays and alarms. The main building blocks unique to ESUs are control input switches, the high-frequency power amplifier and the safety monitor. The first two will be discussed briefly here and the latter will be discussed later.

Control input switches include front panel controls, footswitch controls and handswitch controls. In order to make operating an ESU more uniform between models and manufacturers and to reduce the possibility of operator error, the ANSI/AAMI HF-18 standard makes specific recommendations concerning the physical construction and location of these switches and prescribes mechanical and electrical performance standards. For instance, front panel controls need to have their function identified by a permanent label and their output indicated on alphanumeric displays or on graduated scales; the pedals of foot switches need to be labelled and respond to a specified activation force; and if the active electrode handle incorporates two finger switches, their position has to correspond to a specific function.

Four basic high-frequency power amplifiers are in use currently; the somewhat dated vacuum tube/spark gap configuration, the parallel connection of a bank if bipolar power transistors, the hybrid connection of parallel bipolar power transistors cascaded with metal oxide silicon field effect transistors (MOSFETs) and the bridge connection of MOSFETs. Each has unique properties and represents a stage in the evolution of ESUs. In a vacuum tube/spark gap device, a tuned-plate, tuned-grid vacuum tube oscillator is used to generate a continuous waveform for use in cutting. This signal is introduced to the patient by an adjustable isolation transformer. To generate a waveform for fulguration, the power supply voltage is elevated by a step-up transformer to about 1600 V rms which then connects to a series of spark gaps. The voltage across the spark gaps is capacitively coupled to the primary of an isolation transformer. The RLC circuit created by this arrangement generates a high crest factor, damped sinusoidal, interrupted waveform. One can adjust the output power and characteristics by changing the turns ratio or tap on the primary and/or secondary side of the isolation transformer or by changing the spark gap distance.

In those devices that use a parallel bank of bipolar power transistors, the transistors are arranged in a Class A configuration. The bases, collectors and emitters are all connected in parallel and the collective base node is driven through a current-limiting resistor. A feedback RC network between the base node and the collector node stabilises the circuit. The collectors are usually fused individually before the common node connects them to one side of the primary of the step-up transformer. The other side of the primary is connected to the high-voltage power supply. A capacitor and resistor in parallel to the primary create a resonance tank circuit that generate the output waveform at a specific frequency. Additional elements may be switched in and out of the primary parallel RLC to alter the output power and waveform for various electrosurgical modes. Small-value resistors between the emitters and ground improve the current sharing between transistors. This configuration sometimes requires the use of matched sets of high-voltage power transistors.

A similar arrangement exists in amplifiers using parallel bipolar transistors cascaded with a power MOSFET. This is arrangement is called a hybrid cascade amplifier. In this type of amplifier, the collectors of a group if bipolar transistors are connected, via protection diodes, to one side of the primary of the step-up output transformer. The other side of the primary is connected to the high-voltage power supply. The emitters of two or three bipolar transistors are connected, via current limiting resistors, to the drain of an enhancement mode MOSFET. The source of the MOSFET is connected to ground and the gate of the MOSFET is connected to a voltage-snubbing network driven by a fixed amplitude pulse created by a high-speed MOS driver circuit. The bases of the bipolar transistors are connected, via current control RC networks, to a common variable based voltage source. Each collector and base is separately fused. In cut modes, the gate drive pulse is a fixed frequency and the base voltage is varied according to the power setting. In the coagulation modes, the base voltage is fixed and the width of the pulses driving the MOSFET is varied. This changes the conduction time of the amplifier and controls the amount of energy imparted to the output transformer and its load. In the coagulation modes and in high-power cut modes, the bipolar power transistors are saturated and the voltage across the bipolar/MOSFET combination is low. This translates to high efficiency and low power dissipation.

The most common high-frequency power amplifier in use is a bridge connection of MOSFETs. In this configuration, the drains of a series of power MOSFETs are connected, via protection diodes, to one side of the primary of the step-up output transformer. The drain protection diodes protect the MOSFETs against the negative voltage swings of the transformer primary. The other side of the transformer primary is connected to the high-voltage power supply. The source of the MOSFETs are connected to ground. The gate of each MOSFET has a resistor connected to ground and one to its driver circuitry. The resistor to ground speeds up the discharge of the gate capacitance when the MOSFET is turned on while the gate series resistor eliminates turn-off oscillations. Various combinations of capacitors and/or LC networks can be switched across the primary of the step-up output transformer to obtain different waveforms. In the cut mode, the output power is controlled by varying the high-voltage power supply voltage. In the coagulation mode, the output power is controlled by varying the on time of the gate drive pulse.

AN ESU POWER AMPLIFIER

In order to supply energy of about 400 W to an electrosurgical electrode, a reasonably efficient power amplifier is required. Any waste heat may be dissipated in an aluminium or copper heat sink, sometimes force-cooled with a fan. The problem of dissipating the waste heat in ESU amplifiers is sufficiently difficult that the duration of continuous cutting allowed is limited by the manufacturer's specifications. If the heat is not dissipated from the power transistor chip, junction temperatures in excess of 250°C occur and the device may fail. An example of power amplifier is given in Fig. 18.2. The first stage driver amplifier supplies the base of the power transistor with a peak-to-peak voltage V_{BPP}. An ideal representation of the transistor voltage-current characteristic is given in Fig. 18.3.

The operation of the amplifier is described as follows. When V_B is zero, the transistor is turned off and V_{CE} nearly equals V_{BB}. As V_B increases above the forward base to emitter voltage (0.7 V in silicon), the transistor begins to conduct. When V_B reaches its peak voltage, V_{BPP}, V_{CE} will be nearly zero and the current I_C will equal its peak value I_{CPP}. I_{CPP} induces the peak-to-peak voltage in the active electrode through the $N_1:N_2$ turns ratio of the transformer. A detailed ideal analysis follows to determine the requirements on the components and to compute the amplifier power gain.

When the transistor is fully on, $I_C = I_{CPP}$ and $V_{CE} = 0$. Then, from Fig. 18.2,

$$V_{BB} = I_{CPP} (R_{EQ} + R_{EM})$$

where V_{BB} is the bias voltage, R_{EM} is the emitter bias resistance and

$$R_{EQ} = \left(\frac{N_1}{N_2}\right)^2 R_L \qquad \qquad \dots (18.2)$$

where $R_L = R_E + R_B + R_R$ is the total load resistance on the ESU, called the body-electrode resistance. In the transistor with current gain β,

$$I_{CPP} = \beta I_{BPP}$$

Thus,

$$R_{EQ} + R_{EM} = \frac{V_{BB}}{\beta I_{BPP}} \qquad \qquad ... (18.3)$$

This gives a means of choosing proper resistor values for obtaining a full-swing output for a given available current from the previous stage, I_{BPP}. Usually, however, the voltage output maximum capability of the previous stage V_{BP} is given. It is then necessary to calculate the input impedance Z_{IN} from Fig. 18.2. Kirchhoff's voltage law around the base loop gives

$$V_B = V_{BE} + \beta I_B R_{EM}$$

When $V_B = V_{BPP}$ and $V_{BPP} \gg V_{BE}$ ($V_{BE} = 0.7$ V in silicon), we can usualiy approximate

$$V_{BPP} \approx I_{BPP}\, \beta R_{EM}$$

and

$$R_{EM} \approx \frac{V_{BPP}}{\beta I_{BPP}} \qquad \qquad ... (18.4)$$

Thus, using this equation, one can find the R_{EM} for a given β on the transistor, required to give a full-swing output when V_B is at its peak value, V_{BPP}. Equations (18.2), (18.3) and (18.4) are design equations for the amplifier in Fig. 18.2.

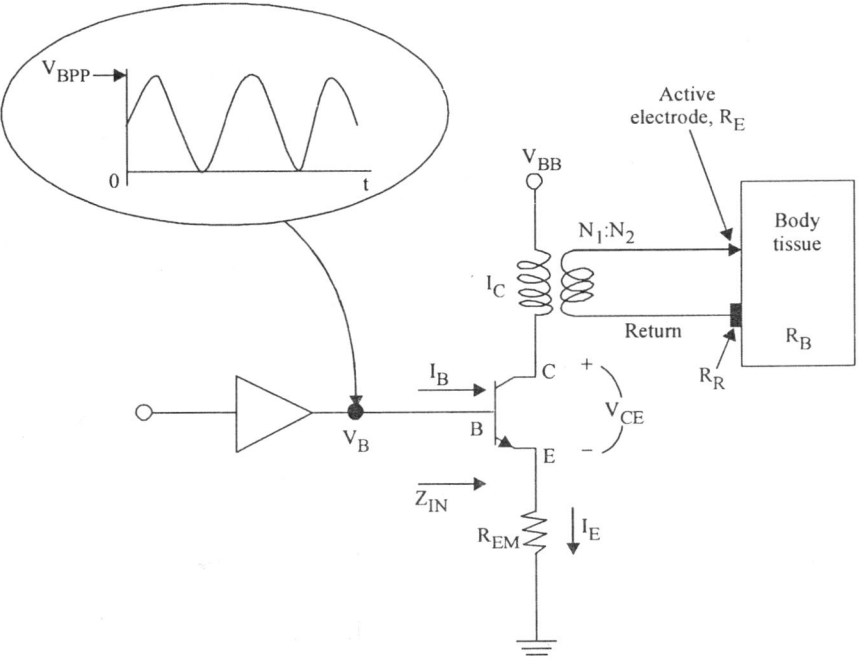

Fig. 18.2. An ESU power amplifier.

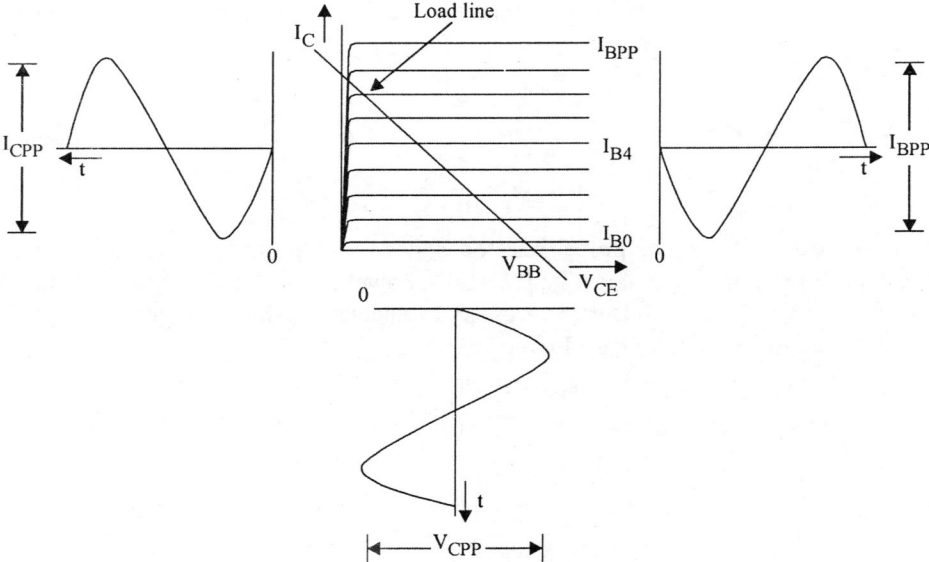

Fig. 18.3. Power transistor voltage-current characteristics.

ACTIVE ELECTRODES

An active blade-type electrode approximately 1 mm thick and 10 mm wide, used for cutting, is illustrated in Fig. 18.4. When the electrode is in the cutting mode, a sinusoidal steady-state oscillating current appears at the tip. If the blade is held a short distance from the skin, a sharply directed spark will be drawn to the skin. The voltage along the blade will have the same value everywhere. Therefore, the electric field intensity, in units of volts per meter, will be strongest at the tip, thus producing a well-defined spark and resulting in a cut. The electrode may also be operated in the coagulation (or coag) mode, produced by a wide spark. The wide spark as shown in Fig. 18.4 may be produced by transients on the electrode, which cause a maximum voltage to appear somewhere other than at the tip. The breakdown electric field intensity would then originate from the maximum voltage region on the blade and produce a spraying effect in the spark. The power for the blade would then be spread over a larger region of skin and would tend to cauterise the tissue and coagulate the blood.

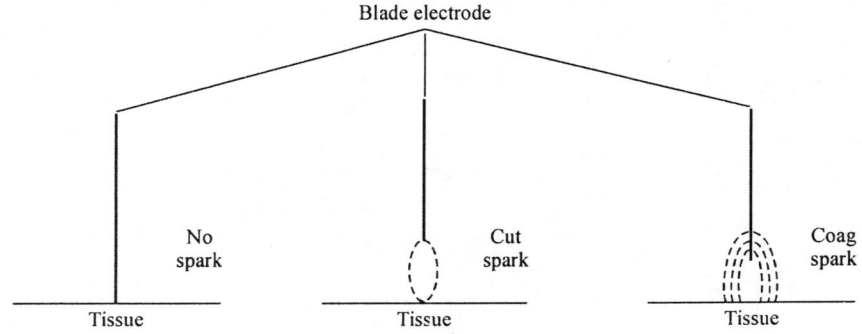

Fig. 18.4. The skin-electrode contact for various ESU modes.

Tissue cauterisation and coagulation can be facilitated by blunting the tip of the electrode, as illustrated in Fig. 18.5. The spark produced by the spherical-tip electrode tends to broaden across the tissue, because there are several equidistant paths from the skin to electrode surface. The air along all such paths tends to break down simultaneously. The hemostat electrode may be used to lift the clamp or grasp tissue, especially a bleeding vessel. The ESU current then would flow broadly through the grasped tissue, causing a coagulation effect. The bipolar electrode is arranged on the tip of a forceps. Each tip has a separate electrical path, one from the ESU active head and one to the patient return. When in use, these two electrodes contact tissue in close proximity to each other. In this case it is not necessary to have a return, ground-plate electrode. With the bipolar electrode, the current density on both electrodes is equally high. Therefore, each electrode may have both a cutting effect and a coagulation effect.

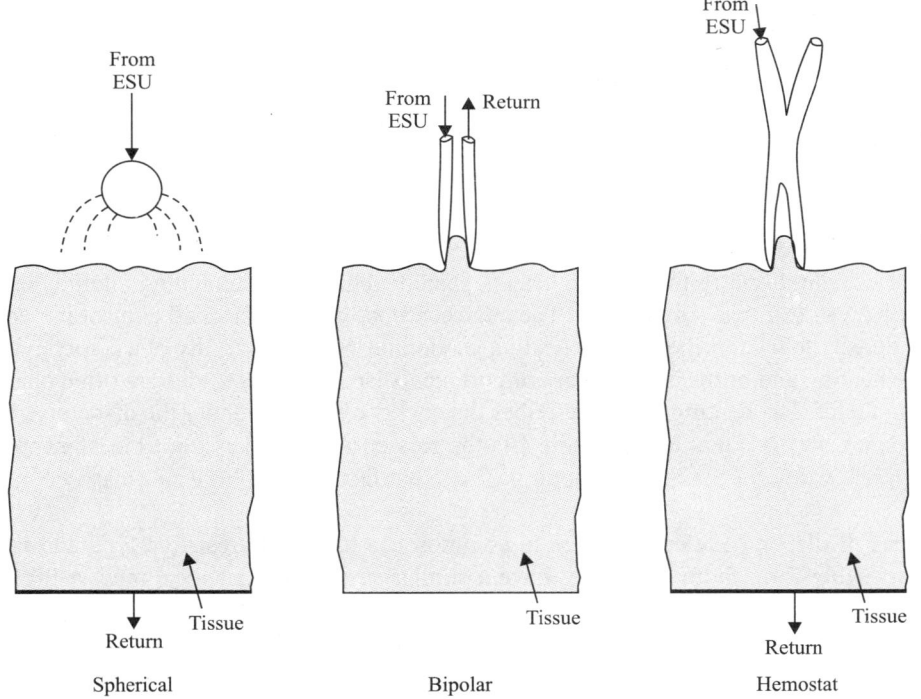

Fig. 18.5. The spherical, bipolar and hemostat electrode connections.

Active Electrode Resistance

The active electrode-to-skin resistance, R_E, varies considerably, depending upon how much of the electrode actually contacts the tissue. This variable is changed or controlled, by the surgeon. It is important to realise that the amount of the power delivered to the tissue for a given ESU instrument voltage depends in turn on this resistance.

An equivalent circuit of the ESU in Fig. 18.6 shows its internal resistance, R_I and R_E, as well as a body resistance, R_B and return electrode resistance, R_R. The power dissipated by each of these resistances determines the cut, coagulation, warming or burning effect at each of the sites.

In accordance with the maximum power rule, the maximum power delivered to the patient occurs when R_E equals the sum of the other resistances of the circuit, $R_I + R_B + R_R$.

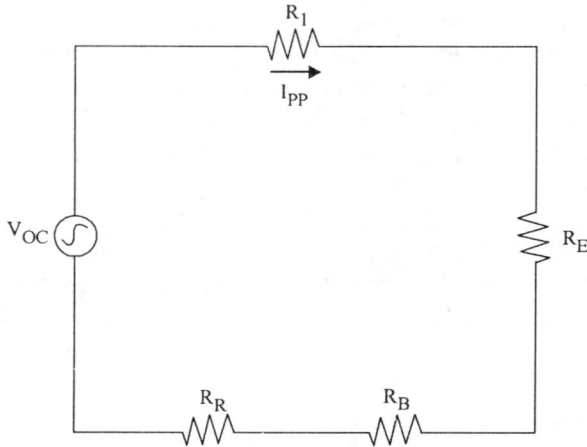

Fig. 18.6. An ESU electrical equivalent circuit.

DISPERSIVE ELECTRODES

The main purpose of the dispersive electrode is to return the high-frequency current to the electrosurgical unit without causing harm to the patient. This is usually achieved by attaching a large electrode to the patient's skin away from the surgical site. The large electrode area and a small contact impedance reduce the current density to levels where tissue heating is minimal. Since the ability of a dispersive electrode to avoid tissue heating and burns is of primary importance, dispersive electrodes are often characterised by their heating factor. The heating factor describes the energy dissipated under the dispersive electrode per Ω of impedance and is equal to I^2t, where I is the rms current and t is the time of exposure. During surgery a typical value for the heating factor is 3 A^2s, but factors of up to 9 A^2s may occur during some procedures.

Two types of dispersive electrodes are in common use today, the resistive type and the capacitive type. In disposable form, both electrodes have a similar structure and appearance. A thin, rectangular metallic foil has an insulating layer on the outside, connects to a gel-like material on the inside and may be surrounded by an adhesive foam. In the resistive type, the gel-like material is made of an adhesive conductive gel, whereas in the capacitive type, the gel is an adhesive dielectric non-conductive gel. The adhesive foam and adhesive gel layer ensure that both electrodes maintain good skin contact to the patient, even if the electrode gets stressed mechanically from pulls on the electrode cable. Both types have specific advantages and disadvantages. Electrode failures and subsequent patient injury can be attributed mostly to improper application, electrode dislodgment and electrode defects rather than to electrode design.

BLOCK DIAGRAM

A generic solid-state ESU block diagram is given in Fig. 18.7, along with example waveforms available at the output electrode for the cut, coag and blend modes of operation. In this circuit the power output of the cut wave form may be up to 400 W into a 500 Ω load. Open-circuit voltages may range from 1000 to 10000 V peak-to-peak. In Fig. 18.7 the coag pulse train is a digital pulse that modulates the RF output according to selected duty cycles as shown in Table 18.4.

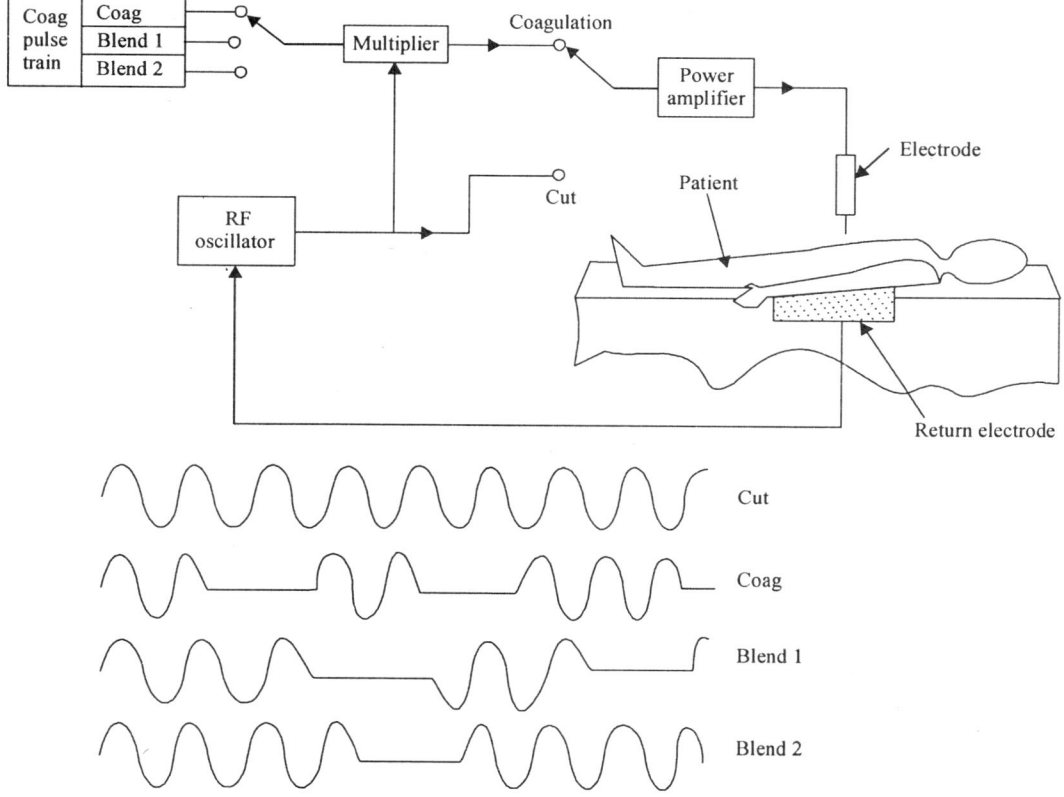

Fig. 18.7. An ESU with cut, coagulation and blend modes and the waveforms of these modes.

Table 18.4. RF output according to selected duty cycle.

Pulse train	Duty cycle(%)	Power (W)
Cut	100	400
Coag	33	132
Blend 1	50	200
Blend 2	75	300

The waveforms are also illustrated for the selected settings. The cut setting is used to cause vapourisation of the cell. The coag setting, on the other hand, heats the tissue, causing relatively deep dehydration and tissue cauterisation. Blend 1 and 2 controls are used by the surgeon along with the power amplifier gain control to create the degree and speed of coagulation desired. The power in the blend settings is selected in fixed, repeatable steps by adjusting the duty cycle of the applied RF waveform. In order to measure the power output of an ESU, as well as its leakage currents, an ESU analyser is used.

The ESU is a high-power device used on patients when they are the most vulnerable and defenseless-during surgery. Safety in its use is therefore of the highest priority. Several safety hints are listed in Table 18.5.

Table 18.5. ESU safety hints.

Do not use in the presence of combustible materials such as flammable anaesthesia agents or flammable disinfection agents

Bowel gas contains explosive methane. Use protective measures during electrosurgery involving the bowel or colon

Low-frequency leakage current may be present in the ESU pencil electrode, presenting a microshock hazard

Check the patient for alternative return paths for the ESU current to avoid burns. Isolate the ESU circuit

Place the dispersive patient electrode as close as possible to the operative site

Avoid placing the dispersive electrode over scar tissue, bony prominences, unshaved hairy areas, metal implants or wet areas

Place the dispersive electrode at right angles to a pacemaker to avoid ESU interference

Rigid-metal dispersive electrodes should only be used on the buttocks, where the weight of the body will maintain good contact

Adhesive disposable electrodes should not be used where the weight of the body would put uneven pressure on the electrode, causing hot spots and possible burns

Be alert to electromagnetic radio frequency interference from the ESU upon monitoring equipment in the vicinity

SINUSOIDAL OSCILLATORS

The ESU requires the use of sinusoidal radio frequency signals. The general form of the sinusoidal oscillator consists of the isolated blocks shown in Fig. 18.8, where K is an amplifier of gain K and β is a feedback element.

The gain of this circuit, $A_V = V_{OUT}/V_1$, is given by the following analysis:

$$V_{OUT} = KV_X = K (V_1 + \beta V_{OUT})$$

Solving for A_V gives

$$A_V = \frac{V_{OUT}}{V_1} = \frac{K}{1 - K\beta} \qquad \text{... (18.5)}$$

Notice in Equation (18.5) that when

$$K\beta = 1 \qquad \text{... (18.6)}$$

the gain A_V becomes infinite. This means that the smallest bit of random noise produces an output voltage when the loop gain $K\beta = 1$.

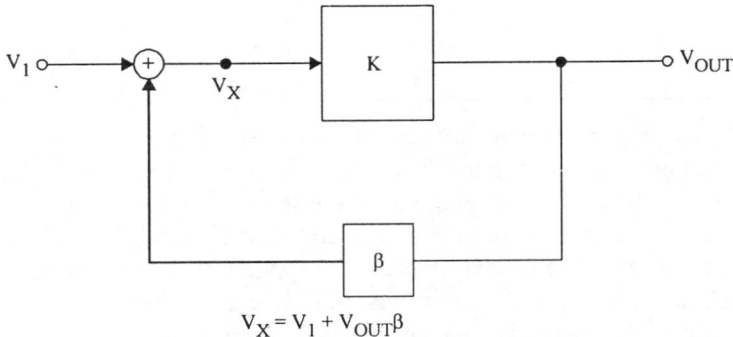

$$V_X = V_1 + V_{OUT}\beta$$

Fig. 18.8. The basic sinusoidal oscillator.

Such an output is self-sustaining because this loop gain equals 1. The circuit therefore oscillates. In this sinusoidal oscillator both K and β may be functions of frequency. When they are, the frequency of oscillation is found by solving Equation (18.6) when the gain expression for K and β are known in terms of frequency and the circuit element values. When this condition holds for only one frequency, the circuit becomes a pure sinusoidal oscillator.

The example oscillator circuit in Fig. 18.9 utilises operational amplifiers and is analysed as follows. The rule for ideal different amplifiers is $V_1 = V_2$. Also, by voltage division, we have for the K side

$$\beta = \frac{V_2}{V_{OUT}} \qquad K = \frac{V_{OUT}}{V_2}$$

and then

$$V_2 = \frac{R_2}{R_1 + R_2} V_{OUT} \qquad\qquad \text{... (18.7)}$$

Again, by voltage division for β we have

$$\beta = \frac{V_1}{V_{OUT}}$$

Then

$$V_1 = \frac{\dfrac{\dfrac{R}{j\omega C} V_{OUT}}{R + \dfrac{1}{j\omega C}}}{R + \dfrac{1}{j\omega C} + \dfrac{\dfrac{R}{j\omega C}}{R + \dfrac{1}{j\omega C}}}$$

Simplifying this gives

$$V_1 = \frac{\dfrac{R}{j\omega C} V_{OUT}}{\left(R + \dfrac{1}{j\omega C}\right)^2 + \dfrac{R}{j\omega C}}$$

Expanding the square yields

$$V_1 = \frac{\dfrac{R}{j\omega C} V_{OUT}}{R^2 - \left(\dfrac{1}{\omega C}\right)^2 + \dfrac{3R}{j\omega C}} \qquad\qquad \text{... (18.8)}$$

Because K, from Equation (18.7), is a real number, the oscillator condition $K\beta = 1$ implies that β must be real as well. To make that happen in Equation (18.8), let

$$\omega C = \frac{1}{R} \qquad \qquad ... (18.9)$$

Substituting this into Equation (18.8) gives

$$\frac{V_1}{V_{OUT}} = \frac{1}{3}$$

Because $V_2 = V_1$ at the input to the different amplifier, Equation (18.7) then gives

$$\frac{R_2}{R_1 + R_2} = \frac{1}{3} \qquad \qquad ... (18.10)$$

The conclusion we draw from this analysis is that the oscillator radian frequency $\omega = 2\pi f$ is computed from equation (18.9) and the choice of R_1 and R_2 is made to satisfy Equation (18.10) in the ideal case. Conversely, equations (18.9) and (18.10) may be taken as the design equations for the sinusoidal oscillator in Fig. 18.9 from which we can compute the component values that produce oscillations at a desired frequency.

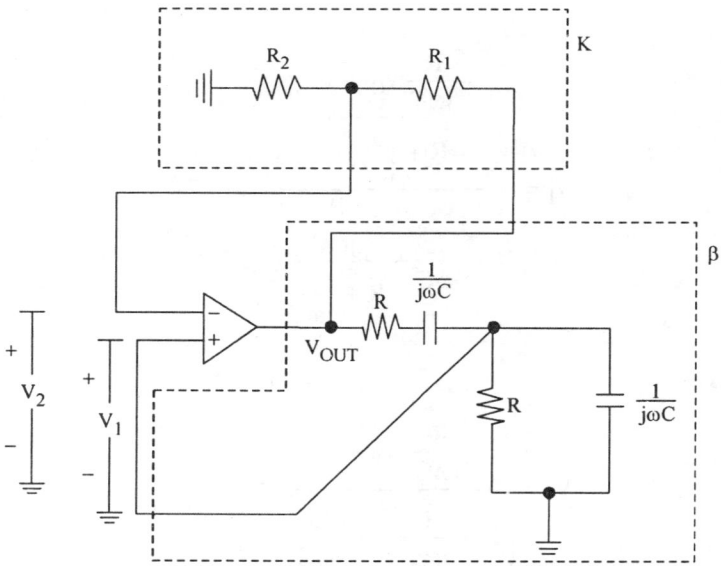

Fig. 18.9. A sinusoidal oscillator circuit.

ESU HAZARDS

Improper use of electrosurgery may expose both the patient and the surgical staff to a number of hazards. By far the most frequent hazards are electric shock and undesired burns. Less frequent are undesired neuromuscular stimulation, interference with pacemakers or other devices, electrochemical effects from direct currents, implant heating and gas explosions.

Current returns to the ESU through the dispersive electrode. If the contact area of the dispersive electrode is large and the current exposure time short, then the skin temperature under the electrode does not rise above 45°C, which has been shown to be the maximum safe temperature. However, to include a safety margin, the skin temperature should not rise more than 6°C above the normal surface temperature of 29–33°C. The current density at any point under the dispersive electrode has to be significantly below the recognised burn threshold of 100 mA/cm^2 for 10 seconds.

To avoid electric shock and burns, the American National Standard for Electrosurgical Devices requires that 'any electrosurgical generator that provides for a dispersive electrode and that has a rated output power of greater than 50 W shall have at least one patient circuit safety monitor'. The most common safety monitors are the contact quality monitor for the dispersive electrode and the patient circuit monitor. A contact quality monitor consists of a circuit to measure the impedance between the two sides of a split dispersive electrode and the skin. A small high-frequency current flows from one section of the dispersive electrode through the skin to the second section of the dispersive electrode. If the impedance between these two sections exceeds a certain threshold or changes by a certain percentage, an audible alarm sounds and the ESU output is disabled.

Patient circuit monitors range from simple to complex. The simple ones monitor electrode cable integrity while the complex ones detect any abnormal conditions that could result in electrosurgical current flowing in other than normal pathways. Although the output isolation transformer present in most modern ESUs usually provides adequate patient protection, some potentially hazardous conditions may still arise. If a conductor to the dispersive electrode is broken, undesired arcing between the broken conductor ends may occur, causing fire in the operating room and serious patient injury. Abnormal current pathways may also arise from capacitive coupling between cables, the patient, operators, enclosures, beds or any other conductive surface or from direct connections to other electrodes connected to the patient. The patient circuit monitoring device should be operated from an isolated power source having a maximum voltage of 12 V rms. The most common device is a cable continuity monitor. Unlike the contact quality monitor, this monitor only checks the continuity of the cable between the ESU and the dispersive electrode and sounds an alarm if the resistance in the conductor is greater than 1 kΩ. Another implementation of a patient circuit monitor measures the voltage between the dispersive electrode connection and ground. A third implementation functions similarly to a ground fault circuit interrupter (GFCI) in that the current in the wire to the active electrode and the current in the wire to the dispersive electrode are measured and compared with each other. If the difference between these currents is greater than a pre-set threshold, the alarm sounds and the ESU is disconnected.

There are other sources of undesired burns. Active electrodes get hot when they are used. After use, the active electrode should be placed in protective holster, if available or on a suitable surface to isolate it from the patient and surgical staff. The correct placement of an active electrode will also prevent the patient and/or surgeon from being burned if an inadvertent activation of the ESU occurs (e.g., someone accidentally stepping on a foot pedal). Some surgeons use a practice called buzzing the hemostat in which a small bleeding vessel is grasped with a clamp or hemostat and the active electrode touched to the clamp while activating. Because of the high voltages involved and the stray capacitance to ground, the surgeon's glove may be compromised. If the surgical staff cannot be convinced to eliminate the practice of buzzing hemostats, the probability of burns can be reduced by use of a cut waveform instead of a coagulation waveform (lower voltage), by maximising contact between the surgeon's hand and the clamp and by not activating until the active electrode is firmly touching the clamp.

Although it is commonly assumed that neuromuscular stimulation ceases or is insignificant at frequencies above 10 kHz, such stimulation has been observed in anaesthetised patients undergoing certain electrosurgical procedures. This undesirable side effect of electrosurgery is generally attributed to non-linear events during the electric arcing between the active electrode and tissue. These events rectify the high-frequency current leading to both DC and low-frequency current components. These current components can reach magnitudes that stimulate nerve and muscle cells. To minimise the probability of unwanted neuromuscular stimulation, most ESUs incorporate in their output circuit a high-pass filter that suppresses DC and low-frequency current components.

The use of electrosurgery means the presence of electric discharge arcs. This presents a potential fire hazard in an operating room where oxygen and flammable gases may be present. These flammable gases may be introduced by the surgical staff (anaesthetics or flammable cleaning solutions) or may be generated within the patients themselves (bowel gases). The use of disposable paper drapes and dry surgical gauge also provides a flammable material that may be ignited by sparking or by contact with a hot active electrode. Therefore, prevention of fires and explosions depends primarily on the prudence and judgement of the ESU operator.

TROUBLESHOOTING AN ESU

Troubleshooting an ESU often begins with a symptom written on a work request, which can sometimes be a rather vague instruction such as 'ESU is broken. Please fix it'. A logical first step to better define the symptom would be to interview the operator, if possible. An alternative is to test the ESU with an electrosurgical analyser. This test equipment can be used to measure output power in all modes of ESU operation. It can also be used to measure the RF leakage to ground, as well as low-frequency currents. It is especially important for the troubleshooter to detect 60-~ leakage currents, because they can cause microshock.

The service manual accompanying the ESU often provides helpful troubleshooting guides. Module-level troubleshooting can be done by following block schematics or diagrams, provided in the manual.

For example, a block diagram of the Valleylab Model SSE4 ESU, shown in Fig. 18.10, can be used as a troubleshooting aid. There are two outputs to the ESU electrode in the figure: The bipolar outputs are on the lower right side of the schematic; the monopolar active output and the patient return are located just above the centre. The keying switches on the electrodes feed into the upper right corner of the schematic. Optical coupling isolates the electrodes, as do transformers on both the monopolar and bipolar electrodes. The patient is completely isolated from unwanted signals generated within the unit. Keying of all ESU functions is controlled by the central processing unit (CPU) of the microprocessor.

The service manual for the SSE4 gives a troubleshooting guide in the form of common symptoms and suggested remedies, stated in terms of the block schematic modules. These modules are keyed to circuit boards that the manufacturer recommendations should be stocked in the hospital as replacement parts. An outline of some symptoms and possible remedies are given below:

1. Symptom: There is no RF output from the monopolar ESU electrode.
2. Possible causes: High-voltage power supply. Fuse blown. Surgical pencil open-circuited.
3. Symptom: There is RF output in all modes except one.
4. Possible causes: If the bipolar mode is at fault, the bipolar control module should be checked. If a monopolar mode has failed, the clock/control module should be checked.
5. Symptom: The power output in the monopolar modes is more than 30 per cent below normal.
6. Possible cause: Some components in the power amplifier stripline and output modules may have failed.

7. Symptom: The display is dead.
8. Possible cause: The low-voltage power supplies may be faulty.

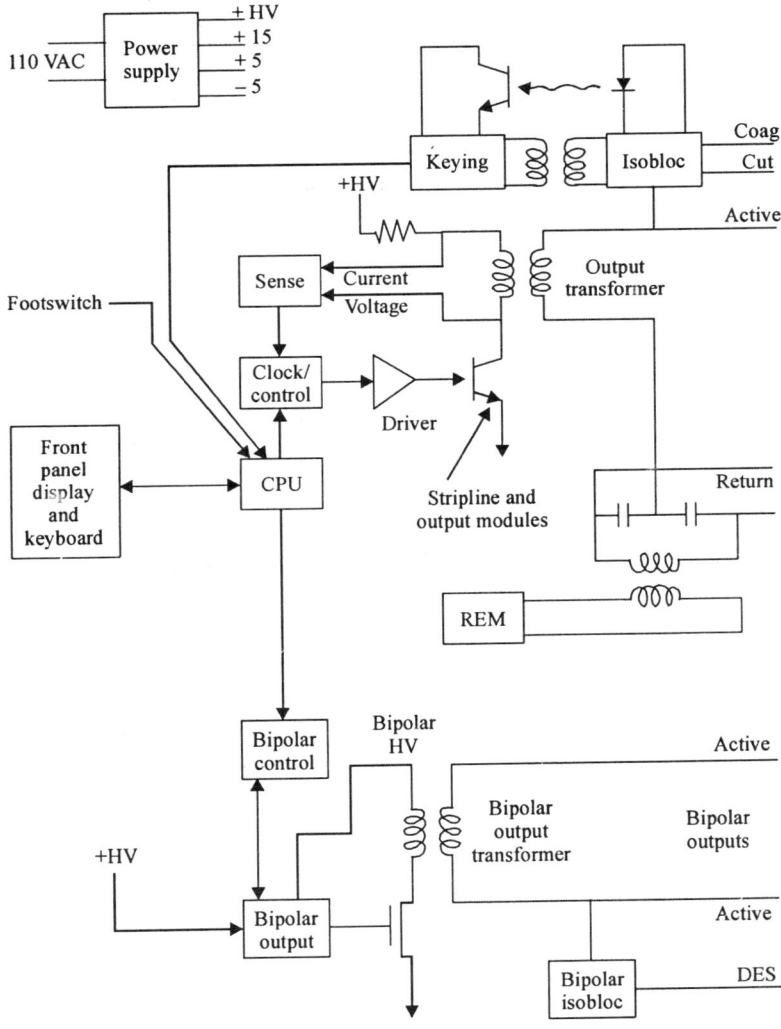

Fig. 18.10. A model SSE4 block diagram.

Troubleshooting Tip

Turn the power off before removing or inserting any circuit board. Otherwise, transients induced may damage the board.

More detailed troubleshooting guides are provided in the service manual, keyed to the unit module schematics. There a symptom is described and a relevant troubleshooting tree is given. The troubleshooting tree lists steps that should be taken in sequence until the fault is located and corrected.

RECENT DEVELOPMENTS

Electrosurgery is being enhanced by the addition of a controlled column of argon gas in the path between the active electrode and the tissue. The flow of argon gas assists in clearing the surgical site of fluid and improves visibility. When used in the coagulation mode, the argon gas is turned into a plasma allowing tissue damage and smoke to be reduced and producing a thinner, more flexible eschar. When used with the cut mode, lower power levels may be used.

Many manufacturers have begun to include sophisticated computer-based systems in their ESUs that not only simplify the use of the device but also increase the safety of patient and operator. For instance, in a so-called soft coagulation mode, a special circuit continuously monitors the current between the active electrode and the tissue and turns the ESU output on only after the active electrode has contacted the tissue. Furthermore, the ESU output is turned off automatically, once the current has reached a certain threshold level that is typical for coagulated and desiccated tissue. This feature is also used in a bipolar mode termed autobipolar. Not only does this feature prevent arcing at the beginning of the procedure, but it also keeps the tissue from being heated beyond 70°C. Some devices offer a so-called power-peak-system that delivers a very short power peak at the beginning of electrosurgical cutting to start the cutting arc. Other modern devices use continuous monitoring of current and voltage levels to make automatic power adjustments in order to provide for a smooth cutting action from the beginning of the incision to its end. Some manufacturers are developing waveforms and instruments designed to achieve specific clinical results such as bipolar cutting tissue lesioning and vessel sealing. With the growth and popularity of laparoscopic procedures, additional electrosurgical instruments and waveforms tailored to this surgical speciality should also be expected.

Increased computing power, more sophisticated evaluation of voltage and current waveforms and the addition of miniaturised sensors will continue to make ESUs more user-friendly and safer.

Chapter 19

Biomedical Lasers

INTRODUCTION

Laser light differs from ordinary light in that it is coherent, which means that all of its light waves are in phase. Laser light is also monochromatic, which means that all of the light waves are of the same frequency. The effect of these two properties is that the light can be very sharply focused, much more sharply than sunlight can be focused with a magnifying glass to burn paper. In fact, laser light can be focused to the size of a living cell. In laser surgery, all of the energy of the beam can be focused on the cell, causing it to vapourise and thereby cutting the tissue. This explains the first major advantage of the laser for the surgery—namely, it is more precise than either the knife (surgical scalpel) or the ESU electrode. Furthermore, the laser beam can be directed down narrow passages, such as are encountered in eye and brain surgery, too small for ESU electrodes or surgical scalpels. These advantages are balanced by the fact that laser surgical units are more expensive, larger and sometimes awkward to manipulate.

Approximately 30 years ago the CO_2 laser was introduced into surgical practice as a tool to photothermally ablate and thus to incise and to debulk, soft tissues. Subsequently, three important factors have led to the expanding biomedical use of laser technology, particularly in surgery. These factors are: (i) the increasing understanding of the wave-length selective interaction and associated effects of ultraviolet-infrared (UV-IR) radiation with biologic tissues, including those of acute damage and long-term healing; (ii) the rapidly increasing availability of lasers emitting (essentially monochromatically) at those wavelengths that are strongly absorbed by molecular species within tissues; and (iii) the availability of both optical fibre and lens technologies as well as of endoscopic technologies for delivery of the laser radiation to the often remote internal treatment site. Fusion of these factors has led to the development of currently available biomedical laser systems.

This chapter briefly reviews the current status of each of these three factors. In doing so, each of the following topics will be briefly discussed:

1. The physics of the interaction and the associated effects (including clinical efforts) of UV-IR radiation on biological tissues.
2. The fundamental principles that underlie the operations and construction of all lasers.
3. The physical properties of the optical delivery systems used with the different biomedical lasers for delivery of the laser beam to the treatment site.

4. The essential physical features of those biomedical lasers currently in routine use ranging over a number of clinical specialities and brief descriptions of their use.
5. The biomedical uses of other lasers used surgically in limited scale or which are currently being researched for applications in surgical and diagnostic procedures and the photosensitised inactivation of cancer tumours.

CO$_2$ LASER

The laser light is generated in the gas laser tube depicted in Fig. 19.1. The tube contains a mixture of carbon dioxide, nitrogen and helium gases at a low pressure maintained by the vacuum pump. In the flow-type laser shown, the gas is continuously changed because the laser process destroys CO_2 molecules that must be replaced and it is supplied by the storage bottle. A DC voltage is applied to the gas. As with most gases, if the voltage is high enough, the gas will break down or ionise and cause a current stream of ions. The stream of ions causes laser action by colliding with the atoms of the gas, causing them to rise to an excited state. An atom in an excited state has some electrons that have moved from lower energy orbits to higher energy orbits, which are unstable. When the atom returns to its stable state, it emits a photon of laser light, at an energy level and frequency specific to the gas. This photon eventually collides with another excited atom and stimulates it to emit a photon of light in phase with it, thus adding to it. The laser light beams travelling along the axis of the tube are reflected by the mirrors at either end, reinforcing the light along the axis and causing it to build in intensity. One of the mirrors in the tube is partially transmitting, thereby allowing the beam to exit the tube and travel along the optical guidance system. Such a system, called the beam manipulator, may consist of hollow tubes articulated by elbows containing lenses and mirrors that direct the laser light around the corners down the centre of the tube. The output of the tube is focused by an output lens system.

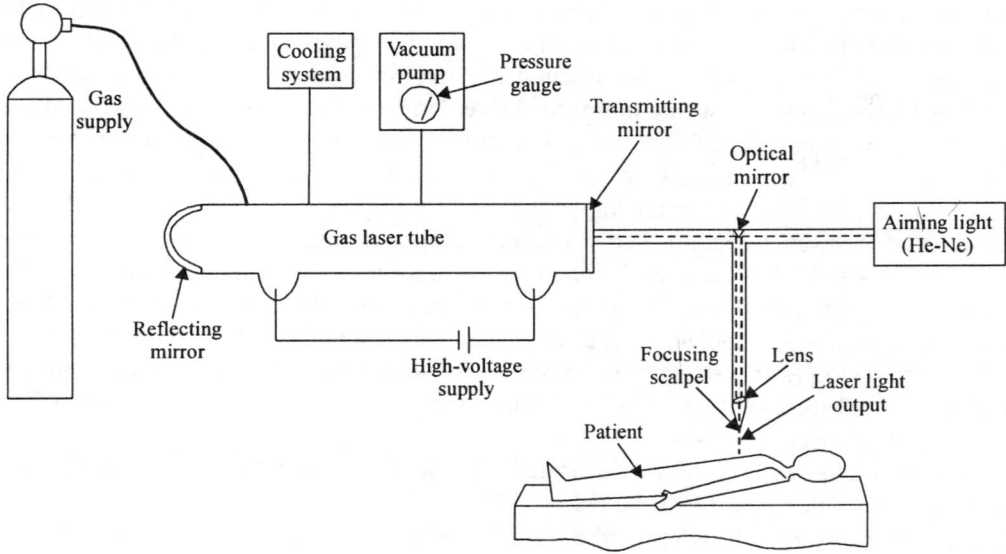

Fig. 19.1. A CO$_2$ laser block diagram.

The focal point of the output beam must be adjusted to fall on the tissues to be cut. The size of the focal point, called the spot diameter, determines the energy density applied to the tissue for a given beam power. The surgeon adjusts the spot diameter with the output lens system. To cut, the beam is adjusted for a small spot diameter; to coagulate, a larger spot diameter is chosen.

The size of the spot must be adjusted before the laser is turned on, in the case of the CO_2 laser, because the light is infrared and thus invisible to the eye. In any case an unfocused beam would cause tissue damage if it were run at high power. Therefore, low-power focusing light, called aiming light, is run through the output lens system to calibrate the focal spot before the high-energy laser light is applied. A low-power helium-neon (He-Ne) laser is often used as an aiming light because it produces visible, red light.

The CO_2 laser emits light at power levels ranging from 20 to 100 W.

ARGON LASER SURGICAL UNIT

Like CO_2, argon is a gas. The argon laser therefore works on basically the same principle as the CO_2 laser. The most distinctive difference is in the wavelength of the laser light emitted. CO_2 emits light primarily at a wavelength of 10.6 µm, in the invisible, infrared range, whereas argon emits laser light at 0.488 µm, blue light and 0.515 µm, green light. The wavelength of laser light gives rise to selective absorption of the light energy by tissue. CO_2 laser light is absorbed by water, which makes up the bulk of tissue and cells and so it is effective at cutting tissue. Argon, however, passes through water without being absorbed, but is absorbed by dark tissue such as haemoglobin or tissue containing melanin. Thus, argon laser light is not so effective in cutting and is used instead to coagulate tissue.

It is used, for example, in retinal re-attachment, because the light beam passes through the vitreous humour and is selectively absorbed by the detached retina, which is thereby re-bonded. The argon laser operates at power levels from 0.01 to 20 W, which is adequate for the coagulation and bonding task.

Nd:YAG LASER

A common crystal laser for medical applications uses an artificial crystal neodymium-doped yttrium aluminium garnet (Nd:YAG). Nd:YAG produces laser light at a wavelength of 1.06 µm. To generate laser light, the crystal is placed between two reflecting mirrors, as shown in Fig. 19.2. An electrical source produces non-coherent light, containing 1.06 µm rays, which is directed toward the Nd:YAG. This light stimulates laser action, as described for the CO_2 laser and is referred to as a light pump. The Nd:YAG laser light can be coupled to the patient through optical fibres somewhat more efficiently that the longer-wavelength CO_2 laser. Optical fibre cooling is achieved by passing air along the fibre's length. The Nd:YAG laser lies between the CO_2 laser and argon laser in its effectiveness at cutting tissue. Because of its visible wavelength, it is nearly as effective as the CO_2 laser in cutting heavily pigmented tissues. Like the CO_2 laser, the Nd:YAG laser can deliver up to 100 W of light energy. This power is produced at about 15 per cent efficiency. Therefore a cooling system is required to dissipate the waste heat.

Since the laser beam can cause damage at considerable distances from the surgical field, it is necessary to observe safety precautions when using it.

INTERACTION AND EFFECTS OF UV-IR LASER RADIATION ON BIOLOGIC TISSUES

Electromagnetic radiation in the UV-IR spectral range propagates within biologic tissues until it is either scattered or absorbed.

Scattering in Biologic Tissue

Scattering in matter occurs only at the boundaries between regions having different optical refractive indices and is a process in which the energy of the radiation is conserved. Since biologic tissue is structurally inhomogeneous at the microscopic scale, e.g., both sub-cellular and cellular dimensions and at the macroscopic scale, e.g., cellular assembly (tissue) dimensions and predominantly contains water, proteins and lipids, all different chemical species, it is generally regarded as a scatterer of UV-IR radiation. The general result of scattering is deviation of the direction of propagation of radiation.

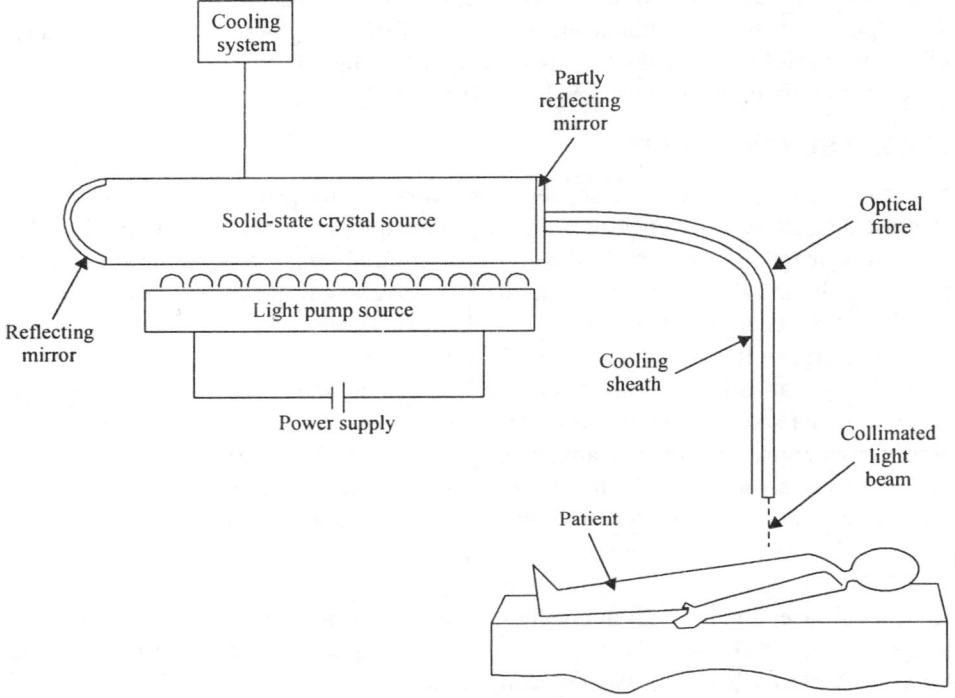

Fig. 19.2. An Nd:YAG laser block diagram.

The deviation is strongest when wavelength and scatterer are comparable in dimension (Mie scattering) and when wavelength greatly exceeds particle size (Rayleigh scattering). This dimensional relationship results in the deeper penetration into biologic tissues of those longer wavelengths which are not absorbed appreciably by pigments in the tissues. This results in the relative transparency of non-pigmented tissues over the visible and near-IR wavelength ranges.

Absorption in Biologic Tissue

Absorption of UV-IR radiation in matter arises from the wavelength-dependent resonant absorption of radiation by molecular electrons of optically absorbing molecular species. Because of the chemical inhomogeneity of biologic tissues, the degree of absorption of incident radiation strongly depends upon its wavelength. The most prevalent or concentrated UV-IR absorbing molecular species in biologic tissues are listed in Table 19.1 along with associated high-absorbance wavelengths. These species include the peptide bonds; the phenylalanine, tyrosine and tryptophan residues of proteins, all of which absorb in the UV range; oxy and deoxyhaemoglobin of blood which absorb in the visible to near-IR range; melanin, which absorbs throughout the UV to near-IR range, which decreasing absorption occurring with increasing wavelength; and water, which absorbs maximally in the mid-IR range. Biomedical lasers and their emitted radiation wavelength values also are tabulated also in Table 19.1. The correlation between the wavelengths of clinically useful lasers and wavelength regions of absorption by constituents of biological tissues is evident. Additionally, exogenous light-absorbing chemical species may be intentionally present in tissues. These include:

1. Photosensitisers, such as porphyrins, which upon excitation with UV-visible light initiate photochemical reactions which are cytotoxic to the cells of the tissue, e.g., a cancer which concentrates the photosensitiser relative to surrounding tissues.
2. Dyes such as indocyanine green which, when dispersed in a concentrate fibrin protein gel can be used to localise 810 nm GaAlAs diode laser radiation and the associated heating to achieve localised thermal denaturation and bonding of collagen to effect joining or welding of tissue.
3. Tattoo pigments including graphite (black) and black, blue, green and red organic dyes.

Table 19.1. UV-IR radiation-absorbing constituent of biological tissues and biomedical laser wavelengths.

| Constituent | Tissue type | Optical absorption | | Laser type | Wavelength, nm |
		Wavelength*, nm	Relative† strength		
Proteins	All				
Peptide bond		<220 (r)	+++++++	ArF	193
Amino acid					
Residues					
Tryptophan		220–290 (r)	+		
Tyrosine		220–290 (r)	+		
Phenylalanine		220–2650 (r)	+		
Pigments					
Oxyhaemoglobin	Blood	414 (p)	+++	Ar ion	488–514.5
	vascular	537 (p)	++	Frequency	532
	tissues	575 (p)	++	Doubled	
		970 (p)	+	Nd:YAG	
		(690–1100) (r)		Diode	810
				Nd:YAG	1064
Deoxyhaemoglobin	Blood	431 (p)	+++	Dy˜	400–700
	vascular tissues	554 (p)	++	Nd:YAG	1064
Melanin	Skin	220–1000 (r)	++++	Ruby	693
Water	All	2.1 (p)	+++	Ho:YAG	2100
		3.02 (p)	+++++++	Er:YAG	2940
		>2.94 (r)	++++	CO_2	10640

* (p): Peak absorption wavelength; (r): wavelength range.

† The number of + signs qualitatively ranks the magnitude of the optical absorbtion.

PENETRATION AND EFFECTS OF UV-IR LASER RADIATION INTO BIOLOGIC TISSUE

Both scattering and absorption processes affect the variations of the intensity of radiation with propagation into tissues. In the absence of scattering, absorption results in an exponential decrease of radiation intensity described simply by Beers law. With appreciable scattering present, the decrease in incident intensity from the surface is no longer monotonic. A maximum in local internal intensity is found to be present due to efficient back-scattering, which adds to the intensity of the incoming beam, for visible light penetrating into the skin for 1.064 μm Nd:YAG laser radiation penetrating into the prostate gland. Thus, the relative contributions of absorption and scattering of incident laser radiation will stipulate the depth in a tissue at which the resulting tissues effects will be present. Since the absorbed energy can be released in a number of different ways including thermal vibrations, fluorescence and resonant electronic energy transfer according to the identity of the absorber, the effects on tissues are in general different. Energy release from both haemoglobin and melanin pigments and from water is by molecular vibrations resulting in a local temperature rise. Sufficient continued energy absorption and release can result in local temperature increases which, as energy input increases, result in protein denaturation (41–65°C), water evaporation and boiling (up to ≃300°C under confining pressure of tissue), thermolysis of proteins, generation of gaseous decomposition products and of carbonaceous residue or char (≥300°C). The generation of residual char is minimised by sufficiently rapid energy input to support rapid gasification reactions. The clinical effect of this chain of thermal events is tissue ablation. Much smaller values of energy input result in coagulation of tissues due to protein denaturation.

Energy release from excited exogenous photosensitising dyes is via formation of free-radical species or energy exchange with itinerant dissolved molecular oxygen. Subsequent chemical reactions following free-radical formation or formation of an activated or more reactive form of molecular oxygen following energy exchange can be toxic to cells with take-up of the photosensitiser.

Energy release following absorption of visible (VIS) radiation by fluorescent molecular species, either endogenous to tissues or exogenous, is predominantly by emission of longer wavelength radiation. Endogenous fluorescent species include tryptophan, tyrosine, phenylalanine, flavins and metal-free porphyrins. Comparison of measured values of the intensity of fluorescence emission from hyperplastic (transformed pre-cancerous) cervical cells to cancerous cervical cells with normal cervical epithelial cells shows a strong potential for diagnostic use in the automated diagnosis and staging of cervical cancer.

EFFECTS OF MID-IR LASER RADIATION

Because of the very large absorption by water of radiation with wavelength in the IR range ≥ 2.0 μm, the radiation of Ho:YAG, Er:YAG and CO_2 lasers is absorbed within a very short distance of the tissue surface and scattering is essentially unimportant. Using published values of the water absorption coefficient and assuming an 80 per cent water content and that the decrease in intensity is exponential with distance the depth in the 'average' soft tissue at which the intensity has decreased to 10 per cent of the incident value (the optical penetration depth) is estimated to be 619, 13 and 170 micrometers, respectively, for Ho:YAG, Er:YAG and CO_2 laser radiation. Thus, the absorption of radiation from these laser sources and thermalisation of this energy results essentially in the formation of a surface heat source. With sufficient energy input, tissue ablation through water boiling and tissue thermolysis occur at the surface. Penetration of heat to underlying tissues is by diffusion alone; thus, the depth of coagulation of tissue below the surface region of ablation is limited by competition between thermal diffusional and the rate of descent of the heated surface impacted by laser radiation during ablation of tissue. Because of this competition, coagulation depths obtained in soft biologic tissues with use of mid-IR laser radiation are typically ≤ 205–500 μm and the ability to achieve sealing of blood vessels leading to haemostatic ('bloodless') surgery is limited.

EFFECTS OF NEAR-IR LASER RADIATION

The 810 nm and 1064 µm radiation, respectively, of the GaAlAs diode laser and Nd:YAG laser penetrate more deeply into biologic tissues than the radiation of longer-wavelength IR lasers. Thus, the resulting thermal effects arise from absorption at greater depth within tissues and the depths of coagulation and degree of hemostasis achieved with these lasers tend to be greater than with the longer-wavelength IR lasers. For example, the optical penetration depths (10 per cent incident intensity) for 810 nm and 1.024-µm radiation are estimated to be $\simeq 4.6$ and $\simeq 8.6$ mm respectively in canine prostate tissue. Energy deposition of 3600 J from each laser onto the urethral surface of the canine prostate results in maximum coagulation depths of $\simeq 8$ and 12 mm respectively using diode and Nd:YAG lasers.

Depths of optical penetration and coagulation in porcine liver, a more vascular tissue than prostate gland, of $\simeq 2.8$ and 9.6 mm, respectively, were obtained with a Nd:YAG laser beam and of 7 and 12 mm respectively with an 810 nm diode laser beam. The smaller penetration depth obtained with 810 nm diode radiation in liver than in prostate gland reflects the effect of greater vascularity (blood content) on near-IR propagation.

EFFECTS OF VISIBLE-RANGE LASER RADIATION

Blood and vascular tissues very efficiently absorb radiation in the visible wavelength range due to the strong absorption of haemoglobin. This absorption underlies, for example, the use of:
1. The argon ion laser (488–514.5 nm) in the localised heating and thermal coagulation of the vascular choroid layer and adjacent retina, resulting in the anchoring of the retina in treatment of retinal detachment.
2. The argon ion laser (488–514.5 nm), frequency-doubled Nd:YAG laser (532 nm) and dye laser radiation (585 nm) in the coagulative treatment of cutaneous vascular lesions such as port wine stains.
3. The argon ion (488–514.5 nm) and frequency-doubled Nd:YAG lasers (532 nm) in the ablation of pelvic endometrial lesions which contain brown iron-containing pigments.

Because of the large absorption by haemoglobin and iron-containing pigments, the incident laser radiation is essentially absorbed at the surface of the blood vessel or lesion and the resulting thermal effects are essentially local.

EFFECTS OF UV LASER RADIATION

Whereas exposure of tissue to IR and visible-light-range energy result in removal of tissue by thermal ablation, exposure to argon fluoride (ArF) laser radiation of 193 nm wavelength results predominantly in ablation of tissue initiated by a photochemical process. This ablation arises from repulsive forces between like-charged regions if ionised protein molecules that result from ejection of molecular electrons following UV photon absorption. Because the ionisation and repulsive processes are extremely efficient, little of the incident laser energy escapes as thermal vibrational energy and the extent of thermal coagulation damage adjacent to the site of the incidence is very limited. This feature and the ability to tune very finely the fluence emitted by the ArF laser so that micrometer depths of tissue can be removed have led to ongoing clinical trials to investigate the efficiency of the use of the ArF laser to selectively remove tissue from the surface of the human cornea for correction of short-sighted vision to eliminate the need for corrective eyewear.

EFFECTS OF CONTINUOUS AND PULSED IR-VISIBLE LASER RADIATION AND ASSOCIATION TEMPERATURE RISE

Heating following absorption of IR-visible laser radiation arises from molecular vibration during loss of the excitation energy and initially is manifested locally within the exposed region of tissue. If incidence of the laser energy is maintained for a sufficiently long time, the temperature within adjacent regions of biologic tissue increases due to heat diffusion. The effect of limiting lateral thermal damage is desirable in the cutting of cornea and sclera of the eye and joint cartilage, all of which are avascular (or nearly so, with cartilage) and the hemostasis arising from lateral tissue coagulation is not required.

GENERAL DESCRIPTION AND OPERATION OF LASERS

Lasers emit a beam of intense electromagnetic radiation that is essentially monochromatic or contains at most a few nearly monochromatic wavelengths and is typically only weakly divergent and easily focused into external optical systems. These attributes of laser radiation depend on the key phenomenon which underlies laser operation, that of light amplification by stimulated emission of radiation, which in turn gives rise to the acronym laser.

In practice, a laser is generally a generator of radiation. The generator is constructed by housing a light-emitting medium within a cavity defined by mirrors which provide feedback of emitted radiation through the medium. With sustained excitation of the ionic or molecular species of the medium to give a large density of excited energy states, the spontaneous and attendant stimulated emission of radiation from these states by photons of identical wavelength (a lossless process), which is amplified by feedback due to photon reflection by the cavity mirrors, leads to the generation of a very large photon density within the cavity. With one cavity mirror being partially transmissive, say 0.1 to 1 per cent, a fraction of the cavity energy is emitted as an intense beam. With suitable selection of a laser medium, cavity geometry and peak wavelengths of mirror reflection, the beam is also essentially monochromatic and very nearly collimated. Identity of the lasing molecular species or laser medium fixes the output wavelength of the laser. Laser media range from gases within a tubular cavity, organic dye molecules dissolved in a flowing inert liquid carrier and heat sink, to impurity-doped transparent crystalline rods (solid state lasers) and semi-conducting diode junctions. The different physical properties of these media in part determine the methods used to excite them into lasing states.

Gas-filled or gas lasers are typically excited by DC or RF electric current. The current either ionises and excites the lasing gas, e.g., argon, to give the electronically excited and lasing Ar^+ ion or ionises a gaseous species in a mixture also containing the lasing species, e.g., N_2, which by efficient energy transfer excites the lasing molecular vibrational states of the CO_2 molecule.

Dye lasers and so-called solid-state lasers are typically excited by intense light from either another laser or from a flash lamp. The excitation light wavelength range is selected to ensure efficient excitation at the absorption wavelength of the lasing species. Both excitation and output can be continuous or the use of a pulsed flashlamp or pulsed exciting laser to pump a solid-state or dye laser gives pulsed output with high peak power and short pulse duration of 1 μs to 1 ms. Repeated excitation gives a train of pulses. Additionally, pulses of higher peak power and shorter duration of approximately 10 ns can be obtained from solid lasers by intracavity Q-switching. In this method, the density of excited states is transiently greatly increased by impeding the path between the totally reflecting and partially transmitting mirror of the cavity interrupting the stimulated emission process. Upon rapid removal of the impeding device (a beam-interrupting or deflecting device), stimulated emission of the very large population of excited lasing states leads to emission of an intense laser pulse. The process can give single pulses or can be repeated to give a pulse train with repetition frequencies typically ranging from 1 Hz to 1 kHz.

Gallium aluminium (GaAlAs) lasers are, as are all semi-conducting diode lasers, excited by electrical current which creates excited hole-electron pairs in the vicinity of the diode junction. Those carrier pairs are the lasing species which emits spontaneously and with photon stimulation. The beam emerges parallel to the function with the plane of the function forming the cavity and thin-layer surface mirrors providing reflection. Use of continuous or pulsed excitation current results in continuous or pulsed output.

BIOMEDICAL LASER BEAM DELIVERY SYSTEMS

Beam delivery systems for biomedical lasers guide the laser beam from the output mirror to the site of action on tissue. Beam powers of up to 100 W are transmitted routinely. All biomedical lasers incorporate a coaxial aiming beam, typically from a HeNe laser (632.8 nm) to illuminate the site of incidence on tissue.

Usually, the systems incorporate two different beam-guiding methods, either (i) a flexible fused silica (SiO_2) optical fibre or light guide, generally available currently for laser beam wavelengths between ≈ 400 nm and ≈ 2.1 µm, where SiO_2 is essentially transparent; and (ii) an articulated arm having beam guiding mirrors for wavelengths greater than circa 2.1 µm (e.g., CO_2 lasers), for the Er:YAG and for pulsed lasers having peak power outputs capable of causing damage to optical fibre surfaces due to ionisation by the intense electric field (e.g., pulsed ruby). The arm comprises straight tubular sections articulated together with high-quality power-handling dielectric mirrors at each articulation junction to guide the beam through each of the sections. Fused silica optical fibres usually are limited to a length of 1–3 m and to wavelengths in the visible-to-low mid-range IR (<2.1 µm), because longer wavelengths of IR radiation are absorbed by water impurities (<2.9 µm) and by the SiO_2 lattice itself (wavelengths >5 µm).

Since the flexibility, small diameter and small mechanical inertia of optical fibres allow their use in either flexible or rigid endoscopes and offer significantly less inertia to hand movement, fibres for use at longer IR wavelengths are desired by clinicians. Currently, researchers are evaluating optical fibre materials transparent to longer IR wavelengths. Material systems showing promise are fused Al_2O_3 fibres in short lengths for use with near-3-micrometer radiation of the Er:YAG laser and Ag halide fibres in short lengths for use with CO_2 laser emitting at 10.6 µm. A flexible hollow Teflon waveguide 1.6 mm in diameter having a thin metal film overlain by a dielectric layer has been reported recently to transmit 10.6 µm CO_2 radiation with attenuation of 1.3 and 1.65 dB/m for straight and bent (5 mm radius, 90° bend) sections, respectively.

Optical Fibre Transmission Characteristics

Guiding of the emitted laser beam along the optical fibre, typically of uniform circulation cross-section, is due to total internal reflection of the radiation at the interface between the wall of the optical fibre core and the cladding material having refractive index n_1 less than that of the core n_2. Total internal reflection occurs for any angle of incidence θ of the propagating beam with the wall of the fibre core such that $\theta > \theta_c$ where

$$\sin \theta_c = \left(\frac{n_1}{n_2} \right)$$

... (19.1)

or in terms of the complementary angle α_c

$$\cos \alpha_c = \left(\frac{n_1}{n_2} \right) \qquad \qquad \text{... (19.2)}$$

For a focused input beam with apical angle α_m incident upon the flat face of the fibre as shown in Fig. 19.3, total internal reflection and beam guidance within the fibre core will occur for

$$NA = \sin(\alpha_m/2) \le \left[n_2^2 - n_1^2 \right]^{0.5} \qquad \qquad \text{... (19.3)}$$

where NA is the numerical aperture of the fibre.

This relationship ensures that the critical angle of incidence of the interface is not exceeded and that total internal reflection occurs. Typical values of NA for fused SiO_2 fibres with polymer cladding are in the range of 0.36–0.40. The typical values of $\alpha_m = 14°$ used to insert the beam of the biomedical laser into the fibre is much smaller than those values (≈ 21–$23°$) corresponding to typical NA values. The maximum value of the propagation angle α typically used in biomedical laser systems is $\approx 4.8°$.

Leakage of radiation at the core-cladding interface of the fused SiO_2 fibre is negligible, typically being ≈ 0.3 dB/m at 400 nm and 0.01 dB/m at 1.064 µm. Bends along the fibre length always decrease the angle of the incidence at the core cladding interface. Bends do not give appreciable losses for values of the bending radius sufficiently large that the angle of incidence θ of the propagating beam in the bent core does not becomes less than θ_c at the core-cladding interface. The relationship given by Levi between the bending radius r_b, the fibre core radius r_o, the ratio (n_2/n_1) of fibre core to cladding refractive indices and the propagation angle α in Fig. 19.3 which ensures that the beam does not escape is

$$\frac{n_1}{n_2} > \frac{1-\rho}{1+\rho} \cos \alpha \qquad \qquad \text{... (19.4)}$$

where $\rho = (r_o/r_b)$. The inequality will hold for all $\alpha \le \alpha_c$ provided that

$$\frac{n_1}{n_2} \le \frac{1-\rho}{1+\rho} \qquad \qquad \text{... (19.5)}$$

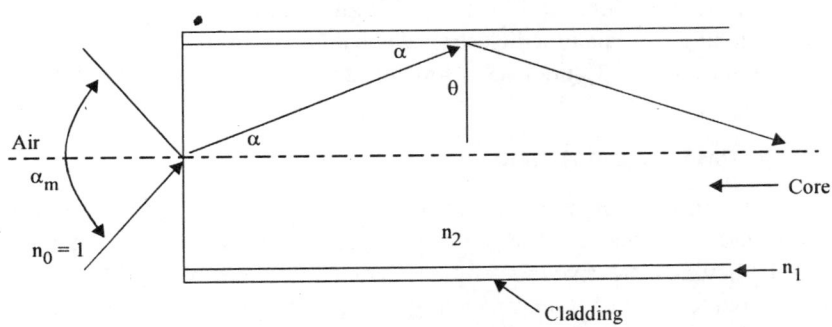

Fig. 19.3. Critical reflection and propagation within an optical fibre.

Thus, the critical bending radius r_{bc} is the value of r_b such that Eq. (19.5) is an equality. Use of Eq. (19.5) predicts that bends with radii ≥ 12, 18 and 30 mm, respectively, will not result in appreciable beam leakage from fibres having 400, 600 and 1000 micron diameter cores, which are typical in biomedical use. Thus, use of fibres in flexible endoscopes usually does not compromise beam guidance.

This relationship ensures that the critical angle of incidence of the interface is not exceeded and that total internal reflection occurs.

Because the integrity of the core-cladding interface is critical to beam guiding, the clad fibre is encased typically in a tough but flexible protective fluoropolymer buffer coat.

Mirrored Articulated Arm Characteristics

Typically two or three relatively long tubular sections or arms of 50–80 cm length make up the portion of the articulated arm that extends from the laser output fixturing to the handpiece, endoscope or operating microscope stage used to position the laser beam onto the tissue proper. Mirrors placed at the articulation of the arms and within the articulated handpiece, laparoscope or operating microscope stage maintain the centration of the trajectory of the laser beam along the length of the delivery system. Dielectric multilayer mirrors routinely are used in articulated devices.

Their low high reflectivity ≤ 99.9 + per cent and power-handling capabilities ensure efficient power transmission down the arm. Mirrors in articulated devices typically are held in kinetically adjustable mounts for rapid stable alignment to maintain beam concentration.

Optics for Beam Shaping on Tissues

Since the rate of heating on tissue and hence rates of ablation and coagulation, depends directly on energy input per unit volume of tissue, selection of ablation and coagulation rates of various tissues are achieved through control of the energy density (J/cm^2 or $W \cdot s/cm^2$) of the laser beam. This parameter is readily achieved through use of optical elements such as discrete focusing lenses placed in the handpiece or rigid endoscope which control the spot size upon the tissue surface or by affixing a so-called contact tip to the end of an optical fibre. These are conical or spherical in shape with diameters ranging from 300–1200 µm and with very short focal lengths. The tip is placed in contact with the tissue and generates a sub-millimeter-sized focal spot in tissue very near the interface between the tip and tissue. One advantage of using the contact tip over a focused beam is that ablation proceeds with small lateral depth of attendant coagulation. This is because the energy of the tightly focused beam causes tissue thermolysis essentially at the tip surface and because the resulting tissue products strongly absorb the beam resulting in energy deposition and ablation essentially at the tip surface. This contrasts with the radiation penetrating deeply into tissue before thermolysis which occurs with a less tightly focused beam from a free lens or fibre. An additional advantage with the use of contact tips in the perception of the surgeon is that the kinesthetics of moving a contact tip along a resisting tissue surface more closely mimics the 'touch' encountered in moving a scalpel across the tissue surface.

Recently a class of optical fibre tips has been developed which laterally directs the beam energy from a silica fibre. These tips, either a gold reflective micromirror or an angled refractive prism, offer a lateral angle of deviation ranging from 35–105° from the optical fibre axis (undeviated beam direction). The beam reflected from a plane micromirror is unfocused and circular in cross-section, whereas the beam from a concave mirror and refractive devices is typically elliptical in shape, fused with distal diverging rays. Fibres with these terminations are currently finding rapidly expanding, large-scale application in coagulation (with 1.064 µm Nd:YAG laser radiation) of excess tissue lining the urethra in treatment of benign prostatic hypertrophy. The capability for lateral beam direction may offer additional utility of these terminated fibres in other clinical specialities.

Features of Routinely Used Biomedical Lasers

Currently four lasers are in routine large-scale clinical biomedical use to ablate, dissect and to coagulate soft tissue. Two, the carbon dioxide (CO_2) and argon ion (Ar ion) lasers, are gas-filled lasers. The other two employ solid-state lasing media. One is the neodymium-yttrium-aluminium-garnet (Nd:YAG) laser, commonly referred to as solid-state laser and the other is the gallium-aluminium arsenide (GaAlAs) semi-conductor diode laser. Salient features of the operating characteristics and biomedical applications of those lasers are listed in Tables 19.2 to 19.5. The operational descriptions are typical of the lasers currently available commercially and do not represent the product of any single manufacturer.

Table 19.2. Operating characteristics of principal biomedical lasers.

Characteristics	Ar ion laser	CO_2 laser
Cavity medium	Argon gas, 133 Pa	10% CO_2, 10% Ne, 80% He; 1330 Pa
Lasing species	Ar+ ion	CO_2 molecule
Excitation	Electric discharge, continuous	Electric discharge, continuous, pulsed
Electric input	208 V_{AC}, 60 A	110 V_{AC}, 15 A
Wall plug efficiency	≈0.06%	≈10%

Characteristics	Nd:YAG laser	GaAlAs diode laser
Cavity medium	Nd-doped YAG	n-p junction, GaAlAs diode
Lasing species	Nd3t in YAG lattice	Hole-electron pairs at diode junction
Excitation	Flashlamp, continuous, pulsed	Electric current, continuous pulsed
Electric input	208/240 V_{AC}, 30 A continuous 110 V_{AC}, 10 A pulsed	110 V_{AC}, 15 A
Wall plug efficiency	≈1%	≈23%

Table 19.3. Output beam characteristics of Ar ion and CO_2 biomedical lasers.

Output characteristics	Argon laser	CO_2 laser
Output power	2–8 W, continuous	1–100 W, continuous
Wavelength(s)	Multiple lines (454.6–528.7 nm), 488, 514.5 dominant	10.6 μm
Electromagnetic wave propagation mode	TEM_∞	TEM_∞
Beam guidance, shaping	Fused silica optical fibre with contact tip or flat-ended for beam emission, lensed handpiece. Slit lamp with ocular lens	Flexible articulated arm with mirrors; lensed handpiece or mirrored microscope platen

Table 19.4. Output beam characteristics of Nd:YAG and GaAlAs diode biomedical lasers.

Output characteristics	Nd:YAG lasers	GaAlAs diode laser
Output power	1–100 W continuous at 1.064 millimicron 1–36 W continuous at 532 nm (frequency doubled with KTP)	1–25 W continuous

(Contd)...

Output characteristics	Nd:YAG lasers	GaAlAs diode laser
Wavelength(s)	1.064 µm/532 nm	810 nm
Electromagnetic wave propagation modes	Mixed modes	Mixed modes
Beam guidance and shaping	Fused SiO_2 optical fibre with contact tip directing mirrored or refracture tip	Fused SiO_2 optical fibre with contact tip or laterally directing mirrored or refracture tip

Table 19.5. Clinical uses of principal biomedical lasers.

Ar-ion laser: Pigmented (vascular) soft-tissue ablation in gynecology; general and oral surgery; otolaryngology; vascular lesion coagulation in dermatology; retinal coagulation in ophthalmology

CO₂ laser: Soft-tissue ablation—dissection and bulk tissue removal in dermatology; gynecology; general, oral, plastic and neurosurgery; otolaryngology; podiatry; urology

Nd:YAG laser: Soft-tissue, particularly pigmented vascular tissue, ablation—dissection and bulk tissue removal—in dermatology; gastroenterology; gynecology; general, arthroscopic, neuroplastic and thoracic surgery; urology; posterior capsulotomy (ophthalmology) with pulsed 1.064 millimicron and ocular lens

GaAlAs diode laser: Pigmented (vascular) soft-tissue ablation—dissection and bulk removal in gynecology; gastroenterology, general surgery and urology; FDA approval for otolaryngology and thoracic surgery pending

Other Biomedical Lasers

Some important biomedical lasers have smaller-scale use or currently are being researched for biomedical application. The following four lasers have more limited scales of surgical use:

1. The Ho:YAG (Holmium:YAG) laser, emitting pulses of 2.1 µm wavelength and up to 4 J in energy, used in soft tissue ablation in arthroscopic (joint) surgery (FDA approved).
2. The Q-switched Ruby ($Cr:Al_2O_3$) laser, emitting pulses of 694 nm wavelength and up to 2 J in energy is used in dermatology to disperse black, blue and green tattoo pigments and melanin in pigmented lesions (not melanoma) for subsequent removal by phagocytosis by macrophages (FDA approved).
3. The flashlamp pumped pulsed dye laser emitting 1 to 2 J pulses at either 577 or 585 nm wavelength (near the 537–577 absorption region of blood) is used for treatment of cutaneous vascular lesions and melanin pigmented lesions except melanoma. Use of pulsed radiation helps to localise the thermal damage to within the lesions to obtain low damage of adjacent tissue.

The following lasers are being investigated for clinical uses.

1. The Er:YAG laser, emitting at 2.94 µm near the major water absorption peak (OH stretch), is currently being investigated for ablation of tooth enamel and dentin.
2. Dye lasers emitting at 630–690 nm are being investigated for application as light sources for exciting dihematoporphyrin ether or benzoporphyrin derivatives in investigation of the efficacy of these photosensitives in the treatment of esophageal, bronchial and bladder carcinomas for the FDA approved process.

Some laser safety tips are listed in Table 19.6.

Table 19.6. Laser safety tips.

Position the laser beam with a low-power aiming light before applying full power

Calibrate the aiming lights to ensure accuracy

(Contd)...

Keep reflective surfaces, which may misdirect the laser beam, away from the surgical field

Cover plastic or rubber tubing with adhesive metal foil to avoid burning by the laser beam

Do not use a laser with flammable anesthetics or in an oxygen concentration above 40 per cent

Use suction to remove laser smoke from the surgical field

Do not allow the laser beam to contact OR personnel

Wear eyeglasses with filters to prevent a reflected laser beam from entering the eyes

Eliminate flammable drapes and cover the windows with opaque material

Place wet sponges around the surgical field to prevent tissue damage if the beam is accidentally misdirected

Chapter 20

Ventilators and Humidifiers

INTRODUCTION

This chapter presents an overview of the structure and function of mechanical ventilators. Mechanical ventilators, which are often also called respirators, are used to artificially ventilate the lungs of patients who are unable to naturally breathe from the atmosphere. The very early devices used bellows that were manually operated to inflate the lungs. Today's respirators employ an array of sophisticated components such as microprocessors, fast response servo valves and precision transducers to perform the task of ventilating the lungs. The changes in the design of ventilators have come about as the result of improvements in engineering the ventilator components and the advent of new therapy modes by clinicians. A large variety of ventilators are now available for short-term treatment of acute respiratory problems as well as long-term therapy for chronic respiratory conditions.

It is reasonable to broadly classify today's ventilators into two groups. The first and indeed the largest group encompasses the intensive care respirators used primarily in hospitals to support patients following certain surgical procedures or assist patients with acute respiratory disorders. The second group includes less complicated machines that are primarily used at home to treat patients with chronic respiratory disorders. The level of engineering design and sophistication for the intensive care ventilators is higher than the ventilators used for chronic treatment. However, many of the engineering concepts employed in designing intensive care ventilators can also be applied in the simpler chronic care units. Therefore, this presentation focuses on the design of intensive care ventilators; the terms respirator, mechanical ventilator or ventilator that will be used from this point on refer to the intensive care unit respirators. At the beginning, the designers of mechanical ventilators realised that the main task of a respirator was to ventilate the lungs in a manner as close to natural respiration as possible. Since natural inspiration is a result of negative pressure in the pleural cavity generated by distention of the diaphragm, designers initially developed ventilators that created the same effect. These ventilators are called negative-pressure ventilators. However, more modern ventilators use pressures greater than atmospheric pressures to ventilate the lungs; they are known as positive-pressure ventilators.

NEGATIVE-PRESSURE VENTILATORS

The principle of operation of a negative-pressure respirator is shown in Fig. 20.1. In this design, the flow of air to the lungs is created by generating a negative pressure around the patient's thoracic cage. The negative pressure moves the thoracic walls outward expanding the intra-thoracic volume and dropping the pressure inside the lungs. The pressure gradient between the atmosphere and the lungs causes the flow of atmospheric air into the lungs. The inspiratory and expiratory phases of the respiration are controlled by cycling the pressure inside the body chamber between a sub-atmospheric level (inspiration) and the atmospheric level (exhalation). Flow of the breath out of the lungs during exhalation is caused by the recoil of thoracic muscles.

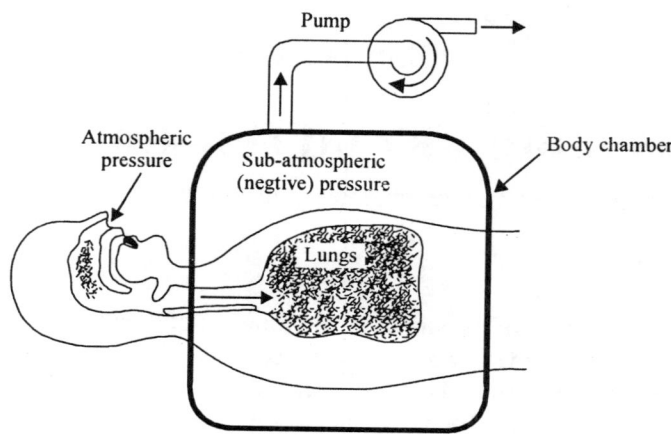

Fig. 20.1. A simplified illustration of a negative-pressure ventilator.

Although it may appear that the negative-pressure respirator incorporates the same principles as natural respiration, the engineering implementation of this concept has not been very successful. A major difficulty has been in the design of a chamber for creating negative pressure around the thoracic walls. One approach has been to make the chamber large enough to house the entire body with the exception of the head and neck. Using foam rubber around the patient's neck, one can seal the chamber and generate a negative pressure inside the chamber. This design configuration, commonly known as the iron lung, was tried back in the 1920s and proved to be deficient in several aspects. The main drawback was that the negative pressure generated inside the chamber was applied to the chest as well as the abdominal wall, thus creating a venous blood pool in the abdomen and reducing cardiac output.

More recent designs have tried to restrict the application of the negative pressure to the chest walls by designing a chamber that goes only around the chest. However, this has not been successful because obtaining a seal around the chest wall (Fig. 20.1) is difficult.

Negative-pressure ventilators also made the patient less accessible for patient care and monitoring. Further, synchronisation of the machine cycle with the patient's effort has been difficult and they are also typically noisy and bulky. These deficiencies of the negative-pressure ventilators have led to the development of the positive-pressure ventilators.

POSITIVE-PRESSURE VENTILATORS

Positive-pressure ventilators generate the inspiratory flow by applying a positive pressure (greater than the atmospheric pressure) to the airways. Figure 20.2 shows a simplified block diagram of a positive-pressure ventilator. During inspiration, the inspiratory flow delivery system creates a positive pressure in the tubes connected to the patient airway, called patient circuit and the exhalation control system closes a valve at the outlet of the tubing to the atmosphere. When the ventilator switches to exhalation, the inspiratory flow delivery system stops the positive pressure and the exhalation system opens the valve to allow the patient's exhaled breath to flow to the atmosphere. The use of a positive pressure gradient in creating the flow allows treatment of patients with high lung resistance and low compliance. As a result, positive-pressure ventilators have been very successful in treating a variety of breathing disorders and have become more popular than negative-pressure ventilators.

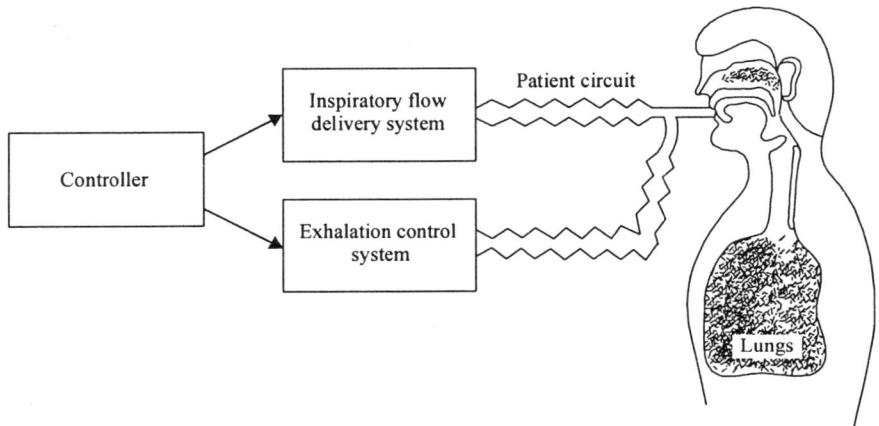

Fig. 20.2. A simplified diagram of the functional blocks of a positive-pressure ventilator.

Positive-pressure ventilators have been employed to treat patients ranging from neonates to adults. Due to anatomical differences between various patient population, the ventilators and their modes of treating infants are different than those for adults. Nonetheless, their fundamental design principles are similar and adult ventilators comprise a larger percentage of ventilators manufactured and used in clinics. Therefore, the emphasis here is on the description of adult positive-pressure ventilators. Also, the concepts presented will be illustrated using a microprocessor-based design example, as almost all modern ventilators use microprocessor instrumentation.

VENTILATION MODES

Since the advent of respirators, clinicians have devised a variety of strategies to ventilate the lungs based on patient conditions. For instance, some patients need the respirator to completely take over the task of ventilating their lungs. In this case, the ventilator operates in mandatory mode and delivers mandatory breaths. On the other hand, some patients are able to initiate a breath and breathe on their own, but may need oxygen-enriched air flow or slightly elevated airway pressure. When a ventilator assists a patient who is capable of demanding a breath, the ventilator delivers spontaneous breaths and operates in spontaneous mode. In many cases, it is first necessary to treat the patient with mandatory ventilation and as the patient's condition improves spontaneous ventilation is introduced; it is used primarily to wean the patient from mandatory breathing.

Mandatory Ventilation

Designers of adult ventilators have employed two rather distinct approaches for delivering mandatory breaths; volume controlled ventilation and pressure controlled ventilation. Volume controlled ventilation, which presently is more popular, refers to delivering a specified tidal volume to the patient during the inspiratory phase. Pressure controlled ventilation, however, refers to raising the airway pressure to a level, set by the therapist, during the inspiratory phase of each breath. Regardless of the type, a ventilator operating in mandatory mode must control all aspects of breathing such as tidal volume, respiration rate, inspiratory flow pattern and oxygen concentration of the breath. This is often labelled as controlled mandatory ventilation (CMV).

Figure 20.3 shows the flow and pressure waveforms for a volume controlled ventilation (CMV). In this illustration, the inspiratory flow waveform is chosen to be a half sinewave. In Fig. 20.3a, t_i is the inspiration duration, t_e is the exhalation period and Q_i is the amplitude of inspiratory flow. The ventilator delivers a tidal volume equal to the area under the flow waveform in Fig. 20.3a at regular intervals $(t_i + t_e)$ set by the therapist. The resulting pressure waveform is shown in Fig. 20.3b. It is noted that during volume controlled ventilation, the ventilator delivers the same volume irrespective of the patient's respiratory mechanics. However, the resulting pressure waveform such as the one shown in Fig. 20.3b, will be different among patients. Of course, for safety purposes, the ventilator limits the maximum applied airway pressure according to the therapist's setting.

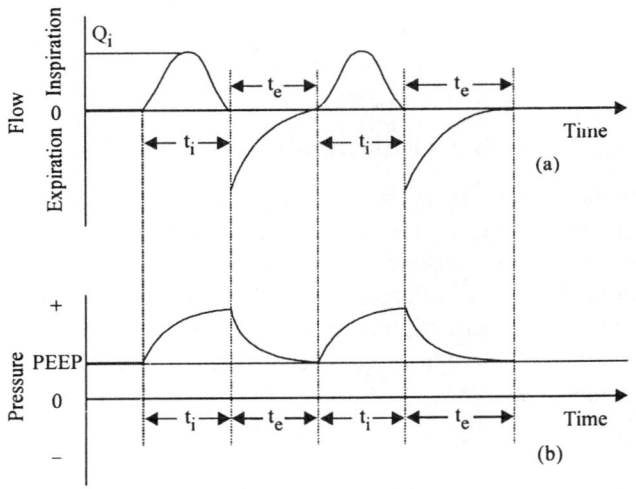

Fig. 20.3. (a) Inspiratory flow for a controlled mandatory volume controlled ventilation breath; and (b) airway pressure resulting from the breath delivery with a non-zero PEEP.

As can be seen in Fig. 20.3b, the airway pressure at the end of exhalation may not end at atmospheric pressure (zero gauge). The positive end expiratory pressure (PEEP) is sometimes used to keep the alveoli from collapsing during expiration. In other cases, the expiration pressure is allowed to return to the atmospheric level.

Figure 20.4 shows a plot of the pressure and flow during a mandatory pressure controlled ventilation. In this case, the respirator raises and maintains the airway pressure at the desired level independent of patient airway compliance and resistance. The level of pressure during inspiration, P_i, is set by the therapist. While the ventilator maintains the same pressure trajectory for patients with different respiratory resistance and compliance, the resulting flow trajectory, shown in Fig. 20.4b, will depend on the respiratory mechanics of each patient.

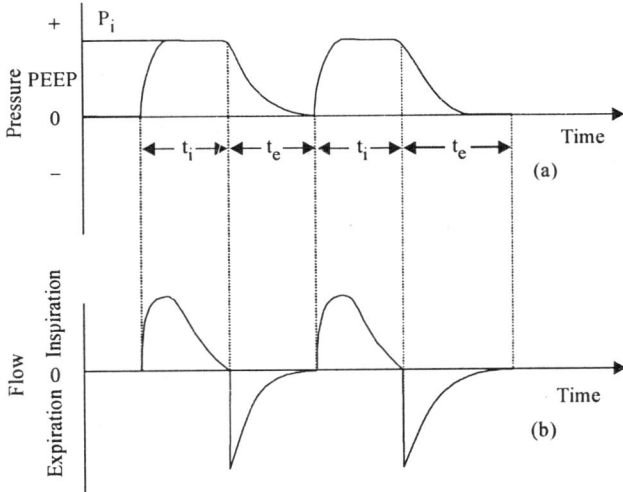

Fig. 20.4. (a) Inspiratory pressure pattern for a controlled mandatory pressure controlled ventilation breath; and (b) airway flow pattern resulting from the breath delivery. Note that PEEP is zero.

In the following, the presentation will focus on volume ventilators, as they are more common. Further, in a microprocessor-based ventilator, the mechanism for delivering mandatory volume and pressure controlled ventilation have many similar main components. The primary difference lies in the control algorithms governing the delivery of breaths to the patient.

Spontaneous Ventilation

An important phase in providing respiratory therapy to a recovering pulmonary patient is weaning the patient from the respirator. As the patient recovers and gains the ability to breathe independently, the ventilator must allow the patient to initiate a breath and control the breath rate, flow rate and the tidal volume. Ideally, when a respirator is functioning in the spontaneous mode, it should let the patient take breaths with the same ease as breathing from the atmosphere. This, however, is difficult to achieve because the respirator does not have an infinite gas supply or an instantaneous response. In practice, the patient generally has to exert more effort to breathe spontaneously on a respirator than from the atmosphere. However, patient effort is reduced as the ventilator response speed increases. Spontaneous ventilation is often used in conjunction with mandatory ventilation since the patient may still need breaths that are delivered entirely by the ventilator. Alternatively, when a patient can breathe completely on his own but needs oxygen-enriched breath or elevated airway pressure, spontaneous ventilation alone may be used.

As in the case of mandatory ventilation, several modes of spontaneous ventilation have been devised by therapists. Two of the most important and popular spontaneous breath delivery modes are described below.

Continuous positive airway pressure (CPAP) in spontaneous mode

In this mode, the ventilator maintains a positive pressure at the airway as the patient attempts to inspire. Figure 20.5 illustrates a typical airway pressure waveform during CPAP breath delivery. The therapist sets the sensitivity level lower than PEEP. When the patient attempts to breathe, the pressure drops below the sensitivity level and the ventilator responds by supplying breathable gases to raise the pressure back to the PEEP level. Typically, the PEEP and sensitivity levels are selected such that the patient will be impelled to exert effort to breathe independently. As in the case of the mandatory mode, when the patient exhales the ventilator shuts off the flow of gas and opens the exhalation valve to allow the exhaled gases to flow into atmosphere.

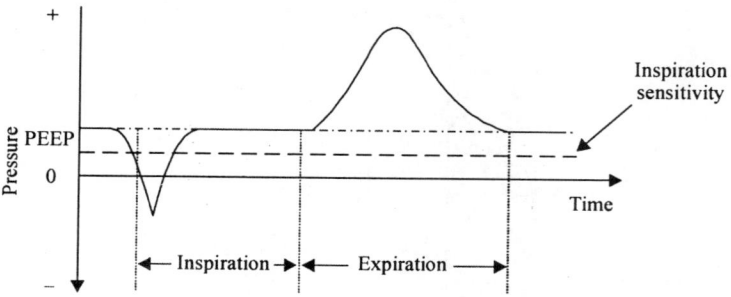

Fig. 20.5. Airway pressure during a CPAP spontaneous breath delivery.

Pressure support in spontaneous mode

This mode is similar to the CPAP mode with the exception that during the inspiration the ventilator attempts to maintain the patient airway pressure at a level above PEEP. In fact, CPAP may be considered a special case of pressure support ventilation in which the support level is fixed at the atmospheric level.

Figure 20.6 shows a typical airway pressure waveform during the delivery of pressure support breath. In this mode, when the patient's airway pressure drops below the therapist-set sensitivity line, the ventilator inspiratory breath delivery system raises the airway pressure to the pressure support level (>PEEP), selected by the therapist. The ventilator stops the flow of breathable gases when the patient starts to exhale and controls the exhalation valve to achieve the set PEEP level.

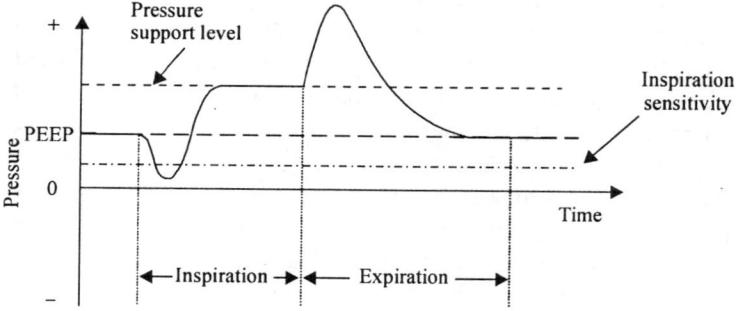

Fig. 20.6. Airway pressure during a pressure support spontaneous breath delivery.

BREATH DELIVERY CONTROL

Figure 20.7 shows a simplified block diagram for delivering mandatory or spontaneous ventilation. Compressed air and oxygen are normally stored in high pressure tanks ($\cong$1400 kPa) that are attached to the inlets of the ventilator. In $\_$ me ventilators, an air compressor is used in place of a compressed air tank. Manufacturers of mechanical respirators have designed a variety of blending and metering devices.

The primary mission of the device is to enrich the inspiratory air flow with the proper level of oxygen and to deliver a tidal volume according to the therapist's specifications. With the introduction of microprocessors for control of metering devices, electromechanical valves have gained popularity. In Fig. 20.7, the air and oxygen valves are placed in closed feedback loops with the air and oxygen flow sensors. The microprocessor controls each valves to deliver the desired inspiratory air and oxygen flows for mandatory and spontaneous ventilation. During inhalation, the exhalation valve is closed to direct all the delivered flows to the lungs. When exhalation starts, the microprocessor actuates the exhalation valve to achieve the desired PEEP level. The airway pressure sensor, shown on the right side of Fig. 20.7, generates the feedback signal necessary for maintaining the desired PEEP (in both mandatory and spontaneous modes) and airway pressure support level during spontaneous breath delivery.

Mandatory Volume Controlled Inspiratory Flow Delivery

In a microprocessor-controlled ventilator (Fig. 20.7), the electronically actuated valves open from a closed position to allow the flow of blended gases to the patient. The control of flow through each valve depends on the therapist's specification for the mandatory breath. That is, the clinician must specify the following parameters for delivery of CMV breaths: (i) respiration rate; (ii) flow waveform; (iii) tidal volume; (iv) oxygen concentration (of the delivered breath); (v) peak flow; and (vi) PEEP, as shown in the lower left side of Fig. 20.7. It is noted that the PEEP selected by the therapist in the mandatory mode is only used for control of exhalation flow; that will be described in the following section. The microprocessor utilises the first five of the above parameters to compute the total desired inspiratory flow trajectory. To illustrate this point, consider the delivery of a tidal volume using a half sinewave as shown in Fig. 20.3.

The ratio of inspiratory to expiratory periods of a mandatory breath is often used for adjusting the respiration rate.

A number of control design strategies may be appropriate for the control of the air and oxygen flow delivery valves. A simple controller is the proportional plus integral controller that can be readily implemented in a microprocessor.

The control structure shown in Fig. 20.7 provides the flexibility of quickly adjusting the percentage of oxygen in the enriched breath gases. That is, the controller can regulate both the total flow and the per cent oxygen delivered to the patient. Since the internal volume of the flow control valve is usually small (<50 ml), the desired change in the oxygen concentration of the delivered flow can be achieved within one inspiratory period. In actual clinical applications, rapid change of per cent oxygen from one breath to another is often desirable, as it reduces the waiting time for the delivery of the desired oxygen concentration. A design similar to the one shown in Fig. 20.7 has been successfully implemented in a microprocessor-based ventilator and is deployed in hospitals around the world.

Pressure Controlled Inspiratory Flow Delivery

The therapist entry for pressure-controlled ventilation is shown in Fig. 20.7 (lower left-hand side). In contrast to the volume-controlled ventilation, the total desired flow is generated by a closed loop controller labelled as airway pressure controller in Fig. 20.7. This controller used the therapist-selected inspiratory pressure, respiration rate and the I:E ratio to compute the desired inspiratory pressure trajectory. The trajectory serve as the controller reference input. The controller then computes the flow necessary to make the actual airway pressure track the reference input.

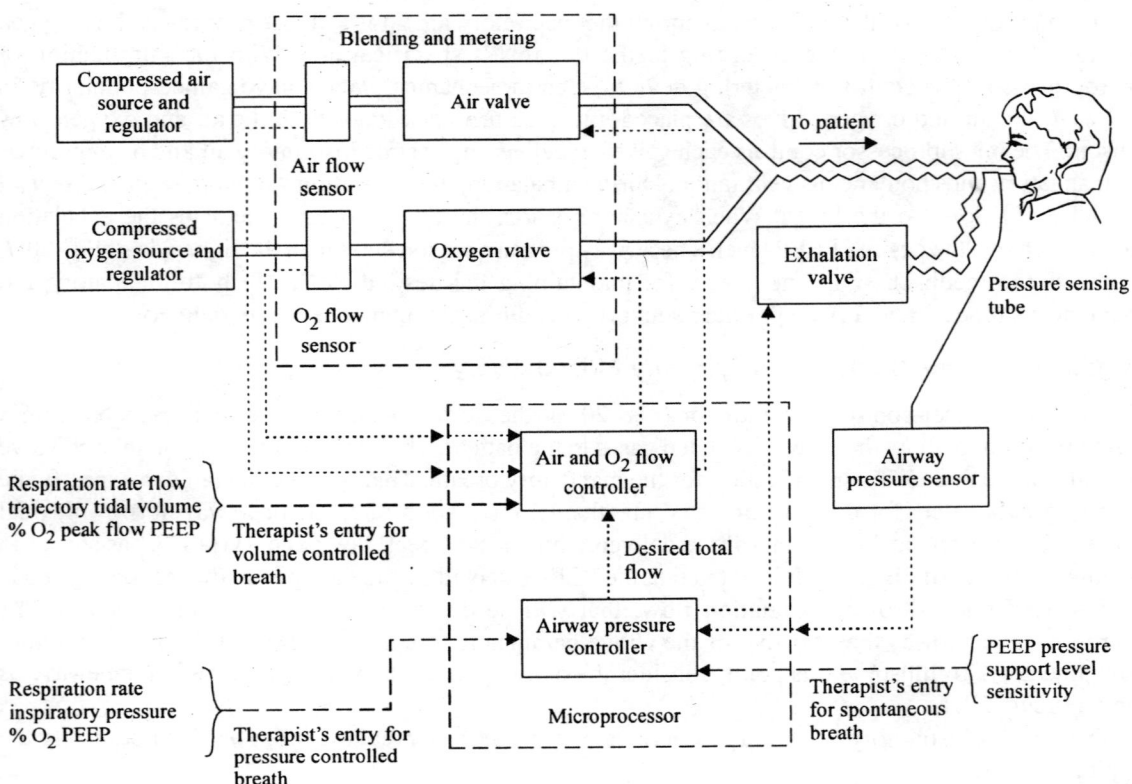

Fig. 20.7. A simplified block diagram of a control structure for mandatory and spontaneous breath delivery.

Expiratory Pressure Control in Mandatory Mode

It is often desirable to keep the patient's lungs inflated at the end of expiration at a pressure greater than atmospheric level. That is, rather than allowing the lungs to deflate during the exhalation, the controller closes the exhalation valve when the airway pressure reaches the PEEP level. When expiration starts, the ventilator terminates flow to the lungs; hence, the regulation of the airway pressure is achieved by controlling the flow of patient exhaled gases through the exhalation valve.

In a microprocessor-based ventilator, an electronically actuated valve can be employed that has adequate dynamic response ($\cong$ 20 ms rise time) to regulate PEEP. For this purpose, the pressure in the patient breath delivery circuit is measured using a pressure transducer (Fig. 20.7). The microprocessor will initially open the exhalation valve completely to minimise resistance to expiratory flow. At the same time, it will sample the pressure transducer's output and start to close the exhalation valve as the pressure begins to approach the desired PEEP level.

Since the patient's exhaled flow is the only source of pressure, if the airway pressure drops below PEEP, it cannot be brought back up until the next inspiratory period. Hence, an overrun (i.e., a drop to below PEEP) in the closed-loop control of PEEP cannot be tolerated.

Spontaneous Breath Delivery Control

The small diameter ($\cong$ 5mm) pressure sensing tube, shown on the right side of Fig. 20.7, pneumatically transmits the pneumatic pressure signal from the patient airway to a pressure transducer placed in the ventilator. The output of the pressure transducer is amplified, filtered and then sampled by the microprocessor. The controller receives the therapist's inputs regarding the spontaneous breath characteristics such as the PEEP, sensitivity and oxygen concentration, as shown on the lower right-hand side of Fig. 20.7. The desired airway pressure is computed from the therapist entries of PEEP, pressure support level and sensitivity. The multiple-loop control structure shown in Fig. 20.7 is used to deliver a CPAP or a pressure support breath. The sensed proximal airway pressure is compared with the desired airway pressure. The airway pressure controller computes the total inspiratory flow level required to raise the airway pressure to the desired level. This flow level serves as the reference input or total desired flow for the flow control loop. Hence, in general, the desired total flow trajectory for the spontaneous breath delivery may be different for each inspiratory cycle. If the operator has specified oxygen concentration greater than 21.6 per cent (the atmospheric air oxygen concentration of the ventilator air supply), the controller will partition the total required flow into the air and oxygen flow rates. The flow controller then uses the feedback signals from air and oxygen flow sensors and actuates the air and oxygen valves to deliver the desired flows. For a microprocessor-based ventilator, the control algorithm for regulating the airway pressure can also be a proportional plus integral controller.

If a non-zero PEEP level is specified, the same control strategy as the one described for mandatory breath delivery can be used to achieve the desired PEEP.

HUMIDIFIERS FOR USE WITH AUTOMATIC LUNG VENTILATORS

The ventilation of a patient for prolonged periods with room air or cylinder gases when the air-conditioning action of the nasal passages is by-passed by an endotracheal or tracheotomy tube is likely to result in a marked drying of bronchial and alveolar secretions. Depletion of this mucosal moisture increases the viscosity of the mucous layer, slows its movement and reduces ciliary action. The build-up of solidifying secretions can significantly affect the airway resistance. In order to avoid these complications, a humidifier is usually attached to the output of the ventilator in order to add water vapour to the inspired gas delivered to the patient (Fig. 20.8).

In the past, the commonest type of humidifier for use with ventilators has been the 'bubbler' type. In principle, this is simply a container of water thermostatically maintained at about body temperature and through which each expired tidal volume from the ventilator is bubbled to pick-up water vapour. British Standard 4494 specifies the operation of humidifiers for use with breathing machines. Over the minute volume range of 5 to 20 litres per minute, the output from the humidifier should contain not less than 53 mg of water vapour per litre (a relative humidity of not less than 75 per cent at 37°C) at the end of a one meter length of 22 mm bore corrugated rubber tubing when the input gas temperature is in the range 10 to 25°C. The gas temperature at the point of entry to the patient must not exceed 39°C at any time and the resistance to flow of the humidifier should not exceed 30 mm of water at a steady flow of 30 litres per minute.

Considerable improvements have been made in the design of bubbler type humidifiers, for example, in the version incorporated in the Type AV3 intensive care ventilator by Philips Medical Systems Ltd. This is a two tank design which has a low and constant compressible volume with a plug-in sterilisable water bath unit. A thermostat controls the water bath temperature and as an additional safeguard, a thermistor senses the temperature of the humidified gas supplied to the patient. This can be set between 27 and 37°C.

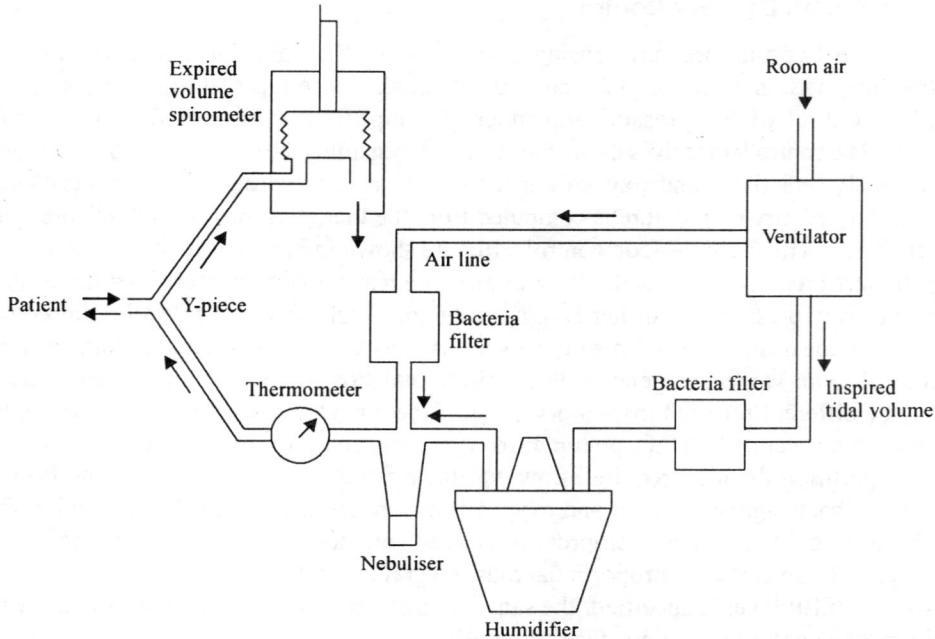

Fig. 20.8. The connection of a humidifier and a nebuliser to a ventilator.

Other forms of humidifier include the 'scent-spray' type. A fine jet of water produced by a vibrator pump and a jewelled orifice is caused to impact on to a metal tube where it forms a fine mist of water vapour which is entrained by the passing tidal volume going to the patient. The humidifier uses a maximum rate of 20 ml of water per hour and it can hold 500 ml.

Assuming that the incoming gas to the humidifier is dry and the water vapour content of the humidified gas is 6 per cent by volume at 37°C, for an 8 litre minute volume the humidifier is supplying 400 ml of water vapour per minute. At 37°C, 1 ml of liquid water is equivalent to 1400 ml of vapour so this represents a consumption of 20 ml of water per minute.

This type of humidifier is compact and can be mounted adjacent to the inspiratory valve which with the expiratory valve may be mounted in a valve block close to the patient. In order to prevent the condensation of water vapour from causing the disk valves to stick, Dräger electrically heat the valve block to 40–45°C. The Dräger Spiromat 661 ventilator is provided with a concentric delivery hose arrangement with the inner tube carrying the humidified air to the patient. This is a heat exchanger system, the warm expired air which surrounds the inner tube helps to prevent condensation of the water vapour contents of the inspired air. The fact that the lumen of the inspiratory hose of a ventilator can be smaller than that of the expiratory hose also led Bushman and Robinson to the design of a double-lumen concentric ventilator hose. In many types of ventilator, the expired gas is returned to the machine and passes through the expiratory port and valve and often a tidal and minute volume measuring device. Since this part of the ventilator is normally at room temperature, a considerable condensation of water vapour may occur when a humidifier is in use. This can cause a light-weight mica disk valve to stick and also give rise to false readings with turbine or vane type volume meters. Hence, it may be necessary to heat these devices to about 45°C to prevent the condensation of water in them or to provide drainage facilities and to employ materials which will not take up water.

A number of ventilators are fitted with ultrasonic humidifiers. Radio frequency power is supplied to a concave piezoelectric transducer made of a ceramic material. This results in the transducer vibrating at an ultrasonic frequency of the order of 1.4 MHz. The concave shape of the ceramic focuses the ultrasonic waves into a container full of sterile water. The resulting intense agitation of the water gives rise to the production of a fine mist of water particles which are claimed to have a close range of drop sizes. This helps to achieve a uniform penetration of the lungs. A powerful ultrasonic humidifier can produce copious amounts of water and care must be taken in its use with patients. One possible regime is to use a bubbler humidifier and an ultrasonic humidifier for alternate hours. Care must also be taken to ensure that any radio frequency field from an ultrasonic humidifier will not effect pacemakers and other apparatus used by the patient.

Nebulisers

Humidifiers, except those of the ultrasonic types, are basically designed to produce a maximum amount of water vapour with a minimum amount of particulate water. This is in contrast to nebulisers which are designed to generate a maximum output of particles of medication in a desired size range. There may be a considerable overlap in function between a humidifier and a nebuliser, the difference often being one of degree. Nebulisers are frequently used in conjunction with a patient-triggered assistor for the administration of drugs such as broncho-dilators in the form of an aerosol. Other forms of aerosol therapy use mucolytic, proteolytic or antibiotic aerosols. A heated aerosol of hypertonic saline, with or without propylene glycol, can be employed for sputum induction of for the removal of thick bronchial plugs.

Chapter 21

Implantable Insulin Delivery Systems

INTRODUCTION

The pathogenesis of long-term complications associated with insulin dependent diabetes mellitus (IDDM) remains a contentious issue between two schools of thought: Accelerated macroangiopathy, microangiopathy and neuropathy are either genetically determined and independent of biochemical derangements or they result from non-genetic metabolic abnormalities. Although proponents of the metabolic theory have gathered impressive clinical evidence, confirmatory data from animal models and demonstrable histologic changes that correlate with metabolic abnormalities, there have also been contradictory reports.

Hyperglycemia is the most important, metabolic abnormality that is potentially responsible for long-term complications. Conventional insulin therapy has been unable to normalise both blood glucose and other metabolic and hormonal abnormalities. Thus new methods of intensified intermittent sub-cutaneous insulin injection (ISII) treatment have been used to achieve normal blood glucose levels in insulin-dependent (type 1) diabetes. This treatment modality requires intensive patient and provider activity, including multiple daily injections of insulin, multiple daily blood glucose self-measurements and frequent clinic visits.

Research using relatively small experimental groups of diabetic patients, studied for a year or less, indicate that intensive ISII can normalise glycosylated haemoglobin levels. In largs non-research patient population, however, the long-term safety and effectiveness of this treatment appear unclear since glycosylated haemoglobin levels are not reduced into the normal range and since significant treatment related complications have been reported.

DRUG DELIVERY DEVICES

One of the principle activities of clinical medicine is the pharmacologic treatment of diseases. Traditionally, this has been carried out by administering drugs and other materials in individual doses by the oral, sub-cutaneous, intramuscular or intravenous route. In some cases, however, these methods of administration are not satisfactory, because drug levels vary from one administration to the next. For drugs the therapeutic levels of which are close to their toxic levels, this type of administration results in either toxic side effects or sub-optimal therapy. Methods of using physical devices to administer drugs continuously within a narrow therapeutic range have been developed to overcome these problems.

Drug Infusion Pumps

Controlled infusion of fluids and drugs is a well-established technique in the hospital. Intravenous (IV) therapy from a gravity-fed fluid reservoir is extensively used in cases ranging from the treatment of severe infections to intensive-care in the operating room and post-operatively. These fluids are frequently routed by gravity-fed through some type of constriction that controls the total amount of fluid administered. Although this method is widely used in hospitals and is relatively inexpensive, it is limited in that careful control of the amount of fluid or drug administered is not possible. In those cases where precise control is necessary, some type of volumetric controller or a complete pumping system must be used.

In the case of a volumetric controller, the amount of fluid administered through a gravity-fed system is carefully regulated. Most clinical intravenous fluid administration sets include a drip chamber where the fluid passes through a fixed-diameter capillary tube and forms drops that drip from the tube into the chamber when they reach a certain volume. The clinician adjusts the flow rate to produce a certain number of drops per unit of time. A simple controller can achieve the same function by photoelectrically observing each drop as it interrupts a light beam passing from a light-emitting diode source to a photodetector such as a phototransistor. A device containing the light source and light detector can be clamped on the drip chamber of a conventional IV administration set and used to control a valve located between the fluid reservoir and the drip chamber. The clinician determines the number of drops required per unit time and sets the controller to deliver drops at the required rate.

Another approach is to use a peristalsis pump such as a roller pump to allow only a certain amount of fluid to pass from a gravity-fed reservoir to the patient. The inside diameter of the tubing and the propagation velocity of the peristalsis wave determine the amount of fluid administered.

There are other methods that can be used to meter the amount of fluid administered. All these systems require some type of electronic control to maintain steady infusion at a fixed, pre-determined rate. Though earlier systems utilised a DC motor to drive a piston pump at a rate determined by a gear system, stepping motors are used today and the angular velocity is controlled by digital electronics. Such a system is illustrated in Fig. 21.1. The object of this system is to provide a series of pulses to the stepping motor at a precise frequency so that it drives the metering pump to supply the fluid at the desired rate. The pulse rate required for the desired infusion rate is set by the operator, who adjusts the rate-setting control. The advantage of using a stepping motor and this system is that the motor advances by a known amount for each applied pulse. Thus, by precisely controlling the number of pulses applied to the stepping motor, it is possible to control precisely its angular displacement. And by precisely controlling the rate at which pulses are applied to the motor, it is possible to control its angular velocity. This degree of control is not possible with open loop analog motors.

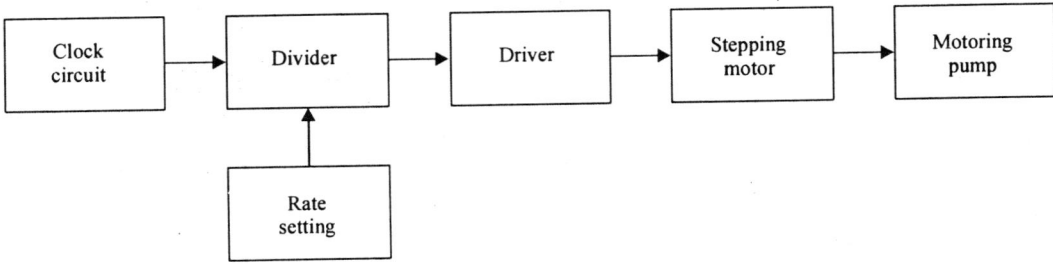

Fig. 21.1. Block diagram of the electronic control system for a fluid or drug delivery pump.

Infusion systems can be used in two general ways. For an open-loop device, the operator sets the desired infusion rate and the fluid or drug is delivered at that rate until the setting is changed. The closed-loop system involves operating the pump in such a way as to keep a physiological variable as close as possible to a desired value. An example of such a system is the use of controlled infusion of the drug sodium nitroprusside, a vasodilator, to control the blood pressure of hypertensive patients during surgery and post-operatively. A pressure sensor measures the blood pressure and this information is fed into a control algorithm that determines the number of pulses sent to the stepping motor—and hence the rate at which it infuses the drug into the patient. Investigators have shown that the automatic control of blood pressure in this way is more efficacious than the manual control of blood pressure via the same chemical agent.

NEW TECHNIQUES OF INSULIN ADMINISTRATION

Islet and Pancreas Transplants

The major advantages of transplantation as an insulin delivery device are that both the source of insulin and the power for its delivery are derived from the blood without the need for external interference and the insulin delivery is controlled by a sophisticated feedback mechanism. Pancreatic islets are relatively easy to transplant, but the problems of isolation, supply and rejection prevent this from becoming even an experimental option at present.

Pancreatic transplantation is becoming more common worldwide. Many of the difficulties are technical and advances in surgical procedure are needed before the operation is suitable for use in people without an immediate life-threatening illness.

External Infusion Devices

External pumps have been widely used in diabetes and the rate of the pump is usually adapted manually according to intermittent blood glucose testing (the open-loop or better the semi-closed-loop system).

Approximately 30 different devices are commercially offered for insulin delivery, most of which are motor-driven syringes. One model supplies the syringes pre-filled as cartridges (Nordisk-infuser). The second pump principle to be encountered is the peristaltic or roller pump. The technical data for each of the various types cannot be discussed here. Instead, reference is made to what currently must be considered the most comprehensive survey on the topic.

With the general trend toward miniaturisation of the devices, the reservoirs (syringes) are reduced more and more in size. Nearly all devices are suitable only for the sub-cutaneous (SC) route. Figure 21.2 represents an example with a long-term reservoir (30 ml) for the central catheter route, currently mostly intraperitoneally (IP).

Implantable Devices

Pumps

The number of companies making implantable devices is lower than those making external devices because of the greater technical complexity.

Devices with fixed rates

The implant commercially for human use at present is a product which is purely mechanical pump. A titanium bellows is filled with the infusion liquid through a pierceable spectrum and is pressurised by means of an evaporating fluid (Freon) (Fig. 21.3). The fluid is driven out through a capillary flow resistor into a suitably placed catheter. The supply rate depends upon the differential pressure between the bellows interior and the catheter tip, the viscosity of the fluid and the fixed dimensions of the capillary. The pressure in the bellows interior varies considerably with the temperature and the level of the fluid. The viscosity is selected as high as possible for insulin infusion to achieve the desired low flow rate with the largest possible capillary lumen (minimising the risk of clogging due to precipitated insulin). Apparently, users of these devices can cope with these fluctuations by taking special precautions measures when flying, mountaineering, sitting in the sauna, having a fever and so on.

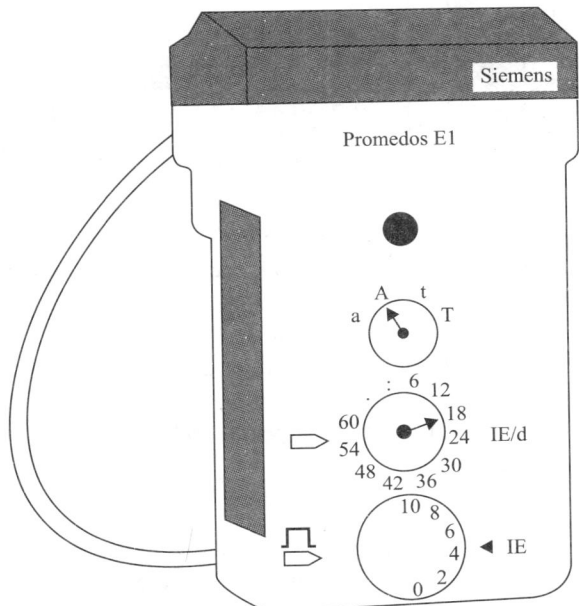

Fig. 21.2. Siemens Promedos E1 external portable insulin pump.

The rates of these devices can be changed only on a long-term basis by replenishment and are therefore only conditionally suitable for diabetes therapy. This statement concerns the commercially available devices.

Devices with controllable rates

These devices are necessarily electromechanical. The information transfer from the external programming or control device takes place electromagnetically or magnetically, storage in the implant occurs electronically. The drug delivery is necessarily a mechanical process.

Sandia laboratory pump

The main difference between it and the Siemens pump is that the Sandia pump has its reservoir outside the pump capsule. To date, only Schade has implanted this pump and no prototypes have been available for testing at other centers.

Siemens pump

This pump was first implanted in a human being in 1981 by Irsigler at Vienna-Lainz. The continued problem of insulin instability seen in animal experimentation has prevented any further human implantation.

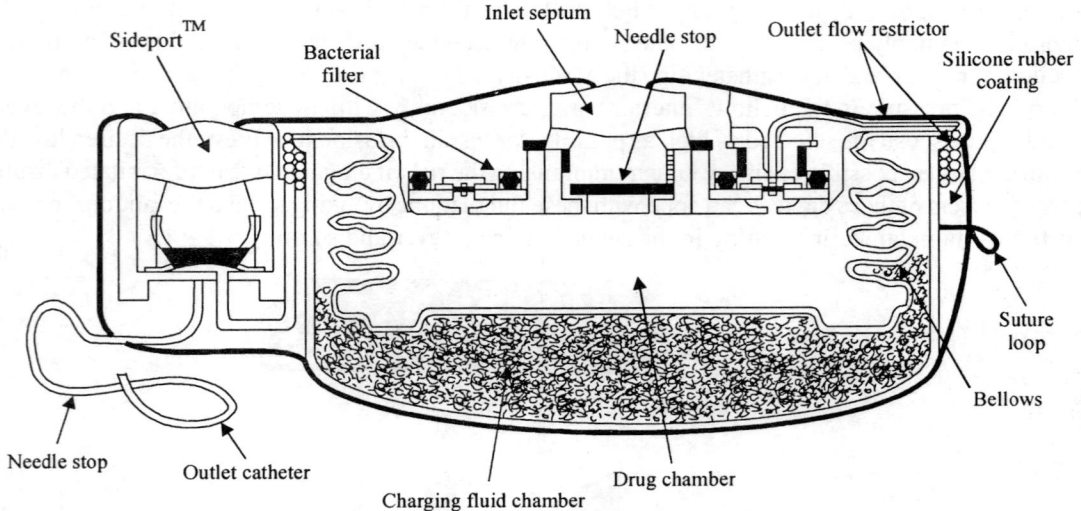

Fig. 21.3. Cross-section through an Infusaid Model 400 fixed-rate implantable pump.

Medtronic pump

This pump was first used in human to deliver morphine and has been implanted in dogs for insulin delivery. Human implantation is planned as soon as problems with insulin aggregation are solved. The medtronic pump works on a peristaltic principle. A special feature is its programmability by patient and physician using a computer terminal.

Pacesetter pump

The Pacesetter (presently minimed) pump (Fig. 21.4) was developed at Johns Hopkins University and noteworthy is the use of the diaphragm. Freon gas is used in the pump to create a negative pressure, so that there is no risk that insulin can leak out into the body. Figure 21.5 shows a cross-section through the Pacesetter's variable rate infusion pump. The infusion rate is set by a telemetry coil from an external programmer which is held over the implanted device during the programming procedure. A battery powers the electronics and telemetry modules and controls the pulsatile pump, which delivers the drug from the medication reservoir to the patient through the catheter. Several pumps have functioned successfully in diabetic dogs for more than three years.

AMBULATORY AND IMPLANTABLE INFUSION SYSTEMS

Miniature infusion pumps have been developed for patients with special therapeutic needs. Insulin pumps that are small enough to be worn by a patient are routinely used to help diabetic patient control their blood glucose. These insulin-delivery systems are currently run open-loop, because there is no reliable, continuously operating glucose sensor available for such a system. The patient controls the rate of infusion, after taking into account his or her activity level, meals and occasional self-administered serum glucose tests.

Miniature pumps that are only slightly larger than an implantable cardiac pacemaker have been developed for implantable drug delivery. These pumps apply a known pressure to a reservoir of the drug and there is a high-resistance connection between the pump and the site where the drug is to be infused, which is usually a vein. This high-resistance connection is generally a long, thin capillary tube that is wound around the periphery of the pump. The constant pressure in the reservoir and the fixed resistance of the tube maintain a steady but slow rate of infusion of the drug into the venous circulation. Implantable pumps, therefore, utilise a concentrated form of the agent to be infused. Nevertheless, it is periodically necessary to re-fill the reservoir. This is done percutaneously by means of a needle that can enter the reservoir and re-fill it without any of the drug leaking into the surrounding tissues. This technique is no more uncomfortable to the patient than receiving an injection.

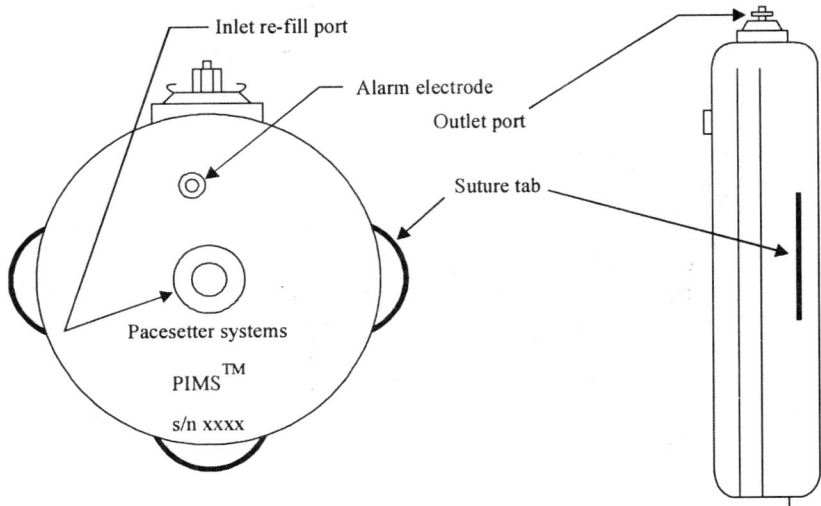

Fig. 21.4. Pacesetter systems, electronically controlled variable-rate implantable infusion pump.

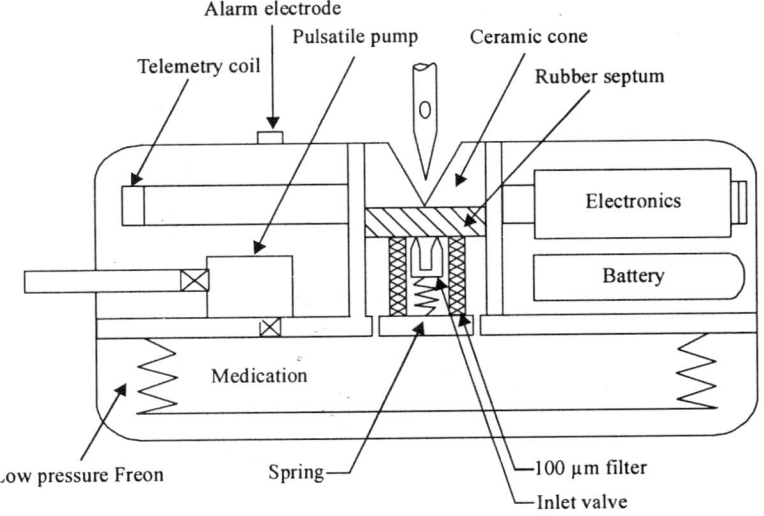

Fig. 21.5. Cross-section through Pacesetter systems, electronically controlled variable rate implantable infusion pump.

Implantable pumps, have also been used for delivering drugs to a specific tissue. This technique has been found useful in cancer chemotherapy, because systemic administration of the cytotoxic agents used would have far more serious side effects than the patient experiences when the agent is administered locally. Implantable closed-loop drug delivery systems are of great interest for biomedical therapy because with the appropriate control algorithm they should be able to imitate the behaviour of malfunctioning organs. The classic example of a closed-loop drug delivery system is the artificial pancreas. This device consists of an implantable pump of the type described in previous paragraphs. This pump, as shown in Fig. 21.6, has a reservoir containing insulin and a control valve that determines the flow rate of insulin into the surrounding tissue from which it is picked up by the circulation.

The valve in turn is controlled by an electronic control system which performs the control algorithm for the device. A glucose sensor determines the body's glucose level and serves as the input device for the control system. Elevated glucose levels cause the pump to dispense increased amounts of insulin, while reduced glucose levels have the opposite effect. Most of these components have been developed in implantable form and miniature closed-loop insulin delivery systems should be quite feasible with the exception of one component: the sensor. Although various investigators have developed glucose sensors that function *in vitro*, reliable miniature *in vivo* sensors capable of measurements for many years are not available. Without this crucial component, the implantable artificial pancreas is constrained to being a dream for the future.

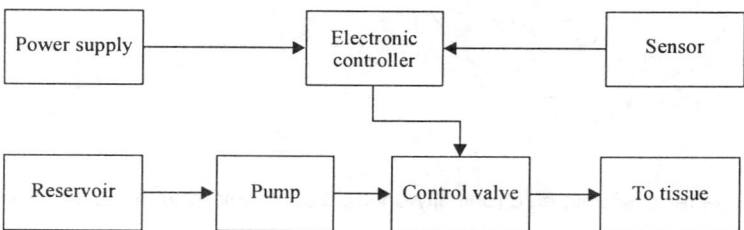

Fig. 21.6. A block diagram of an implantable artificial pancreas showing the major components of the system.

Long-term drug delivery from passive devices has been demonstrated and utilised in some products. The basic principle has been described and reduced to practice by Langer and consists of a polymer matrix in which the drug is dispersed that is implanted in tissue. The drug slowly leaches from this material and is taken up by the capillaries in the surrounding tissue whereupon it is dispersed throughout the body by the cardiovascular system. By choosing appropriate materials and forming them in a specific shape, the drug can be leached out to give a desired level in the body appropriate for the therapeutic situation. An example of such a device is a thin polymer cylinder that can be injected beneath the skin and slowly leaches the hormone progesterone to provide contraceptive protection lasting several months in women. Even though these devices do not require electronic control system and they must operate open-loop, they have several clinical advantages due to their simplicity.

Access ports

Access ports are totally implanted sub-cutaneous reservoirs, with or without catheter, which give access to central routes of transcutaneous drug administration (intravascular, intrathecal, intraperitoneal, etc.). All alternative for IP insulin delivery is the sub-cutaneous peritoneal access device (SPAD). As the name implies, no transcutaneous tubing, requiring dressing and carrying the risk of infection, is introduced periluminally and patients do not wear external pumps. Administration of insulin is by the multiple injection techniques over the moderately larger surface of the dome (8 cm^2) and into the extraperitoneal reservoir or bowl of the device (Fig. 21.7). This access device is surgically implanted supraumbilically in the midline so that it will remain clear of potentially irritating clothing, especially belts.

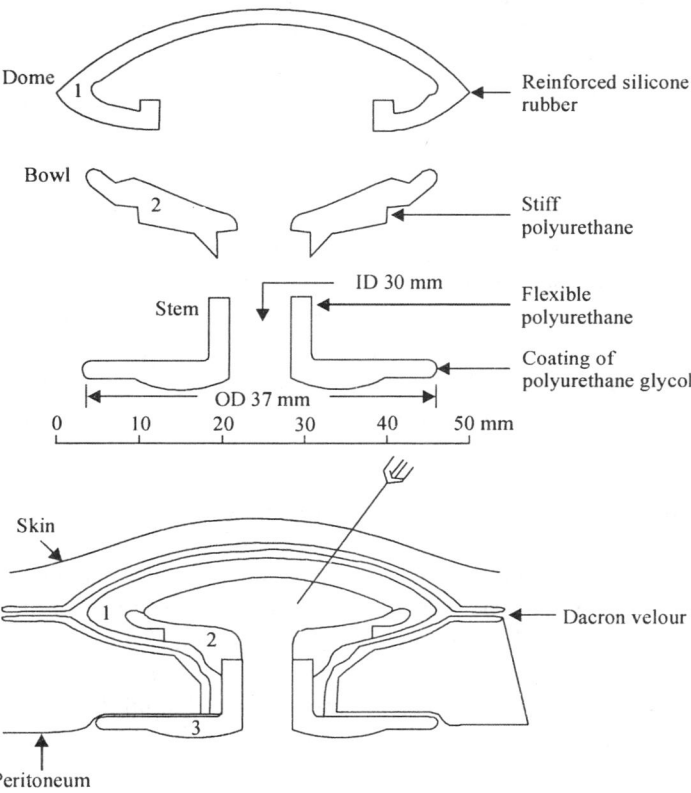

Fig. 21.7. Sub-cutaneous peritoneal access device.

The only constraining advice offered patients is that they avoid sports involving heavy bodily contact such as American football; otherwise there are no restraints on lifestyle whatsoever. In common with almost all other investigation using the peritoneal route for insulin delivery or other purposes, the major complication has been obstruction of the access device, usually caused by mesothelial overgrowth. Improved long-term maintenance of the access device (once-monthly flushing with 30 ml saline) and the evolution of a surgery for relief of obstructions have assisted in the actuarial survival rate for access device. But the most important progress followed animal experiments using IP implants of different materials to improve the IP biocompatibility of the SPADs, beginning with standard polyurethane, then silicone and finally polyethylene-glycol polyurethane, which is manufactured in-house and is used to coat the pellethane IP flange.

In conclusion, several types of devices are now available for more exact and controlled administration of insulin than by the usual syringe injections.

ALTERNATE ROUTES

Sub-cutaneous Route

Although reduced compared with conventional injections, local degradation of insulin persists after subcutaneous infusion and is still variable, resulting in a 20–50 per cent unpredictable loss of activity in certain individuals. Moreover, the kinetics of resorption are not greatly different from those of sub-cutaneous injections. A mean delay of 136 minutes for the plasma insulin peak following a 1 hour square wave of 6 units and a persistent hyperinsulinemia 4 hours after the bolus, under a 1-U/hour basal infusion, were observed. The peak delay is shortened by 15–30 minutes if the bolus is given over a few minutes. However, the return to baseline is in any case sluggish, approximately 6–8 hours.

Efficiency

The superiority of continuous SC insulin infusion (CSII) over injections has been questioned. CSII is probably ineffective in brittle and insulin-resistant diabetes because it does not by-pass the sub-cutaneous tissue, the poor resorption of which is probably involved in the mechanism of such forms of diabetes. CSII is probably superior to injections in highly insulin-sensitive, low-dose-requiring patients (pancreatectomised, hypophysectomised diabetics). In the average diabetic patient, it seems that CSII may be superior to twice-daily conventional insulin injections but not to multiple-dose programmes.

Feasibility

The technique of CSII is easy to handle and does not require sophisticated pumps or highly stable insulin because the reservoirs and catheters are changed frequently.

The risks and problems are limited to accidental under or overdosage and local sub-cutaneous reactions. However, long-term acceptability is poorer than expected, with a significant dropout rate. Unverifiable intermittent disconnections from the pump must also be accounted for.

Finally, it is recommend the sub-cutaneous route for CSII only in non-brittle, insulin-dependent but poorly controlled diabetes and only if the patient wishes to avoid multiple injections or fixed mealtimes. This route is definitely not adapted to feedback-controlled systems.

Intravenous (IV) Route

Physiology

The physiology of intravenously infused insulin was extensively investigated in the 1970s because it was the route for insulin from the artificial pancreas. The IV infusion gives the fastest insulin response: Plasma insulin reaches its maximum and returns to baseline values in <30 minutes following a bolus. However, this route invariably produces hyperinsulinemia.

Efficiency

The efficiency of the intravenous route has been proven, even in the most severe forms of diabetes. However, this advantage is balanced by the risk of rapid glucose rise in the case of pump discontinuation and rapid glucose fall during physical exercise.

Feasibility

The procedure for catheter insertion in a central vein is difficult and not innocuous. Technical requirements and patient constraints with portable intravenous pumps are as important as with the intraperitoneal route. The risks of infection can be minimised by severe aseptic precautions, but not the risk of catheter obstruction by blood clotting, which was the cause of termination of the authors' only two chronic intravenous catheters after eight and six months of constant infusion. However, results with totally implanted devices appear more encouraging and about half of the devices currently implanted in human are connected to a chronic IV catheter.

Peritoneal Route for Insulin Infusion

Since 1980 it was suggested to treat brittle type-I diabetics with pumps using the intraperitoneal (IP) route for insulin infusion. Based on various research experiences and those reported in the literature, this section reviews the arguments for choosing this route for implantable insulin pumps.

Route of insulin resorption

The portal system connects the liver, the gut and the pancreas into a unique relationship which permits nutrient homeostasis. In a pilot study Schade and Eaton reported a near-50 per cent portal resorption of intraperitoneally infused insulin. Others have reported a significant porto peripheral insulin gradient similar to normals. However, Schade and Eaton recently reported no difference between sub-cutaneous and intraperitoneal routes regarding hepatic output suppression and peripheral captation of glucose. It was found in acute and chronic human studies a significant decrease of the insulin requirements when compared with sub-cutaneous injections and infusion. Thus it appears that further studies are needed to confirm that peritoneal insulin is primarily portally absorbed.

Portal insulin kinetics

It has been shown that fasting plasma-free insulin values were near or below normal with IP infusion, in contrast with the hyperinsulinemia usually seen with SC and IV insulin. Insulin dynamics following a bolus was also near normal, with peak times after 60–75 minutes for a square-wave bolus and 30–60 minutes for instant bolus. The return to basal values is delayed (3 hours) but in any case is more rapid than with sub-cutaneous infusion. It must be noted that plasma insulin kinetics varies with the position of the catheter in the abdomen, the lower basal and peak values being obtained with low-placed catheters. However, those variations do not influence significantly the day-to-day ambulatory equilibrium of the patients.

Depot effect of intraperitoneal insulin

Plasma glucose decreases during physical exercise under IP infusion, although less than under SC infusion. Other researchers did not find any significant decrease with IP and surprisingly, did find a clear decrease under IV infusion. Hepp and Piwernetz compared the glucose control obtained with an artificial pancreas using intravenous and intraperitoneal infusion. Although more variable and difficult to obtain, glucose values could be controlled during IP infusion using modified IV algorithms. However, depot effect may conversely have some advantages: blood glucose may escape less abruptly if insulin is discontinued abruptly. Plasma insulin steady-state may be satisfactorily maintained even with pumps functioning with basal rate pulse intervals instead of continuous flow, although those should not exceed 1 hour.

Access facilities

A simple blind-needle techniques to insert an IP catheters for portable pumps has been developed. This procedure could be adapted to implantable pumps. If the pump is placed SC in the lateral abdomen, the two procedures (pump and catheter insertions) could be done relatively simply under local anaesthesia.

In the same way, we have repaired external IP catheters on several occasions under minilaparoscopy and local anaesthesia (adhesiolysis, cut-off of obstructed extremity). This technique can be easily applied to implantable pumps, allowing the catheter to remain in place in case of problems, as if it were intravenous.

Efficacy of diabetes control

It was found during a three month randomised study using one month each of IV, SC and IP infusion in six patients that IV and IP routes are superior to SC in minimising mean values and variations of blood glucose. Insulin requirements are lowest with IP infusion.

Personal long-term results on our 80 IP-infused (representing more than 200 patient-years of continuous ambulatory infusion) are of the same magnitude. It was thus decided to use the IP route for our only experience with the implantable insulin pump in a patient. The pump functioned satisfactorily during 1.5 year, with a near-normalisation of blood glucose. Others have confirmed the superiority of IP versus SC infusion, especially on the most difficult cases (i.e., brittle diabetics). However, IP does not seem superior to IV infusion. About half of the pumps implanted in human are connected to chronic IP catheters. Blood metabolite and hormone (other than glucose and insulin) responses to SC or IP insulin infusion have been studied using short-term protocols only. Although conflicting, these studies show a failure to normalise all metabolites and hormones by peripheral insulin delivery (notably, lactates and hydroxybutyrate are still elevated), whereas CIPII demonstrates improved results with an almost normal pattern of all metabolites and hormones.

Local-Regional tolerance

The risks of infection are low with portable IP pumps and lower again with implantable devices compared with the risks of phlebitis and septicemia with IV infusion. Cases of secondary general or local amyloidosis (presence of plasma amyloid protein) have been reported with long-term insulin infusion. However, this does not seem to depend on the route but on the aggregating properties of the infused insulin. Moreover, we did not suspect clinically or visually (during occasional laparascopies for catheter obstruction) amyloidosis in any of our cases, although organ biopsies were not done. However, the major problem is the frequent occurrence of catheter obstruction (10 per cent of our catheters) by intra and periluminal fibrin growth, with formation of peritoneal adhesions along the catheters or fibrin nodes at their tips. This phenomenon appeared after a mean of 16 months and seemed more frequent with short catheters (10 cm). This important problem occurred with different types of insulin catheters and implantable pumps. We are currently evaluating the effect of the geometry of the catheter (diameter, configuration, etc.) on the incidence of obstruction. Thus we conclude that even if the IP route is theoretically and practically the best adapted to insulin infusion via portable and implantable pumps, it will be superior to the IV route only when the problem of catheter-peritoneum reactions is solved or minimised.

Chapter 22

Essentials of Anaesthesia Delivery

INTRODUCTION

The intent of this chapter is to provide an introduction to the practice of anaesthesiology and to the technology currently employed. The practice of anaesthesia includes more than just providing relief from pain. In fact, pain relief can be considered a secondary facet of the speciality. In actuality, the modern concept of the safe and efficacious delivery of anaesthesia requires consideration of three fundamental tenets, which are ordered here by relative importance:

1. Maintenance of vital organ function.
2. Relief of pain.
3. Maintenance of the 'internal milieu'.

The first, maintenance of vital organ function, is concerned with preventing damage to cells and organ systems that could result from inadequate supply of oxygen and other nutrients. The delivery of blood and cellular substrates is often referred to as perfusion of the cells or tissues. During the delivery of an anaesthetic, the patient's 'vital signs' are monitored in an attempt to prevent inadequate tissue perfusion. However, the surgery itself, the patient's existing pathophysiology, drugs given for the relief of pain or even the management of blood pressure may compromise tissue perfusion. Why is adequate perfusion of tissues a higher priority than providing relief of pain for which anaesthesia is named? A rather obvious extreme example is that without cerebral perfusion or perfusion of the spinal cord, delivery of an anaesthetic is not necessary. Damage to other organ systems may result in a range of complications from delaying the patient's recovery to diminishing their quality of life to premature death.

In other words, the primary purpose of anaesthesia care is to maintain adequate delivery of required substrates to each organ and cell, which will hopefully preserve cellular function. The second principle of anaesthesia is to relieve the pain caused by surgery. Chronic pain and suffering caused by many disease states is now managed by a relatively new sub-speciality within anaesthesia, called Pain Management.

The third principle of anaesthesia is the maintenance of the internal environment of the body, for example, the regulation of electrolytes (sodium, potassium, chloride, magnesium, calcium, etc.), acid-base balance and a host of supporting functions on which cellular function and organ system communications rest.

The person delivering anaesthesia may be an anaesthesiologist (physician specialising in anaesthesiology), an anaesthesiology physician assistant (a person trained in a medical school at the masters level to administer anaesthesia as a member of the care team lead by an anaesthesiologist) or a nurse anaesthetist (a nurse with Intensive Care Unit experience that has additional training in anaesthesia provided by advanced practice nursing programmes). There are three major categories of anaesthesia provided to patients: (i) general anaesthesia; (ii) conduction anaesthesia; and (iii) monitored anaesthesia care.

General anaesthesia typically includes the intravenous injection of anaesthetic drugs that render the patient unconscious and paralyse their skeletal muscles. Immediately following drug administration a plastic tube is inserted into the trachea and the patient is connected to an electropneumatic system to maintain ventilation of the lungs. A liquid anaesthetic agent is vapourised and administered by inhalation, sometimes along with nitrous oxide, to maintain anaesthesia for the surgical procedure. Often, other intravenous agents are used in conjunction with the inhalation agents to provide what is called a balanced anaesthetic.

Conduction anaesthesia refers to blocking the conduction of pain and possibly motor nerve impulses travelling along specific nerves or the spinal cord. Common forms of conduction anaesthesia include spinal and epidural anaesthesia, as well as specific nerve blocks, for example, auxillary nerve blocks. In order to achieve a successful conduction anaesthetic, local anaesthetic agents such as lidocaine, are injected into the proximity of specific nerves to block the conduction of the electrical impulses. In addition, sedation may be provided intravenously to keep the patient comfortable while he/she is lying still for the surgery.

Monitored anaesthesia care refers to monitoring the patient's vital signs while administering sedatives and analgesics to keep the patient comfortable and treating complications related to the surgical procedure. Typically, the surgeon administers topical or local anaesthetics to alleviate the pain.

In order to provide the range of support required, from the paralysed mechanically ventilated patient to the patient receiving monitored anaesthesia care, a versatile anaesthesia delivery system must be available to the anaesthesia care team. Today's anaesthesia delivery system is composed of six major elements:

1. The primary and secondary sources of gases (O_2, air, N_2O, vacuum, gas scavenging and possibly CO_2 and helium).
2. The gas blending and vapourisation system.
3. The breathing circuit (including methods for manual and mechanical ventilation).
4. The excess gas scavenging system that minimises potential pollution of the operating room by anaesthetic gases.
5. Instruments and equipment to monitor the function of the anaesthesia delivery system.
6. Patient monitoring instrumentation and equipment.

The traditional anaesthesia machine incorporated elements 1, 2, 3 and more recently 4. The evolution to the anaesthesia delivery system adds elements 5 and 6. In the text that follows, references to the 'anaesthesia machine' refer to the basic gas delivery system and breathing circuit as contrasted with the 'anaesthesia delivery system' which includes the basic 'anaesthesia machine' and all monitoring instrumentation.

ANAESTHESIA MACHINES

A special case of a controlled drug delivery system is the anaesthesia machine. This device enables anaesthesiologists and anaesthetists to administer volatile anaesthetic agents to patients in the operating room through their lungs. There are three sections to the typical anaesthesia machine. The first is the gas supply and delivery system. Here oxygen and nitrous oxide from central hospital sources or small storage cylinders on the anaesthesia machine are mixed in the desired proportions. Flow-meters indicate the amount of each gas that is delivered and the operator can adjust the flow rate to get the desired ratio and total volume.

The second section of the anaesthesia machine is the vapouriser. In this section, pure oxygen or an oxygen-nitrous oxide mixture from the gas delivery system is bubbled through or passed over the volatile anaesthetic agent in the liquid phase. The amount of anaesthetic agent given is related to the flow rate of the gas through the vapouriser. The anaesthesiologist or anaesthetist controls this rate by adjusting the valves in the plumbing system and measuring, by means of flow-meters, the flow through the vapouriser and the amount of gas that by-passes it.

The final section of the anaesthesia machine is the patient breathing circuit. This section is responsible for delivery of the anaesthesia-producing gases to the patient and removal of expired gases coming from the patient. This portion of the system is a closed circuit. That is, the gas administered to the patient is introduced via a one-way (check) valve through one section of tubing and the expired gas passes through a different section of tubing, again via a one-way valve. Thus, the expired gas is separated from the inspiratory line. The expired gas is passed through a carbon dioxide absorber to remove the carbon dioxide and is re-introduced into the inspiratory line. A reservoir bag is connected in the circuit to provide low-pressure gas storage and to enable the anaesthesiologist or anaesthetist to assist in ventilating the patient when necessary. Expiratory gas can also be removed from the patient breathing circuit and passed through a scavenging system to remove the anaesthetic agent before the gas is vented to the atmosphere. The patient breathing circuit can be connected to a ventilator for those patients who need assistance in ventilation.

GASES USED DURING ANAESTHESIA AND THEIR SOURCES

Most inhaled anaesthetic agents are liquids that are vapourised in a device within the anaesthesia delivery system. The vapourised agents are then blended with other breathing gases before flowing into the breathing circuit and being administered to the patient. The most commonly administered form of anaesthesia is called a balanced general anaesthetic and is a combination of inhalation agent plus intravenous analgesic drugs. Intravenous drugs often require electromechanical devices to administer an appropriately controlled flow of drug to the patient.

Gases needed for the delivery of anaesthesia are generally limited to oxygen (O_2), air, nitrous oxide (N_2O) and possibly helium (He) and carbon dioxide (CO_2). Vacuum and gas scavenging lines are also required. There needs to be secondary sources of these gases in the event of primary failure or questionable contamination. Typically, primary sources are those supplied from a hospital distribution system at 345 kPa (50 psig) through gas columns or wall outlets. The secondary sources of gas are cylinders hung on yokes on the anaesthesia delivery system.

Oxygen

Oxygen provides an essential metabolic substrate for all human cells, but it is not without dangerous side effects. Prolonged exposure to high concentrations of oxygen may result in toxic effects within the lungs that decrease diffusion of gas into and out of the blood and the return to breathing air following prolonged exposure to elevated O_2 may result in a debilitating explosive blood vessel growth in infants. Oxygen is usually supplied to the hospital in liquid form (boiling point of $-183°C$), stored in cryogenic tanks and supplied to the hospital piping system as a gas. The efficiency of liquid storage is obvious since 1 litre of liquid becomes 860 litres of gas at standard temperature and pressure. The secondary source of oxygen within an anaesthesia delivery system is usually one or more E cylinders filled with gaseous oxygen at a pressure of 15.2 MPa (2200 psig).

Air (78 per cent N₂, 21 per cent O₂, 0.9 per cent Ar, 0.1 per cent Other Gases)

The primary use of air during anaesthesia is as a diluent to decrease the inspired oxygen concentration. The typical primary source of medical air (there is an important distinction between 'air' and 'medical air' related to the quality and the requirements for periodic testing) is a special compressor that avoids hydrocarbon based lubricants for purposes of medical air purity. Dryers are employed to rid the compressed air of water prior to distribution throughout the hospital. Medical facilities with limited need for medical air may use banks of H cylinders of dry medical air. A secondary source of air may be available on the anaesthesia machine as an E cylinder containing dry gas at 15.2 MPa.

Nitrous Oxide

Nitrous oxide is a colourless, odourless and non-irritating gas that does not support human life. Breathing more than 85 per cent N_2O may be fatal. N_2O is not an anaesthetic (except under hyperbaric conditions), rather it is an analgesic and an amnestic. There are many reasons for administering N_2O during the course of an anaesthetic including: enhancing the speed of induction and emergence from anaesthesia; decreasing the concentration requirements of potent inhalation anaesthetics (i.e., halothane, isoflurane, etc.) and as an essential adjunct to narcotic analgesics. N_2O is supplied to anaesthetising locations from banks of H cylinders that are filled with 90 per cent liquid at a pressure of 5.1 MPa (745 psig). Secondary supplies are available on the anaesthesia machine in the form of E cylinders, again containing 90 per cent liquid. Continual exposure to low levels of N_2O in the workplace has been implicated in a number of medical problems including spontaneous abortion, infertility, birth defects, cancer, liver and kidney disease and others. Although there is no conclusive evidence to support most of these implications, there is a recognised need to scavenge all waste anaesthetic gases and periodically sample N_2O levels in the workplace to maintain the lowest possible levels consistent with reasonable risk to the operating room personnel and cost to the institution. Another gas with analgesic properties similar to N_2O is xenon, but its use is experimental and its cost is prohibitive at this time.

Carbon Dioxide

Carbon dioxide is colourless and odourless, but very irritating to breathe in higher concentrations. CO_2 is a by-product of human cellular metabolism and is not a life-sustaining gas. CO_2 influences many physiologic processes either directly or through the action of hydrogen ions by the reaction:

$$CO_2 + H_2O \leftrightarrow H_2CO_3 \leftrightarrow H^+ + HCO_3^-$$

Although not very common in the US today, in the past CO_2 was administered during anaesthesia to stimulate respiration that was depressed by anaesthetic agents and to cause increased blood flow in otherwise compromised vasculature during some surgical procedures. Like N_2O, CO_2 is supplied as a liquid in H cylinders for distribution in pipeline systems or as a liquid in E cylinders that are located on the anaesthesia machine.

Helium

Helium is a colourless, odourless and non-irritating gas that will not support life. The primary use of helium in anaesthesia is to enhance gas flow through small orifices as in asthma, airway trauma or tracheal stenosis. The viscosity of helium is not different from other anaesthetic gases (Table 22.1) and is therefore of no benefit when airway flow is laminar. However, in the event that ventilation must be performed through abnormally narrow orifices or tubes which create turbulent flow conditions, helium is the preferred carrier gas. Resistance to turbulent flow is proportional to the density rather than viscosity of the gas and helium is an order of magnitude less dense than other gases. A secondary advantage of helium is that it has a large specific heat relative to other anaesthetic gases and therefore can carry the heat from laser surgery out of the airway more effectively than air, oxygen or nitrous oxide. Physical properties of currently available volatile anaesthetic agents are shown in Table 22.2.

Table 22.1. Physical properties of gases used during anaesthesia.

Gas	Molecular wt.	Density (g/l)	Viscosity (cp)	Specific heat (KJ/kg°C)
Oxygen	31.999	1.326	0.0203	0.917
Nitrogen	28.013	1.161	0.0175	1.040
Air	28.975	1.200	0.0181	1.010
Nitrous oxide	44.013	1.836	0.0144	0.839
Carbon dioxide	44.01	1.835	0.0148	0.850
Helium	4.003	0.1657	0.0194	5.190

Table 22.2. Physical properties of currently available volatile anaesthetic agents.

Agent generic name	Boiling point (°C at 760 mmHg)	Vapour pressure (mmHg at 20°C)	Liquid density (g/ml)	MAC* (%)
Halothane	50.2	243	1.86	0.75
Enflurane	56.5	175	1.517	1.68
Isoflurane	48.5	238	1.496	1.15
Desflurane	23.5	664	1.45	6.0
Sevoflurane	58.5	160	1.51	2.0

* Minimum alveolar concentration is the per cent of the agent required to provide surgical anaesthesia to 50 per cent of the population in terms of a cummulative dose response curve. The lower the MAC, the more potent the agent.

GAS BLENDING AND VAPOURISATION SYSTEM

The basic anaesthesia machine utilises primary low pressure gas sources of 345 kPa (50 psig) available from wall or ceiling column outlets and secondary high pressure gas sources located on the machine as pictured schematically in Fig. 22.1. Tracing the path of oxygen in the machine demonstrates that oxygen comes from either the low pressure source or from the 15.2 MPa (2200 psig) high pressure yokes via cylinder pressure regulators and then branches to service several other functions. First and foremost, the second stage pressure regulator drops the O_2 pressure to approximately 110 kPa (16 psig) before it enters the needle valve and the rotameter type flowmeter. From the flowmeter O_2 mixes with gases from other flowmeters and passes through a calibrated agent vapouriser where specific inhalation anaesthetic agents are vapourised and added to the breathing gas mixture. Oxygen is also used to supply a reservoir canister that sounds a reed alarm in the event that the oxygen pressure drops below 172 kPa (25 psig). When the oxygen pressure drops to 172 kPa or lower, then the nitrous oxide pressure sensor shut-off valve closes and N_2O is prevented from entering its needle valve and flowmeter and is therefore eliminated from the breathing gas mixture. In fact, all machines built in the US have pressure sensor shut-off valves installed in the lines to every flowmeter, except oxygen, to prevent the delivery of hypoxic gas mixture in the event of an oxygen pressure failure. Oxygen may also be delivered to the common gas outlet or machine outlet via a momentary normally closed flush valve that typically provides a flow of 65 to 80 litres of O_2 per minute directly into the breathing circuit. Newer machines are required to have a safety system for limiting the minimum concentration of oxygen that can be delivered to the patient to 25 per cent. The flow paths for nitrous oxide and other gases are much simpler in the sense that after coming from the high pressure regulator or the low pressure hospital source, gas is immediately presented to the pressure sensor shut-off valve from where it travels to its specific needle valve and flowmeter to join the common gas line and enter the breathing circuit.

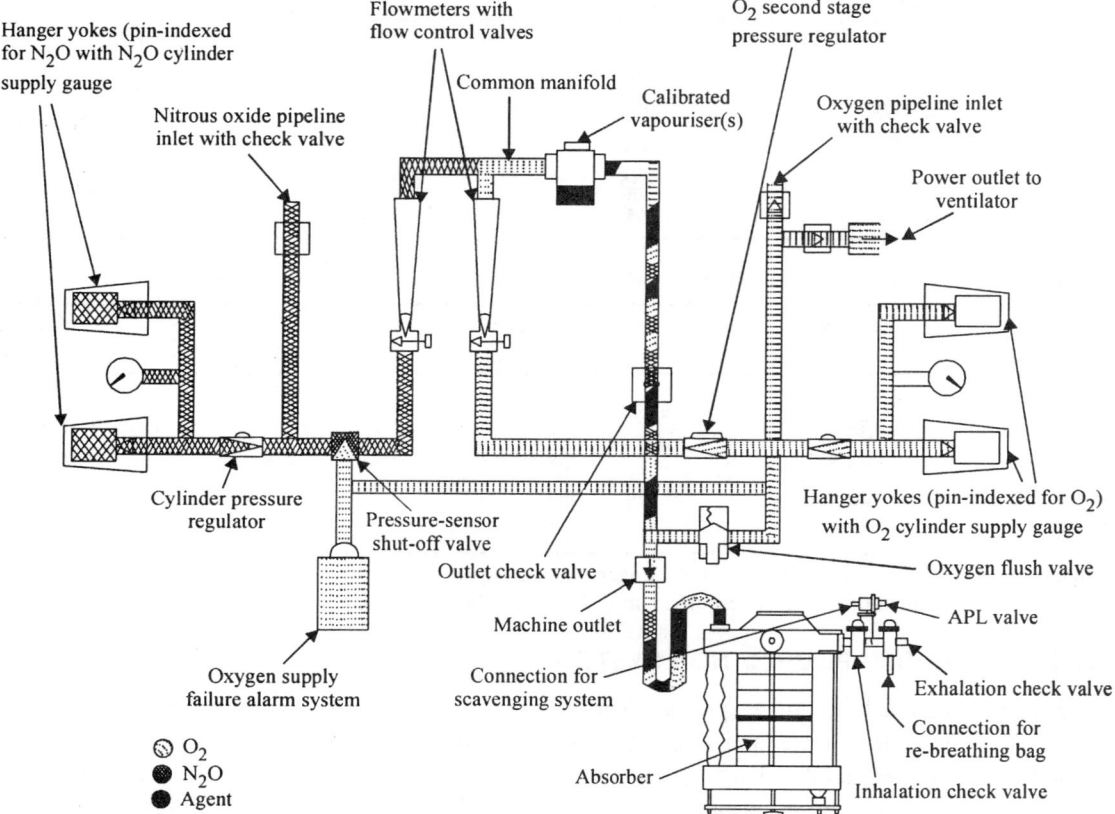

Fig. 22.1. Schematic diagram of gas piping within a simple two-gas (oxygen and nitrous oxide) anaesthesia machine.

Currently all anaesthesia machines manufactured in the US use only calibrated flow-through vapourisers, meaning that all of the gases from the various flowmeters are mixed in the manifold prior to entering the vapouriser. Any given vapouriser has a calibrated control knob that, once set to the desired concentration for a specific agent, will deliver the concentration to the patient. Some form of interlock system must be provided such that only one vapouriser may be activated at any given time. Figure 22.2 schematically illustrates the operation of a purely mechanical vapouriser with temperature compensation. This simple flow-over design permits a fraction of the total gas flow to pass into the vapourising chamber where it becomes saturated with vapour before being added back to the total gas flow.

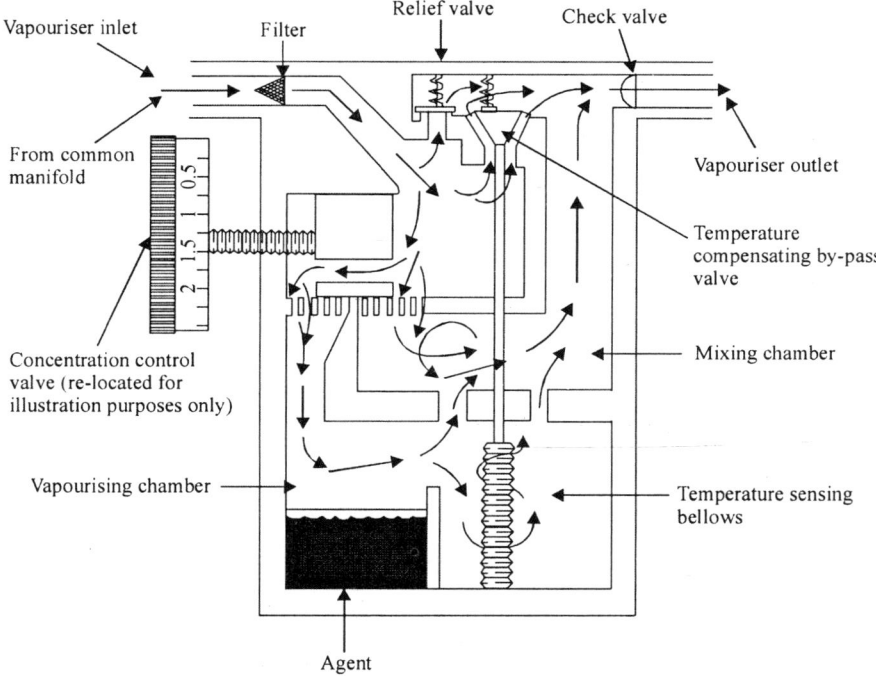

Fig. 22.2. Schematic diagram of a calibrated in-line vapouriser that uses the flow-over technique for adding anaesthetic vapour to the breathing gas mixture.

Since vapourisation is an endothermic process, anaesthetic vapourisers must have sufficient thermal mass and conductivity to permit the vapourisation process to proceed independent of the rate at which the agent is being used.

BREATHING CIRCUITS

The concept behind an effective breathing circuit is to provide an adequate volume of a controlled concentration of gas to the patient during inspiration and to carry the exhaled gases away from the patient during exhalation. There are several forms of breathing circuits which can be classified into two basic types; (i) open circuit, meaning no re-breathing of any gases and no CO_2 absorber present; and (ii) closed circuit, indicating presence of CO_2 absorber and some rebreathing of other gases. Figure 22.3 illustrates the Lack modification of a Mapleson open circuit breathing system. There are no valves and no CO_2 absorber. There is great potential for the patient to re-breath their own exhaled gases unless the fresh gas inflow is 2 to 3 times the patient's minute volume. Figure 22.4 illustrates the most popular form of breathing circuit, the circle system, with oxygen monitor, circle pressure gauge, volume monitor (spirometer) and airway pressure sensor. The circle is a closed system or semi-closed when the fresh gas inflow exceeds the patient's requirements. Excess gas evolves into the scavenging device and some of the exhaled gas is re-breathed after having the CO_2 removed. The inspiratory and expiratory valves in the circle system guarantee that gas flows to the patient from the inspiratory limb and away from the patient through the exhalation limb. In the event of a failure of either or both of these valves, the patient will re-breath exhaled gas that contains CO_2, which is a potentially dangerous situation.

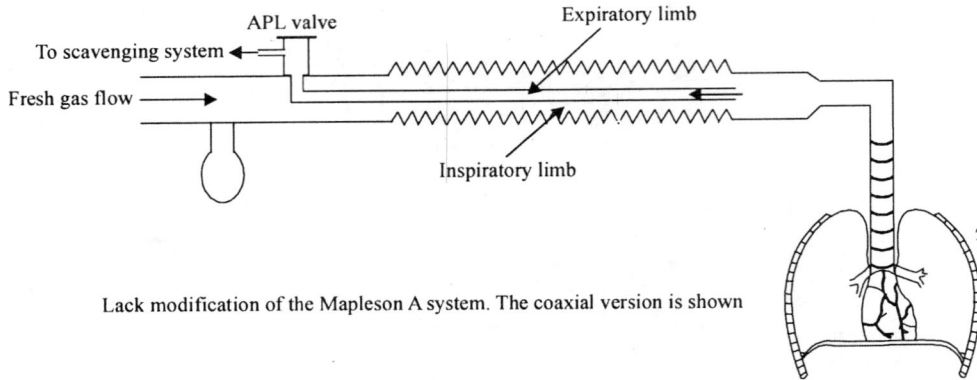

Lack modification of the Mapleson A system. The coaxial version is shown

Fig. 22.3. An example of an open circuit breathing system that does not use unidirectional flow valves or contain a carbon dioxide absorbent.

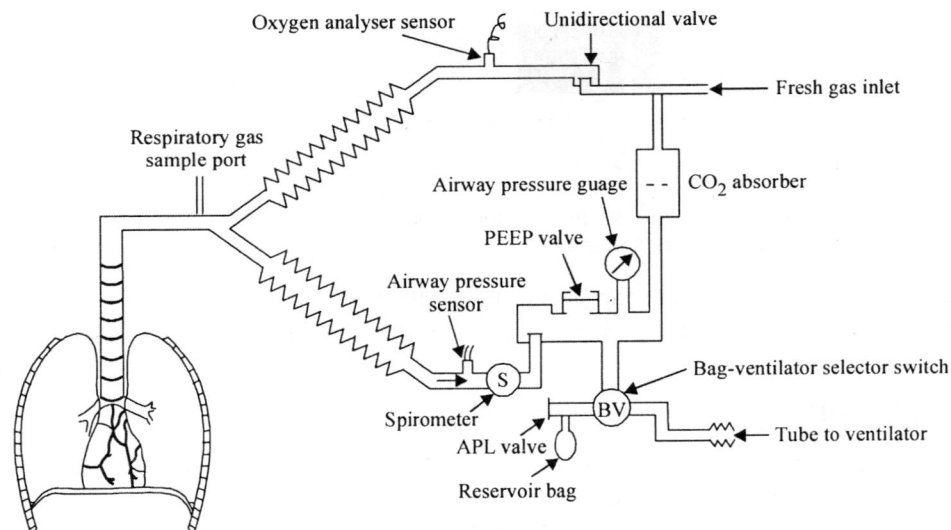

Fig. 22.4. A diagram of a closed circuit circle breathing system with unidirectional valves, inspired oxygen sensor, pressure sensor and CO_2 absorber.

There are two forms of mechanical ventilation used during anaesthesia: (i) volume ventilation, where the volume of gas delivered to the patient remains constant regardless of the pressure that is required; and (ii) pressure ventilation, where the ventilator provides whatever volume to the patient that is required to produce some desired pressure in the breathing circuit.

Volume ventilation is the most popular since the volume delivered remains theoretically constant despite changes in lung compliance. Pressure ventilation is useful when compliance losses in the breathing circuit are high relative to the volume delivered to the lungs.

Humidification is an important adjunct to the breathing circuit because it maintains the integrity of the cilia that line the airways and promote the removal of mucus and particulate matter from the lungs. Humidification of dry breathing gases can be accomplished by simple passive heat and moisture exchangers inserted into the breathing circuit at the level of the endotracheal tube connectors or by elegant dual servo electronic humidifiers that heat a reservoir filled with water and also heat a wire in the gas delivery tube to prevent rain-out of the water before it reaches the patient. Electronic safety measures must be included in these active devices due to the potential for burning the patient and the fire hazard.

GAS SCAVENGING SYSTEMS

The purpose of scavenging exhaled and excess anaesthetic agents is to reduce or eliminate the potential hazard to employees who work in the environment where anaesthetics are administered, including operating rooms, obstetrical areas, special procedures areas, physician's offices, dentist's offices and veterinarian's surgical suites. Typically more gas is administered to the breathing circuit than is required by the patient, resulting in the necessity to remove excess gas from the circuit. The scavenging system must be capable of collecting gas from all components of the breathing circuit, including adjustable pressure level valves, ventilators and sample withdrawal type gas monitors, without altering characteristics of the circuit such as pressure or gas flow to the patient. There are two broad types of scavenging systems as illustrated in Fig. 22.5: the open interface is a simple design that requires a large physical space for the reservoir volume and the closed interface with an expandable reservoir bag and which must include relief valves for handling the cases of no scavenged flow and great excess of scavenged flow.

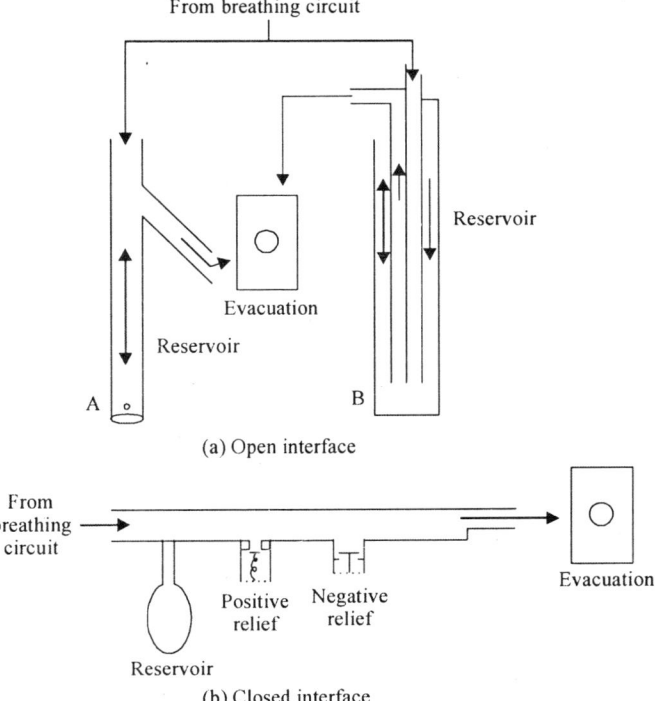

Fig. 22.5. Examples of open and closed gas scavenger interfaces. The closed interface requires relief valves in the event of scavenging flow failure.

Trace gas analysis must be performed to guarantee the efficacy of the scavenging system. The National Institutes of Occupational Safety and Health (NIOSH) recommends that trace levels of nitrous oxide be maintained at or below 25 parts per million (ppm) time weighted average and that halogenated anaesthetic agents remain below 2 ppm.

MONITORING THE FUNCTION OF THE ANAESTHESIA DELIVERY SYSTEM

The anaesthesia machine can produce a single or combination of catastrophic events, any one of which could be fatal to the patient:

1. Delivery of a hypoxic gas mixture to the patient.
2. The inability to adequately ventilate the lungs by not producing positive pressure in the patient's lungs, by not delivering an adequate volume of gas to the lungs or by improper breathing circuit connections that permit the patient's lungs to receive only re-breathed gases.
3. The delivery of an overdose of an inhalational anaesthetic agent.

Monitoring Equipment

The necessary monitoring equipment to guarantee proper function of the anaesthesia delivery system include at least:

1. Inspired oxygen concentration monitor with absolute low level alarm of 19 per cent.
2. Airway pressure monitor with alarms for:
   (a) Low pressure indicative of inadequate breathing volume and possible leaks.
   (b) Sustained elevated pressures that could compromise cardiovascular function.
   (c) High pressures that could cause pulmonary barotrauma.
   (d) Sub-atmospheric pressure that could cause collapse of the lungs.
3. Exhaled gas volume monitor.
4. Carbon dioxide monitor (capnography).
5. Inspired and exhaled concentration of anaesthetic agents by any of the following:
   (a) Mass spectrometer.
   (b) Raman spectrometer.
   (c) Infrared or other optical spectrometer.

A mass spectrometer is a very useful cost-effective device since it alone can provide capnography, inspired and exhaled concentrations of all anaesthetic agents, plus all breathing gases simultaneously (O_2, N_2, CO_2, N_2O, Ar, He, halothane, enflurane, isoflurane, desflurane and suprane). The mass spectrometer is unique in that it may be tuned to monitor an assortment of exhaled gases while the patient is asleep, including: (i) ketones for detection of diabetic ketoacidosis; (ii) ethanol or other marker in the irrigation solution during transurethral resection of the prostate for early detection of the TURP syndrome, which results in a severe dilution of blood electrolytes; and (iii) pentanes during the evolution of a heart attack, to mention a few.

Sound monitoring principles require: (i) earliest possible detection of untoward events (before they result in physiologic derangements); and (ii) specificity that results in rapid identification and resolution of the problem. An extremely useful rule to always consider is 'never monitor the anaesthesia delivery system performance through the patient's physiologic responses'. That is, never intentionally use a device like a pulse oximeter to detect a breathing circuit disconnection since the warning is very late and there is no specific information provided that leads to rapid resolution of the problem.

MONITORING THE PATIENT

The anaesthetist's responsibilities to the patient include: providing relief from pain and preserving all existing normal cellular function of all organ systems. Currently the latter obligation is fulfilled by monitoring essential physiologic parameters and correcting any substantial derangements that occur before they are translated into permanent cellular damage. The inadequacy of current monitoring methods can be appreciated by realising that most monitoring modalities only indicate damage after an insult has occurred, at which point the hope is that it is reversible or that further damage can be prevented.

Standards for basic intraoperative monitoring of patients undergoing anaesthesia, that were developed and adopted by the American Society of Anesthesiologists, became effective in 1990. Standard I concerns the responsibilities of anaesthesia personnel, while Standard II requires that the patient's oxygenation, ventilation, circulation and temperature be evaluated continually during all anaesthetics. The following list indicates the instrumentation typically available during the administration of anaesthetics.

Electrocardiogram	Non-invasive or invasive blood pressure
Pulse oximetry	Temperature
Urine output	Nerve stimulators
Cardiac output	Mixed venous oxygen saturation
Electroencephalogram (EEG)	Transesophageal echo cardiography (TEE)
Evoked potentials	Coagulation status

Blood gases and electrolytes (P_{O_2}, P_{CO_2}, pH, BE, Na^+, K^+, Cl^-, Ca^{++} and glucose)

Mass spectrometry, Raman spectrometry or infrared breathing gas analysis

Control of Patient Temperature

Anaesthesia alters the thresholds for temperature regulation and the patient becomes unable to maintain normal body temperature. As the patient's temperature falls even a few degrees toward room temperature, several physiologic derangements occur: (i) drug action is prolonged; (ii) blood coagulation is impaired; and (iii) post-operative infection rate increases. On the positive side, cerebral protection from inadequate perfusion is enhanced by just a few degrees of cooling. Proper monitoring of core body temperature and forced hot air warming of the patient is essential.

Monitoring the Depth of Anaesthesia

There are two very unpleasant experiences that patients may have while undergoing an inadequate anaesthetic: (i) the patient is paralysed and unable to communicate their state of discomfort and they are feeling the pain of surgery and are aware of their surroundings; and (ii) the patient may be paralysed, unable to communicate and is aware of their surroundings, but is not feeling any pain. The ability to monitor the depth of anaesthesia would provide a safeguard against these unpleasant experiences. However, despite numerous instruments and approaches to the problem it remains elusive. Brain stem auditory evoked responses have come the closest to depth of anaesthesia monitoring, but it is difficult to perform, is expensive and is not possible to perform during many types of surgery. A promising new technology, called bi-spectral index (BIS monitoring) is purported to measure the level of patient awareness through multivariate analysis of a single channel of the EEG.

Anaesthesia Computer-Aided Record Keeping

Conceptually, every anaesthetist desires an automated anaesthesia record keeping system. Anaesthesia care can be improved through the feedback provided by correct record keeping, but today's systems have an enormous overhead associated with their use when compared to standard paper record keeping. No doubt that automated anaesthesia record keeping reduces the drudgery of routine recording of vital signs, but to enter drugs and drips and their dosages, fluids administered, urine output, blood loss and other data requires much more time and machine interaction than the current paper system. Despite attempts to use every input/output device ever produced by the computer industry from keyboards to bar codes to voice and handwriting recognition, no solution has been found that meets wide acceptance. Tenants of a successful system must include:

1. The concept of a user transparent system, which is ideally defined as requiring no communication between the computer and the clinician (far beyond the concept of user friendly) and therefore that is intuitively obvious to use even the most casual users.
2. Recognition of the fact that educational institutions have very different requirements from private practice institutions.
3. Real time hard copy of the record produced at the site of anaesthetic administration that permits real time editing and notation.
4. Ability to interface with a great variety of patient and anaesthesia delivery system monitors from various suppliers.
5. Ability to interface with a large number of hospital information systems.
6. Inexpensive to purchase and maintain.

Alarms

Vigilance is the key to effective risk management, but maintaining a vigilant state is not easy. The practice of anaesthesia has been described as moments of shear terror connected by times of intense boredom. Alarms can play a significant role in re-directing one's attention during the boredom to the most important event regarding patient safety, but only if false alarms can be eliminated, alarms can be prioritised and all alarms concerning anaesthetic management can be displayed in a single clearly visible location.

Ergonomics

The study of ergonomics attempts to improve performance by optimising the relationship between people and their work environment. Ergonomics has been defined as a discipline which investigates and applies information about human requirements, characteristics, abilities and limitations to the design, development and testing of equipment, systems and jobs. This field of study is only in its infancy and examples of poor ergonomic design abound in the anaesthesia workplace.

Simulation in Anaesthesia

Complete patient simulators are hands-on realistic simulators that interface with physiologic monitoring equipment to simulate patient responses to equipment malfunctions, operator errors and drug therapies. There are also crisis management simulators. Complex patient simulators, which are analogous to flight simulators, are currently being marketed for training anaesthesia personnel. The intended use for these complex simulators is currently being debated in the sense that training peole to respond in a preprogrammed way to a given event may not be adequate training.

Chapter 23

Lung, Blood Gas and Dialysis Machines

INTRODUCTION

According to one definition, respiration is the exchange of gases between the external environment and the blood. In human this exchange takes place in small sacs in the lungs called alveoli. These sacs are the point of exchange between the outside environment and the blood as oxygen comes into the body and carbon dioxide waste products leave it. Pulmonary function tests are used to assess the efficacy of this process. Unfortunately, though, no one single test will give all of the information that is required. In place of a comprehensive test, there is instead a collection of tests that can be considered together where appropriate.

The lungs in human are elastic bags or sacs located in the body's thoracic cavity. The right lung has three lobes or sections while the left lung has two since it must allow room for the heart. In the back of the throat, there is a little 'trap door' called the epiglottis and this prevents liquids or food from entering the respiratory system. Following this is the trachea, which branches into two further tubes, called the left and right bronchi.

Breathing is allowed by pressure dyamics and the thoracic musculature, primarily the diaphram, that allows the volume of the thoracic cavity to expand. Since this cavity is a closed system, expansion of its volume creates what is essentially a slight negative pressure. Atmospheric pressure forces air in through the mouth and the elastic lungs expand.

The ability of the lungs to expand and contract is measured by a factor called lung compliance and this is expressed as the derivative dV/dp, where V is the volume of the lungs and p is the intra-alveolar pressure. This pressure, incidentally, varies from a positive pressure of about three torr to a negative pressure of approximately the same magnitude over the inspiration/expiration cycle.

Pulmonary function is dependent upon many factors that include the properties of the mouth, all of the air tubes, the condition of the musculature and the compliance of the lungs. Some of these parameters can be assessed by examination and analysis of certain volume changes during specific phases of the respiratory cycle. Figure 23.1 shows a graph of various volumes relating to respiration. Normal breathing of a resting subject is shown in the figure as the resting tidal volume (RTV). The graph shows the normal changes in lung volume due to regular resting respiration. There are several other features of this waveform that will prove of interest: expiratory reserve volume (ERV), residual volume (RV), total lung capacity (TLC), inspiratory capacity (IC), vital capacity (VC) and functional residual capacity (FRC). These can be defined as follows:

1. ERV—this volume measurement is the amount of gas that can be expired under maximum effort after completing an inspiration/expiration cycle. This is defined as the volume change from the negative half of the tidal volume waveform and a maximum effort expiration.
2. RV—this is the volume of the gases remaining in the lungs after a maximum effort exhalation. The patient is forced to breath out as much air as possible.
3. TLC—this is the maximum amount of air the lungs can hold after a maximum effort inspiration. TLC is the sum of two other factors, RV and VC.
4. IC—the inspiratory capacity is the volume of gas that could be inhaled if a maximal inspiration effort is made. Measurement is made from the end of a normal resting respiration cycle, the low point on the tidal volume feature of the waveform in Fig. 23.1.
5. IRC—the inspiratory reserve capacity after normal inspiration at rest.
6. VC—vital capacity is the difference between total lung capacity and residual volume. It can be expressed as the total volume change when a maximum inspiration is followed immediately by a maximum expiration.
7. FRC—this measurement determines the amount of air remaining in the lungs when a normal respiration expiration has occurred. It can be expressed as the total volume change between zero and the inspiratory capacity minimum point.

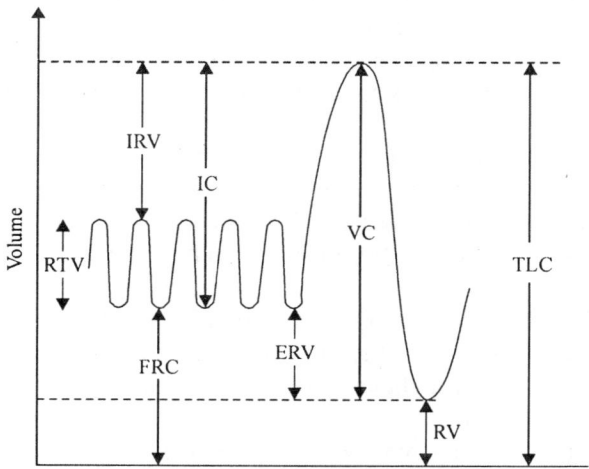

Fig. 23.1. Graph showing the various types of respiratory volume in human.

Another test often made in pulmonary laboratories is the minute volume. This is the volume of air taken into the lungs during one minute of normal respiration. The minute volume can be determined on paper by multiplying together the tidal volume and the patient's respiration rate in breaths per minute. In electronic equipment this can also be found by integrating the volume flow signal.

SPIROMETERS

All lung volumes can be measured on an instrument called a spirometer, of which several different types are common. One of the most common of the recording spirometers is known as the bell or water spirometer (Fig. 23.2). The bell is inverted in a tank of water and counterweighted so that atmospheric pressure and the weight tending to force the bell to move up is exactly counteracted by the weight of the bell tending to force itself down.

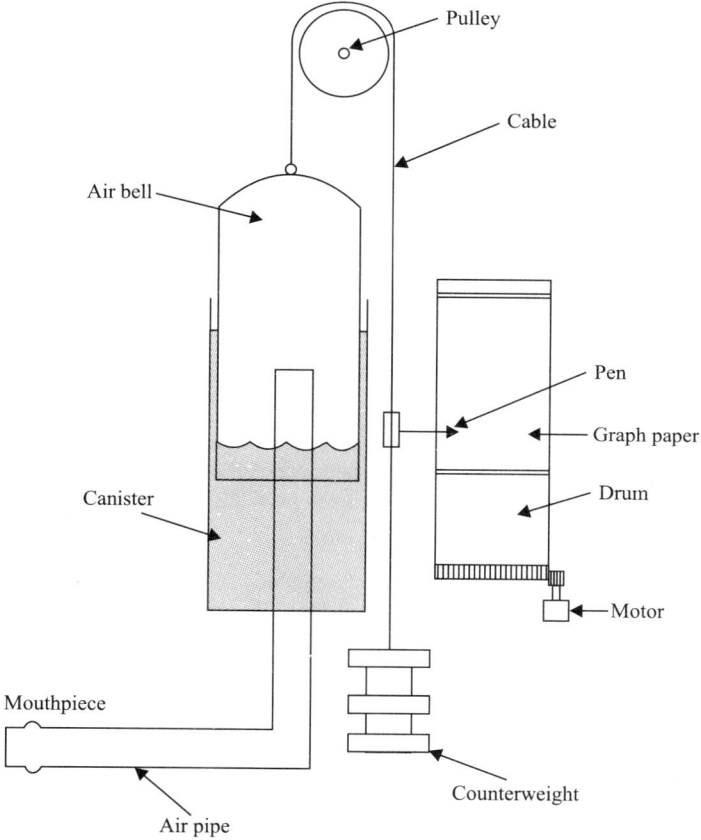

Fig. 23.2. Water-displacement or 'diving bell' spirometer.

The cable supporting the bell passes by the chart of a drum recorder, called a kymograph. When the spirometer is at rest, only atmospheric pressure affects the air inside of the bell, so the chart recorder pen remains at zero.

The patient is seated and the mouthpiece positioned so that he can breath into it. The patient's nose is blocked with a small clip so that air cannot escape by passing through the nostrils. When the patient exhales air into the mouthpiece, this increases the amount of gas inside the bell. The bell then rises in order to allow the air pressure inside to be at equilibrium with the atmospheric pressure. This motion causes the pen attached to the support cable to fall, scribing a line on the chart paper. Similarly, when the patient inhales, air pressure in the bell decreases, the bell's weight forces it to fall and this causes the pen to rise. Two bell sizes are common, 9 and 13.5 litres, but the smaller is probably the more common of the two. The kymograph is usually a multispeed design that can move the chart at speeds of 32, 160 or 1900 millimetres per minute. Not shown but also included in the spirometer system will be a carbon dioxide absorber.

An alternate version of this instrument uses a slide-operated, linear potentiometer with its wiper terminal ganged to the support cable, in place of a pen, to generate an electrical signal that is proportional to volume. This signal can be processed, if desired, to yield several other parameters or it can be fed directly to the chart recorder.

Another type of mechanical spirometer is the bellows type. This is often seen on respirators or other breathing assistance devices. A cannister containing a bellows is connected into the air system in such a way as to catch the expired air. The displacement of the bellows tells an observer how much air volume was exhaled. A scale in units of volume (e.g., cubic centimetres) is painted or etched onto the side of the plastic cannister. In some cases, the rod driving the bellows is ganged to a potentiometer as in the previous case to derive an electrical signal that is proportional to volume. A small magnet attached to the drive rod passes a coil concentric to the rod to create a magnetic field that changes as the patient breathes. This field interacts with the coil to generate an electrical signal that varies with the respiration. A timer circuit is re-set every time the magnet generates a signal, but will sound an alarm if allowed to time out.

An ultrasonic spirometer was once available and used a transducer such as shown in Fig. 23.3. The transducer has a pair of obliquely mounted piezoelectric crystal transducers. These are used to generate ultrasonic waves that are fired across the path taken by the inspiratory and expiratory gases breathed by the patient. One transducer is pulsed while the other acts as the receiver. A determination of the time of travel in the downstream direction is thus obtained. Next, the situation is reversed and the other transducer is pulsed so the upstream transmission time is obtained. This information is then used by the instrument to calculate the flow volume, respiration rate, etc.

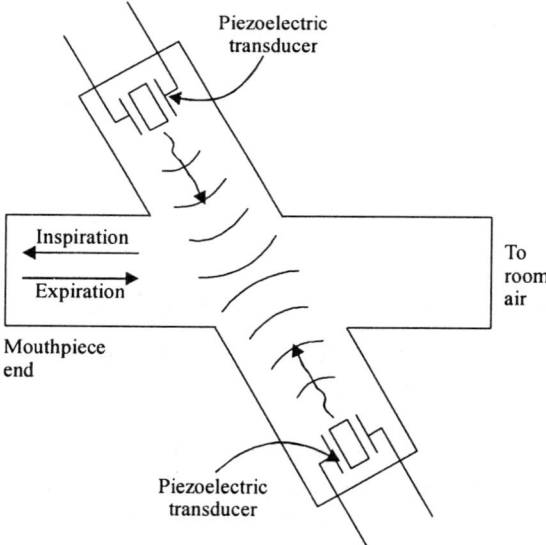

Fig. 23.3. Construction of an ultrasonic transducer for an electronic spirometer. The transducers are both used for transmit and receive in order to accurated measure the Doppler shift due to air speed.

GAS MEASUREMENTS

Pulmonary function laboratories can measure both pulmonary gases and blood gases. We will, discuss the techniques used to measure the partial pressures of oxygen (O_2) and carbon dioxide (CO_2) in inhaled and expired gases.

Measurement of oxygen concentration is made easier by the fact that oxygen is among the few molecules that will respond to a magnetic field. A special transducer is constructed so that oxygen passes through two coils of nickel wire. One of these coils is in the field of a permanent magnet, but both are part of a bridge circuit. The coil in the magnetic field experiences a varying flux because of the oxygen flow and this causes a varying bridge current to flow.

The measurement of carbon dioxide is made easier by the fact that CO_2 has infrared absorption properties. The relative CO_2 concentration in the patient's exhaled gas can therefore be calculated by measuring the infrared properties of the gas and comparing them with those of a known calibration gas that has either zero or a calibrated amount of CO_2 present. These calibration gases can be purchased from local bottled-gas suppliers or can be made up in-house if proper facilities are at hand.

KIDNEY DIALYSIS MACHINES

Human kidneys have two principal functions. They eliminate waste products from the blood and assist in the control of certain elements in the body. Renal failure is fatal unless artificial means of fulfilling the kidney's functions is provided.

The method currently in favour is called dialysis, shown in a highly simplified diagram in Fig. 23.4. The patient will have a by-pass inserted between a vein and an artery of the arm (called an A-V shunt). This tube is kept from clotting by the passage of blood. When it is time to dialyse—on the average of two or three times a week—the by-pass is removed and tubing to and from the dialysis machine is attached to open ends. Blood from the arterial side of the A-V shunt is passed through a peristaltic pump (Fig. 23.5) to a disposable coil filter, which is semi-permeable to H_2O and certain crystalloid substances but non-permeable to most of the large molecules and colloids found in the blood.

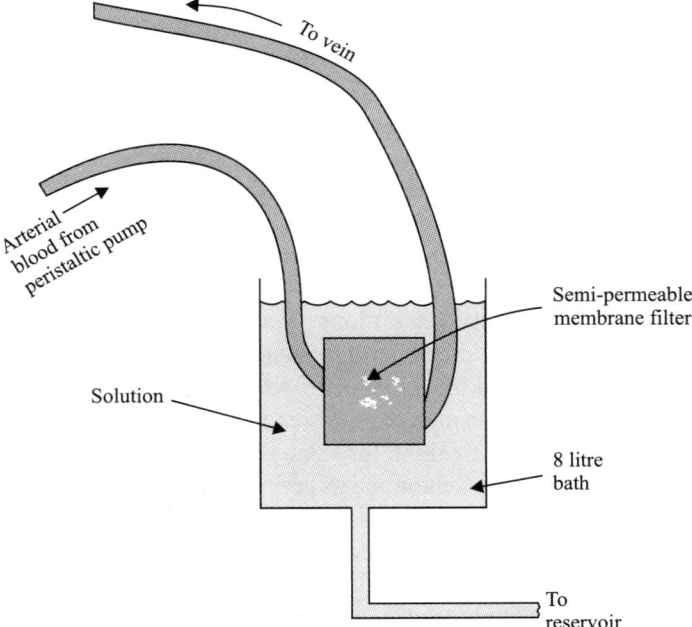

Fig. 23.4. Diagram of a renal dialysis machine.

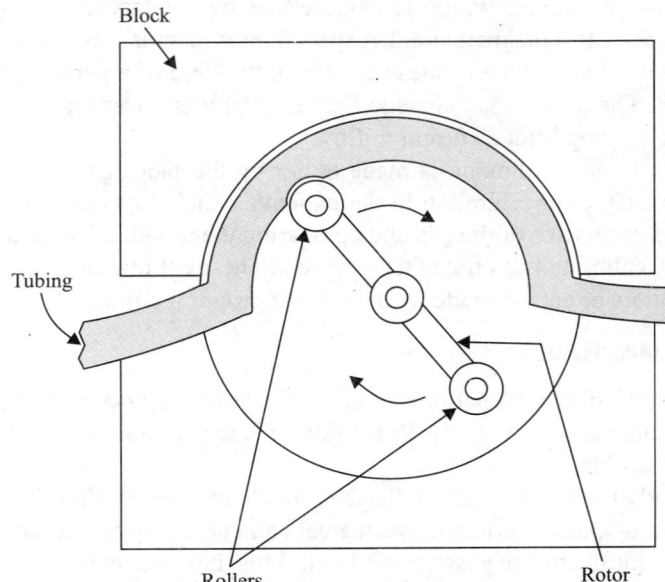

Fig. 23.5. Operation of a peristaltic pump. Fluid, such as blood, passes through the plastic tubing. The nylon rollers on the ends of the rotor arms gently push fluid forward. This is a single-rotor design, but multirotor types are also found. Speed is approximately 20 rpm.

This filter assembly is immersed in a bath containing elements in concentrations similar to those actually found in the blood. These are, for example, magnesium, sodium, calcium, glucose, salts, etc. The concentration of these constituents are adjusted to cause osmotic pressure to force the unwanted substances out of the blood line and into the 8 litre bath. Fluid in this bath is recirculated several times and is then replaced by fluid from a 120 litre reservoir.

Although not shown in this simplified drawing, there are also several safety features and controls that are either part of or peripherally related to the kidney machine. A pressure alarm, for example, is used to warn of a break in the lines from the patient. Such an alarm could turn off the machine as well as alert the staff of an impending catastrophy. There are also temperature regulators and controls provided.

The kidney dialysis machine is both in and of itself a 'wet environment' and so must come under some rather stringent electrical safety regulations. The use of ground fault interrupters (GFI) is recommended because the dialysis fluid can get into some of the electrical circuits and create ground-line currents from the case in excess of the 5 mA 'safe' level.

Many of the machines in current use may require some modification in order to bring them up to the standards met by more recent designs. It might, for example, be necessary to replace some of the regular AC power outlets and plugs of both the machine and its peripherals with rubber-covered or other waterproof types. Most older machines used regular outlets and plugs as might be found on any electronic equipment.

A bonnet over the filter bath was also used in older machines to protect against electrical shorts due to splashing water. This appears to be faulty logic, though, because it does not account for the fact that the machines can be operated without the bonnets—and they will be operated in that manner if the bonnets are broken or get misplaced. Also, it does not take into account the tendency of people to become careless with the garden hose used to fill the 120 litre reservoir. Where this is a problem, contact your local electrical (not electronic) supplier for rubber or neoprene waterproof outlets.

Be sure to examine the electrical cable bringing power from the wall outlet to the machine. If it is regular black rubber, have it replaced with a waterproof neoprene cable. In one installation it was found that machines awaiting servicing or cleaning would be pushed aside with the AC power cable laying in the still full 120 litre reservoir. The electrolytes in that reservoir can impregnate the insulation of the wire and create a dangerous low-resistance situation. Replacement of the cable with a waterproof type is deemed appropriate.

Preventive maintenance is even better than educating the users to watch out for the cable because a hospital might have a very high turnover rate of personnel, requiring a constant in-service education regiem. It is also true that Murphy's law and the normal perversity of the universe tend to keep at least 10 per cent of the people from 'getting the word'. Since 10 per cent never get the word even if present when given, it is wise to re-design their environment to prevent their lack of awareness (or ignorance, when one doesn't care to be charitable) from causing trouble.

In normal repair operations it is wise to stock certain items. These include switches, bulbs, fuses and other small electrical or electronic items, as appropriate. Also keep pump motors, pump impellers (water pumps), drain solenoid assemblies and any control regulators. Where lack of service has been a problem in the locality (as it often is), you may become more than a little surprised at the mechanical dexterity and repair ability of the nurses who operate this equipment. After all, although some time may be available, repair is essential because a kidney machine is life support equipment and must work properly.

SOME FINAL ADVICE

Several pointers are in order for the prospective medical equipment technician. One is to be always alert to possibilities for learning. New situations come up all of the time and you will not want to be caught unaware. It is necessary that you adapt a really professional attitude toward the work. In medical electronics it can be considerably more serious and can cost somebody their life. It is wise to present a positive image to the nurses, technicians and physicians who use the equipment.

Become used to writing things down. This will take on two forms. One, carry a pocket notebook and jot down any equipment complaint that you will have to remedy later. This will not only keep your memory jogged, it will result in a high overall level of confidence from your medical and nursing customers. Also, keep extensive records of all equipment repairs, safety inspections and examinations. Your administration will require the records for accreditation or licensure inspections and in case of a malpractice suit. Even your own efforts may be subject to such a suit, so you will want to keep the records up-to-date to show your competence and good faith.

HEMODIALYSIS

One of the most important prosthetic devices in modern medicine is the artificial kidney, which is periodically connected to the circulatory systems of uremic patients to remove metabolic waste products from their blood. A general scheme for the operation of this device is shown in Fig. 23.6.

There are two basic units in a hemodialysis system: the exchanger and the dialysate delivery system. The exchanger consists of the dialysis chamber itself, which is a compartment containing the patient's blood and a compartment containing the dialysate. These two compartments are separated by a semi-permeable membrane that allows the waste components in the blood to diffuse through to the dialysate, which carries them away.

There are three basic types of exchangers in use. The coil dialyser consists of a tube made of the semi-permeable membrane material wound into a coil, in such a way that the dialysate can be circulated between individual turns of it. This is the most commonly used type of dialyser. It has the limitation that the coil must be fairly long to provide a large effective surface area for mass transport and it thus imposes a relatively high resistance to the flow of blood. For this reason and to maintain effective blood flow, it is necessary to put a pump in series with the arterial blood supply to increase the pressure. However, the increased pressure improves the ultrafiltration rate of the membrane. It is important in this unit that the dialysate also be forcibly circulated to ensure rapid mixing. Because fresh dialysate must be available to the surface of the membrane throughout the coil, a pump is necessary for the dialysate as well.

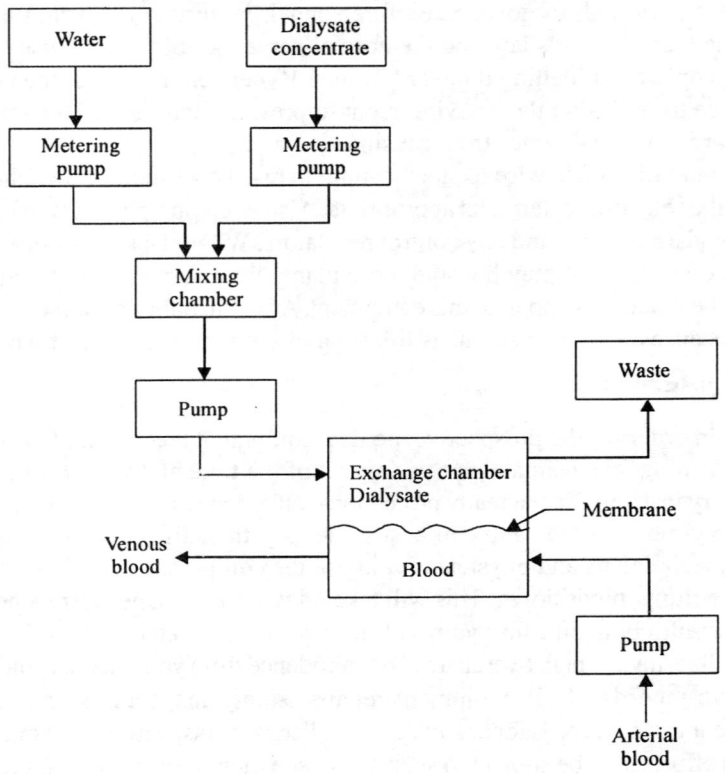

Fig. 23.6. An artificial kidney. The dialysate delivery system in this unit mixes dialysate from a concentrate before pumping it through the exchange chamber.

The second type of exchanger used in artificial-kidney systems is the parallel-plate dialyser. It is constructed similarly to a multilayer parallel-plate capacitor, with the plates made of semi-permeable-membrane material. Blood is circulated between pairs of plates and the dialysate is circulated between the other plates. Each plate thus serves as a membrane between dialysate and blood. The blood flows in thin sheets to maximise the surface-to-volume ratio for the dialyser.

The third type of exchange apparatus is the hollow-fibre kidney. This consists of from 10000 to 15000 hollow fibres, with an internal diameter of approximately 0.2 mm and a length of approximately 150 mm, connected in parallel. The blood flows in the lumen of the fibres while the dialysate surrounds them. The walls of the fibres serve as the semi-permeable membrane. The dialysate is pumped through the space surrounding the fibres to achieve the most efficient exchange.

The remainder of the artificial kidney consists of the dialysate-delivery system. The dialysate is made up of water with various solutes added. Either it is prepared in a batch and pumped through the dialysis chamber or (in applications in which large amounts of dialysate are used) a concentrated solution of the solutes is made and automatically mixed with pure water to achieve the correct concentration (Fig. 23.6). Metering pumps administer the correct amount of dialysate concentrate and water into a mixing chamber to produce the dialysate, which is then pumped through a dialysis chamber, where it picks up the metabolic waste products. It is then discarded.

As in the case of the cardiovascular prostheses, the hemodialysis apparatus does not require any electronic instrumentation to function. However, in using this device with patients, the clinician finds that several pieces of electronic instrumentation greatly aid in its application and operation. Because only a membrane separates the patient's blood from the dialysate, it is important that any leaks in the membrane be detected immediately before serious losses of blood occur. In some cases, in fact, dialysate can leak into the patient's circulatory system. The blood is usually at a higher pressure than the dialysate, so loss of blood is the hazard of major concern. The dialysate is a clear liquid and the presence of blood in it can be detected as a colourimetric or optical density change; thus optical systems are used to detect leaks. In addition, instruments monitor the pressure in the blood compartment to detect rapidly any abnormalities, such as major leaks or clotting phenomena, that might change the pressure.

The gross concentration of electrolytes of the dialysate is also monitored by electronic instrumentation. Because the solute is made up of electrolytes, the overall concentration of these in the dialysate is determined by impedance techniques. Thus, by measuring the conductivity of the dialysate in the mixing chamber, instruments can detect any major abnormalities in concentration before the dialysate enters the dialysis chamber.

Another problem common to both hemodialysis units and the pump oxygenator is that air bubbles cannot be tolerated in the blood that re-enters the patient: This produces air emboli that may be life-threatening. Thus it is important that some type of bubble detector be included in the path of the blood before it re-enters the body. If bubbles are detected, the blood pump is turned off until the technician operating the dialyser solves the problem.

SECTION IV
Special Topics

Chapter 24

Hospital Equipment Safety

INTRODUCTION

A hospital is more than simply a building in which health care is delivered. It is a high-tech centre that must be superbly organised in order to operate effectively. A typical modern community hospital contains more than 3000 pieces of medical equipment used by hundreds of physicians, health care workers, other staff and even the patients themselves. In order to avoid electrical shock, burns, excessive radiation, toxic exposure, fire, explosion and other hazards, many of the devices must be handled with extreme care. Serious accidents can be kept to a minimum if hospital personnel are properly trained to exercise caution, if regulations and procedures are strictly adhered to.

The objective in this chapter is to alert health care professionals to existing hazards and to describe the various means available to provide protection against them.

ELECTRICAL HAZARDS OF MEDICAL INSTRUMENTS

One of the main hazards connected with the use of medical equipment is electrical shock. The physiological effects of electrical current on the body, macroshock as the undesirable effects of a current greater than 5 mA at 60 cycles applied to the surface of the body. These effects range from discomfort and pain to tissue injury, heart fibrillation and death if a vital body part, such as the heart or respiratory centre, is affected. A macroshock to a limb of a technician repairing equipment may also cause secondary injury, such as cuts on the hand as the person pulls away from the equipment. Or worse, a fall could results, if the technician were on a ladder while being jolted by an electrical current. Microshock is defined as the undesirable effects of a current greater than 10 µA applied directly to the heart. Microshock can cause a heart fibrillation and can result in a patient's death. It is, however, a hazard only to patients who are in a critical-care situation, because the current must be applied directly to the heart.

Shock is defined in terms of current because the voltage is caused by wide variation in skin resistance among individuals and among differing clinical situations. For example, the skin resistance at 60 cycles may vary from 93 kΩ down to 200 Ω, depending on the condition, as indicated in Table 24.1.

All electrical and electronic devices in the hospital are sources of potentially harmful current. Most of this equipment is energised by the building wiring. Therefore, an understanding of the shock hazards begins with a discussion of this wiring. The electrical power bus consists of three wires as shown in Fig. 24.1: a hot wire H at 110 or 220 V, 60 cycle, usually colour-coded black; a neutral wire N, usually colour-coded white, connected to ground through a pipe embedded in the earth and a ground wire G, usually colour-coded green. The neutral wire carrier the return current from the equipment loads and normally carries the same current as the hot lead. The G-wire is connected to the external parts of the equipment to bleed away any leakage that may occur and to prevent the external parts from acquiring a high voltage in case of a short or fault in the circuit. It normally carries very small current, though in fault situations it may cause large currents.

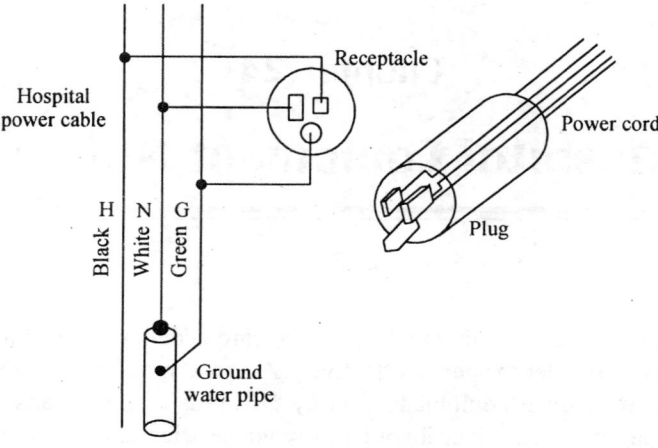

Fig. 24.1. A power bus.

Macroshock Hazards

Macroshock occurs more often with two-wire systems than with three-wire systems (Fig. 24.2). With two-wire equipment it is always dangerous to get between the hot H and neutral N wires. Touching H and N wires simultaneously with two limbs can direct currents through vital organs of circulation and respiration. Because N wires are internally grounded, touching H and G wire can produce macroshock. In some commercial equipment, such as inexpensive AC/DC radios, which are often brought to the hospital by patients, the power-cord plug may be reversed so that the hot lead becomes attached to the chassis. In this case, a macroshock hazard exists when the chassis and ground are touched simultaneously.

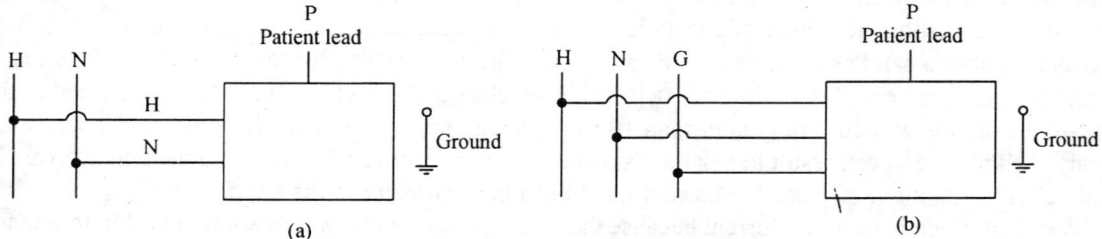

Fig. 24.2. Power bus connections to (a) two-wire; and (b) three-wire equipment.

Figure 24.3 illustrates additional hazardous situations that results from faults that may occur in the equipment. In part (a) the H lead shorts to the patient lead P. Thus, a macroshock results if the patient touches ground or the chassis. In part (b) the hot wire H and neutral N are reversed because the two-wire plug has been reversed. A grounded patients is therefore shocked upon touching the chassis.

In part (c) the H wire is shorted to the chassis, causing the shock configuration shown as the patient touches either neutral or ground and the chassis. In part (d) the neutral wire accidentally shorts to the equipment case leading to a shock situation of H to chassis or H to ground. If the H line faults to N, no shock occurs unless the patient touches H or N and ground.

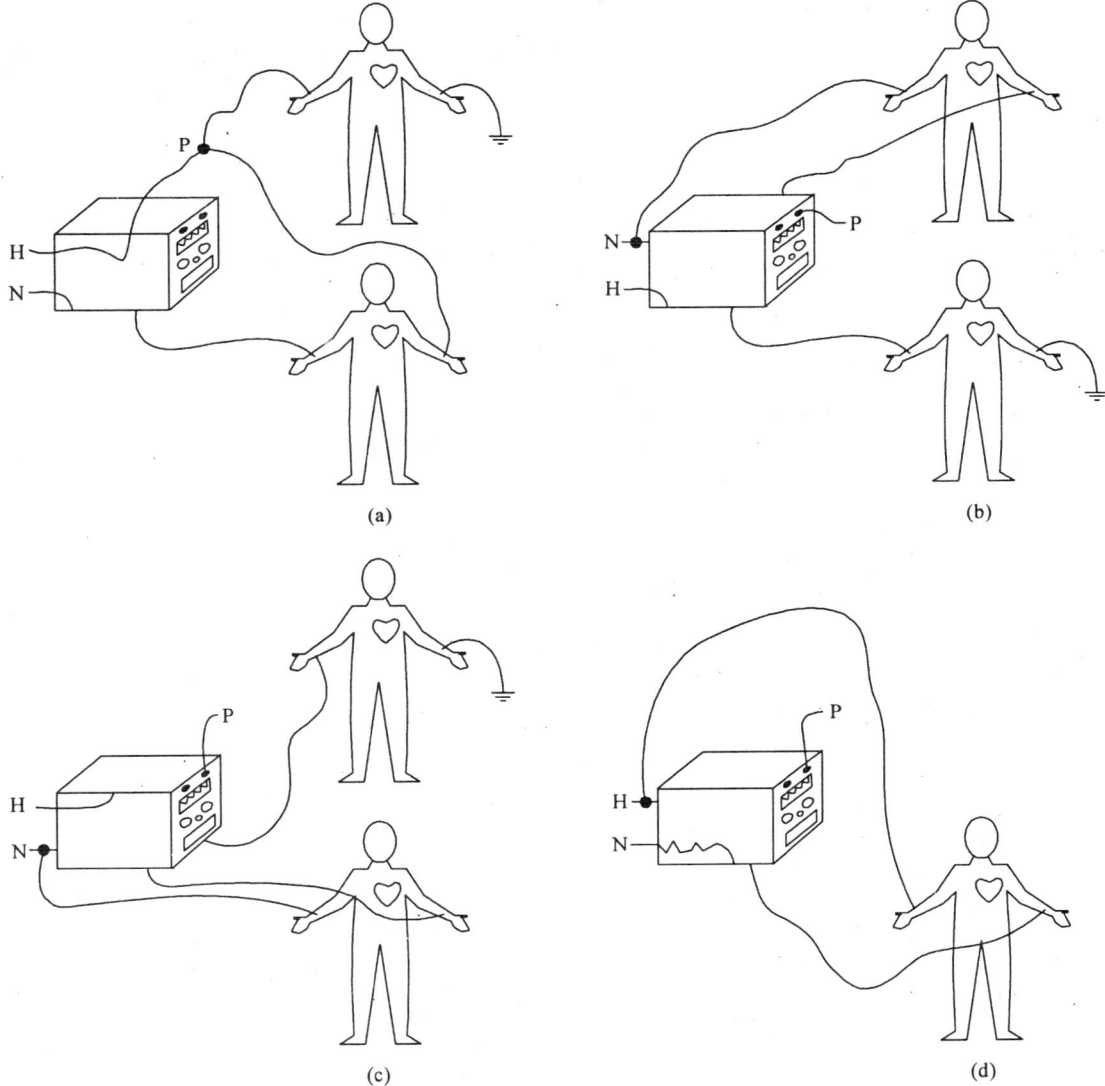

(a) (b) (c) (d)

Fig. 24.3. Macroshock situations other than touching H and N or H and G wires for two-wire units.

The primary defense against the hazards of a two-wire plug is to add a third ground wire, as shown in Fig. 24.2b. This wire is usually connected to the chassis of the equipment and ensures that it will not rise to a high voltage. Another method is to double-insulate the chassis—that is, to place a layer of insulation between the circuit-board chassis and the equipment case exposed to the user. To prevent a hot chassis on this type of equipment, two-prong plugs have prongs of different sizes so they cannot be reversed.

The addition of a ground wire protects against the hazards of high voltage on the chassis. Assuming the equipment is not faulty, the only macroshock danger occurs when a person gets between the hot lead and ground, neutral or chassis. Of course, when the third wire faults (is broken) the hazards of the two-wire equipment are once again present, except for plug reversal, which is prevented by the shape of the three-prong plug. Other macroshock hazard faults would occur if the hot lead were to short to the patient lead, as illustrated in Fig. 24.4a or in the double-faults case, if the hot lead were to short to the chassis with the ground lead open, as illustrated in Fig. 24.4b.

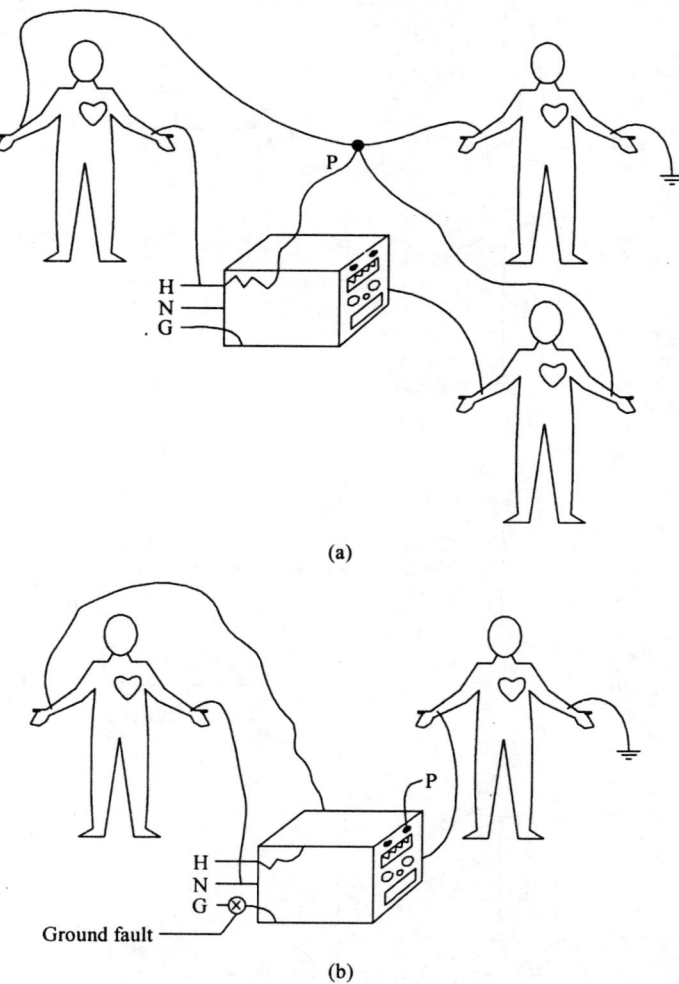

(a)

(b)

Fig. 24.4. Macroshock situations other than touching H and N or H and G for three-wire units.

Microshock Hazards

Microshock occurs when a current applied to the heart causes depolarisations to originate from sites other than the sinoatrial (SA) node of the heart. The resulting fibrillations can impair circulation and can ultimately be fatal.

Microshock is apt to occur if the heart receives currents above 10 µA. The conditions leading to such a situation include all of those that induce macroshock, as discussed previously. Additional conditions (Fig. 24.5) include the leakage of current and slight elevations of the chassis voltage resulting from high power-line current.

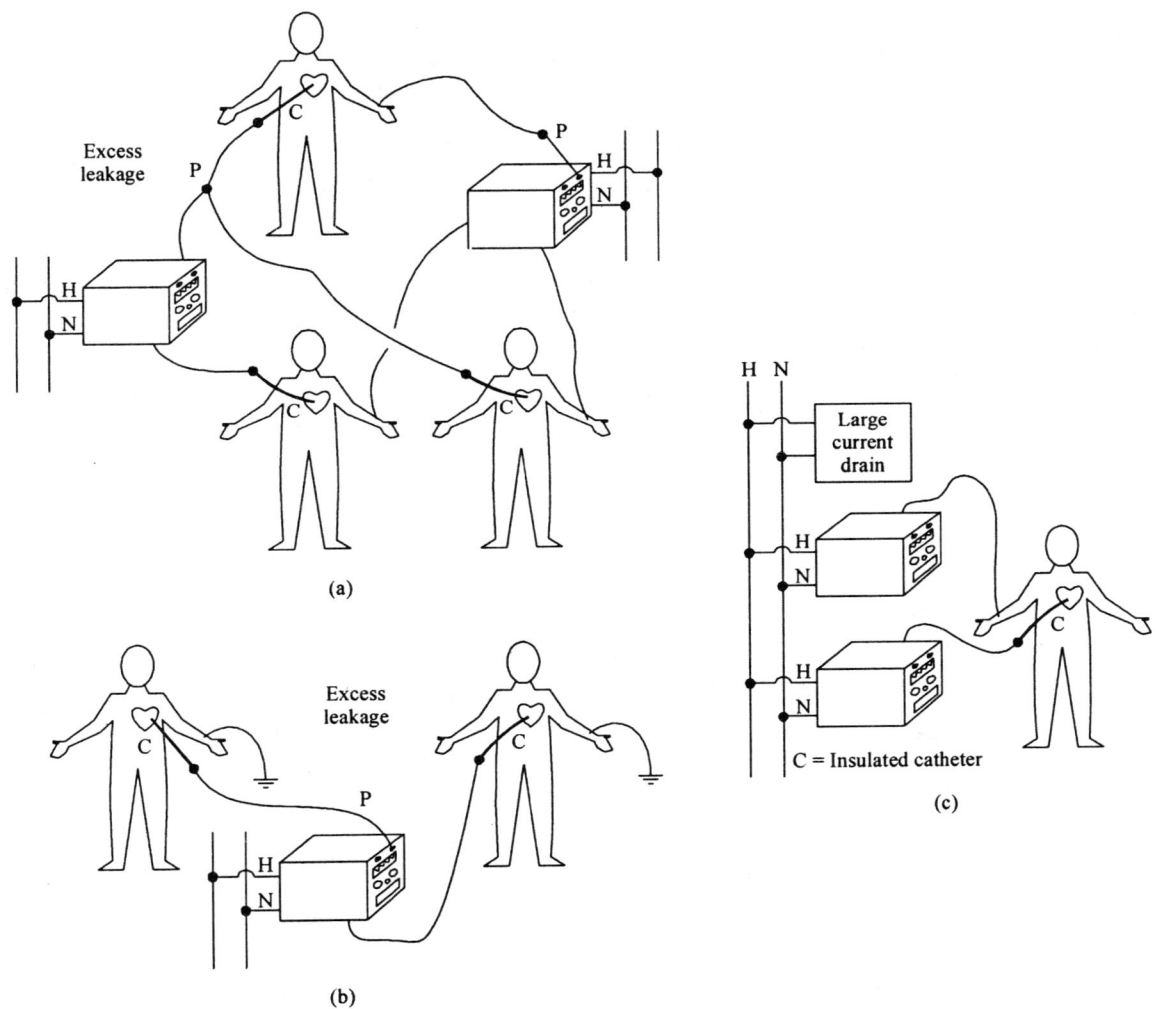

Fig. 24.5. Microshock situations other than those illustrated in Fig. 24.3 for two-wire units.

Leakage current is caused by inductive, capacitive or resistive coupling of electronic circuit currents to the chassis or the patient lead on equipment. Inductive coupling may exist in the power supply transformer or between the windings of equipment motors and the chassis or lead. Likewise, circuit wires and the metal of the equipment could form a capacitive coupling. Resistive coupling of current from the circuit arises from dirt, oil or fluids that may get into the equipment and cause a conductive pathway.

Figures 24.5a and 24.5c illustrate the microshock hazard that occurs when a person gets between two pieces of equipment. The chassis voltages between the two-pieces of two-wire equipment could be considerable because of power-line currents in the different power buses that cause leakage current and elevate chassis voltage. This effect is virtually eliminated by the third wire in three-wire equipment.

Furthermore, leakage currents from the patient leads need to be considered. Protection against the effects of leakage current is achieved by periodically inspecting equipment and measuring the leakage current. Figure 24.5c illustrates the case in which elevated chassis voltage could be caused by large currents existing in the power bus. For example, a ventilation fan may draw over 10A. Equipment that operates safely with the fan turned off could acquire an elevated voltage when the fan was turned on. To guard against this, a third wire is added to ground the chassis of the equipment, as illustrated in Fig. 24.6a. Even with the third wire, the leakage hazard still exists. For this reason, periodic inspection of leakage currents in medical equipment is a necessity.

Two subtle faults can occur that introduce microshock faults into three-wire equipment. First, the ground wire or neutral wire may break. Since the power cord is vulnerable to metal fatigue from being moved around and to abuse, breakage in the cord is not rare. Therefore, periodic inspection of the power cord is a necessity. Figure 24.6a illustrates microshock hazards due to a broken ground wire. Elevated voltage may exist between the chassis and ground or between the two pieces of equipment that are sufficient to cause a microshock in a catheterised patient.

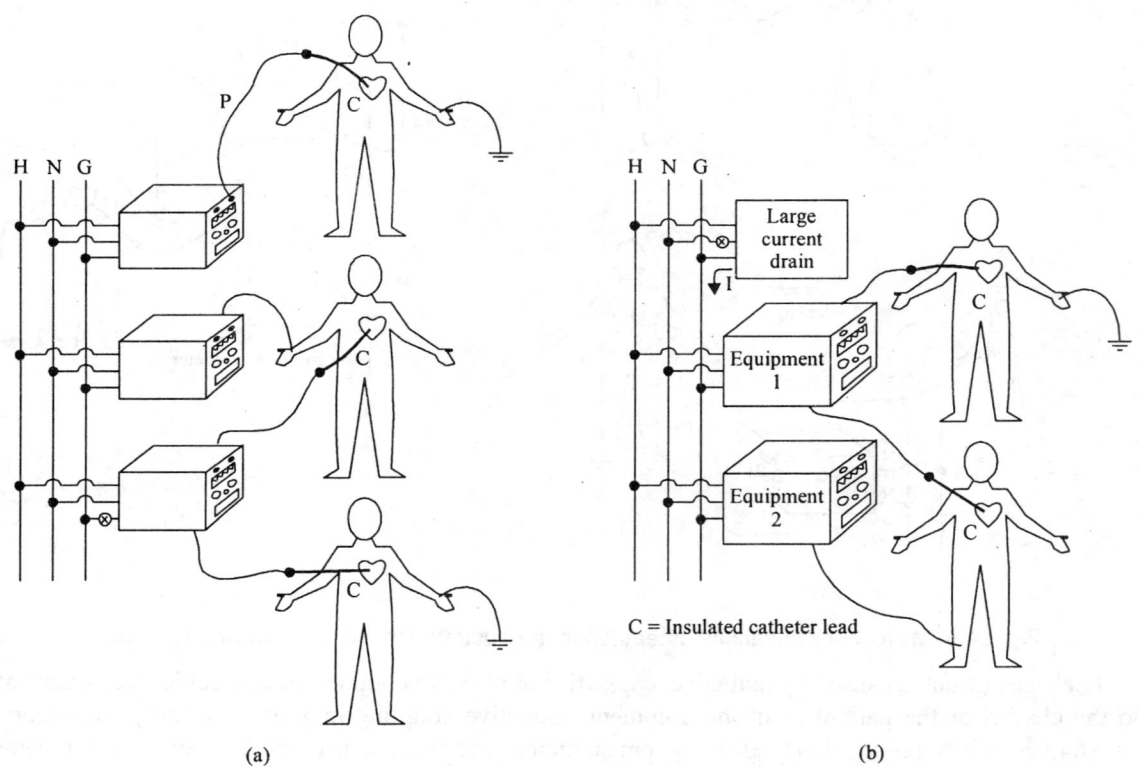

(a)

(b)

Fig. 24.6. Microshock situations other than those illustrated in Fig. 24.4 for three-wire units.

Second, as Fig. 24.6b illustrates, a microshock hazard may result from a fault in equipment not used in patient care. For example, suppose an air conditioning unit opens in the neutral and uses the ground lead to supply the large current needed to drive it. This is the case of a neutral fault that occurs while the ground wire remains intact. This fault would pour a large current into the ground lead. Two medical equipment units attached to this ground could have elevated voltage between their chassis. In this case, the medical equipment would have tested normal and the elevated voltage constituting a microshock situation would be due to equipment outside the medical area. To protect against this situation, the medical circuits may be isolated from such large-current equipment. As a last defence, however, the user may shunt the two pieces of equipment with a ground wire connected exclusively between the units attached to a catheterised patient.

DEVICES TO PROTECT AGAINST ELECTRICAL HAZARDS

Several devices are available to protect patients and health care workers from hazardous electrical currents. These range from devices to protect against high-voltage macroshock hazards to procedures that minimise the probability that a microshock will occur.

Ground Fault Interrupter

A ground fault interrupter (GFI) protects against a shock that occurs if a person touches the hot lead with one hand and the ground with the other. The GFI opens the power lead if the hot lead current differs by more than approximately 2 mA from the neutral lead current for a duration of longer than 0.2 second. The GFI shown in Fig. 24.7 consists of a magnetic coil on which the hot lead and the neutral lead are wound with the same number of turns, but in opposite directions. When the system is normal, I_N is equal to I_H and the magnet flux, ϕ, in the coil due to these currents cancels. Under this condition, the sensing coil does not have a voltage induced in it. However, when the hot lead faults or is touched by a person, the fault current I_F is shunted to ground. Then we have

$$I_N = I_H - I_F$$

and I_H is not equal to I_N. Under this fault condition the corresponding fluxes in the coil are unequal and a net flux exists in the coil. This induces a voltage into the sensing amplifier. If the current I_F exceeds 2 mA for 0.2 second, the relay opens the line and prevents a macroshock from injuring the person, as well as preventing further damage to the equipment. The GFI can be conveniently mounted in the power receptacle. It is required in wet areas.

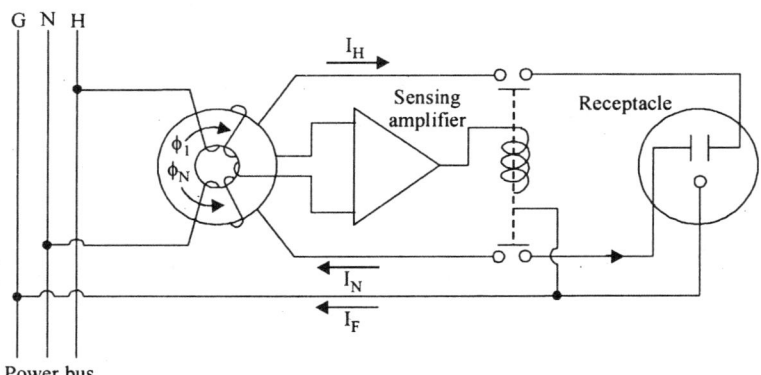

Fig. 24.7. Ground fault interrupter.

Isolation Transformer

The isolation transformer provides a second means of protecting against an H-lead to G-lead macroshock. It also prevents sparks when the H lead touches ground, a particularly important protection in an explosive or flammable environment, such as when flammable anaesthetics or excessive oxygen is present. Figure 24.8a clearly shows that a fault such as a short circuit from either secondary lead of the transformers to ground will carry no current. Therefore, a secondary lead to ground spark or shock is prevented.

However, when the isolation transformer is in use and equipment is plugged into the secondary, the stray capacitance and input impedance of the hardware tend to make a conductive path to ground. This reduces the isolation by completing the circuit from either secondary lead to ground and then to the other secondary lead. If a fault should now occur on the secondary, a hazardous current could flow.

Line Isolation Monitor

A line isolation monitor (LIM) puts a relatively large impedance from either secondary lead through an ammeter to ground of the isolation transformer. If there is a conductive path through the equipment shown in Fig. 24.8b, the meter in the LIM will read a current. The meter on the LIM is calibrated to read what current would flow through a short-circuit fault if it should occur from either secondary to ground. This number will vary according to the leakage in the equipment attached to the secondary and any faults that may exist between the secondary leads and ground. An alarm in the LIM is usually set off when it is calculated that a short-circuit fault between a secondary lead and ground would draw 2 to 5 mA of current. This alarm merely indicates that the back-up system has failed and the equipment is no longer isolated. It does not mean that the dangerous currents are already flowing. Therefore, if the equipment is critically needed, the LIM alarm may, sometimes, justifiably be overridden.

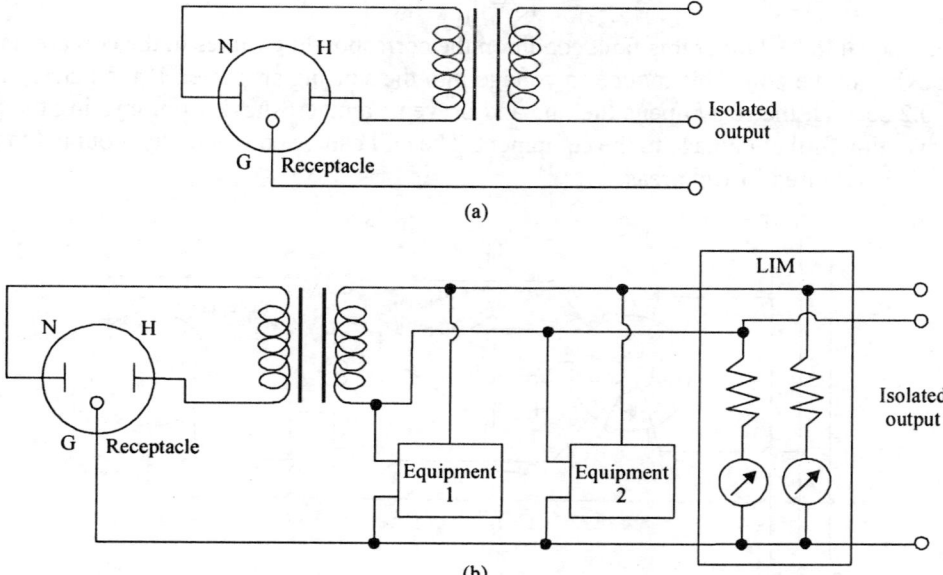

Fig. 24.8. (a) An isolation transfomer; and (b) an isolation transformer connected to a line isolation monitor and other equipment.

Receptacle Tester

The LIM and GFI are permanently attached to the power lines in order to warn of potential hazards or to open the circuit when hazardous current flows. Other types of equipment are available for inspecting equipment and circuits for hazardous conditions. For example, the receptacle tester may be inserted in the power receptacle to check for defects in the wiring, such as polarity reversals, shorts or opens. Light-emitting diodes (LEDs) in series with a directional diode and a limiting resistor R are used to give a coded indication of a receptacle fault. If the receptacle is normal, the LEDs in Fig. 24.9 will all be OFF when H is negative. However, when H is positive, LEDs 1 and 3 go ON, blinking at 60 times as second. The observer will perceive both LEDs 1 and 3 as being ON steadily in this case, since the time response of the eye will cause the blinks to merge. Also, 2 will be perceived as OFF. An H to G short will turn all LEDs OFF, as will an open H lead. The light responses for several fault states possible in the figure are as follows:

Possible wiring defect	LED state		
	1	2	3
Normal	ON	OFF	ON
H to G short	OFF	OFF	OFF
H, N reversed	OFF	ON	ON

The receptacle also needs to be tested for the grasping tension it exerts on the plug and the device for this is the receptacle contact tester, which consists of a plug blade attached to a spring scale. As the plug is retracted from the receptacle, the scale is read to ensure that the tension it is required to overcome exceeds approximately 8 oz.

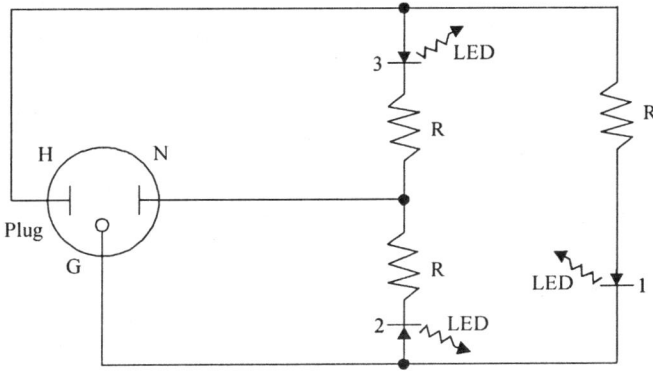

Fig. 24.9. A power receptacle tester.

Electrical Safety Analyser Equipment

The equipment discussed in the processing section is mostly used as protection against macroshock. The safety analyser, as illustrated by the block diagram in Fig. 24.10, is primarily used to test medical equipment for leakage currents that can cause microshock to patients. The safety analyser is calibrated by placing switch S_5 in the calibrate position while adjusting the meter for 1 µA. The equipment under test (EUT) is plugged into the safety analyser. To measure the chassis to ground leakage on the EUT, S_4 is opened while S_1 is in position 1, S_2 is in position 2 and S_3 is opened. The ground leakage is then also measured with the hot and neutral leads reversed by means of switch S_1. Switch S_2 may then be moved to position 1 to measure the leakage current in the patient lead P_1. The leakage current between patient leads when the hot lead is applied to one of the P-leads is measured when S_3 is closed.

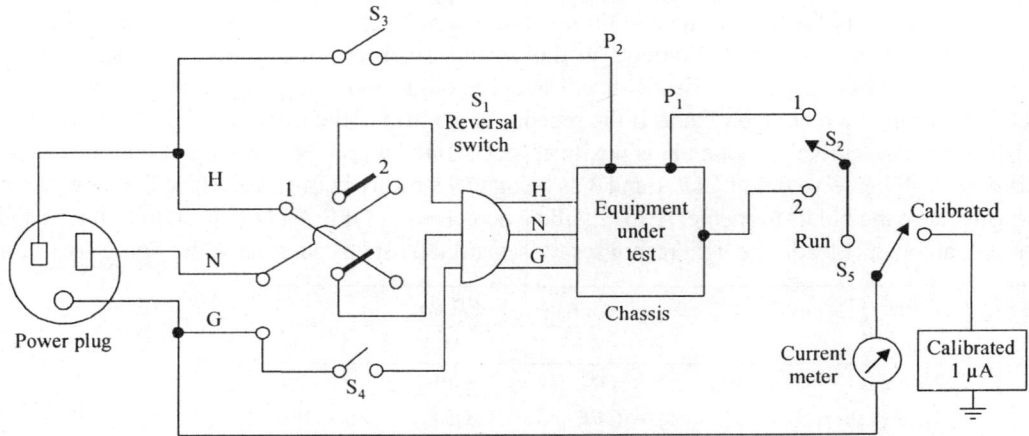

Fig. 24.10. Block diagram of a generic safety analyser.

AN EQUIPMENT SAFETY PROGRAMME

The clinical engineering department in a hospital should take responsibility for establishing an equipment safety programme. Such a programme should conform to safety regulations established by government agencies and professional organisations. The programme is necessary to ensure the safety of patients and health care workers in the hospital. Specific regulations must be met in order to secure accreditation and license to operate.

The instrumentation described in the preceding sections is used to make safety tests and to ensure safety in the hospital. Here we present a sample programme in order to discuss the issues involved. A specific safety programme would need to be geared to a particular clinical situation and would of course differ from that described here.

Hospital Regulations

The many instruments, medicines and procedures used to deliver health care in a hospital for the benefit of patients may also present hazards. In order to protect patients and health care workers, hospital regulations have been developed to cope with hazards of electricity, radiation, magnetism, toxics, infectious agents, pressure, flame, heat, explosion and energy interruptions.

Legally enforceable regulations are issued by various government agencies: (i) Occupational Safety and Jealth Administration (OSHA), founded in 1971; and through the Federal Drug Administration (FDA) the Medical Device Amendments of 1976 to the Food, Drug and Cosmetic Act. Both of these mechanisms arose as a result of the increased environmental awareness during the 1970s. In addition, local building codes for fire, electrical and structural safety are enforced in hospitals.

Furthermore, voluntary regulations are issued by civic and professional groups for the protection of the public and the professions. Although such regulations are not always legally enforceable, they are effective because failure to comply may result in a withdrawal of third-party funding and insurance, a damaged reputation, a loss of professional staff and a loss of clients. In some cases, voluntary regulations are the only rules in a evidence, because the cost of rigid enforcement cannot be justified in terms of the risk involved. This, coupled with the fact that voluntary regulations do work, makes voluntary compliance all the more important. Furthermore, when these regulations are adopted as local building codes, they acquire the force of law.

Inspections of Equipment

The frequency of electrical safety inspections generally depends upon the degree of vulnerability of the equipment user and patient to hazards associated with the equipment. In general care areas, tests are done every years.

In wet areas, where the patient's skin resistance is likely to be low, tests are done every six months. In critical areas, where the skin might be penetrated in surgery by a catheter or a needle or injury, tests are also done every six months.

Equipment testing begins with concern for the integrity of the power system. A receptacle tester, as discussed in the previous section, is used to test for power-line opens, shorts or wiring errors. In order to prevent excessive leakage current and shock hazards, medical instrumentation either has a power cord with a three-prong plug or is double-insulated.

Double-insulated equipment has its hot and neutral power leads connected to electronics insulated from the chassis and the chassis insulated from the external case of the equipment. With these provisions, the power-cord leakage should test less than 100 µA. Existing equipment in the hospital may have a power-cord leakage as high as 500 µA. These cases need to be documented to ensure safe use of such equipment.

Specifications on hospital equipment to be used in patient areas typically take into account that a 5 mA current applied through the surface of the body is dangerous and that currents in excess of 10 µA applied to a catheterised heart can be dangerous.

Leakage currents are measured with the safety analyser. A typical set of leakage current values that meet specifications of equipment safe to use in patient areas is given in Table 24.2. The leakage of the individual patient lead, the leakage of all leads together and the chassis leakage are measured with the AC line power normally connected to the equipment. The driven patient leads are connected to the power line in order to determine how much current the 120 V would drive through them. Equipment used outside the patient's vicinity may exhibit as much as 500 µA leakage current.

Table 24.2. Leakage current values for equipment used with patient.

Description	Leakage current (µA)
Individual patient lead	10
Driven patient lead	20
Current between patient leads	50
All patient leads connected together	100
Chassis leakage to ground	100

The leakage current specifications on hospital equipment are a function of the current frequency due to the high-frequency effects. The leakage current specifications follow the Equation:

$$I = I_{lk}{}^{f}$$

$$\dots (24.1)$$

where I is the leakage current allowed at a frequency f, given in kHz. I_{lk} is the leakage current for frequencies below 1 kHz.

Leakage currents in equipment may be measured with a safety analyser.

Emergency Power Systems

The power is occasionally interrupted by severe weather such as high winds, lightning, snow and ice. In less-developed countries, power outages are common, sometimes lasting for several hours during the business day. Uninterrupted power, however, is necessary for many modern medical instruments, among them artificial blood circulators, ventilators, operating room equipment, intensive care units, external pacemakers, kidney dialysis machines and artificial hearts. Injury to patients relying on any of these devices would obviously occur if the power were to fail for an extended period.

To protect against such interruptions, hospitals use two independent sources of power. An in-house emergency power source may consist of an internal combustion engine driving an electrical generator. The time it takes for the emergency source to switch on when an outage occurs is typically less than 10 seconds. The reliability of the emergency power system should be ensured by exercising the emergency generator for 30 minutes every 30 days and by inspecting batteries on the engine every seven days. Other causes of power interruption, such as ground fault interrupters, should not turn off critical equipment but should have automatic re-set systems with alarms to warn of hazards or else have back-up systems.

Oxygen Safety

A widely used gas in the hospital, oxygen must be handled carefully, because it supports flame and fire, is stored at high pressure and can be toxic when misused.

In order to prevent fire and explosion with oxygen, the ambient temperature where the gas is used or stored should be kept below 130°F. As a rule of thumb, one can ordinarily just keep skin contact with a surface at that temperature. A second precaution is to keep any flammable substance out of the oxygen system, including flammable gases. Oil must be kept off the oxygen system valves, because it is highly combustible in the presence of oxygen. As a safety precaution, if the valves become frozen from high-pressure gas release, for example, a flame torch must not be used to thaw them; wet rags would provide a safe alternative. Many materials normally resistant to flame will burn in an oxygen-rich atmosphere. Examples include human tissue, body oils, silicon rubber, oil-based cosmetics, polyvinyl chloride, alcohols, acetone, asbestos-containing paint, glass epoxy compounds, tent canopies and suction tubing. Since some of these materials are invariably present in the hospital—for example, in oxygen tents, on respirators and near anaesthesia machines—it is essential to eliminate sources of ignition in the oxygen-enriched atmosphere. Common sources of ignition that must be kept away from oxygen are open flame, static electricity burning tobacco, electric radiant heaters, electric shavers, electric bed controls, hair dryers, remote TV controls and telephones. Hearing aids, external pacemakers and other equipment worn by patients can also be sources of ignition. Of course, any other potential sources of ignition should likewise be eliminated.

Safety in the Operating Room

The operating room (OR) is carefully designed and maintained to protect the patient from hazards including fire, explosion, mechanical injury, toxic overdose, anoxia and infection. Many of these hazards arise from anaesthesia and surgery.

Protection against infection is achieved by sterilisation. Surgeons and surgical assistants scrub their hands and arms, wear sterile gloves, gowns, caps, masks and foot coverings. The operation room has sterile regions where the patient, instruments for surgery and anaesthesia machine are located. The periphery of the operating room is usually a non-sterile area where equipment and technicians who do not come in contact with the patient are located. Personnel confined to this region also wear gowns, caps, masks and foot coverings, but do not need to scrub.

Instruments may be sterilised in the OR with either steam, ethylene oxide gas or a liquid, glutamic aldehyde. Steam sterilisation may be done under pressure to produce superheated steam temperatures up to 144°C. After treatment for approximately 15 minutes, the instruments are dried at high temperatures. The resulting temperature stress, which may be damaging to the instruments, may be avoided by sterilising at low temperatures with ethylene oxide (ETO) gas. Although the temperature in this treatment may be reduced below 60°C, exposure time is increased to several hours. Careful ventilation of the ETO from the instruments is then necessary since the gas is hazardous.

Anaesthetics and anaesthesia delivery equipment also present safety hazards. An example block diagram of an anaesthesia machine appears in Fig. 24.11. The anaesthetic, in this case nitrous oxide (N_2O), is mixed with oxygen and fluorocarbons and then delivered to the patient on the inspiration cycle. Exhalation passes through a one-way valve, through a CO_2 absorber and is delivered again to the patient. The anaesthetic is constantly monitored and adjusted for the correct mixture. A portion of the anaesthetic is exhausted and usually delivered to the outside through vent ducts.

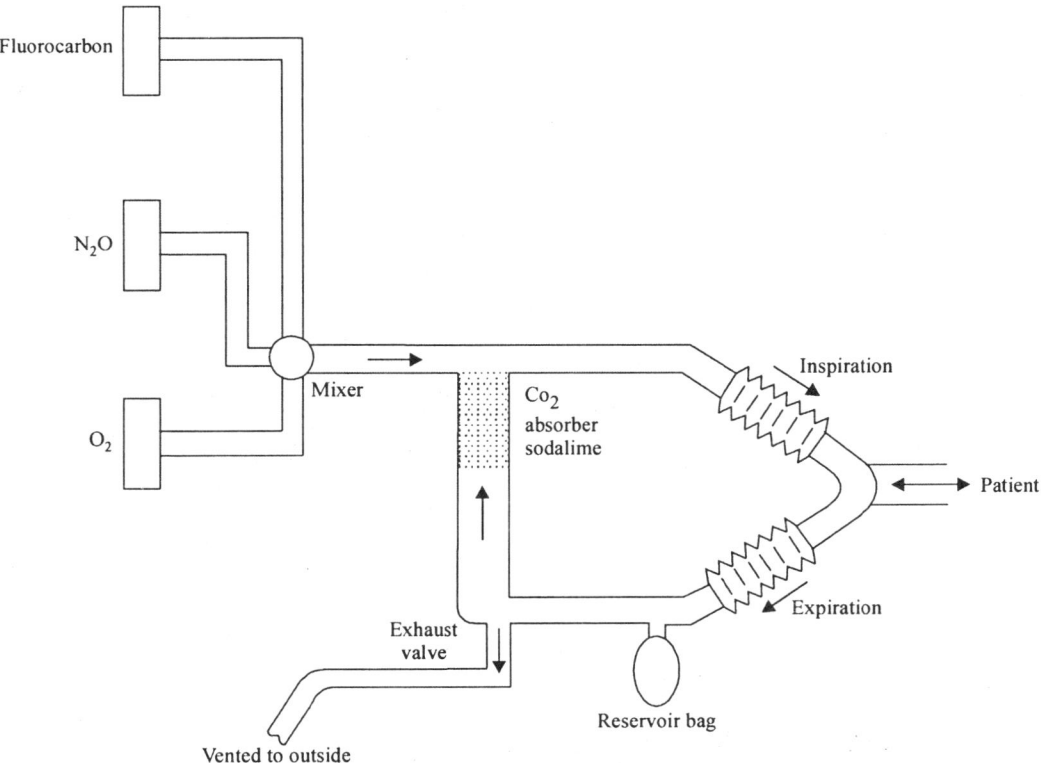

Fig. 24.11. An anaesthesia machine.

The most commonly used anaesthetic is nitrous oxide, used in combination with fluorocarbons such as halothane, enflurane or methoxyflurane. These are non-flammable but should not be vented into the OR, since they may have deleterious effects on OR personnel. Although flammable anaesthetics such as ether and cyclopropane are no longer in common use, operating rooms are still designed to avoid fire hazards from these anaesthetics. Any oxygen-enriched atmosphere, especially at elevated pressures, justifies continued caution.

Hazards of Gases

Before the 1970s gases were exhausted into the OR. Now waste gases are drawn through an exhaust ventilator to the outside.

The OR is specifically designed to provide protection against fire from flammable gas, toxic effects of anaesthesia that may escape inadvertently into the atmosphere and the dangers of electrical spark ignition and shock. To monitor operating room personnel for exposure to toxic material, a dosimetry indicator, such as that illustrated in Fig. 24.12, may be used.

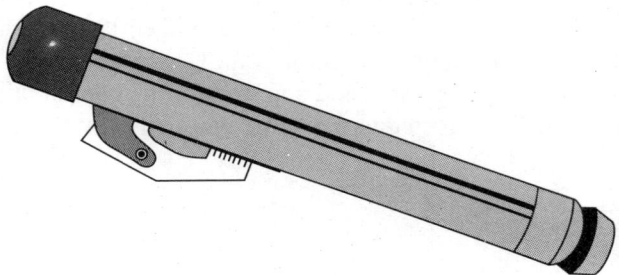

Fig. 24.12. A pocket chemical dosimetry device.

The ventilating system of the OR usually produces a positive pressure to sweep contaminated air out through doors, openings and exhaust vents. It also regulates the temperature and humidity.

To reduce the probability of flame due to sparks, the humidity should be kept above 50 per cent; in non-flammable areas it may be allowed to drop to 30 per cent. Since oxygen and most flammable anaesthetics are heavier than air, they tend to sink to the floor. Exhaust vents in the OR are therefore mounted within three inches of the floor, which helps to keep dangerous gas from reaching the faces of people working there. The air inlet is near the OR ceiling and ventilation should exceed eight air changes per hour. In general, the ventilating system should keep the toxic and flammable gases in the OR below five feet.

To keep explosive gas out of contact with electrical outlets in the OR, since sparks may be created when power cords are plugged in or pulled out, outlets are placed five feet above the floor. Furthermore, all switches and wires are enclosed in screens to prevent ignition due to sparks. Hot spots, such as fixed lighting, are located more than eight feet above the floor. To guard against sparks that could cause a fire from static charges induced by shoes, clothing and equipment, a conductive floor with a resistance of less than 1 megohm should be installed in an OR qualified for flammable anaesthetics. This high resistance conductive path bleeds off any build-up of static charge.

The resistance of the floor is specified to be an average greater than 25 kΩ, measured with an electrode 2.5 inches in diameter and at no point should it be less than 10 kΩ. The lower limit on the resistance offers protection against macroshock to OR personnel by limiting shock current should they come in contact with a high voltage.

An isolation transformer is used to maintain an open circuit between the ground and the return path of currents in the electrical equipment. This reduces the probability that a spark will be created by faults in the equipment. It also reduces the possibility that operating room personnel who wear conductive clothing will receive shocks.

Because of the gas hazards in the OR, personnel must be careful to avoid bringing in any objects that might be sources of ignition or static charges.

All portable equipment in the OR should be labelled for 'flammable' or 'non-flammable' use. Electrosurgical units or lasers are not to be used with flammable anaesthetics, because they cut with a spark; neither are appliances such as portable drills. Portable X-ray machines require special approval for use with flammable anaesthetics. Equipment with hot spots is either permanently mounted above the five-foot level in the OR or mounted on portable devices that keep it above that level.

Any foot treadle switch should be explosion-proof unless non-flammable anaesthetics are being used and it should be splash-proof. Flexible power cords may sometimes be used in the OR when the extension receptacles are permanently attached to equipment.

To further prevent static sparks, all accessory devices should be either conductive or antistatic, if the use of conductive materials is impractical. For example, antistatic sheets should be used, as should conductive footwear with a resistance of less than 500 kΩ to prevent sparks. Sparks from hot wires coming into contact with ground may be avoided by use of an isolation transformer, isolating the OR power currents.

Before 1950, the anaesthetics in use, primarily chloroform and diethyl ether, were flammable. It was then that the previously mentioned techniques to protect against fire in the OR were developed. With the introduction of non-flammable anaesthesia, the requirement to use these techniques was sometimes relaxed. However, in cases where an oxygen-rich environment exists, such as in pressure chambers, at other than atmospheric pressure, the fire hazard returns and fire safety precautions should be taken. Other common flammable substances found in the hospital are aldehydes, ketones, esters, benzene, toluene and oils. Other flammable gases include cyclopropane, ethyl chloride and ethylene. Therefore, precautions against fire hazards are always prudent. Halothane is used in the OR to reduce the flammbility of anaesthetics. The common non-flammable anaesthetic nitrous oxide is toxic. Clinical personnel should not breathe air containing more than 5 parts per million (ppm) and the temperature of exposed surfaces in its presence should be below 130°F. Ethylene oxide, another toxic gas used for sterilising procedures in the OR had an exposure limit of less than 50 ppm in 1982, but this was changed to 2 ppm in 1987.

Pressure Chambers

High-pressure facilities, called hyperbaric chambers, are used in medical procedures to facilitate oxygen transfer in the blood. The partial pressure of oxygen in the blood, P_{O_2}, is greatly increased when the patient is placed in a hyperbaric chamber. For example, in a 100 per cent oxygen atmosphere, P_{O_2} increases from 650 mmHg to 200 mmHg as the pressure increases from 1 to 3 atmospheres (atm). This allows the use of blood with less haemoglobin when large quantities of blood are required.

Under conditions of 100 per cent oxygen at 3 atm, the danger of fire is acute. Thus, a hyperbaric chamber should have a non-combustible floor and be equipped with fire extinguishers and fire detectors. Flameproof clothing and conductive footwear are required, as are individual breathing supplies for occupants. One is cautioned not to introduce cotton, wool, synthetic fabrics, flammable hairspray or skin oil into the environment. X-ray and electrosurgical equipment are not allowed in these chambers. In general, the chamber must be rated safe for 100 per cent oxygen at 3 atm of pressure.

PREVENTIVE MAINTENANCE

Preventive maintenance is done on medical equipment to make sure that it is safe and in proper working order. The inspections necessary to ensure that safety specifications are met are a part of the preventive maintenance procedure. Furthermore, equipment should be inspected to ensure that it is calibrated accurately. Physicians use the output data from medical equipment to make diagnoses and to prescribe treatment of disease, so inaccurate data from the equipment can clearly lead to serious mistakes. Preventive maintenance can protect a patient by reducing the likelihood of these mistakes.

Preventive maintenance procedures are recommended by the manufacturers of equipment and are usually given in the equipment service manual. Every biomedical equipment shop should have a programme of regular preventive maintenance that goes beyond the basic safety checks described in the previous section.

The frequency of preventive maintenance depends on how vital the instrumentation is and on the frequency of observed failures. Preventive maintenance of equipment used to maintain vital functions such as patient blood circulation or breathing should be more frequent than that of equipment that does not come in contact with the patient. Also, if a particular kind of equipment is observed to fail frequently, it should be scheduled for more frequent inspections.

In spite of all precautions taken, however, equipment will fail. In fact, certain parts of equipment are wearing parts and like automobile tyres, must be changed periodically. X-ray tubes, chemical electrodes and air filters are examples of wearing parts in medical equipment. In any case, when the equipment becomes inoperative, it is necessary to do troubleshooting and repair.

A LOGICAL APPROACH TO TROUBLESHOOTING

Troubleshooting is done either by analysis based on circuit theory or by re-call of previous cases, sometimes called the case-study approach. These are two different logical processes that can be used to fix broken equipment.

The case-study approach would be used if a piece of equipment were known to have a chronic or repetitive, problem. In this case one would naturally check to see if it had reoccurred before looking for other problems. This is an example of the approach often used by physicians in diagnosing disease. Equipment repair records are used to systematically store such information. The records form a database that can be accessed with the shop computer as an aid to troubleshooting.

The other basic method of troubleshooting uses logical analysis of given evidence. In this procedure data relating to the problem is gathered and used to isolate the cause analytically. Because circuit theory is basic to the design of medical equipment, it could, in principle, be used to deduce every problem with the hardware. However, that process may be more complicated than is necessary. A systematic approach to troubleshooting uses both methods, analysis and re-call.

A flow diagram outlining logical steps to troubleshooting is presented in Fig. 24.13. In troubleshooting you would follow the steps indicated until the problem is identified. At whatever step this happens, you would skip down to step 25, fix the equipment and assess the need for future preventive maintenance.

Step one in the diagram implies that in troubleshooting, all available resources should be used. This begins with assessing the environment. Is there an emergency or a hazard involved? It is important also to interview the person who reported the problem and to use diplomacy and tact so that issues of personal blame do not arise. Others who have been involved with the equipment may also be interviewed.

Equipment is organised at various levels, the most complex being the system level. A system consists of units. Each unit might be a different type of equipment such as an electrocardiograph or a pressure monitor. Each unit consists of modules that perform particular functions within the equipment. One module may consist of a transducer and another the signal processing section of the unit. The modules consist of circuit boards and discrete elements and circuit boards themselves consist of discrete elements. The troubleshooting process is the effort to find the discrete element or elements that have failed. The logical process described here is to start at the system level and work down to the discrete element.

At the system level, interconnecting cables, which are vulnerable to breakage, loosening and corrosion, should be checked early in the troubleshooting process. It is then necessary to isolate the sub-system unit that may be causing the problem.

At the unit level, patient cables and other cables attached to the equipment should be checked. At this point you may want to refer to the equipment service manual for equipment troubleshooting aids. Many medical instruments display error message that aid in troubleshooting. Sometimes these appear automatically; other times self-testing procedures must be externally executed. At this point (step 11 in the figure) it will be necessary to open the equipment casing, if the trouble has not been located. After a visual and tactile assessment, it is good policy again to check the cables. One good test of a cable is to invert it in its connector, if possible. If the symptoms of the problems change, the cable is probably bad.

Troubleshooting at the circuit-board level is facilitated if the equipment block diagram provided in the service manual is used as a guide. Troubleshooting flowcharts are often provided to expedite the process. Data for problem analysis may be gathered from designated test points. The equipment's maintenance history may give some clue. Further information may be obtained by telephoning the manufacturer's representative, who should have a broad perspective on the kinds of problems that the equipment may be susceptible to. As indicated in step 22, this data can be used to isolated the problem either to a particular board or to an ancillary component that is often too large or that gets too hot to be attached to a board because of heat sink requirements.

If a particular circuit board has been found to be the source of the problem, it may be replaced by a board known to be good. Before a board swap is made, however, a visual inspection should be performed to look for any evidence of short circuits or overheating. Checks should be made for power supply over-voltage, which could damage a new board. Antistatic spray should be used to prevent damage due to static charge build-up. Circuit boards are expensive and all precautions should be taken not to damage them during troubleshooting procedures.

If a board swap does not correct the problem or change the symptoms, the old board should be put back and the analysis process should be continued.

When a circuit board has been found to be faulty, component-level troubleshooting should be done. This involves detailed signal tracing, voltage and resistance measurements and use of the equipment schematic showing interconnections between the individual components. This task is sometimes highly specialised. Before it is undertaken, a decision has to be made either to fix the board in house or to send it back to the manufacturer. This depends on the complexity of the board, how it is manufactured and the cost of one option versus the other. Since shipping circuit boards is easily done and the manufacturer may have specialists who can fix the board most economically, this option should always be considered.

When the source of the problem is discovered, the repair procedure will involve systematic disassembling and re-sembling of the equipment. To disassemble the equipment, number each part as you remove it. Then to reassemble, replace the parts in the reverse order, in order to be sure you are putting all the parts back together correctly.

Equipment repair requires manual dexterity and an ability to solder parts. After the troubleshooting and repair procedures have been completed, the need for future preventive maintenance of the equipment should be assessed.

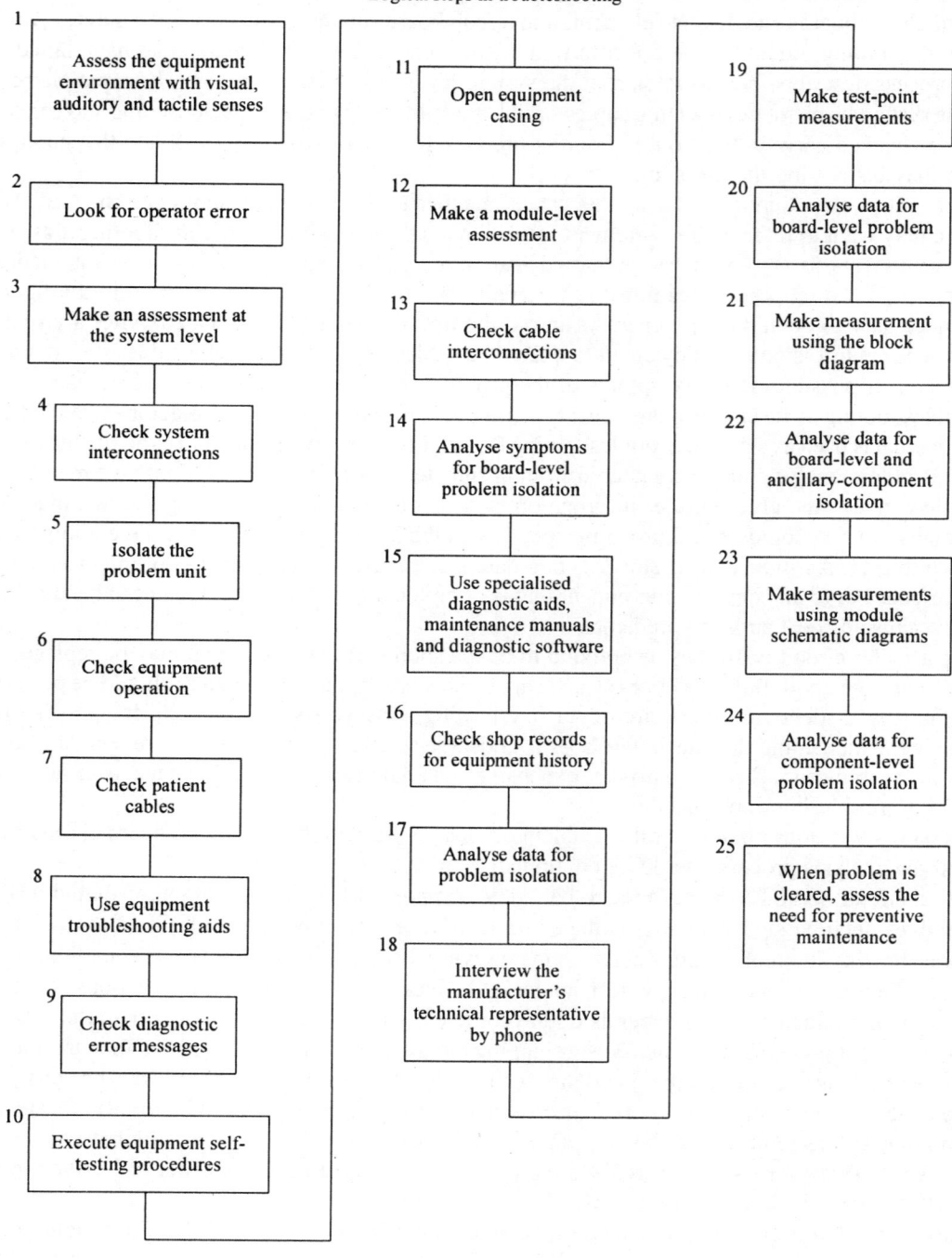

Fig. 24.13. A general troubleshooting flowchart.

Chapter 25

Computer Application in Biomedical Instrumentations

INTRODUCTION

The modern digital computer is well known to nearly everyone in our culture because it is so utterly widespread. The computer is, however, a relatively new technology in that it did not exist prior to World War II. Although there were programmable 'analytic engines' that were based on mechanical devices, the concept of the digital computer had to await the development of electronic switches that could carry on the switching functions that are required in a computer at ultrahigh speeds.

Although companies like IBM and certain advanced universities worked on computers in the 1930s, it took necessities of war to stimulate the development of the computer. The first practical computers were developed under the auspices of military and naval authorities who needed fire control computations for their big guns. The calculations for a large cannon are not very difficult on the mathematical scale of things, but they have to be made and are 'labour intensive' (as the saying goes). The computer could make the calculations based on inputs from observers, the number of rounds fired (barrels warp as they heat) and other factors and then direct the crew where to point the gun.

The early computer pioneers were divided into two camps. On the one hand, some of them wanted to build special-purpose computers that were optimised for a specific job (like artillery). But the other faction, in one of the greatest insights and most far-reaching visions of the twentieth century, decided to build a programmable digital computer. The concept is simple, but at the time it was revolutionary: a single processor that would obey instructions that were stored in memory bank (along with data). By writing a program, that is, a set of instructions that tell the computer what to do, the user could make the same machine do a lot of different chores.

The microcomputer has literally revolutionised medical (and other) instrument and control system design. Where designers were once strictly analog engineers, the instrument designer today has to be a synergist who can integrate the principles of the sensor selection, analog circuit design, computer hardware selection and/or design and software. Today, even small instruments are based on microcomputer chips and for that reason we are going to consider these devices in some detail.

DATA BASE MANAGEMENT (DBM)

Computer-based database management systems (DBMSs) have evolved rapidly over the last few years. Essentially, they are used for entry, storage, processing and retrieval of information through the application of computer technology. They consist of one or more data files, the software programs that create, update or delete these files and the necessary hardware (personal, mini or mainframe computer). Figure 25.1 is a block diagram of a simple DBMS.

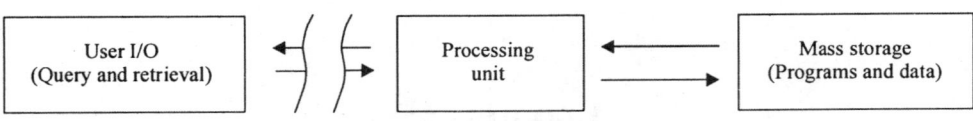

Fig. 25.1. A simple DBMS.

Advantages and Disadvantages of a DBMS

A primary advantage of automated DBMSs, when compared with manual systems, is the speed with which information can be entered, stored, manipulated and retrieved. Manual record-keeping systems, however, prevail to this day in institutional or office-based medical practices. They provide, in most cases, relatively rapid data storage mechanisms. (It is easy and requires little skill to file a report manually in a cabinet.) However, the manual processing retrieval of information that consists of handwritten records in patient charts, as is often the case in clinical research, may in many instances be slow, inaccurate and frustrating. Through the use of a DBMS, a large institution can ensure that information is centrally maintained so that it can be shared by many users, thus avoiding redundancy and possible inconsistencies. At the same time, dedicated files containing data of interest to only one user can still be maintained locally in specific areas of application. In addition, an automated DBMS ensures data integrity, consistency and security to a much greater extent than manual record keeping.

The main disadvantages associated with a DBMS compared with manual record keeping are the higher cost, the need for more comprehensive training of users and the dependence on complex hardware.

Faced with the need to implement a DBMS, a potential user is offered two main alternatives: the development of an in-house system or the acquisition of a commercial package.

IN-HOUSE SYSTEMS

In-house DBMSs can be tailored to the specific needs of an institution, department within the institution or a medical office. In the hospital environment such systems require the close co-operation of the departments involved and a data-processing facility. An in-house programming staff is desirable. A system can then be designed for the specific needs of the users, although its capacity for expansion may be limited. The in-house approach is not the best for a medical office or an institution with limited manpower resources. In a hospital setting, a typical computer-based database may include personal and demographic information on in-patients and out-patients, usually entered in a data file at the time of a person's admission to the hospital or visit to an out-patient department. Additional records may be entered into the same or other data files during the course of a patient's hospital stay and during subsequent hospitalisations or visits to the out-patient department. These records may originate in various ancillary departments (such as clinical laboratory radiology, pharmacy, central services, dietary and business office) and may consist of physicians' orders, requests for tests or treatments, reports from laboratories or other hospital departments, business office charges, information needed by insurance companies or government agencies and so on. Creation, addition, storage, retrieval, modification and eventual deletion of patient records are functions performed by the DBMS and controlled by its users. Figure 25.2 illustrates the interactions that take place in a typical hospital DBMS.

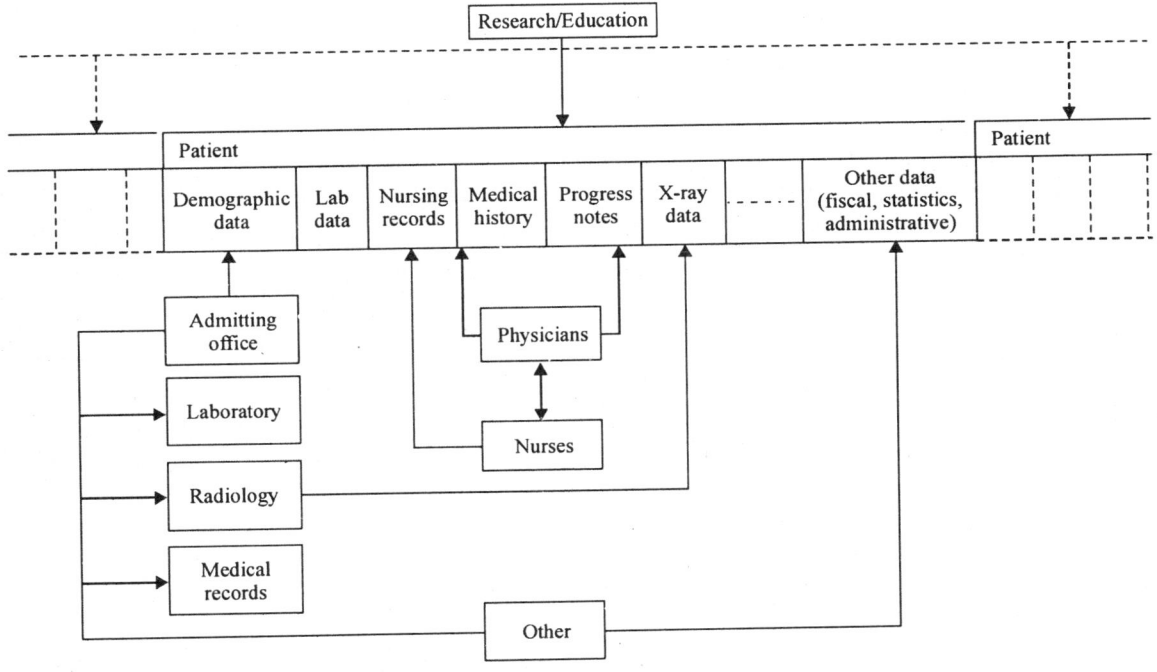

Fig. 25.2. Interactions affecting a patient database.

COMMERCIALLY AVAILABLE SYSTEMS

Commercially available DBMSs have become increasingly sophisticated in recent years. Entry, review and modification of information can take place interactively. Printed reports can be produced by a variety of devices from portable printers to graphic hard-copy hardware. DBMSs now offer sorting of records on one or more keys, in ascending or descending order and other forms of information processing without the need for special application programs.

Many DBMSs can be used by individuals with little or no knowledge of computer technology after they acquire a certain amount of training. This includes learning to use a query language, which is many cases closely resembles a natural language. Furthermore, the use of data dictionaries simplifies access to the information stored in the database. A dictionary consists of one-time entries that describe the attributes of data and files contained in the database. In most cases the database administrator(s) (one or more individuals) is responsible for the identification of information to be included in a database, its storage or display format, the length of time it should be preserved, users who should be allowed to access it and so on.

DESIRABLE FEATURES

Careful consideration should be paid to the functionality of any DBMS whether it is an in-house project or a commercial turnkey package. The following features are highly desirable in a medical environment.

1. Any piece of information should enter the DBMS only once. A patient should not be asked the same question more than once; name, address, social security number and other demographic or personal data should be entered into the system at admission time and should not have to be re-entered by laboratory, radiology, pharmacy or other departments. Data entered at one point should instantaneously be available to all need-to-know areas, avoiding redundant entry which is obviously inefficient and invites inconsistencies.
2. Any incorrect action should generate a reaction. Failure to make a necessary entry or the entry of erroneous data should generate an immediate reaction by the system itself or a later reaction by another user (i.e., a request for an X-ray examination should not be accepted by the system if height and weight have not been entered by nursing personnel into the patient's record). This rule prevents most human errors of omission or commission.
3. User accountability should be built into the system. Any transaction taking place in the DBMS, including entering, updating, transferring or deleting records, should take place in such a way that date, time, place and responsible person can be identified.
4. New needed data should be derived from existing primary data whenever possible. For example, patient's data of birth do not change but their ages at subsequent hospitalisations do.
5. Checks for logically impossible errors should be implemented whenever possible. Manual entry of systolic blood pressure of 160 mm Hg for an actual reading of 140 mm Hg cannot be logically prevented, but an entry of 350 mm Hg should immediately generate an error message to the user since most manometers read a maximum of 300 mm Hg.
6. Data should be independent of application programs using the DBMS. Modifications to existing programs or the addition of new ones to the environment using a DBMS should not affect data structures or elements.
7. Data should be independent of users. Adding or removing DBMS users from the environment should not affect data structures or elements.
8. Users and programs should be able to share data. A comprehensive DBMS permits multiple user access to the data files through a number of different application programs.
9. Updates to one record by a user should not make it necessary for other records in the database to be updated manually by the user.

SPECIFIC MEDICAL APPLICATIONS

Both commercial and special-purpose in-house medical DBMSs have proliferated in recent years and it is anticipated that their usage will increase as hardware costs decrease, as software becomes more sophisticated and as user acceptance grows. Large medical databases have been created and continue to increase in size in areas of application such as:

1. Creation, maintenance and update of medical records.
2. The evaluation of the long-term results of coronary artery by-pass surgery.
3. The acquisition, storage and retrieval of long-term electrocardiographic monitoring data.
4. Registries for neurological disorders.
5. Tumour registries and others.

ACCESS CONTROL

The confidentiality of medical records must be preserved. Although it is virtually impossible to prevent all unauthorised access to any database, efforts should be made to that effect. This includes attention to the placement of remote stations or other input/output devices, the use of passwords, access codes or user identification mechanisms, limiting access to hard-copy devices, printing and reviewing logs and audit trails, restricting user access to specific data files and so on. Particularly vulnerable to intrusion are those databases that can be accessed through telephone data lines.

BACK-UP AND REMOTE STORAGE

The data contained in a medical database are vital to the institution or the medical office and their safety and integrity must be preserved. Critical data files, shared by many users and updated frequently, should be backed up on removable storage media (magnetic tape, disks, etc.) at regular and frequent intervals. Less critical files should be backed up at intervals dictated by the frequency of updates to those files. In addition, a standard operating procedure should be instituted whereby weekly or monthly back-up files are created and stored in removable storage media, kept preferably at a location remote from the institution or office. Thus a fire, flood or other natural disaster cannot cause total loss of the information.

COMPUTERISED CRITICAL CARE UNITS

A critical care unit is an area in a hospital where highly trained personnel and sophisticated equipment are concentrated to take care of a limited number of actually or potentially severely ill patients. Special units may be known as general intensive care units or labelled according to the type of patients treated. Thus we have medical, surgical, neurological, respiratory or pediatric intensive care units. Coronary care units, recovery rooms, telemetry monitoring areas, burn and trauma units are also critical care areas. Physicians trained to work in these units are commonly referred to as 'intensivists'. Likewise, nursing personnel permanently assigned to these units undergo specialised training.

Computers are now commonplace in critical care areas in both large and small hospitals. They cover a wide range of applications, from the microprocessor that controls specialised bedside and nurses desk monitoring equipment to the mini or mainframe computer that is part of either a dedicated critical care system or an integrated overall hospital-wide information facility. Figure 25.3 represents a commonly seen special care unit arrangement, consisting of (i) microprocessor-controlled patient monitoring hardware with bedside and nursing-desk scopes and controls, as well as hard-copy functions; and (ii) remote computer stations, usually video display terminals (VDT) communicating through a central mainframe installation with ancillary departments, other patient care areas and business and financial offices.

The first attempts at computer-assisted patient monitoring in critical care areas took place in the 1960s. Some of the early applications were based on electrocardiographic waveform analysis and attempted to establish the morphologic diagnosis of myocardial ischemia or injury, conduction defects or chamber enlargement. Other developments focusing on the automated recognition of cardiac arrhythmias followed but had limited success and to this day arrhythmia interpretation by computer remains an elusive goal since technology has not yet equalled the human mind in recognising complex patterns.

Today it is unusual to find drug infusion devices. ECG and blood pressure monitors, intraaortic balloon assist pumps or other critical care unit devices that are not controlled by microprocessors. Many of these new devices also have built-in communication controllers that allow them to transfer information to and/or be controlled by, an external computer system. A microprocessor-controlled bedside physiologic monitoring unit in a coronary care unit can be used. It is primarily used to acquire, display and transmit a patient's heart rate, electrocardiogram and arterial blood pressure, but additional parameters can be incorporated. Built-in audible and visual alarms alert the staff if pre-set upper or lower limits are exceeded in any monitoring channel.

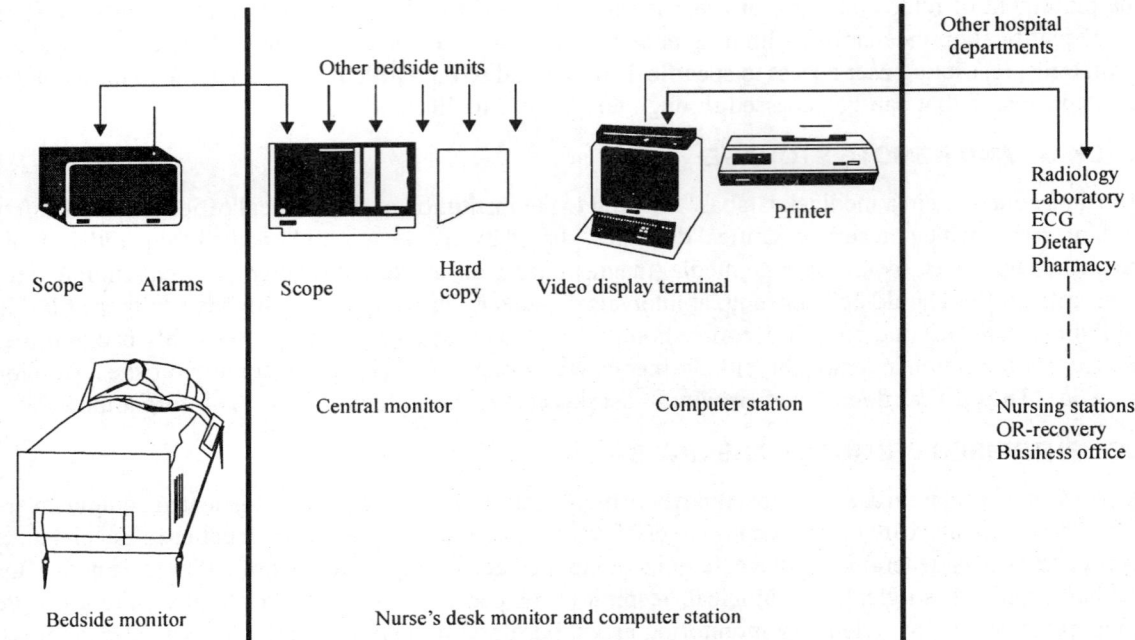

Fig. 25.3. Diagram of a typical critical care unit arrangement consisting of microprocessor controlled bedside and central-station monitors, complemented by a computer station.

With the advancement of technology, personal computers and even small hand-held computers have become popular because they offer powerful processing tools in small and relatively inexpensive packages. Permanent printed records can be maintained since many of these small systems accept compatible hard-copy devices. Programs are available that accept as input hemodynamic and blood gas information to calculate and print a patient's hemodynamic profile. Other programs control infusion of drugs or blood, perform cardiac output and drug dosage calculations, help manage the treatment of acid-base disorders or assist in hyperalimentation therapy. These small dedicated computers allow, in some cases, transfer of information to a larger central system if this is available.

In a typical intensive care unit organisation in the foreground, a remote computer station tied to a central hospital-wide-information system is complemented by a portable desktop printer. On top of the station, a computer-controlled device with sound and light alarms alerts the staff when critical laboratory results arrive or when blood needed for a transfusion becomes available. In the background, a microprocessor controlled, multichannel, central monitoring station displays information simultaneously available at the patient's bedside.

In addition to automated bedside monitoring, computer technology is used in special care units for acquisition, storage and processing of patient information needed for determination and reporting of trends, requesting and reporting ancillary department tests or procedures and administrative functions such as inventory control and billing. These uses result in the elimination of manual tasks, improve accuracy, eliminate redundant bookkeeping and reduce the possibility of human errors. Figure 25.4 illustrates the complementing functions in a special care unit of both the physiologic monitoring hardware and the centralised mainframe-based hospital information system.

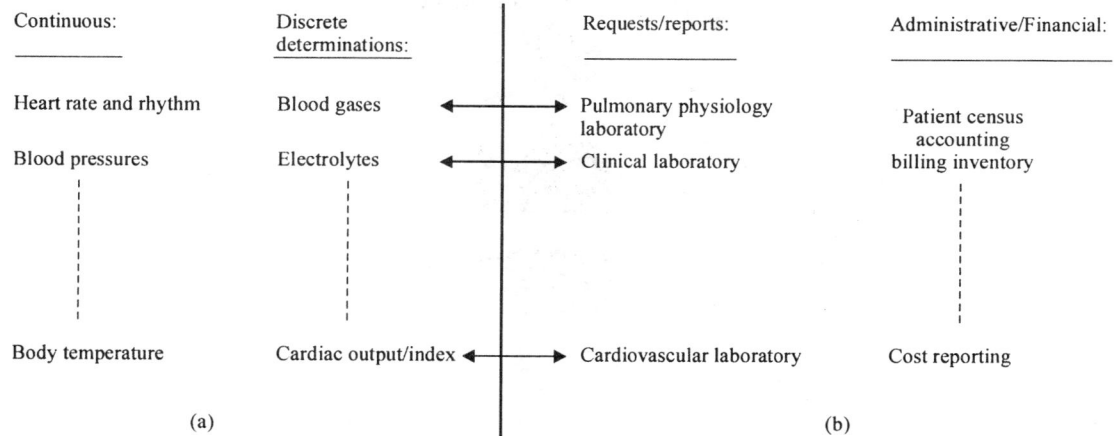

Continuous:	Discrete determinations:	Requests/reports:	Administrative/Financial:

Heart rate and rhythm   Blood gases ←→ Pulmonary physiology laboratory

Patient census accounting

Blood pressures   Electrolytes ←→ Clinical laboratory

billing inventory

Body temperature   Cardiac output/index ←→ Cardiovascular laboratory

Cost reporting

(a)   (b)

Fig. 25.4. Functional interactions between physiologic monitoring in special care areas and departments served by a hospital-wide, computer-based information system. (a) Physiologic monitoring; and (b) information system.

PLANNING AND DESIGNING A COMPUTERISED CRITICAL CARE UNIT

Experience has shown that a computer system can help to reduce the length of stay of a patient in a special care area. In this age of increased awareness of the cost of providing high technology health care, this fact results in better utilisation of the resources in the unit and lower costs can be expected. Those individuals involved in the process of planning, designing and activating a state-of-the-art critical care unit incorporating advances in computer technology may want to follow the steps outlined below. However, every institution presents a different environment and therefore, individual designs will probably be significantly personalised.

1. A planning committee including medical and nursing staff members as well as high-level administrative personnel should be established. Delegating the task of planning a project of this magnitude to lower-level management may not produce satisfactory results.

2. A comprehensive evaluation of existing and projected patient care needs should be undertaken to determine specifications for the special care unit in question. Some of these specifications may be determined by existing facilities and/or budgetary constraints. A state-of-the-art unit should incorporate the capability to acquire and process signals representing biological variables as continuous functions of time (physiological monitoring), as well as acquisition, storage, processing and recall of discrete patient information. If no centralised computer system is available in the institution, the a small dedicated special care system may be realistic approach. On the other hand, if a comprehensive hospital information system is currently available, as is the case in many institutions throughout the country, then a major objective should be the integration of a special care unit into the central system.

3. When considering automation in the unit, a decision must be made early in the planning process whether to obtain a commercial turnkey hardware-software package, as opposed to the in-house development of a dedicated microprocessor or minicomputer-based special care unit system. If a mainframe central installation is available, a link to it should be considered in either case. Figure 25.5 lists several approaches to linking a mainframe-based hospital information system and a dedicated local or satellite computer.

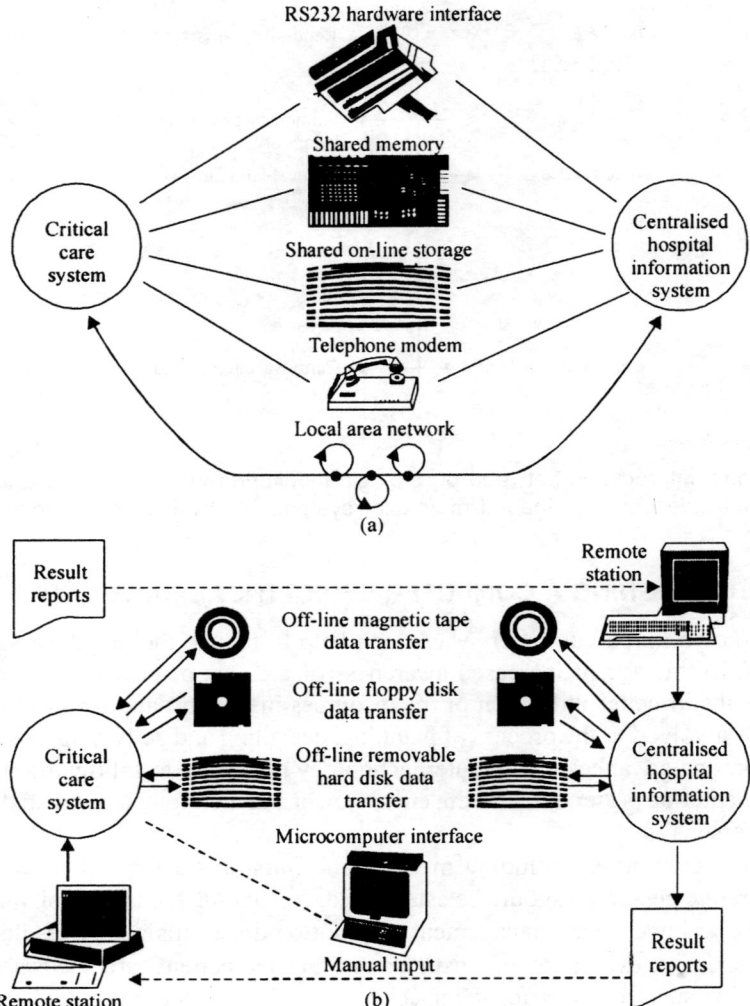

Fig. 25.5. Direct (a) and indirect (b) approaches to establishing communications between a dedicated special care system and a central mainframe-based hospital information system.

The choice of one of these approaches may depend to a large degree on existing facilities, equipment, staff and experience. In-house developed computer systems have the advantages of being designed and built according to the needs and desires of the staff and afford the ability to make changes as they become necessary, sometimes on short notice. One disadvantage of the in-house approach is that the development time may be long and therefore, personnel costs may be high. Commercially available turnkey systems, on the other hand, are usually ready for production work once installation is completed and development time and costs are substantially lower. However, modifications to the system to meet existing institutional policies or procedures, if needed, may be expensive or not possible. This rigidity of design entails, in many cases, modifications in policies or procedures to conform to a somewhat inflexible, commercial package.

These decisions may not be simple but should be based on the approach that best suits the present and future needs in the existing hospital environment. In any case, provisions should be included during the planning stages for future implementation or expansion of capabilities for automated entry, communication, archiving, processing and reporting of information.

4. Whether acquiring a commercial package or designing an in-house system, the administrative aspects of the operation of the special care units should not be neglected. A special care unit package should provide administrative services (or interact with any existing system that already provides them). These should include, but not be limited to, inventory control, patient charges, bed use and cost analysis information with daily, weekly and/or yearly reports and appropriate audit trails.

5. Once the new computerised techniques for data acquisition, storage, processing and reporting become established, usually after a suitable 'paralleling' period, the old manual methods should be discontinued. However, contingency procedures based on the old methods should be established, documented and tested frequently in the event of an equipment breakdown or other computer system failures.

6. If not already available, an uninterruptible power supply (UPS) should be included as an integral part of the state-of-the-art special care unit. A UPS system should provide power to all computer systems in the unit, if the normal AC service is interrupted. Many computer storage devices are volatile (i.e., random-access memory chips) and do not retain information if the power is interrupted, even for a fraction of second. Therefore, there is a real potential for losing critical patient information obtained during spontaneous clinical events that cannot be reproduced. UPS systems are available in many configurations and capacities depending on the particular electrical service required. Typically, they include a utility-fed rectifier that supplies DC power to a set of batteries and an inverter that provides clean, transient-free AC power to the equipment. The batteries provide back-up during short power failures (minutes) or until the hospital emergency generators take over in case of longer outages.

The actual design of the state-of-the-art critical care unit follows the planning stages and should be a multidisciplinary task. Physicians, nurses, architects, clinical and/or biomedical engineers, data processing personnel and systems engineers should integrate the design team.

Often, too little thought is given to the practical aspects of the room layout, including computer cabling and connections and the design and placement of computer terminal cabinets. These items are often ignored until after the room is already under construction or completed. Many potential problems can be eliminated by building an actual full-size prototype of the proposed critical care area to ensure optimum placement and accessibility of all monitors, computer-related equipment and other necessary devices. Particular attention should be paid to the location of the patient's bed and the space surrounding it, as well as to other pieces of furniture in the room (Fig. 25.6). Thus potential design problems can be resolved before construction actually starts.

SELECTION OF MONITORING EQUIPMENT

There are always questions regarding the number and types of biological variables that should be continuously monitored on special care unit patients. In most institutions, the choice is dictated largely by the capabilities and limitations of the monitoring systems commercially available at any given time. The recent trend towards the use of multiple modular components that may be combined in variable configurations by simply replacing a box in a monitor chassis offers much more versatility than the fixed two, three or four-channel monitors of a few years ago. Table 25.1 lists some commonly monitored physiologic variables.

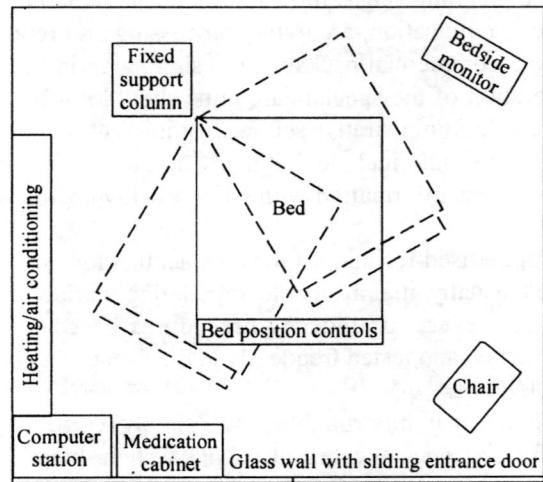

Fig. 25.6. Special care unit layout incorporating a pivoting bed designed to permit maximum accessibility to the patient in the event of an emergency. The support column contain cables and connectors for sensors, oxygen and vacuum lines, computer cables, electrical power outlets and so forth.

Table 25.1. Parameters commonly monitored in a critical care unit.

Electrocardiogram (ECG)—one or more leads
Blood pressure: arterial, central venous
Body temperature
Cardiac output
Blood gases and blood PH
Respiration—(rate and volume)
Serum electrolytes
Electroencephalogram (EEG)—one or two leads
Urinary output
Drainage—chest or abdominal tubes
Fluid intake—oral, intravenous infusion

It is desirable for potential users to become familiar with the technical terminology on equipment specification sheets. These specifications usually describe the actual capabilities of the equipment much more clearly and in more detail than do aggressive sales persons or colourful, eye-catching sales literature. If an in-house biomedical engineering department is available, it should evaluate this information and help the medical and nursing staffs interpret it. Table 25.2 shows a typical specification sheet. Determining what systems are available may require a comprehensive review of the scientific and trade literatures as well as calls and site visits to vendors and users for detailed information. It is recommended that a firm understanding of the capabilities and limitations of any system be established before pricing and contracts are considered. It should be stressed that the selection process should include site visits to institutions that have used or are using equipment similar to that being considered. This should include visits to institutions not in the vendor's reference list. User's level of satisfaction should be noted and equipment performance parameters should be investigated: mean time between failures, mean time to repair, parts availability, vendor response time and so on. Table 25.3 provides a general check list of some of the criteria that should be applied before actually purchasing or leasing computer-based monitoring equipment from any vendor.

Table 25.2. Partial list of specifications for a typical commercial bedside ECG amplifier.

Input impedance:	10 MΩ @ 15 Hz
CMRR:	80 dB
Calibration:	1 mV = 10 mm deflection
Upper frequency limit:	450 Hz (–3 dB)
Linearity tolerance:	1/– 1% in +/– 1.5 V output
Line noise filter:	60 Hz interference reduced by >18 dB
Somatic interference filter:	Attenuation to 25 Hz
Drain:	+/–550 mA
Dimensions:	9.5″ × 12.6″ × 15.7″
Weight:	10.3 lb

Table 25.3. Some of the criteria commonly used for evaluation of monitoring equipments.

Scope size, shape and weight

Number of display channels

Interchangeable modular amplifiers for heart rate, pressures, temperature, etc.

Audible and/or visible alarms

Digital display visibility

Local and/or remote hard copy capabilities

Trend display and trending time periods

Bedside and central nursing station displays

Interface for mainframe and/or local computer system

Ease of maintenance and repairs; availability of spare parts

Vendor-provided training, upgrades and other support

Estimated time to obsolescence of equipment

Certain facts about the vendors being considered should be known early in the evaluation process. These include the vendor's reputation among users of their equipment, the availability of local or conveniently located sales and service personnel, the financial situation and length of existence of these companies and related information.

The warranties supplied with the equipment should be screened very carefully as to extent and limitations. Warranties on electronic equipment often do not extend beyond 90 days. Sometimes warranties are extended by the vendor, especially if large quantities of equipment are being purchased and a service (often called maintenance) contract is signed between the institution and the vendor. If only a 90-day warranty is offered, the equipment should be adequately tested within the warranty period. This can easily be overlooked, especially if the equipment is being purchased for a new facility and arrives before the facility is activated. Finally, it should be noted that the successful implementation of critical care unit systems rests not only on the adequacy of the hardware and software but also on the human component. Users, including physicians, nurses and the technicians, should not only be involved in the selection process, but should receive comprehensive hands-on training in the use of the equipment before and during the actual implementation phase.

MONITORING BY COMPUTER OF PARTICULAR VARIABLES

Arterial Blood Pressure

The blood pressure waveform might be sampled at a rate of 100 per second and the program establishes two time 'windows' at pre-set intervals from the preceding R-wave of the ECG in which it looks for the systolic maximum and the diastolic minimum. Alternatively, a pre-processor can be used to provide outputs on a beat-by-beat basis proportional to the systolic, diastolic and mean pressures.

Ectopic Beats

The ECG could be sampled at 250 or 300 samples per second and the R-waves detected on a basis of their amplitude and the steepness of the downslope. The data points can then be searched again to give the R-wave widths and logic statements in the program used to sort the beats into various categories such as normal, premature, wide, late, premature and wide. The searching of this amount of data uses a lot of computer time and hence it is more effective to use a pre-processor to generate the R-R intervals and R-wave widths. Figures 25.7a and 25.7b, illustrates the use of this pre-processor to monitor the transient ectopic beats consequent upon the intravenous injection of atropine and the use of a beta adrenergic drug to terminate a run of ectopic beats.

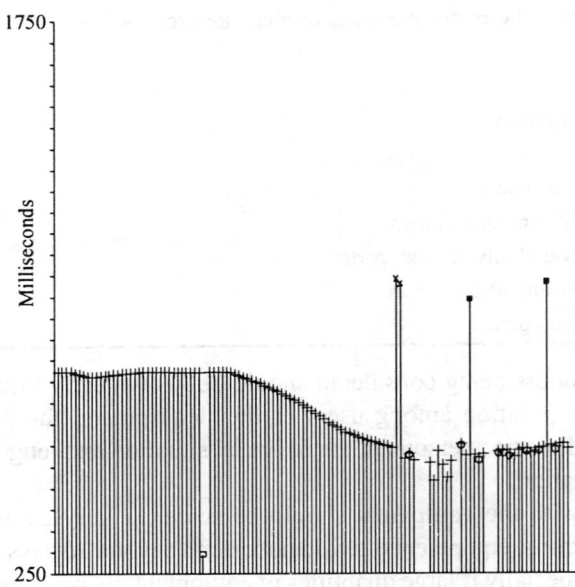

Fig. 25.7a. The use of an analogue pre-processor to identify ectopic beats consequent upon an intravenous injection of atropine.

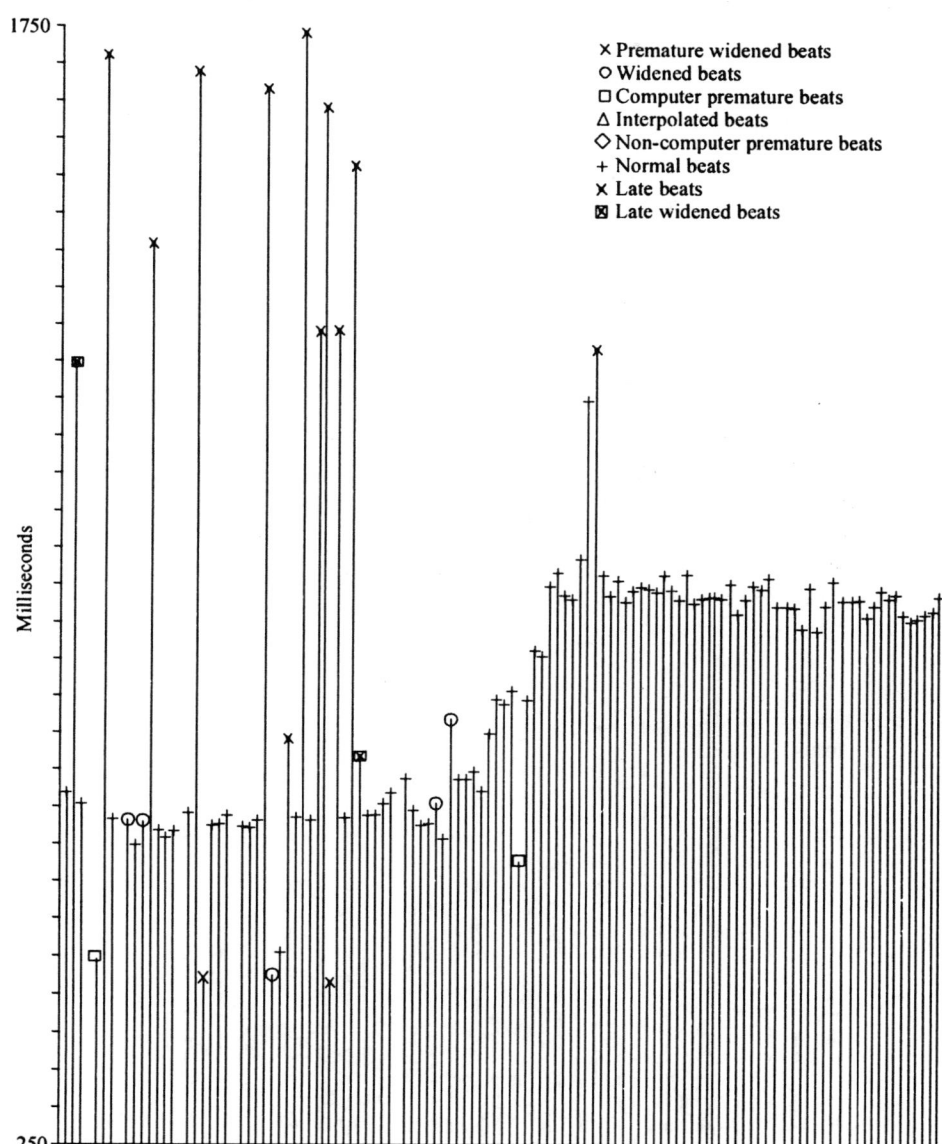

Fig. 25.7b. A similar plot of 128 successive R-R intervals, but showing the action of the drug propanalol is suppressing cardiac arrhythmias.

The occurrence of ectopic beats can be displayed in a variety of ways, for example, plots of successive R-R intervals, Figs. 25.8a and 25.8b, histograms of R-R intervals, Fig. 25.8c or scatter plots, Fig. 25.8d in which alternate R-R intervals are plotted on the X and Y axes of a graph. With a sinus rhythm, the plots should lie within an oval area, but ectopic beats of different origins will form clusters away from the 45° line. Cox has described an efficient pre-processing computer program for the sorting of ectopic beats which is being successfully used in coronary care units.

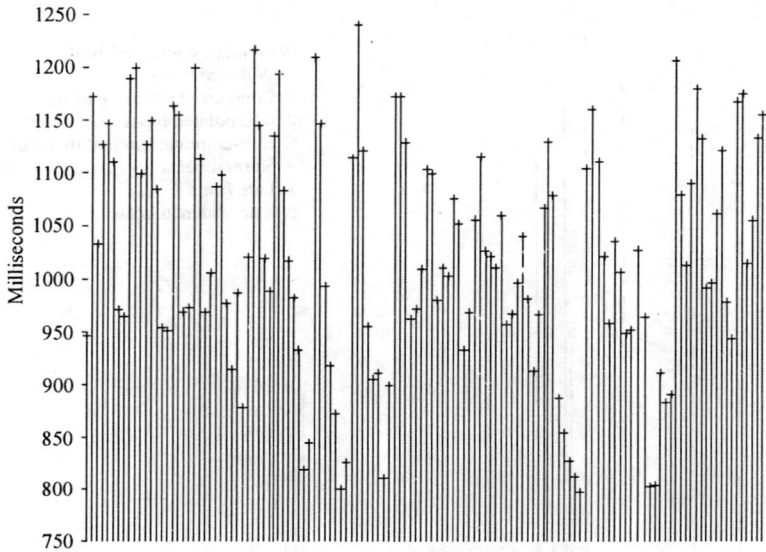

Fig. 25.8a. A plot of 128 successive R-R intervals from a fit young man with a marked sinus arrhythmia, alternate intervals being plotted on the X and Y axes.

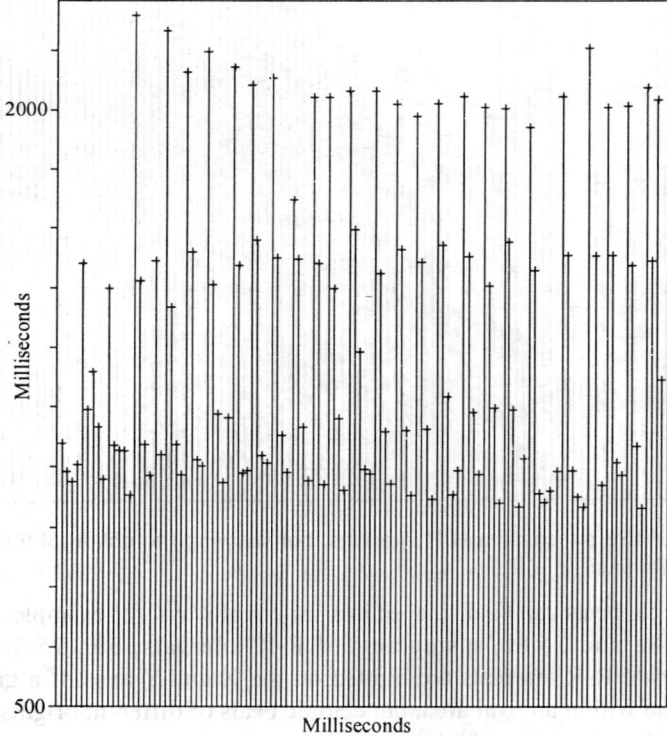

Fig. 25.8b. A similar plot to Fig. 25.8a but for a patient with three competing rhythms.

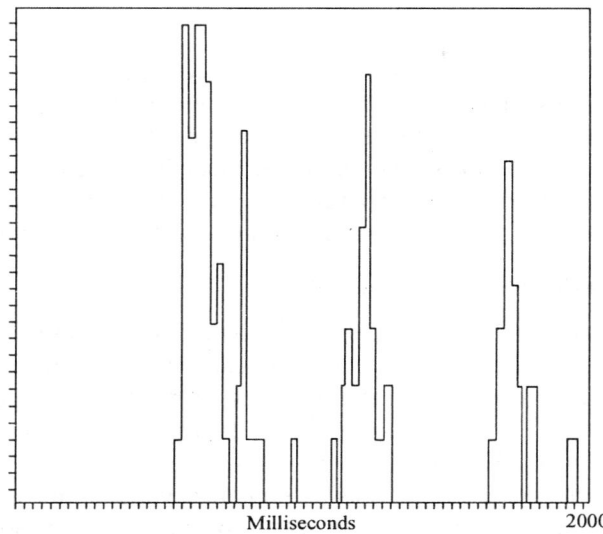

Fig. 25.8c. Histogram of the 128 R-R intervals shown in Fig. 25.8b.

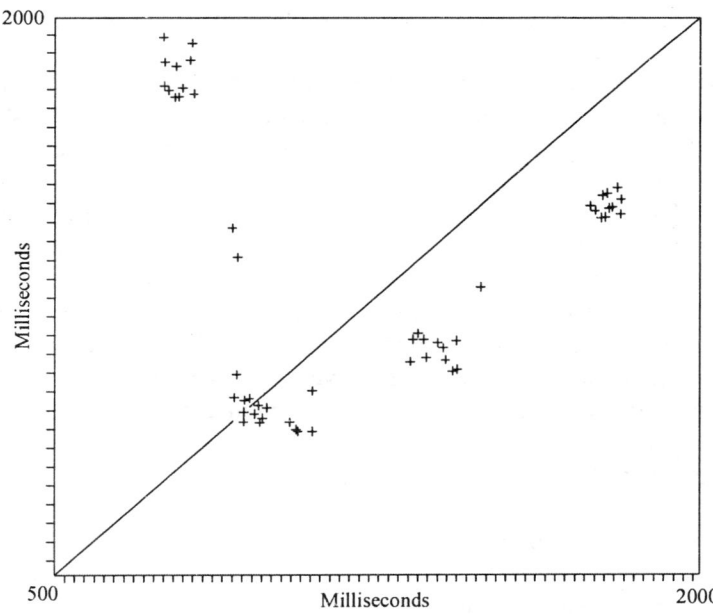

Fig. 25.8d. Scatter plot of the R-R intervals shown in Fig. 25.8b.

Respiratory Rate

Respiratory rate can be monitored indirectly from the pressure fluctuations observed on the central venous pressure or from the variations in the height of the R-waves of the ECG.

Cardiac Output

In the case of the dye dilution technique where re-circulation occurs, it can usually be assumed that the downslope of the dye curve is a simple exponential function from 70 per cent of the peak concentration down to 40 per cent. If the shape of the curve is known from the start of its description to the time at which the concentration has fallen to 40 per cent of the peak then it is possible to forecast the complete area of the curve which would be present if re-circulation did not occur. If less accuracy is tolerable there are a number of approximation methods available for calculating the area under the curve.

Respiratory Mechanics and Ventilator Management

A detailed account of a computer-based patient monitoring system which amongst other variables monitored tidal volume, minute volume, respiratory rate, 'total' compliance of the ventilatory system, non-elastic airway resistance, work of inspiration during positive-pressure breathing, oxygen uptake, respiratory quotient, alveolar ventilation and the ratio of dead space-to-tidal volume is that of Osborn. Hilberman and others have described a phase method of the calculation of respiratory mechanics with a digital computer. Rosner and Caceres discuss the computer analysis of expiratory volume-time curves obtained from a spirometer when a patient breathes maximally or makes a forced expiration. Some of the parameters which can be obtained are the maximum voluntary ventilation and the forced vital capacity, the time to exhale the forced vital capacity, the time of the maximum instantaneous expiratory flow rate, the forced expiratory velocities at 0.5, 0.75, 1 and 3 seconds and the flow rates over the periods 25–75 per cent, 25–50 per cent and 50–75 per cent of the forced vital capacity.

It is also possible to use a pneumotachograph connected to the computer rather than a spirometer. The computer produces a plot of instantaneous expired flow rate versus time. The shape of the curve provides an indication of whether obstructive and/or restrictive abnormalities are present. A restrictive abnormality implies an interference with lung expansion due to pulmonary, pleural or chest wall disease. It is characterised by a reduction in the forced vital capacity with the maintenance of normal expiratory flow rates (peak expiratory flow rate, forced expiratory volume at 1 second and the maximum mid-expiratory flow rate). An obstructive abnormality implies that there is a generalised airway obstruction. This is characterised by a reduction in the expiratory flow rates (forced expiratory volume at 1 second, maximum mid-expiratory flow rate and peak expiratory flow rate). The forced vital capacity may stay normal but it often becomes reduced in the case of a severe obstruction.

The computer can calculate both the patient's actual and predicted values for:
Forced vital capacity (FVC) in litres
Forced expiratory volume at 1 second (FEV1) in litres
FEV1/FVC
Forced expiratory volume at 3 seconds (FEV3) in litres
FEV3/FVC
Peak expiratory flow rate (PEFR) l/second
Maximum mid-expiratory flow rate (MMFR) l/second
Inspiratory capacity in litres
The FEV1 provides useful information about the prognosis in chronic obstructive lung disease. The MMFR provides an assessment of airway resistance and is of use in the detection of early obstructive lung disease. The PEFR is not such a good index of airway obstruction but is affected by factors important to the production of a good cough.

Menin describe a computer program for use with time-sharing terminals. Information is provided about the patient, his respiratory functions and arterial blood gases. The computer generates the patient's respiratory profile and provides a narrative statement of the patient's respiratory condition. It can suggest the optimum ventilator settings for weaning a patient from a ventilator.

Electroencephalograms

The requirements for EEG analysis during patient monitoring are much simpler than the analyses performed by computer for example, in the case of a patient suspected of having epilepsy. Normally only one or two leads are monitored. The use of the Fast Fourier Transform has made it feasible to perform on-line frequency analysis of the EEG. Carrie has given a technique for the analysis of transient EEG abnormalities. Although frequency analysis is particularly suitable for performance on a digital computer, there remains a need for some technique of characterising changes in the wave shape of the EEG and also of providing some degree of data reduction. Hjorth has proposed three descriptors of the EEG. The 'activity' provides a measure of the mean power in the wave over a certain period. The 'mobility' yields a measure of the average slope of the wave as a number of amplitude standard deviations per unit of time whilst the complexity indicates how much the variability of the slope of the EEG signal exceeds that of a comparable sinewave. Hjorth has developed hybrid pre-processing circuitry which will generate the three descriptors in real-time for feeding into a computer. Sufficient clinical evidence is not yet available to indicate the value of this descriptor approach.

Blood pH and Blood-Gas Calculations

Maas and others have described a computer program based on a mini-computer for the calculation of blood acid-base balance parameters. Neff has developed a computer-assisted electrode system for the measurement of blood pH, P_{O_2}, P_{CO_2}, sodium and potassium.

Computer Interpretation of ECG's

The shortage of trained medical staff skilled in the reporting of ECG's is forcing attention on the use of real-time computer systems for the interpretation of ECG's. Program have been written for the analysis of the conventional 12-lead scalar electrocardiogram and the 3-lead vector electrocardiogram. It is becoming usual to employ an ECG trolley which can record 4 groups of 3 scalar leads, each group being approximately 2.5 or 5 seconds in duration followed by 10 seconds of the three vector leads giving a total transmission time of 22 seconds. By means of either the hospital's internal telephone service or a dialled public line, the trolley at the bedside can be connected to the computer. Patient identification data is first sent to the computer by means of a bank of digital switches and then the ECG is transmitted. The interpretation is sent back to a silent thermal printer in the hospital via a conventional digital telephone data link, usually within a few minutes.

Systolic Time Intervals and Myocardial Contractility

When it is required to monitor cardiac function, apart from monitoring cardiac output, a computer can be used to follow changes occurring in systolic time intervals. For this, in addition to an arterial blood pressure waveform, it is necessary to have available a phonocardiogram and an ECG. When a direct recording via a pressure transducer of the arterial pressure is not available, a carotid artery pulse transducer may be used to provide a non-invasive indication of the pulse waveform. The left ventricular ejection time (LVET) is defined as the time interval between the systolic upstroke of the blood pressure waveform and the incisura of the dichrotic notch. The total electromechanical time of the cardiac contraction is taken as the time interval between the onset of the QRS complex of the ECG and the first fast component of the second heart sound of the phonocardiogram. This is the $Q-S_2$ interval. The pre-ejection period (PEP) is taken as the difference between $(Q-S_2)$ and LVET. Reitan found that $1/(PEP)^2$ correlated well with the peak ascending aortic blood flow acceleration which is an index of myocardial contractility, whilst Blackburn found a high correlation between $1/(PEP)^2$ and cardiac output during the administration of carbon dioxide to patients. Blackburn has assumed that PEP is minimally affected by heart rate and changes in afterload. Reitan took $1/(PEP)^2$ to be a good index of the state of myocardial contractility. During a Valsalva manoeuvre, both afterload and heart rate change and so it is likely that both LVET and PEP would change. These changes could result from either a change in the pre-load or in the inotropic state-of-the-heart or of both factors. But, in the blocked Valsalva responses Blackburn also found marked changes occurring in PEP. Since the circulatory reflexes were then inactive, Blackburn felt that the PEP changes resulted from pre-load changes. Blackburn described an analogue pre-processor for calculating PEP. Other possible non-invasive indices of the heart's inotropic state are the ratios P_d/PEP and PEP/LVET where P_d is the diastolic pressure. If S_1-S_2 is the time interval between the first and second heart sounds, the isovolumic contraction time (ICT) is given by (S_1-S_2)—LVET. An indication of the order of magnitude of these quantities can be provided by measurements taken from a 40 year old female, body weight 71.2 kg, who was having a vaginal hysterectomy under halothane, nitrous oxide, oxygen anaesthesia.

Arterial halothane concentration 5.9 mg/100 ml
Cardiac output 5.7 l/min
Arterial blood pressure 82/42 mm Hg
PEP 96 ms
LVET 420 ms
P_d/PEP 438 mm Hg ms^{-1}
S_1-S_2 468 ms
ICT 48 ms
$Q-S_1$ 48 ms
PEP/LVET 0.23
$1/(PEP)^2$ 109
Heart rate 66 beats per minute
Heather index 12.2 (ohms/s)/s = ohms s^{-2}

The Heather index is the ratio of the peak rate change of thoracic electrical impedance during systole in ohms per second to the time interval between the onset of the preceding QRS complex and the attainment of the peak dZ/dt. The Heather index is taken to represent an index of cardiac performance.

Which index to choose as a monitor of the inotropic state-of-the-heart is by no means clear, but in patient's with intact circulatory reflexes current investigations suggest that it is worthwhile using a digital computer to plot on-line values of $1/(PEP)^2$ or the PEP/LVET ratio. Weissler found that in normal subjects the PEP/LVET ratio tends to remain within narrow limits (mean 0.345, S. D. 0.036 in the basal state). The PEP/LVET was found to be increased among patients with heart disease. The differences in the ratio provided a clear separation of subjects with heart disease from normals. The ratio correlated well with cardiac output and stroke volume and provided a simplified semi-quantitative measure of the circulatory impairment in arteriosclerotic and hypertensive heart disease and in primary myocardial disease. Weissler state that evidence current favours the hypothesis that a defect in the contractive performance of the ventricle is primarily responsible for the altered systolic time intervals in heart failure.

Talley found in dogs that PEP may be used as an index of myocardial contractility in situations where the left ventricular end-diastolic pressure is constant or does not vary systematically. They also showed that internal and external measurements of PEP correlated well at left ventricular end-diastolic pressures of less than 12 mm Hg, but increasingly diverged at higher levels of end-diastolic pressure.

Computer Training of Coronary Care Unit Nurses

Warner describes an interesting use of an intensive care digital computer system in providing a teaching aid for coronary care unit nurses. The program simulates the rhythm disturbances a patient with an acute episode of ischaemic heart disease might develop while he was in the coronary care unit. The computer can generate any one of 15 arrhythmias as an ECG on a cathode ray tube. External electrical noise can be simulated by the computer and added to the ECG in the form of mains hum, muscle tremour or the suggestion of a loose electrode. A message is displayed on the screen indicating that three forms of action can be taken: (i) a drug can be given; (ii) a procedure can be carried out; or (iii) more information can be obtained concerning the patient's condition. The nurse has first to diagnose the patient's condition. Once this has been established the nurse might choose to administer digitalis, vasopressors, atropine, isoprenalin, lidocaine, procainamide and quinidine. If she chooses a procedure such as cardioversion, carotid sinus pressure or the use of a pacemaker this is entered by depressing a numbered key. If noise is present it can be cleared by pressing the 'check electrodes' key. After each therapeutic decision is made and the appropriate action taken a transition to a new condition will occur. The program keeps a running score based on the appropriateness of the nurse's decisions and displays this. If no decision is made after two to four sweeps of the oscilloscope's timebase the patient's condition will change again based on the expected natural course of the patient's condition. If no treatment is commenced promptly in conditions such as ventricular fibrillation or hypercalaemia, the patient's death is announced. At any point in the program, the user can call for a chart giving the course of events displayed to date, the blood pressure at the time of each arrhythmia and an indication of whether the patient had been given digitalis. The chart will also indicate the treatment chosen together with the optimum treatment.

TENTATIVE CONCLUSIONS CONCERNING THE VALUE OF COMPUTER-BASED PATIENT MONITORING SYSTEMS

The doctor in charge of implementation of a computer-based patient monitoring system should have charge of the patients and staff in the areas where the system operates and should have a full-time commitment to the operation. The system must be compatible with the existing functioning of the clinical location and should aim to provide a solution to a real problem. Particular attention must be paid to its initial reliability as this will seriously affect the system's subsequent acceptance. A good systems engineer should be available to iron out technical difficulties as they arise.

It seems likely that a computer monitoring system will allow the earlier stabilisation of a patient's condition and that whilst it will not significantly reduce the number of nurses required it will reduce the time they need to spend in taking readings. If computer monitoring reduced the stay of a patient in the ICU by one day and this was offset by an extra day in an ordinary ward, the cost of the monitoring would approximately balance the savings made in the room and ancillary charges.

Chapter 26

Clinical Laboratory: Separation, Spectral and Non-Spectral Methods

INTRODUCTION

The purpose of the clinical laboratory is to analyse body fluids and tissues for specific substances of interest and to report the results in a form which is of value to clinicians in the diagnosis and treatment of disease. A large range of tests has been developed to achieve this purpose. Four terms commonly used to describe tests are accuracy, precision, sensitivity and specificity. An accurate test, on average, yields true values. Precision is the ability of a test to produce identical results upon repeated trials. Sensitivity is a measure of how small an amount of substance can be measured. Specificity is the degree to which a test measures the substance of interest without being affected by other substances which may be present in greater amounts.

The first step in many laboratory tests is to separate the material of interest from other substances. This may be accomplished through extraction, filtration and centrifugation. Another step is derivatisation, in which the substance of interest is chemically altered through addition of reagents to change it into a substance which is easily measured. For example, one method for measuring glucose is to add o-toluidine which, under proper conditions, forms a green-coloured solution with an absorption maximum at 630 nm. Separation and derivatisation both improve the specificity required of good tests.

SEPARATION METHODS

Centrifuges are used to separate materials on the basis of their relative densities. The most common use in the laboratory is the separation of cells and platelets from the liquid part of the blood. This requires a relative centrifugal force (RCF) of roughly 1000 gram (1000 times the force of gravity) for a period of 10 minutes. Relative centrifugal force is a function of the speed of rotation and the distance of the sample from the centre of rotation as stated in Eq. 26.1.

$$\text{RCF} = \left(1.12 \times 10^{-5}\right) r \left(\text{rpm}\right)^2 \qquad \qquad \text{... (26.1)}$$

where RCF = relative centrifugal force in gram and r = radius in cm.

Some mixtures require higher gram-loads in order to achieve separation in a reasonable period of time. Special rotors contain the sample tubes inside a smooth container, which minimises air resistance to allow faster rotational speeds. Refrigerated units maintain the samples at a cool temperature throughout long high-speed runs which could lead to sample heating due to air friction on the rotor. Ultracentrifuges operate at speeds on the order of 10,00,000 rpm and provide relative centrifugal forces of up to 60,00,000 gram. These usually require vacuum pumps to remove the air which would otherwise retard the rotation and heat the rotor.

CHROMATOGRAPHIC SEPARATIONS

Chromatographic separations depend upon the different rates at which various substances moving in a stream (mobile phase) are retarded by a stationary material (stationary phase) as they pass over it. The mobile phase can be a volatilised sample transported by an inert carrier gas such as helium or a liquid transported by an organic solvent such as acetone. Stationary phases are quite diverse depending upon the separation being made, but most are contained within a long, thin tube (column). Liquid stationary phases may be used by coating them onto inert packing materials. When a sample is introduced into a chromatographic column, it is carried through it by the mobile phase. As it passes through the column, the substances which have greater affinity for the stationary phase fall behind those with less affinity. The separated substances may be detected as individual peaks by a suitable detector placed at the end of the chromatographic column.

Gas Chromatography

The most common instrumental chromatographic method used in the clinical laboratory is the gas-liquid chromatograph. In this system the mobile phase is a gas and the stationary phase is a liquid coated onto either an inert support material, in the case of a packed column or the inner walls of a very thin tube, in the case of a capillary column. Capillary columns have the greatest resolving power but cannot handle large sample quantities. The sample is injected into a small heated chamber at the beginning of the column, where it is volatilised if it is not already a gaseous sample. The sample is then carried through the column by an inert carrier gas, typically helium or nitrogen. The column is completely housed within an oven. Many gas chromatographs allow for the oven temperature to be programmed to slowly increase for a set time after the sample injection is made. This produces peaks which are spread more uniformly over time.

Four detection methods commonly used with gas chromatography are thermal conductivity, flame ionisation, nitrogen/phosphorus and mass spectrometry. The thermal conductivity detector takes advantage of variations in thermal conductivity between the carrier gas and the gas being measured. A heated filament immersed in the gas leaving the chromatographic column is part of a Wheatstone bridge circuit. Small variations in the conductivity of the gas cause changes in the resistance of the filament, which are recorded. The flame ionisation detector measures the current between two plates with a voltage applied between them. When an organic material appears in the flame, ions which contribute to the current are formed. The NP detector or nitrogen/phosphorus detector, is a modified flame ionisation detector (see Fig. 26.1) which is particularly sensitive to nitrogen and phosphorus-containing compounds.

Mass spectrometry (MS) provides excellent sensitivity and selectivity. The concept behind these devices is that the volatilised sample molecules are broken into ionised fragments which are then passed through a mass analyser that separates the fragments according to their mass/charge (m/z) ratios. A mass spectrum, which is a plot of the relative abundance of the various fragments versus m/z, is produced. The mass spectrum is characteristic of the molecule sampled. The mass analyser most commonly used with gas chromatographs is the quadrupole detector, which consists of four rods that have DC and RF voltages applied to them. The m/z spectrum can be scanned by appropriate changes in the applied voltages. The detector operates in a manner similar to that of a photomultiplier tube except that the collision of the charged particles with the cathode begins the electron cascade, resulting in a measurable electric pulse for each charged particle captured. The MS must operate in a high vacuum, which requires good pumps and a porous barrier between the GC and MS, that limits the amount of carrier gas entering the MS.

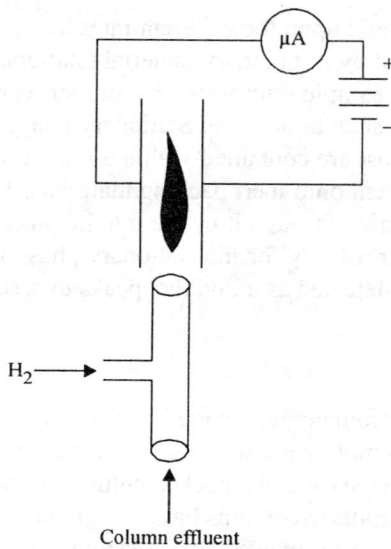

Fig. 26.1. Flame ionisation detector. Organic compounds in the column effluent are ionised in the flame, producing a current proportional to the amount of the compound present.

High-Performance Liquid Chromatography

In liquid chromatography, the mobile phase is liquid. High-performance liquid chromatography (HPLC) refers to system which obtain excellent resolution in a reasonable time by forcing the mobile phase at high pressure through a long thin column. The most common pumps used are pistons driven by asymmetrical cams. By using two such pumps in parallel and operating out of phase, pressure fluctuations can be minimised. Typical pressures are 350–1500 psi, though the pressure may be as high as 10000 psi. Flow rates are in the 1–10 ml/min range.

A common method for placing a sample onto the column is with a loop injector, consisting of a loop of tubing which is filled with the sample. By a rotation of the loop, it is brought in series with the column and the sample is carried onto the column. A UV/visible spectrophotometer is often used as a detector for this method. A mercury arc lamp with the 254 nm emission isolated is useful for detection of aromatic compounds, while diode array detectors allow a complete spectrum from 190 nm to 600 nm in 10 msec. This provides for detection and identification of compounds as they come off the column. Fluorescent, electrochemical and mass analyser detectors are also used.

Basis for Spectral Methods

Spectral methods rely on the absorption or emission of electromagnetic radiation by the sample of interest. Electromagnetic radiation is often described in terms of frequency or wavelength. Wavelengths are those obtained in a vacuum and may be calculated with the formula

$$\lambda = c/v \qquad \qquad ... (26.2)$$

where,

λ = wavelength in meters

c = speed of light in vacuum (3×10^8 m/s)

v = frequency in Hz

The frequency range of interest for most clinical laboratory work consists of the visible (390–780 nm) and the ultraviolet or UV (180–390 nm) ranges. Many substances absorb different wavelengths preferentially. When this occurs in the visible region, they are coloured. In general, the colour of a substance is the complement of the colour it absorbs, e.g., absorption in the blue produces a yellow colour. For a given wavelength or bandwidth, transmittance is defined as

$$T = \frac{I_t}{I_i} \qquad \qquad ... (26.3)$$

where,

T = transmittance ratio (often expressed as per cent)

I_i = incident light intensity

I_t = transmitted light intensity

Absorbance is defined as

$$A = \log_{10} 1/T \qquad \qquad ... (26.4)$$

Under suitable conditions, the absorbance of a solution with an absorbing compound dissolved in it is proportional to the concentration of that compound as well as the path length of light through it. This relationship is expressed by Beer's law:

$$A = abc \qquad \qquad ... (26.5)$$

where,

A = absorbance

a = a constant

b = path length

c = concentration

A number of situations may cause deviations from Beer's law, such as high concentration or mixtures of compounds which absorb at the wavelength of interest. From an instrumental standpoint, the primary causes are stray light and excessive spectral bandwidth. Stray light refers to any light reaching the detector other than light from the desired pass-band which has passed through sample. Source of stray light may include room light leaking into the detecton chamber, scatter from the cuvette and undesired fluorescence. A typical spectrophotometer consists of a light source, some form of wavelength selection and a detector for measuring the light transmitted through the samples. There is no single light source that covers the entire visible and UV spectrum. The source most commonly used for the visible part of the spectrum is the tungsten-halogen lamp, which provides continuous radiation over the range of 360 to 950 nm. The deuterium lamp has become the standard for much UV work. It covers the range from 220–360 nm. Instruments which cover the entire UV/visible range use both lamps with a means for switching from one lamp to the other at a wavelength of approximately 360 nm (Fig. 26.2).

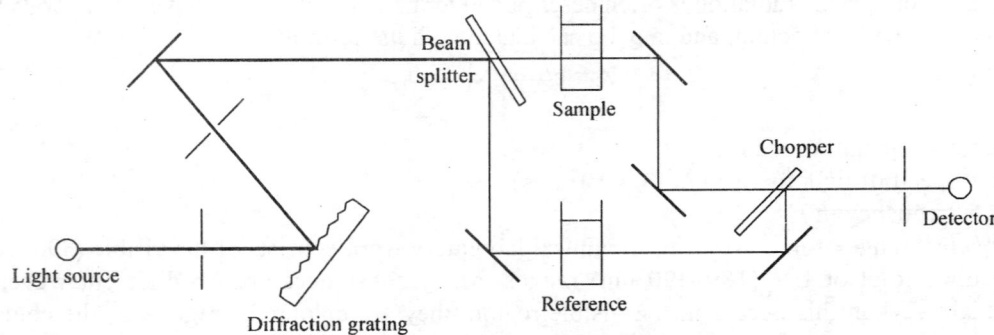

Fig. 26.2. Dual-beam spectrophotometer. The diffraction grating is rotated to select the desired wavelength. The beam splitter consists of a half-silvered mirror which passes half the light while reflecting the other half. A rotating mirror with cut-out sections (chopper) alternately directs one beam and then the other to the detector.

Wavelength selection is accomplished with filters, prisms and diffraction gratings. Specially designed interference filters can provide bandwidths as small as 5 nm. These are useful for instruments which do not need to scan a range of wavelengths. Prisms produce a non-linear dispersion of wavelengths with the longer wavelengths closer together than the shorter ones. Since the light must pass through the prism material, they must be made of quartz for UV work. Diffraction gratings are surfaces with 1000–3000 grooves/mm cut into them. They may be transmissive or reflective; the reflective ones are more popular since there is no attenuation of light by the material. They produce a linear dispersion. By proper selections of slit widths, pass bands of 0.1 nm are commonly achieved.

The most common detector is the photomultiplier tube, which consists of photosensitive cathode that emits electrons in proportion to the intensity of light striking it (Fig. 26.3). A series of 10–15 dynodes, each at 50–100 volts greater potential than the preceding one, produce an electron amplification of 4–6 per stage. Overall gains are typically a million or more. Photomultiplier tubes respond quickly and cover the entire spectral range. They require a high voltage supply and can be damaged if exposed to room light while the high voltage is applied.

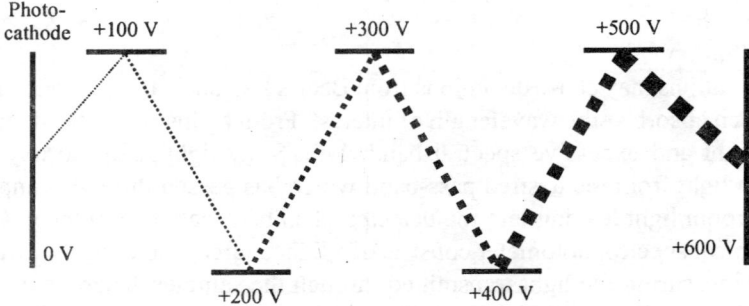

Fig. 26.3. Photomultiplier tube. Incident photons cause the photocathode to emit electrons which collide with the first dynode which emits additional electrons. Multiple dynodes provide sufficient gain to produce an easily measurable electric pulse from a single photon.

Fluorometry

Certain molecules absorb a photon's energy and then emit a photon with less energy (longer wavelength). When the re-emission occurs in less than 10^{-8}s, the process is known as fluorescence. This physical process provides the means for assays which are 10–100 times as sensitive as those based on absorption measurements. This increase in sensitivity is largely because the light measured is all from the sample of interest. A dim light is easily measured against a black background, while it may be lost if added to an already bright background. Fluorometers and spectrofluorometers are very similar to photometers and spectrophotometers but with two major differences. Fluorometers and spectrofluorometers use two monochrometers, one for excitation light and one for emitted light. By proper selection of the band-pass regions, all the light used to excite the sample can be blocked from the detector, assuring the detector sees only fluorescence. The Other difference is that the detector is aligned off-axis, commonly at 90°, from the excitation source. At this angle, scatter is minimal, which helps ensure a dark background for the measured fluorescence. Some spectrofluorometers use polarisation filters both on the input and output light beams, which allows for fluorescence polarisation studies (Fig. 26.4). An intense light source in the visible-to-UV range is desirable. A common source is the xenon or mercury arc lamps, which provide a continuum of radiation over this range.

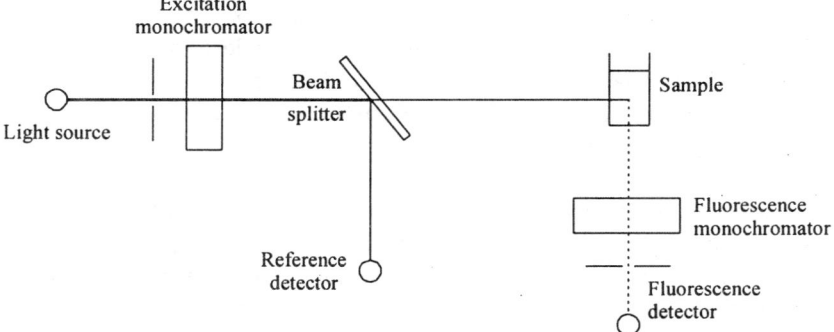

Fig. 26.4. Spectrofluorometer. Fluorescence methods can be extremely sensitive to the low background interference. Since the detector is off-axis from the incident light and a second monochromator blocks light of wavelength illuminating the sample virtually no signal reaches the detector other than the desired fluorescence.

Flame Photometry

Flame photometry is used to measure sodium, potassium and lithium in body fluids. When these elements are heated in a flame they emit characteristic wavelengths of light. The major emission lines are 589 nm (yellow) for sodium, 767 nm (violet) for potassium and 671 nm (red) for lithium. An atomiser introduces a fine mist of the sample into a flame. For routine laboratory use, a propane and compressed air flame is adequate. High quality interference filters with narrow pass-bands are often used to isolate the major emission lines. The narrow band-pass is necessary to maximise the signal-to-noise ratio. Since it is impossible to maintain stable aspiration, atomisation and flame characteristics, it is necessary to use an internal standard of known concentration while making measurements of unknowns. In this way the ratio of the unknown sample's emission to the internal standard's emission remains stable even as the total signal flucturates. An internal standard is usually an element which is found in very low concentration in the sample fluid. By adding a high concentration of this element to the sample, its concentration can be known to a high degree of accuracy. Lithium, potassium and cesium all may be used as internal standards depending upon the particular assay being conducted.

Atomic Absorption Spectroscopy

Atomic absorption spectroscopy is based on the fact that just as metal elements have unique emission lines, they have identical absorption lines when in a gaseous or dissociated state. The atomic absorption spectrometer takes advantage of these physical characteristics in a clever manner, producing an instrument with approximately 100 times the sensitivity of a flame photometer of similar elements. The sample is aspirated into a flame, where the majority of the atoms of the element being measured remain in the ground state, where they are capable of absorbing light at their characteristic wavelengths. An intense source of exactly these wavelengths is produced by a hollow cathode lamp. These lamps are constructed so that the cathode is made from the element to be measured and the lamps are filled with a low pressure of argon or neon gas. When a current is passed through the lamp, metal atoms are sputtered off the cathode and collide with the argon or neon in the tube, producing emission of the characteristic wavelengths. A monochromator and photodetector complete the system.

Light reaching the detector is a combination of that which is emitted by the sample (undesirable) and light from the hollow cathode lamp which was not absorbed by the sample in the flame (desirable). By pulsing the light from the lamp either by directly pulsing the lamp or with a chopper and using a detector which is sensitive to AC signals and insensitive to DC signals, the undesirable emission signal is eliminated. Each element to be measured requires a lamp with that element present in the cathode. Multielement lamps have been developed to minimise the number of lamps required. Atomic absorption spectrophotometers may be either single beam or double beam; the double-beam instruments have greater stability.

There are various flameless methods for atomic absorption spectroscopy in which the burner is replaced with a method for vapourising the element of interest without a flame. The graphite furnace which heats the sample to 2700°C consists of a hollow graphite tube which is heated by passing a large current through it. The sample is placed within the tube and the light beam is passed through it while the sample is heated.

Turbidimetry and Nephelometry

Light scattering by particles in solution is directly proportional to both concentration and molecular weight of the particles. For small molecules the scattering is insignificant, but for proteins, immunoglobulins, immune complexes and other large particles, light scattering can be an effective method for the detection and measurement of particle concentration. For a given wavelength λ of light and particle size d, scattering is described as Raleigh, (d < λ/10), Raleigh-Debye (d $\approx$ λ) or Mie (d > 10λ). For particles that are small compared to the wavelength, the scattering is equal in all directions. However, as the particle size becomes larger than the wavelength, the scattering is equal in all directions. However, as the particle size becomes larger than the wavelength of light, it becomes preferentially scattered in the forward direction. Light-scattering techniques are widely used to detect the formation of antigen-antibody complexes in immunoassays. When light scattering is measured by the attenuation of a beam of light through a solution, it is called turbidimetry. This is essentially the same as absorption measurements with a photometer except that a large pass-band is acceptable. When maximum sensitivity is required a different methods is used—direct measurement of the scattered light with a detector placed at an angle to the central beam. This method is called nephelometry. A typical nephelometer will have a light source, filter, sample cuvette and detector set at an angle to the incident beam (Fig. 26.5).

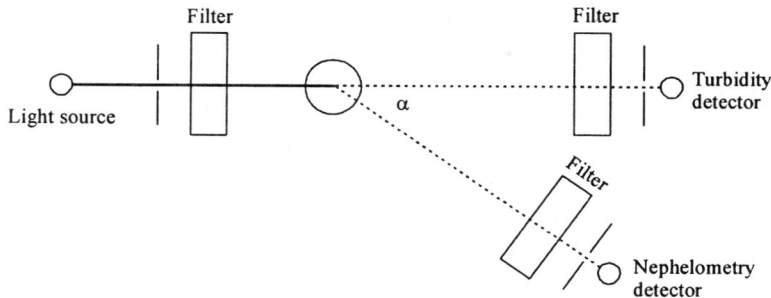

Fig. 26.5. Nephelometer. Light scattered by large molecules is measured at an angle α away from the axis of incident light. The filters select the wavelength range desired and block undesired fluorecnce. When α = 0, the technique is known as turbidimetry.

CLINICAL LABORATORY: NON-SPECTRAL METHODS AND AUTOMATION

Particle Counting and Identification

The Coulter principle was the first major advance in automating blood cell counts. The cells to be counted are drawn through a small aperture between two fluid compartments and the electric impedance between the two compartments is monitored (see Fig. 26.6). As cells pass through the aperture, the impedance increases in proportion to the volume of the cell, allowing large number of cells to be counted and sized rapidly. Red cells are counted by pulling diluted blood through the aperture. Since red cells greatly outnumber white cells, the contribution of white cells to the red cell count is usually neglected. White cells are counted by first destroying the red cells and using a more concentrated sample.

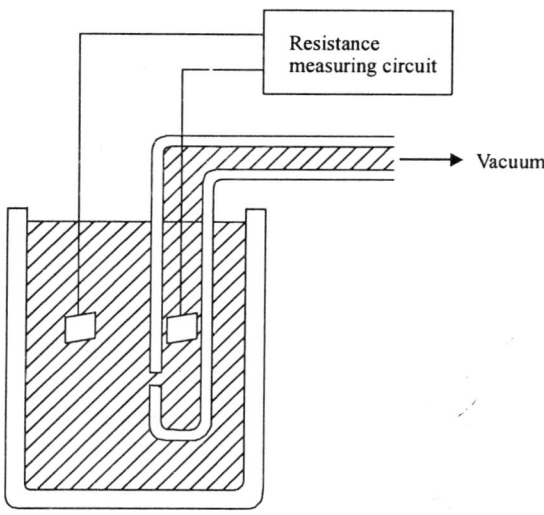

Fig. 26.6. Coulter method. Blood cells are surrounded by an insulating membrane, which makes them non-conductive. The resistance of electrolyte-filled channel will increase slightly as cells flow through it. This resistance variation yields both the total number of cells which flow through the channel and the volume of each cell.

Modern cell counters using the Coulter principle often use hydrodynamic focusing to improve the performance of the instrument. A sheath fluid is introduced which flows along the outside of a channel with the sample stream inside it. By maintaining laminar flow conditions and narrowing the channel, the sample stream is focused into a very thin column with the cells in single file. This eliminates problems with cells flowing along the side of the aperture or sticking to it and minimises problems with having more than one cell in the aperture at a time.

Flow cytometry is a method for characterising, counting and separating cells which are suspended in a fluid. The basic flow cytometer uses hydrodynamic focusing to produce a very thin stream of fluid containing cells moving in single file through a quartz flow chamber (Fig. 26.7). The cells are characterised on the basis of their scattering and fluorescent properties. This simultaneous measurement of scattering and fluorescence is accomplished with a sophisticated optical system that detects light from the sample both at the wavelength of the excitation source (scattering) as well as at longer wavelengths (fluorescence) at more than one angle. Analysis of these measurements produces parameters related to the cells' size, granularity and natural or tagged fluorescence. High-pressure mercury or xenon arc lamps can be used as light sources, but the argon laser (488 nm) is the preferred source for high-performance instruments.

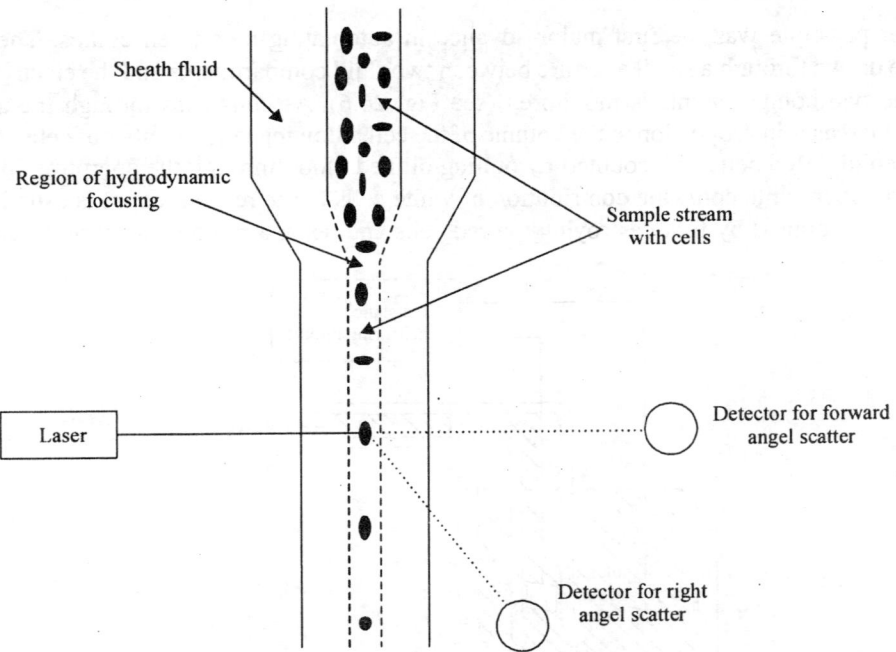

Fig. 26.7. Flow cytometer. By combining hydrodynamic focusing, state-of-the-art optics, fluorescent labels and high-speed computing, large numbers of cells can be characterised and sorted automatically.

One of the more interesting features of this technology is that particular cells may be selected at rates that allow collection of quantities of particular cell type adequate for further chemical testing. This is accomplished by breaking the outgoing stream into a series of tiny droplets using piezoelectric vibration. By charging the stream of droplets and then using deflection plates controlled by the cell analyser, the cells of interest can be diverted into collection vessels.

The development of monoclonal antibodies coupled with flow cytometry allows for quantitation of T and B cells to assess the status of the immune system as well as characterisation of leukemias, lymphomas and other disorders.

Electrochemical Methods

Electrochemical methods are increasingly popular in the clinical laboratory, for measurement not only of electrolytes, blood gases and pH but also of simple compounds such as glucose. Potentiometry is a method in which a voltage is developed across electrochemical cells as shown in Fig. 16.8. This voltage is measured with little or no current flow.

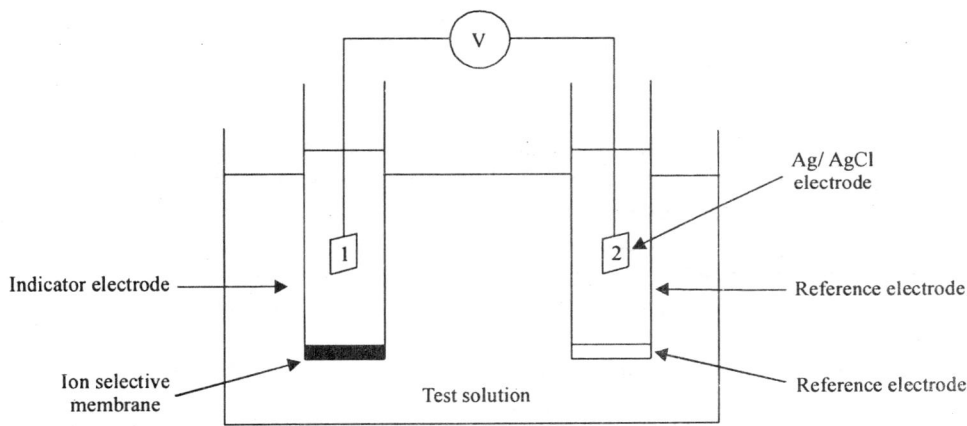

Fig. 26.8. Electrochemical cell.

Ideally, one would like to measure all potentials between the reference solution in the indicator electrode and the test solution. Unfortunately there is no way to do that. Interface potentials develop across any metal-liquid boundary, across liquid junctions and across the ion-selective membrane. The key to making potentiometric measurements is to ensure that all the potentials are constant and do not vary with the composition of the test solution except for the potential of interest across the ion-selective membrane. By maintaining the solutions within the electrodes constant, the potential between these solutions and the metal electrodes immersed in them is constant. The liquid junction is a structure which severely limits bulk flow of the solution but allows free passage of all ions between the solutions. The reference electrode commonly is filled with saturated KCl, which produces a small, constant liquid-junction potential. Thus, any change in the measured voltage (V) is due to a change in the ion concentration in the test solution for which the membrane is selective.

The potential which develops across an ion-selective membrane is given by the Nernst Equation:

$$V = \left(\frac{RT}{zF}\right) \ln \frac{a_2}{a_1} \qquad \text{... (26.6)}$$

where,

R = gas constant = 8.314 J/K · mol

T = temperature in K

z = ionisation number

F = Faraday constant = 9.649×10^4 C/mol

a_n = activity of ion in solution n

When one of the solutions is a reference solution, this equation can be re-written in a convenient form as

$$V = V_0 + \frac{N}{z} \log_{10} a \qquad \qquad \qquad ... (26.7)$$

where,

V_0 = a constant voltage due to reference solution

N = Nernst slope $\approx$ 59 mV/decade at room temperature

The actual Nernst slope is usually slightly less than the theoretical value. Thus, the typical pH meter has two calibration controls. One adjusts the offset to account for the value of V_0 and the other adjusts the range to account for both temperature effects and deviations from the theoretical Nernst slope.

Ion-Specific Electrodes

Ion-selective electrodes use membranes which are permeable only to the ion being measured. To the extent that this can be done, the specificity of the electrode can be very high. One way of overcoming a lack of specificity for certain electrodes is to make multiple simultaneous measurement of several ions which include the most important interfering ones. A simple algorithm can then make corrections for the interfering effects. This technique is used in some commercial electrolyte analysers. A partial list of the ions that can be measured with ion-selective electrodes includes H^+ (pH), Na^+, K^+, Li^+, Ca^{++}, Cl^-, F^-, NH_4^+ and CO_2.

NH_4^+ and CO_2 are both measured with a modified ion-selective electrode. They use a pH electrode modified with a thin layer of a solution (sodium bicarbonate for CO_2 and ammonium chloride for NH_4^+) whose pH varies depending on the concentration of ammonium ions or CO_2 it is equilibrated with. A thin membrane holds the solution against the pH glass electrode and provides for equilibration with the sample solution. Note that the CO_2 electrode in Fig. 26.9 is a combination electrode. This means that both the reference and indicating electrodes have been combined into one unit. Most pH electrodes are made as combination electrodes.

The Clark electrode measures pO_2 by measuring the current developed by an electrode with an applied voltage rather than a voltage measurement. This is an example of amperometry. In this electrode a voltage of approximately –0.65V is applied to a platinum electrode relative to a Ag/AgCl electrode in an electrolyte solution. The reaction:

$$O_2 + 2H^+ + 2e^- \longrightarrow H_2O_2$$

proceeds at a rate proportional to the partial pressure of oxygen in the solution. The electrons involved in this reaction form a current which is proportional to the rate of the reaction and thus to the pO_2 in the solution.

Radio-active Methods

Isotopes are atoms which have identical atomic number (number of protons) but different atomic mass numbers (protons + neutrons). Since they have the same number of electrons in the neutral atom, they have identical chemical properties. This provides an ideal method for labeling molecules in a way that allows for detection at extremely low concentrations. Labeling with radioactive isotopes is extensively used in radioimmunoassays where the amount of antigen bound to specific antibodies is measured. The details of radio-active decay are complex, but for our purposes there are three types of emission from decaying nuclei: alpha, beta and gamma radiation. Alpha particles are made up of two neutrons and two protons (helium nucleus). Alpha emitters are rarely used in the clinical laboratory. Beta emission consists of electrons or positrons emitted from the nucleus. They have a continuous range of energies up to a maximum value characteristic of the isotope. Beta radiation is highly interactive with matter and cannot penetrate very far in most materials. Gamma radiation is a high-energy form of electromagnetic radiation. This type of radiation may be continuous, discrete or mixed depending on the details of the decay process. It has greater penetrating ability than beta radiation. (See Fig. 26.10).

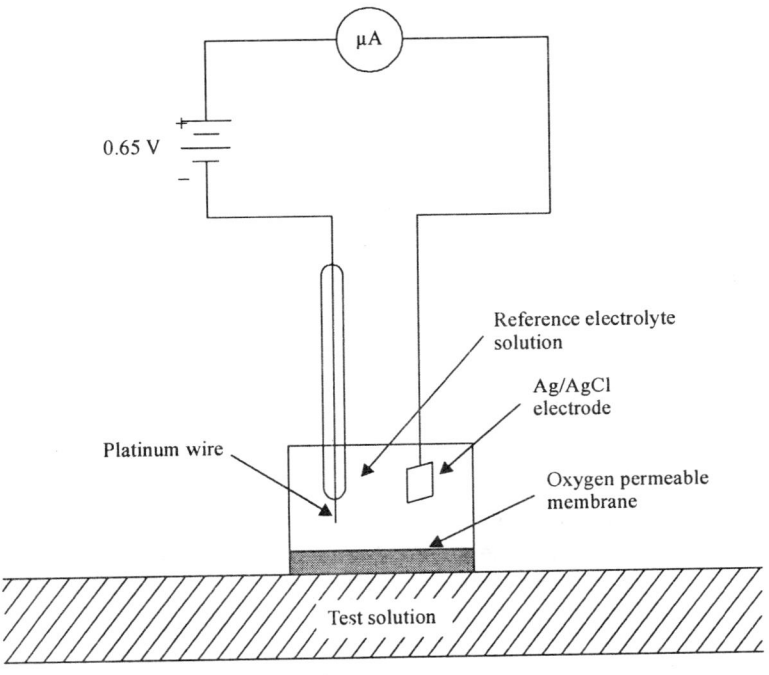

Fig. 26.9. Clark electrode.

The kinetic energy spectrum of emitted radiation is characteristic of the isotope. The energy is commonly measured in electron volts (eV). One electron volt is the energy acquired by an electron falling through a potential of 1 volt. The isotopes commonly used in the clinical laboratory have energy spectra which range from 18 keV–3.6 MeV.

The activity of a quantity of radioactive isotope is defined as the number of disintegrations per second which occur. The usual units are the curie (Ci), which is defined as 3.7×10^{10} dps and the becquerel (Bq), defined as 1 dps. Specific activity for a given isotope is defined as activity per unit mass of the isotope. The rate of decay for a given isotope is characterised by the decay constant λ, which is the proportion of the isotope which decays in unit time. Thus, the rate of loss of radioactive isotope is governed by the equation.

$$\frac{dN}{dt} = -\lambda N \qquad \text{... (26.8)}$$

where, N is the amount of radioactive isotope present at time t.

The solution to this differential equation is:

$$N = N_0 e^{-\lambda t} \qquad \ldots (26.9)$$

It can easily be shown that the amount of radioactive isotope present will be reduced by half after time

$$t_{1/2} = \frac{0.693}{\lambda} \qquad \ldots (26.10)$$

This is known as the half-life for the isotope and can vary widely; for example, carbon-14 has a half-life of 5760 years and iodine-131 has a half-life of 8.1 days.

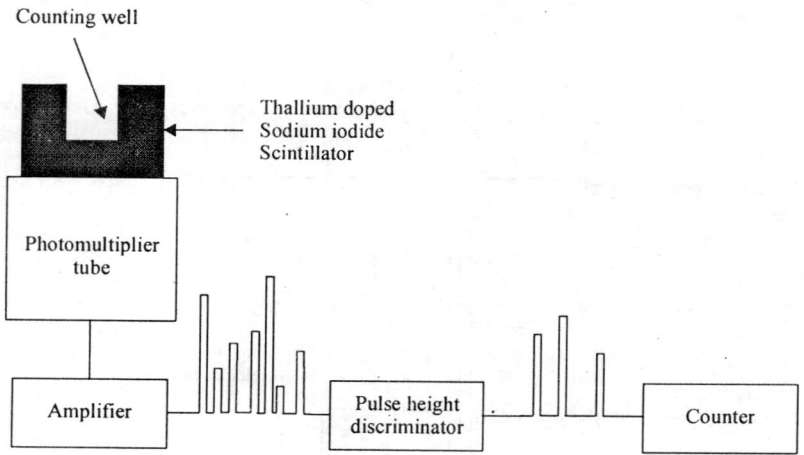

Fig. 26.10. Gamma counted. The intensity of the light flash produced when a gamma photon interacts with a scintillator is proportional to the energy of the photon. The photomultiplier tube converts these light flashes into electric pulses which can be selected according to size (gamma energy) and counted.

The most common method for detection of radiation in the clinical laboratory is by scintillation. This is the conversion of radiation energy into photons in the visible or near-UV range. These are detected with photomultiplier tubes.

For gamma radiation, the scintillating crystal is made of sodium iodide doped with about 1 per cent thallium, producing 20 to 30 photons for each electron-volt of energy absorbed. The photomultiplier tube and amplifier circuit produce voltage pulses proportional to the energy of the absorbed radiation. These voltage pulses are usually passed through a pulse-height analyser which eliminates pulses outside a preset energy range (window). Multichannel analysers can discriminate between two or more isotopes if they have well-separated energy maxima. There generally will be some spill down of counts from the higher energy isotopes into the lower-energy isotope's window, but this effect can be corrected with a simple algorithm. Multiple well detectors with up to 64 detectors in an array are available which increase the throughput for counting systems greatly. Counters using the sodium iodide crystal scintillator are referred to as gamma counters or well counters.

The lower energy and short penetration ability of beta particles requires a scintillator in direct contact with the decaying isotope. This is accomplished by dissolving or suspending the sample in a liquid fluor. Counters which use this technique are called beta counters or liquid scintillation counters.

Liquid scintillation counters use two photomultiplier tubes with a coincidence circuit that prevents counting of events seen by only one of the tubes. In this way, false counts due to chemiluminescence and noise in the phototube are greatly reduced. Quenching is a problem in all liquid scintillation counters. Quenching is any process which reduces the efficiency of the scintillation counting process, where efficiency is defined as

$$\text{Efficiency} = \text{Counts per minute/decays per minute} \qquad \dots (26.11)$$

A number of techniques have been developed that automatically correct for quenching effects to produce estimates of true decays per minute from the raw counts. Currently there is a trend away from beta-emitting isotopic labels, but these assays are still used in many laboratories.

Coagulation Timers

Screening for and diagnosis of coagulation disorders is accomplished by assays that determine how long it takes for blood to clot following initiation of the clotting cascade by various reagents. A variety of instruments have been designed to automate this procedure. In addition to increasing the speed and throughput of such testing, these instruments improve the reproducibility of such tests. All the instruments provide precise introduction of reagents, accurate timing circuits and temperature control. They differ in the method for detecting clot formation. One of the older methods still in use is to dip a small metal hook into the blood sample repeatedly and lift it a few millimeters above the surface. The electric resistance between the hook and the sample is measured and when fibrin filaments form, they produce a conductive pathway which is detected as clot formation. Other systems detect the increase in viscosity due to fibrin formation or the scattering due to the large polymerised molecules formed. Absorption and fluorescence spectroscopy can also be used for clot detection.

Osmometers

The colligative properties of a solution are a function of the number of solute particles present regardless of size or identity. Increased solute concentration causes an increase in osmotic pressure and boiling point and a decrease in vapour pressure and freezing point. Measuring these changes provides information on the total solute concentration regardless of type. The most accurate and popular method used in clinical laboratories is the measurement of freezing point depression. With this method, the sample is supercooled to a few degrees below 0°C while being stirred gently. Freezing is then initiated by vigorous stirring. The heat of fusion quickly brings the solution to a slushy state where a equilibrium exists between ice and liquid, ensuring that the temperature is at the freezing point. This temperature is measured. A solute concentration of 1 osmol/kg water produces a freezing point depression of 1.858°C. The measured temperature depression is easily calibrated in units of milliosmols/kg water.

The vapour pressure depression method has the advantage of smaller sample size. However, it is not as precise as the freezing point method and cannot measure the contribution of volatile solutes such as ethanol. This method is not used as widely as the freezing point depression method in clinical laboratories.

Osmolality of blood is primarily due to electrolytes such as Na^+ and Cl^-. Proteins with molecular weights of 30000 or more atomic mass units (amu) contribute very little to total osmolality due to their smaller numbers (a single Na^+ ion contributes just as much to osmotic pressure as a large protein molecule). However, the contribution to osmolality made by proteins is of great interest when monitoring conditions leading to pulmonary edema. This value is known as colloid osmotic pressure or oncotic pressure and is measured with a membrane permeable to water and all molecules smaller than about 30000 amu. By placing a reference saline solution on one side and the unknown sample on the other, an osmotic pressure is developed across the membrane. This pressure is measured with a pressure transducer and can be related to the true colloid osmotic pressure through a calibration procedure using known standards.

Automation

Improvements in technology coupled with increased demand for laboratory test as well as pressures to reduce costs have led to the rapid development of highly automated laboratory instruments. Typical automated instruments contain mechanisms for measuring, mixing and transport of samples and reagents, measurement systems and one or more microprocessors to control the entire system. In addition to system control, the computer systems store calibration curves, match test results to specimen IDs and generate reports. Automated instruments are dedicated to compete blood counts, coagulation studies, microbiology assays and immunochemistry, as well as high-volume instruments used in clinical chemistry laboratories. The chemistry analysers tend to fall into one of four classes: continuous flow, centrifugal, pack-based and dry-slide-based systems. The continuous flow systems pass successive samples and reagents through a single set of tubing, where they are directed to appropriate mixing, dialysing and measuring stations. Carry-over from one sample to the next is minimised by the introduction of air bubbles and wash solution between samples.

Centrifugal analysers use plastic rotors which serve as reservoirs for samples and reagents and also as cuvettes for optical measurements. Spinning the plastic rotor mixes, incubates and transports the test solution into the cuvette portion of the rotor, where the optical measurements are made while the rotor is spinning.

Pack-based systems are those in which each test uses a special pack with the proper reagents and sample preservation devices built-in. The sample is automatically introduced into as many packs as tests required. The packs are then processed sequentially.

Dry chemistry analysers use no liquid reagents. The reagents and other sample preparation methods are layered onto a slide. The liquid sample is placed on the slide and after a period of time the colour developed is read by reflectance photometry. Ion-selective electrodes have been incorporated into the same slide format.

There are a number of technological innovations found in many of the automated instruments. One innovation is the use of fibreoptic bundles to channel excitation energy toward the sample as well as transmitted, reflected or emitted light away from the sample to the detectors. This provides a great deal of flexibility in instrument layout. Multiwavelength analysis using a spinning filter wheel or diode array detectors is commonly found. The computers associated with these instruments allow for innovative improvements in the assays. For instance, when many analytes are being analysed from one sample, the interference effects of one analyte on the measurement of another can be predicated and corrected before the final report is printed.

Trends in Laboratory Instrumentation

Predicting the future direction of laboratory instrumentation is difficult, but there seem to be some clear trends. Decentralisation of the laboratory functions will continue with more instruments being located in or around ICUs, operating rooms, emergency rooms and physician offices. More electrochemistry-based tests will be developed. The flame photometer is already being replaced with ion-selective electrode methods. Instruments which analyse whole blood rather than plasma or serum will reduce the amount of time required for sample preparation and will further encourage testing away from the central laboratory. Dry reagent methods increasingly will replace wet chemistry methods. Radioimmunoassays will continue to decline with the increasing use of method for performing immunoassays that do not rely upon radioisotopes such as enzyme-linked fluorescent assays.

Glossary

Accretion. Growth or enlargement.

Accuracy. The degree to which the average value of repeated measurements approximate the true value being measured.

Active electrode. Electrode used for achieving desired surgical effect.

Alpha radiation. Particulate radiation consisting of a helium nucleus emitted from a decaying nucleus.

Amnion. Thin membranous structure around fetus.

Amniotic. Pertaining to the amnion.

Amperometry. Measurements based on current flow produced in an electrochemical cell by an applied voltage.

Angstrom. Unit of length, 1 angstrom = 10^{-10} meters.

Aorta. Great artery carrying blood from the left ventricle of the heart to the rest of the body.

Aortic. Pertaining to the aorta.

Arborisations. Form resembling a tree.

Arrhythmia. Alteration in the rhythm.

Arteriole. One of the small twigs of the artery that becomes a capillary.

Artifacts. Erroneous lines or marks on a graph or gram. An error in a test result.

Atria. See atrium.

Atrioventricular. Located between the upper and lower chamber of the heart.

Atrium. Upper chamber of the heart.

Auricle. Chamber of the heart that receives blood from the veins. See atrium.

Autonomic. Action that is independent of free volition.

Aveolus. Air sac or cell in the lungs.

Axon. Long, thin portion of a nerve cell that carries the impulse away from the main section of the cell.

Beer-Lambert law. Principle stating that the optical absorbance of a substance is proportional to both the concentration of the substance and the pathlength of the sample.

Beta radiation. Particulate radiation consisting of an electron or positron emitted from a decaying nucleus.

Bioelectric. Electrical activity pertaining to a living cell.

Biophysical. Branch of science that applies the concepts of physical science to biology.

Brachial. Relating or pertaining to the arm.

Bradycardia. Slow heart rate.

Bronchus. Tube leading from trachea to either left or right lung.

Bronci. See bronchus.

Capillaries. Smallest blood vessels in the body.

Cardiac. Pertaining to the heart.

Cardiology. Study of the heart and its diseases.

Cardiovascular. Relating to the circulatory system.

Catheter. Small tube that is inserted into the body to permit injection of medications, to allow the vessel or passage open or to permit withdrawal of fluids.

Cell. Smallest object capable of life.

Cephalic. Pertaining to the head or skull.

Cerebellum. Large dorsal brain structure.

Cerebrum. Anterior portion of the brain.

Coagulation. Solidification of proteins accompanied by tissue whitening.

Colligative properties. Physical properties that depend on the number of molecules present rather than on their individual properties.

Common mode rejection ratio (CMRR). The ratio between the amplitude of a common mode signal and the amplitude of a differential signal that would produce the same output amplitude or as the ratio of the differential gain over the common-mode gain: $CMRR = G_D/G_{CM}$. Expressed in decibels, the common mode rejection is $20 \log_{10} CMRR$. The common mode rejection is a function of frequency and source-impedance unbalance.

Continuous positive airway pressure (CPAP). A spontaneous ventilation mode in which the ventilator maintains a constant positive pressure, near or below PEEP level, in the patient's airway while the patient breathes at will.

Cornea. Transparent covering of the center portion of the eye.

Cortex. Outer layer of tissue on an organ.

Cortical. Pertaining to the cortex.

Cranium. Portion of the skull containing the brain.

Curare. Drug that produces muscular relaxation.

Cytochromes. Heme-containing proteins found in the membranes of mitochondria and required for oxidative phosphorylation, with characteristic optical absorbance spectra.

Cytoplasm. The matter inside a cell, except for the nucleus.

Defibrillator. An electrical device used to deliver a shock to stop fibrillation of the heart.

Dendrite. Portion of the nerve cell that conducts impulses toward the cell.

Depolarised. State of being partially or totally non-polar.

Desiccation. Drying of tissue due to the evaporation of intracellular fluids.

Diastole. Expansion of the chambers of the heart so that they may fill with blood.

Dicrotic. Double humped waveform.

Dispersive electrode. Return electrode at which no electrosurgical effect is intended.

Dorsal. Situated near or toward the back.

Dysfunctional haemoglobins. Those haemoglobin species that cannot reversibly bind oxygen (carboxyhaemoglobin, methemoglobin and sulfhaemoglobin).

ECG. Electrocardiograph.

Ectopic. Located in other than normal position.

EEG. Electroencephalogram.

Electrocardiogram. Tracing of the electrical signals produced by the heart.

Electrocardiograph. Machine for making electrocardiogram.

Electrode. Conductor used to make electrical contact between a wire and a conductive surface, such as human skin.

Electrodermograph. Recorder for measuring galvanic skin resistance.

Electroencephalogram. Recording of electrical signals produced by the brain.

Electroencephalograph. Machine for making electroencephalograms.

Electrogastrogram. Recording of simultaneous electrical and physical activity of the stomach.

Electrolyte. A solution in which electrical current is due to ionic mobility.

Electromyogram. Recording of electrical activity of skeletal muscles.

Electromyograph. Machine for making electromyograms.

Embolus. Abnormal solid or gaseous particle in the blood stream.

Embryo. Undeveloped stage of fetus.

EMG. Electromyograph; electromyogram.

Extracellular. Outside of the cells.

Extracorporeal. Outside of the body.

Fluorescence. Emission of light by an atom or molecule following absorption of a photon by greater energy. Emission normally occurs within 10^{-8} of absorption.

Fulguration. Random discharge of sparks between active electrode and tissue surface in order to achieve coagulation and/or desiccation.

Functional saturation. The ratio of oxygenated haemoglobin to total non-dysfunctional haemoglobins (oxyhaemoglobin plus deoxyhaemoglobin).

Gamma radiation. Electromagnetic radiation emitted from an atom undergoing nuclear decay.

Hemisphere. Half of a spherical object.

Homogeneous. Of the same sort.

Hydrodynamic focusing. A process in which a fluid stream is first surrounded by a second fluid and then narrowed to a thin stream by a narrowing of the channel.

Hypoxia. Inadequate oxygen supply to tissues necessary to maintain metabolic activity.

Infarct. Area of necrotic tissue due to loss of blood perfusion.

Inhomogeneity. Not homogenous.

Intracellular. Inside of the cell.

Ion. Atom or molecule that carries an electrical charge, either positive or negative.

Iris. Coloured portion of the eye behind the cornea.

Isoelectric. Having the same electric charge so cannot produce an electrical current.

Isolation mode rejection ratio (IMRR). The ratio between the isolation voltage, V_{ISO} and the amplitude of the isolation signal appearing at the output of the isolation amplifier or as isolation voltage divided by output voltage V_{OUT} in the absence of differential and common mode signal: $IMRR = V_{ISO}/V_{OUT}$.

Isothermal. A body with the same temperature in all portions.

Isotopes. Atoms with the same number of protons but differing numbers of neutrons.

Isotropic. Having the same properties in all directions.

Latency. Apparent inacitivity.

Lobe. Rounded portion of an organ.

Lumen. The hollow portion of a tubular organ.

Mandatory mode. A mode of mechanically ventilating the lungs where the ventilator controls all breath delivery parameters such as tidal volume, respiration rate, flow waveform, etc.

Manometer. Device used to determine gas pressures.

Membrane. A thin layer of tissue.

Metabolism. The total of all processes required for an organism to live.

Micron. Unit of length, 10^{-6} meters.

Mitochondria. Small granules or rods.

Mitral stenosis. Narrowing of the oriface between left atria and ventricle.

Multivariate analysis. Empirical models developed to relate multiple spectral intensities from many calibration samples to known analyte concentrations, resulting in an optimal set of calibration parameters.

Myocardium. A muscle layer of the heart.

Myograph. Instrument for measurement of muscular contraction.

Necrosis. Death of tissue or cells.

Nephelometry. Measurement of the amount of light scattered by particles suspended in a fluid.

Neuron. Nerve cell.

Nucleus. Central structure (as in cells and atoms).

Occipital. Relating or pertaining to the rear portion of the head.

Operational amplifier (op-amp). A very high gain DC-coupled differential amplifier with single-ended output, high voltage gain, high input impedance and low output impedance. Due to its high open-loop gain, the characteristics of an op-amp circuit only depend on its feedback network. Therefore the integrated circuit op-amp is an extremely convenient tool for the realisation of linear amplifier circuits.

Organ. Group of specialised cells that perform a specific task or function.

Orthogonal. At right angles or normal to.

Oximetry. The determination of blood or tissue oxygen content, generally by optical means.

Parietal. Pertaining to the upper rear portion of the head.

Patient circuit. A set of tubes connecting the patient airway to the outlet of a respirator.

Permeable. Ability to pass through pores.

Peroneal. Pertaining to the outer side of the lower leg.

Piezoelectric. Electrical activity due to flexure of a crystal.

Plasma. The liquid portion of blood.

Plethysmography. Recording of volume changes due to blood flow.

Pneumatic. Pertaining to or operated by gases, especially air.

Pneumograph. Measuring instrument for recording volume changes in the thorax due to respiration.

Pneumotachygraph. Instrument to measure respiration rate.

Positive end expiratory pressure (PEEP). A therapist-selected pressure level for the patient airway at the end of expiration in either mandatory or spontaneous breathing.

Posterior. Pertaining to the rear.

Potentiometry. Measurement of the potential produced by electrochemical cells under equilibrium conditions with no current flow.

Precision. A measure of test reproducibility.

Pressure controlled ventilation. A mandatory mode of ventilation where during the inspiration phase of each breath, a constant pressure is applied to the patient's airway independent of the patient's airway resistance and/or compliance respiratory mechanics.

Pressure support. A spontaneous breath delivery mode during which the ventilator applies a positive pressure greater than PEEP to the patient's airway during inspiration.

Protoplasm. Substance of water, inorganic and proteinaceous material making up the parts of the cell.

Psychogalvanic. Electrical activity produced by mental stress.

Pulmonary. Pertaining to the lungs.

Pulse oximetry. The determination of functional oxygen saturation of pulsatile arterial blood by ratiometric measurement of tissue optical absorbance changes.

Pupil. Variable-size aperture in the center of the eye.

Radical. Group of atoms that can be replaced by a single atom.

Radioisotope. Artificially produced radioactive element.

Retina. Light-sensitive membrane in the eye.

Rheobase. Smallest electrical current that will produce stimulation.

Sagittal. Pertaining to or parallel to the midline of the body.

Scalp. Skin of the head covered by hair.

Scintillation. The conversion of the kinetic energy of a charged particle or photon to a flash of light.

Semi-permeable. Permeable to certain substances.

Sensitivity. A measure of how small an amount of concentration of an analyte can be detected.

Serum. The liquid portion of blood remaining after clotting has occurred.

Sinoatrial node. Collection of heart cells that functions as the natural pacemaker.

Sinus. Irregular cavity.

Specificity. A measure of how well a test detects the intended analyte without being 'fooled' by other substance in the sample.

Sphygmomanometer. Blood pressure measurement apparatus.

Spirometer. Measuring instrument for determining respiratory air volume.

Spontaneous mode. A ventilation mode in which the patient initiates and breathes from the ventilator supplied gas at will.

Spray. Another term for fulguration. Sometimes this waveform has a higher crest factor than that used for fulguration.

Stereotaxic. Precision positioning.

Synapse. Junction where impulse transmits from one nerve cell to another.

Systemic. Affecting the entire body.

Systole. Period during which the heart contracts.

Tachycardia. Excessively fast heart rate.

Thermistor. Electrical component that exhibits resistance changes due to temperature changes.

Thermocouple. Device that creates a voltage proportional to temperature.

Thoracic. Pertaining to the thorax.

Thorax. Section of the body between abdomen and neck.

Thrombus. Clot of blood remaining at its site of origin.

Tibia. Large, innermost bone of the leg.

Tissue. Collection of similar cells that perform a specific function or take a similar form.

Torso. Trunk of the body.

Trachea. Main tube passing air from outside world to the lungs.

Transducer. Device that converts energy from one form to another for purposes of measurement or control. In this context, the energy converted to is usually electrical.

Turbidimetry. Measurement of the attenuation of a light beam due to light lost to scattering by particles suspended in a fluid.

Ulnar. Pertaining to the larger bone of the human forearm.

Utero. Latin dative for uterus.

Uterus. Organ in the female for protection and nourishment of the embryo.

Vasoconstrictors. Agents that narrow the blood vessels.

Vasomotor. Agent affecting the size of a blood vessel.

Ventricle. Lower chambers of the heart.

Venule. Small vein connected to the capillaries.

Viable. Able to live.

Volume controlled ventilation. A mandatory mode of ventilation where the volume of each breath is set by the therapist and the ventilator delivers that volume to the patient independent of the patient's airway resistance and/or compliance respiratory mechanics.

Appendices

SYMBOLS

This list gives single-letter symbols for quantities, without sub-scripts or modifiers.

Symbol	Quantity	Symbol	Quantity
a	Absorptivity	m	Average number
a	Activity	m	Mass
a	Coefficient	m	Slope
a	Lead vector	M	Mass
A	Absorbance	M	Measured values
A	Area	$\overline{M}$	Modulation
A	Coefficient	M	Cardiac vector
A	Gain	n	Number
A	Per cent	n	Refractive index
b	Coefficient	N	Noise equivalent bandwidth
b	Intercept	N	Number
B	Coefficient	N	Turns ratio
B	Per cent	p	Change in pressure
B	Viscous friction	p	Probability
B	Magnetic flux density	P	Power
c	Coefficient	P	Pressure
c	Specific heat	P	Projection
c	Velocity of sound	q	Charge
C	Capacitance	q	Rate of heat
C	Compilance	q	Change in volume flow
C	Concentration	Q	Heat content
C	Contrast	Q	Volume flow
d	Derivative	r	Correlation coefficient

(Contd...)

Symbol	Quantity	Symbol	Quantity
d	Diameter	r	Radius
d	Distance	r	Resistance/length
D	Density	R	Range
D	Detector responsivity	R	Ratio
D	d/dt	R	Resistance
D	Diameter	S	Standard deviation
D	Diffusing capacity	S	Modulation transfer function
D	Distance	S	Saturation
E	emf	S	Slew rate
E	Energy	S	Source output
E	Exposure	t	Thickness
E	Irradiance	t	Time
E	Modulus of elasticity	T	Interval
f	Force	T	Temperature
f	Frequency	T	Transmittance
f	Function	u	Velocity
F	Filter transmission	u	Work function
F	Flow	U	Molar uptake
F	Force	v	Voltage
F	Fraction	v	Change in volume
F	Molar fraction	V	Voltage
g	Conductance/area	V	Volume
G	Conductance	W	Power
G	Form factor	W	Weight
G	Gauge factor	W	Weighting factor
G	Gain	x	Constant
h	Height	x	Distance
H	Feedback gain	x	Input
i	Current	X	Chemical species
I	Current	X	Effort variable
I	Intensity	X	Value
j	$+(-1)^{1/2}$	y	Constant
J.	Number of standard deviations	y	Output
k	Constant —	Y	Admittance
k	Piezoelectric constant	Y	Flow variable
K	Constant	Y	Value
K	Number	z	Distance
K	Sensitivity	Z	Atomic number

(Contd...)

Symbol	Quantity	Symbol	Quantity
K	Solubility product	Z	Impedance
K	Spring constant		
L	Inductance		
L	Inertance		
L	Length		
L	Line-source response		

GREEK LETTERS

Symbol	Quantity
α	Polytropic constant
α	Thermistor coefficient
α	Thermoelectric sensitivity
β	Thermistor constant
Δ	Deviation
ϵ	Emissivity
ϵ	Dielectric constant
ζ	Damping ratio
η	Viscosity
θ	Angle
Λ	Logarithmic decrement
λ	Wavelength
μ	Attenuation coefficient
μ	Mobility
μ	Permeability
μ	Poisson's ratio
ν	Frequency
ρ	Density
ρ	Mole density
ρ	Resistivity
σ	Conductance
σ	Conductivity/distance
σ^2	Variance
τ	Time constant
ϕ	Number of photons
ϕ	Phase shift
ϕ	Divergence
Φ	Potential
ω	Frequency

APPENDIX II

Abbreviations

A/D	Analog-to-digital
ACD	Annihilation coincidence detection
AEC	Automatic exposure control
B B B	Blood brain barrier
BGO	Bismuth germanate
BOLD	Blood oxygen level dependent
CBF	Cerebral blood flow
CCD	Charge coupled device
$CMRO_2$	Cerebral metabolic rate of oxygen
CNR	Contrast-to-noise ratio
CR	Computed radiography
CSF	Cerebrospinal fluid
CSI	Chemical shift imaging
CT	Computed tomography
CTDI	Computed tomography dose index
CW	Continuous wave
CZT	Cadmium lead telluride
DNA	Deoxyribonucleic acid
DOF	Depth-of-focus
DQE	Detective quantum efficiency
DR	Digital radiography
DSA	Digital subtraction angiography
DTPA	Diethylenetriaminepentaacetic acid
EPI	Echo planar imaging
ESF	Edge spread function
FDG	Fluorodeoxyglucose
FID	Free induction decay
FLASH	Fast low angle shot
fMRI	Functional magnetic resonance imaging
FOV	Field-of-view
FPD	Flat-panel detector
FWHM	Full-width-at-half-maximum
GI	Gastrointestinal
HSA	Human serum albumin
HOCM	High osmolarity contrast media
HVL	Half value layer
IVP	Intravenous pyelogram
kV_p	Accelerating voltage
LED	Light-emitting diode
LOCM	Low osmolarity contrast media

LSF	Line spread function
MAA	Macroaggregated albumin
MIP	Maximum intensity projection
MRA	Magnetic resonance angiography
MRI	Magnetic resonance imaging
MSE	Mean squared error
MTF	Modulation transfer function
NEX	Number of excitations
NFB	Near-field boundary
NMR	Nuclear magnetic resonance
OD	Optical density
PC	Phase contrast
PET	Positron emission tomography
PHA	Pulse height analyser
PMT	Photomultiplier tube
PRESS	Point resolved spectroscopy
PRR	Pulse repetition rate
PSF	Point spread function
PSPMT	Position sensitive photomultiplier tube
PVDF	Polyvinylidine difluoride
PZT	Lead zirconate titanate
QF	Quality factor
RBC	Red blood cell
RES	Reticuloendothelial system
RF	Radiofrequency
ROC	Receiver operating curve
ROI	Region-of-interest
SATA	Spatial average temporal average
SD	Standard deviation
SNR	Signal-to-noise ratio
SPECT	Single photon emission computed tomography
SPIO	Superparamagnetic iron oxide
SPTA	Spatial peak temporal average
TDC	Time-domain correlation
TFT	Thin-film transistor
TGC	Time-gain compensation
TOF	Time-of-flight

APPENDIX III

MEDICAL TERMINOLOGY

Common Prefixes

A medical term has several basic components, one of which is a prefix. Prefixes always precede word roots. The root is the foundation of a word or its element. For example, the element or word root 'gastr-' means stomach. By putting another element in front of the word root, the meaning of the root word is altered, becoming more specific, for example. Thus, by adding the element 'epi-' (meaning 'above') as a prefix to the word 'gastric' ('pertaining to the stomach'), the new medical term 'epigastric', meaning 'pertaining to the region above the stomach,' is formed.

The following alphabetical list includes fifty of the most common prefixes used in medical terminology and their meanings.

Prefix	Meaning	Prefix	Meaning
a-, an-	not, without		
ab-	away from	dia-	through, complete
ad-	toward	dys-	bad, painful, difficult
ana-	up, apart	ec-, ecto-	out, outside
ante-	before, forward	en-, endo-	in, within
anti-	against	epi-	above, upon, on
auto-	self	eu-	good, well
bi-	two	ex-	away from, out
brady-	slow	hemi-	half
cata-	down	hyper-	excessive, beyond
con-	with, together	hypo-	deficient, under
contra-	against, opposite	in-	not, in
de-	down, lack of		
dia-	through, complete		
dys-	bad, painful, difficult		
ec-, ecto-	out, outside		
en-, endo-	in, within		
epi-	above, upon, on		
eu-	good, well		
ex-	away from, out		
hemi-	half		
hyper-	excessive, beyond		
hypo-	deficient, under		
in-	not, in		
infra-	below, inferior	poly-	many
inter-	between	post-	after, behind
macro-	large	pre-, pro-	before, in front of
mal-	bad	pseudo-	false

(Contd...)

Prefix	Meaning	Prefix	Meaning
meso-	middle	re-	back
meta-	change, beyond	retro-	behind, back
micro-	small	semi-	half
pan-	all	sub-	under
para-	near, beside, abnormal	supra-	above
		syn-, sym-	together, with
per-	through	tachy-	fast
peri-	surrounding	trans-	across
polio-	gray matter of brain or spinal cord	ultra-	beyond, excess

Common Suffixes

Suffixes are a basic component of medical words. Suffixes are always at the endings of words, following prefixes and word roots or elements. They often described the conditions of a part of the body or an action involving a body part. For instance, in the word and '-gram" (meaning 'record') is the suffix.

The following alphabetical list includes fifty of the most commonly used medical suffixes and their meanings.

Suffix	Meaning	Suffix	Meaning
-algia	pain	-graphy	process of recording
-cele	hernia	-itis	inflamation
-centesis	surgical puncture	-logy	study of
-clysis	irrigation, washing	-lysis	destruction,
-coccus	berry-shaped bacterai		breakdown
-cyte	cell	-malacia	softening
-dynia	pain	-megaly	enlargement
-ectasis	stretching, dilation	-oma	turnoer
-ectomy	removal, excision	-opsy	to view
-emesis	vomiting	-osis	condition (usually
-emia	blood condition		abnormal)
-genesis	condition of, forming	-pathy	disease
-gram	record of	-penia	deficiency
-graph	instrument for recording	-pepsia	digestion
-pexy	fixation, putting in place	-sclerosis	hardening
		-scope	instrument for examination
-phagia	eating, swallowing		
-phobia	fear	-spasm	a sudden, violet in-
-plasia	develapment, formation		voluntary muscular contraction
-plasty	surgical repair	-stalasis	contraction

(Contd...)

Suffix	Meaning	Suffix	Meaning
-poiesis	formation	-stasis	stopping, controlling
-ptosis	drooping, sagging	-stenosis	tightening, stricture
-ptysis	spitting	-stomy	new opening
-rrhagia,		-theraphy	treatment
-rrhage	bursting forth of blood	-tome	cutting instrument
		-tomy	incision, section
-rrhaphy	suture	-tresia	opening
-rrhea	flow, discharge	-traphy	nourishment, development
-rrhexis	rupture		

TERMINOLOGY OF GENERAL ANATOMY

The following terms pertain to the body as a whole.

Body cavities: Some of the important viscera (internal organs) are found in the following body cavities.

Cavity	Organs
Cranial	Brain
Thoracic	Lungs, heart, trachea, aorta
Abdominal	Stomach, intestines, spleen, gallbladder, liver, pancreas
Pelvic	Urinary bladder, urethra, ureters, uterus, vagina
Spinal	Spinal cord nerves

The cranial and spinal cavities are called dorsal because of their location on the back portion of the body. The thoracic, abdominal and pelvic cavities are considered ventral because of their location on the front or belly side of the body.

The thoracic and abdominal cavities are separated by a muscular partition called the diaphragm.

The abdomen is also divided into six anatomical regions. These divisions are used in describing anatomically the regions in which organs and structures are found:

Hypochonadriac	–	Two upper lateral regions beneath the ribs.
Epigastric	–	Region of the stomach.
Lumbar	–	Two middle lateral regions.
Umbilical	–	Region of the navel or umbilicus.
Hypogastric	–	Lower middle region below the umbilicus.
Iliac or inguinal	–	Two lower lateral regions.

Anatomical Division of the Back

Cervical	Neck region
	7 cervical vertebrae
Thoracic	Chest
	12 thoracic vertebrae
Lumbar	Loin or flank
	5 lumbar vertebrae
Sacral	Sacrum
	5 fused bones
Coccygeal	Coccyx (tailbone)
	4 fused pieces

The spinal column (vertebrae) is made of bone tissue; the spinal cord (nerves running through the column) is made up of nerve tissue. Between each pair of vertebrae is found a piece of cartilage called a disk, which acts as a shock absorber.

POSITIONAL AND DIRECTIONAL TERMS

Afferent	–	Leading toward a structure
Efferent	–	Leading away from a structure
Anterior (ventra)	–	The front of the body
Posterior (dorsal)	–	The back of the body
Central	–	Pertaining to the centre
Deep	–	Away from the surface
Superficial	–	Near the surface
Distal	–	Away from the beginning of the structure
Proximal	–	Pertaining to the beginning of a structure
Inferiro (caudal)	–	Away from the head
Superior (cephalic)	–	Pertaining to the head
Lateral	–	Pertaining to the side
Medical	–	Pertaining to the middle
Supine	–	Lying on the back
Prone	–	Lying on the belly

Planes of the Body

Frontal	–	Vertical plane dividing the body into anterior and posterior portions.
Sagittal	–	Vertical plane that divides the body lengthwise into right and left halves
Transverse	–	The plane that runs across the body horizontally, dividing the body into upper and lower portions

TERMINOLOGY OF CIRCULATION

There are three main types of blood vessels in the body:
1. Arteries are large blood vessels that lead oxygenated blood away from the heart to all parts of the body.
2. Capillaries are very thin-walled vessel that carry oxygenated blood from arteries to the cells of the body.
3. Veins, which have thinner walls than arteries, conduct the waste-filled blood from the tissues back towards the heart.

The heart pumps blood through two systems of circulation. In pulmonary circulation, blood circulates between the heart and the lungs. Non-oxygenated blood circulates from the right atrium (upper chamber of the heart) into the right ventricle (lower chamber) into the pulmonary artery and from there to the lungs. Here the oxygen-deficient blood is re-oxygenated and expels carbon dioxide. The newly oxygenated blood then flows into the pulmonary vein, back to the left side of the heart (left atrium and left ventricle), from which it is pumped into the aorta and out into the body through the systemic circulation.

Two highly important arteries are the coronary arteries, which branch off from the aorta above the heart. A myocardial infarction (heart attack) may occur if these arteries are blocked by a blood clot.

There are two phases to the heartbeat. Diastole occurs when the walls of the heart chambers relax and blood flows into the heart through the veins. Systole occurs next as the heart chamber walls contact to pump blood into the pulmonary artery and the aorta. The cardiac cycle of relaxation and filling, then contracting and pumping, takes about 0.9 second and occurs between 70 and 80 times a minute. The heart pumps about two and a half ounces of blood with each contraction; that is to say, about five quarts a minute or 75 gallons and hour.

TERMINOLOGY OF RESPIRATION

There are actually two processes involved in respiration: external respiration, in which oxygen is inhaled into the lungs from the outside environment and internal respiration, the exchange of the gases oxygen and carbon dioxide at the tissue cell level.

In the process of respiration, air (oxygen) is inspired (inhaled) through these nose, pharynx (throat), larynx (voice box) and tracheas (windpipe). The tracheas divides in the two bronchi (branches), each of which leads into a lung. The bronchi branch into bronchioles, at the end of which are air sacs called alveoli. The gases oxygen and carbon dioxide are exchanged between the alveoli and the capillaries. The alveoli then carry the waste carbon dioxide back through the lungs to be expired (exhaled).

The lungs are divided into lobes; the right lung is divided into three lobes, the light lung into only two. The apex is the upper part of the lung, the hilum is the midline area (for the entrance and exit of blood vessels, nerves and bronchial tubes) and the base is the lower area. The lungs are lined with smooth membrane called an pleura in an airless sac called the pleural cavity. Between the lungs is the mediastinum, a thick wall enclosing the heart, aorta, oesophagus and bronchial tubes.

TERMINOLOGY OF THE NERVOUS SYSTEM

There are two major classifications of the nervous system, the central nervous system and the peripheral nervous system. The central nervous system is made up of the brain and the spinal corn, each covered by three protective membranes called the meninges. The outermost of he three membranes, the dura mater, is a tough, resilient membrane. The second layer surrounding the brain and spinal cord is the arachnoid membrane, so called because of its weblike structure. The third layer of the meanings, that closest to the brain and spinal cord, is the pia mater, a soft, delicate layer that provides the brain with a rich blood supply. The brain is also called the encephalon and consists of three parts, the cerebrum, the cerebellum and the brain steam. The outer layer of the brain is called the cerebral cortex, the centre of intellectual functions. The cerebellum regulates the co-ordination of muscular movements and is the centre for balance. In the brain steam, the thalamus is a relay station for sensory impulse. The hypothalamus controls body temperature and centres for appetite, thirst, sleep, feelings and sexual drive. The medulla oblongata connects the spinal cord with the rest of the brain and contains important centres for regulating internal body activities such as respiration, heartbeat and the dilation of the blood vessels. In the brain is a system of cavities called ventricles in which cerebrospinal fluids is generated. This fluid surrounds both brain and spinal cord and helps to protect them from stress.

The peripheral nervous system is made up of motor and sensor nerve fibres and these peripheral nerves branch and lead to all of the organs of the body. The motor nerve fibres control muscles and glands, while sensory fibres carry information about various parts of the body to the central nervous system. The motor pathways move outward from the brain and spinal cord and are called efferent. The sensory pathways, moving inward toward the brain and spinal cord, are called afferent.

The functions of the body that are not voluntarily controlled (by a conscious act of the will) are regulated by the autonomic nervous system. Examples of these functions are circulation, digestion, excretion and glandular functions. The autonomic nervous system is made up of the two motor systems that work in opposition to each other, the sympathetic and parasympathetic systems. Thus, if the nerve impulses are stimulated by the sympathetic nervous system—for example, if the heart rate increases—the parasympathetic system will bring about a state of equilibrium (homeostasis) by slowing down the heart rate.

TERMINOLOGY OF SENSORY ORGANS

The sensory organs receive information from the environment and pass it on to the brain. The major sensory organs are the eye and the ear; other sensors include the skin, taste buds and olfactory organs.

The visual sense comes to the brain through the eye, whose wall is composed of three layers. The sclera, the outermost layer, includes the transparent cornea. The middle layer, the choroid, is a membrane merging with the iris, the coloured part of the eye surrounding the pupil. Behind the iris is the crystalline lens, whose ciliary muscles adjust its shape and thickness. These changes in the shape of the lends aid in the refraction or bending of light rays. This refractive power is called accommodation. The innermost layer is the retina, the sensitive nerve layer of the eye.

As light energy in the form of waves travels through the eye, it is refracted or bent, by the cornea, the lens and various eye fluids, so that it focuses on the retina's receptor cells called rods and cones. The perception of the colour depends on the cone cells, while rod cells function better in dim light. The rods and cones are connected to the optic nerve, fibres from which lead to the brain.

In the ear, sound waves are received waves are received by the external ear (auditory canal) and are transmitted to the eardrum (tympanic membranae), then through the middle ear by means of three small bones called the malleus, the incus and the stapes. The membrane called the oval window separates the middle from the inner ear. The inner ear, also called the labyrinth, leads to the cochlea, filled with special fluids called perilymph and endolymph through the which the vibrations travel. The receptors located in the cochlea relay the sound waves to auditory nerve fibres, which end in the auditory centre of a the brain.

Another important function of the ear is the maintenance of the pressure of air in the middle ear to the pressure to air in the outside environment. This is done by means of the eustachian tube, which communicates with the pharynx.

The sense of balance is located in the inner ear (three semi-circular canals filled with lymph). Sensitive hair cells fluctuate in response to head movements, thus sending nerve impulses to the brain to ensure that equilibrium is maintained.

Somatic sensors react to touch, pressure, warmth, cold and pain. Tough receptors are most closely spaced on fingertips, lips and the tip of the tongue. Pressure receptors are located in the sub-cutaneous and deeper senses. Temperature senses (heat and cold receptors) have separate nerve fibre connections. Thus, a warm object will stimulate only the heat receptors, while a cool object will affect only cold terminals.

Pain sensors are known as free nerve endings (branching of nerve fibre). They protect the body from damage so there is little adaptation (adjustment) with continued stimulation.

The olfactory organ is located in the upper part of the nasal cavity, where its primary purposes is the interpretation of smell, which is closely related to the sense of taste.

The sense of taste involves receptors in the tongue (tip, border and base) known as taste buds. There are four basis tastes: sweet, sour, bitter and salty. Taste perception is limited to dissolved substances.

APPENDIX IV

ELECTRICAL PRECAUTIONS

Electrical precautions to be taken with patients having completely implanted cardiac pacemakers

Patients with completely implantable pacemakers may for the most part be treated as electrically completely normal (or general category patients) with the following exceptions:

Electrosurgery (surgical diathermy)

During the use of electrosurgery the surgeon should be particularly alert for disturbances in cardiac rhythm. Monitoring of the arterial pulse and electrocardiogram is recommended. The electrocardioscope tracing is likely to be obliterated when the diathermy is operating but should be watched carefully after each episode of diathermy.

Radiotherapy

Cobalt gamma radiation is preferable for pacemaker patients to radiation produce by electrical particle accelerators. The large alternating magnetic fields and intense radiation which may be produced by the latter devices can interfere with pacemaker function. Where treatment by particle accelerators in unavoidable continuous monitoring of the electrocardiogram is required.

Nursing and personal care

1. Electric shavers should not be used to shave the skin over the pacemaker.
2. Patients may use electric shavers for normal cosmetics purposes.
3. Patients may use the bedside call button.
4. Patients may use and electric bed.

Nurses should watch for the usual signs of pacemaker malfunction including bradycardia, tachycardia and dizziness.

Rehabilitation

Short wave physical medicine diathermy is not recommended for cardiac pacemaker patients. Hazards include electromagnetic interference with pacemaker function and the induction heating of metallic pacemaker parts.

Electrical stimulation procedures are also not recommended. If they are used the physician should be alert for disturbances in cardiac rhythm.

Patients with externalised wires—with or without pacemakers—or cardiac catheters (critical category)

Patients with externalised wire or other electrical conductors leading into the thorax, in the region of the heart, are particularly vulnerable to electric shock. The following precautions are required:
1. The patient shall be in a non-electric bed.
2. Only cardiac monitors and other patient care equipment attached to the patient meeting the hospital classification of the critical category (IEC types CF) (CSA type 3) shall be used with the patient. All pieces of equipment meeting these specifications are marked with a green sticker.

3. Externalised conductors are to be insulated with flexible plastic tubing or should be made of insulated with flexible plastic tubing or should be made of insulated wire. They should be taped to the skin. Uninsulated pacemaker terminals should be taped to the skin after they have been covered with electrical tape or an equivalent insulator. (Medical adhesive tape is not a satisfactory insulator). No bare wire is ever to touch the patient's skin directly. Conductive leads are to be labelled to show the site of insertion, e.g., ventricle, atrium, earth.
4. Rubber gloves are to be worn when handling externalised conductors. Those handling externalised wires must avoid contact with an electrically operated devices including lights, monitors, X-rays equipment, foot switches, inhalation therapy equipment, communications and entertainment equipment.
5. Provided the foregoing precautions are followed, the patient may used any equipment normally found in this room. Only battery operated entertainment equipment or approved television units are allowed.
6. The patient may use an electric shaver if the nurses determine that the wires are properly insulated.
7. The patient may use his hospital bedside call-bell if all other requirements are met.
8. If a patient is to be transferred, the charge nurse in the original unit is responsible for informing the charge nurse and/or private duty nurse in the receiving unit of the presence of externalised wires and the precautions that are necessary.

   The nurse in the receiving unit will call the hospital Engineering Department to check the newly assigned room to be sure that all equipment, beds, monitors, etc., are properly earthed before the patient is transferred to that room.

Patients Connected to External Cardiac Pacemakers

The external demand pacemakers should not be operated within ten feet (3.3 m) of a television set, electrical calculating machine or diathermy equipment. Where the use of equipment likely to produce electrical interference is mandatory, the responsible physician should determine whether the external pacemaker can be effective in the asynchronous mode (fixed rate).

Apparent Difficulty with Pacemaker

1. Any malfunction or apparent difficulty with the pacemaker should be reported immediately to the responsible floor resident (houseman), the cardiology resident (registrar) and the Department of Medical Engineering or Medical Physics as appropriate.
2. Any malfunction of the patient care equipment should be immediately reported to the Medical Engineering Department or Medical Physics Department as appropriate.
3. Any electrical leads with broken plugs, worn cables or damaged outlets must be reported to the Plant and Maintenance Department (Hospital Engineer's Department) immediately.

References

Webser, J.G., *Biomedical Instrumentation*, Wiley, New York.

Joseph Carr, *Biomedical Equipment use, Maintenance and Management,* Prentice Hall, New York.

Jacob Kline, *Handbook of Biomedical Engineering*, Academic Press, Inc., London.

Kimmich, H.P., *Encyclopedia of Medical Devices and Instrumentation*, Wiley, New York.

Joseph, S., *Biomedical Engineering,* Academic Press, Inc., London.

Donald. L. Wise, *Bio-instrumentation and Biosensors,* Marcel Dekker, Inc., New York.

Plonsey, R., *Bioelectric Phenomena,* Mcgraw-Hill, New York.

Bracewell, R., *The Fourier Transform and Its Application*, Mcgraw-Hill, New York.

Christensen, D.A., *Ultrasound Bio-instrumentation*, Wiley, New York.

Foster, M.A., *Magnetic Resonance in Medicine and Biology*, Pergamon, New York.

Hine, G.S., *Instrumentation in Nuclear Medicine*, Academic Press, New York.

Wells, P.N.T., *Ultrasonics in Clinical Diagnosis*, Harper & Row, New York.

Cook, A.M., *Therapeutic Medical Devices*, Prentice Hall, New York.

Cobbold, R.C., *Transducers for Biomedical Measurement*, Wiley, New York.

Fry, F.J., *Ultrasound: Its Application in Biology and Medicine*, Elsevier, New York.

Geddes, L.A., *Principles of Applied Biomedical Instrumentation*, Wiley, New York.

Lion, K.S., *Elements of Electronics and Electrical Instrumentation*, Mcgraw-Hill, New York.

Janta, J., *Principles of Chemical Sensors*, Plenum, New York.

Murray, R.W., *Chemical Sensors and Microinstrumentation,* American Chemical Society, Washington D.C.

Payne, J.P., *Pulse Oximetry*, Prentice Hall, New York.

Ferris, C.D., *Introduction to Bioelectrodes*, Plenum, New York.

Miller, H.A., *Biomedical Electrode Technology*, Academic Publishers, New York.

Rogers, D.F., *Ventilators and Humidifiers*, Wiley, New York.

Berenson, C., *Application of Computer in Biomedical Engineering*, Harper & Row, New York.

Faulk, B.F., *Clinical Laboratory Instruments*, Prentice Hall, New York.

James, A.N., *Biomedical Sensors and Chemical Sensors*, Academic Press, Inc., London.

Jolles, Z.E., *Therapeutic Equipment*, Harper & Row, New York.

Index